Handbook on Optimizing Patient Care in Psychiatry

This handbook examines current mental health research, challenges in patient care, and advances in clinical psychiatry with the aim of improving approaches toward the screening of at-risk individuals, facilitating access to care, and supervising rehabilitation.

Combining evidence-based research with clinical case studies, international experts provide detailed, holistic insights into our understanding of mental disorders through biological, social, interpersonal, and economical lenses. Models of intervention, prevention, and treatment are provided, along with methods for continued care and patient advocacy. Finally, experts analyse the future of psychiatric research and mental healthcare. Readers will gain greater understanding of the finer nuances of handling psychiatric cases and a holistic perspective of optimizing patient care within this field.

This innovative book contributes to the development of community management of various psychiatric disorders and will be of interest to case managers, mental health workers, doctors, nurses, and many more.

Dr. Amresh Shrivastava is a professor emeritus of psychiatry at Western University and a scientist of mental health at Lawson Health Research Institute, located in London, Ontario, Canada. His areas of focus include suicide prevention, early intervention, and complex mental disorders. He has served as an editor, reviewer, and member of the editorial board of psychiatric journals and published original research reviews, book chapters, and academic and non-fiction academic books.

Dr. Avinash De Sousa is a consultant psychiatrist who is an avid writer and researcher with over 800 papers in national and international journals. He juggles his time between his teaching assignments and private practice and also enjoys being part of new research projects that investigate novel areas in psychiatry and psychology.

Dr. Nilesh Shah is a professor and head at the Department of Psychiatry, Lokmanya Tilak Municipal Medical College, Mumbai, and is an ardent teacher and researcher and an often-invited speaker and lecturer at various national and international conferences.

Handbook on Optimizing Patient Care in Psychiatry

Edited by
Amresh Shrivastava,
Avinash De Sousa and
Nilesh Shah

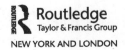

NEW YORK AND LONDON

Cover image: Getty Image

First published 2023
by Routledge
605 Third Avenue, New York, NY 10158

and by Routledge
4 Park Square, Milton Park, Abingdon, Oxon, OX14 4RN

Routledge is an imprint of the Taylor & Francis Group, an informa business

© 2023 Taylor & Francis

The right of Amresh Shrivastava, Avinash De Sousa and Nilesh Shah to be identified as the authors of the editorial material, and of the authors for their individual chapters, has been asserted in accordance with sections 77 and 78 of the Copyright, Designs and Patents Act 1988.

All rights reserved. No part of this book may be reprinted or reproduced or utilised in any form or by any electronic, mechanical, or other means, now known or hereafter invented, including photocopying and recording, or in any information storage or retrieval system, without permission in writing from the publishers.

Trademark notice: Product or corporate names may be trademarks or registered trademarks, and are used only for identification and explanation without intent to infringe.

Library of Congress Cataloging-in-Publication Data
Names: Shrivastava, Amresh, editor. | De Sousa, Avinash, editor. | Shah, Nilesh, editor.
Title: Handbook on optimizing patient care in psychiatry / edited by Amresh Shrivastava, Avinash De Sousa, Nilesh Shah.
Description: New York, NY : Routledge, 2023. | Includes bibliographical references and index.
Identifiers: LCCN 2022018337 (print) | LCCN 2022018338 (ebook) |
  ISBN 9780367140687 (hardback) | ISBN 9780367141158 (paperback) |
  ISBN 9780429030260 (ebook)
Subjects: LCSH: Psychiatry.
Classification: LCC RC435 .H76 2023 (print) | LCC RC435 (ebook) |
  DDC 616.89—dc23/eng/20220512
LC record available at https://lccn.loc.gov/2022018337
LC ebook record available at https://lccn.loc.gov/2022018338

ISBN: 978-0-367-14068-7 (hbk)
ISBN: 978-0-367-14115-8 (pbk)
ISBN: 978-0-429-03026-0 (ebk)

DOI: 10.4324/9780429030260

Typeset in Minion
by Apex CoVantage, LLC

Contents

List of Contributors — x

Optimizing Patient Care in Psychiatry – Preface — xvii
AMRESH SHRIVASTAVA, AVINASH DE SOUSA AND NILESH SHAH

Section 1 Concept and Scope of Optimization of Patient Care in Psychiatry — 1

1. Educational Strategies to Optimise Patient Care in Psychiatry — 3
   JANET ALLISON AND MIKE AKROYD

2. Optimising Patient Care in Psychiatry – Focus on Quality of Life — 18
   SANDEEP GROVER AND SWAPNAJEET SAHOO

3. Optimising Patient Care in Psychiatry With Sound Mental Health Legislation — 33
   BRENDAN D. KELLY, GAUTAM GULATI AND RICHARD M. DUFFY

4. Improving Patient Outcomes by Integration of Public Health and Mental Health — 42
   SWATEJA NIMKAR

5. Building Resilience at a Community and Family Level for Care in Psychiatry — 50
   YASH ACCHAPALIA AND AVINASH DE SOUSA

Section 2 Specific Strategies for Management — 63

6. Comprehensive Management of Violence Against Women: Putting WHO Recommendations Into Practice — 65
   SALMI RAZALI, DINA TUKHVATULLINA, DARIA SMIRNOVA

7	Mental Health Access to the Unreached Using Mobile Mental Health PRAKASH B. BEHERE, SWAROOPA LUNGE PATIL, DEBOLINA CHOWDHURY, ANIRUDDH P. BEHERE AND RICHA YADAV	79
8	Optimising Patient Care When Working With Children of Patients With Mental Illness SANDEEP GROVER AND ABHISHEK GHOSH	84
9	Forensic Risk Assessment and Management of Community Case Managed Clients ANIKET BANSOD AND AKSHATA MULMULE	91
10	Optimizing Patient Care in Sexual Dysfunction in Severe Mental Illness SHIVANANDA MANOHAR, SUMAN S. RAO, T.S. SATHYANARAYANA RAO	100
11	Optimising Patient Care in Psychiatry With Autonomy and Choice RICHARD M. DUFFY, DESHWINDER S. SIDHU AND BRENDAN D. KELLY	110
12	Neurocognitive Rehabilitation Program for People With Mild Cognitive Impairment – "Memory Clinic" VICTOR SAVILOV, OLGA KARPENKO, MARAT KURMYSHEV, GEORGE KOSTYUK	124
13	Huntington's Disease as a Multi-System Disorder: Current "Must Know" for Better Patient Management SVETLANA KOPISHINSKAIA, MARIIA KOROTYSH, SERGEY SVETOZARSKII, MIKHAIL SHERMAN, IVAN VELICHKO, PAUL CUMMING AND DARIA SMIRNOVA	134

Section 3 High-Risk Groups 149

14	Optimizing Patient Care in Psychiatry – Bipolar Mood Disorder RITEEKA DESHPANDE AND ANUJA BENDRE	151
15	Optimising Patient Care – Pharmacogenetics in the Management of Addictions EVGENY KRUPITSKY, ELVINA AKHMETOVA, DINA TUKHVATULLINA, DARIA SMIRNOVA, PAUL CUMMING AND AZAT ASADULLIN	155
16	Optimizing Patient Care in Psychiatry – Behavioral Addictions ELVIN LUKOSE	169
17	Optimizing Patient Care in Psychiatry – Eating Disorders AVINASH DE SOUSA AND SHOROUQ MOTWANI	180

18	Optimising Patient Care in Psychiatry – Homeless Mentally Ill Patients ADARSH TRIPATHI, AATHIRA J. PRAKASH	191
19	Challenges in Community Psychiatry – Farmer Suicides and Their Survivors PRAKASH B. BEHERE, SHRUTI AGARWAL, DEBOLINA CHOWDHURY, ANIRUDDH P. BEHERE AND RICHA YADAV	198
20	Optimizing Patient Care in Psychiatry – Geriatric Psychiatry ELVIN LUKOSE AND HEENA MERCHANT PANDIT	204
21	Optimizing Patient Care in Psychiatry – Borderline Personality Disorder SAYURI PERERA	216
22	Optimising Patient Care in Dementia SHABBIR AMANULLAH, SHIVA K. SHIVAKUMAR, CATRIN THOMAS, SARMISHTHA BHATTACHARYYA AND SWAR SHAH	233
23	Optimizing Patient Care in Attenuated Psychosis Syndrome NIKITA NALAWADE AND AVINASH DE SOUSA	247
24	Optimising Patient Care in Psychiatry – Anxiety Disorders PRERNA KHAR, VINYAS NISARGA AND PRAJAKTA PATKAR	258
25	Optimizing Patient Care in Sleep Disorders KARISHMA RUPANI AND SHILPA ADARKAR	273
26	Optimizing Patient Care in Psychiatry – OCD and Habit Disorders JAVED ATHER SIDDIQUI AND SHAZIA FARHEEN QURESHI	286
27	Optimizing Patient Care in Alcohol Dependence Using Disulfiram Therapy POOJA KAPRI, AVINASH DE SOUSA	292
28	Optimising Patient Care Using Naltrexone for Opioid Use Disorders COLIN BREWER	300
29	Optimizing Patient Care – Suicide Prevention PAUL S. LINKS	317
30	Optimising Patient Care in Psychiatry – Focus on Consultation Liaison Psychiatry PARIJAT ROY AND AVINASH DE SOUSA	333
31	Differential Awareness of Some Psychiatric Presentations TAREK OKASHA	341

Section 4   Innovations in the Model of Care — 355

32 Optimising Patient Care in Psychiatry Using Cognitive Behaviour Therapy — 357
PRAGYA LODHA

33 Optimising Patient Care in Psychiatry With Policy and Practice of ECT in Malaysia — 371
CHEE KOK YOON

34 Rehabilitation and Case Management Using Cognitive Remediation Therapy — 376
AKSHATA MULMULE AND ANIKET BANSOD

35 Optimizing Patient Care With Effective Psychotherapeutic Interventions — 384
TANYA MALIK AND URVEESHA NIRJAR

36 Telepsychiatry as a Means to Optimizing Psychiatric Care — 395
MARY V. SEEMAN

37 Smartphone Technology to Optimize Psychiatric Care in the Community — 405
BONIFACE HARERIMANA AND CHERYL FORCHUK

38 Optimizing School Mental Health Services — 415
AVINASH DE SOUSA

39 Optimising Patient Care in Psychiatry – Focus on Forensic Psychiatry — 421
JASON QUINN, AJAY PRAKASH, JARED SCOTT AND ARUN PRAKASH

40 Optimising Patient Care in the Community Using Psychopharmacology — 436
SHOROUQ MOTWANI AND SAGAR KARIA

41 Chronic Mental Illness and Experience of the Richmond Fellowship Programme — 442
S. KALYANASUNDARAM, PRATHIKSHA SHUKLA AND LATA HEMCHAND

42 Innovative Community Mental Health Approaches From Across the Globe — 457
PRAGYA LODHA

43 Optimizing Patient Care in Psychiatry – Child and Adolescent Psychiatry — 465
ANWESHAK DAS AND JAYASHREE DAS

44	Community Psychiatry – the Argentina Experience ERIC H. WAINWRIGHT AND GUSTAVO E. TAFET	475
45	Optimising Assessment Using the House Tree Person Test PRAGYA LODHA AND AVINASH DE SOUSA	481
46	Challenges in Patient Care in the Aftermath of an Epidemic and Pandemic EFI TSOMAKA AND KONSTANTINOS N. FOUNTOULAKIS	495
47	Optimizing Psychiatric Care Using Functional Neuroimaging SUVARNA BADHE AND AVINASH DE SOUSA	515
48	Personalized Psychiatry of Psychoneurological Diseases: From Theory to Clinical Practice REGINA F. NASYROVA, NIKOLAY G. NEZNANOV, NATALIA A. SHNAYDER	524
49	Exploring fNIRS Potential as an Investigational Tool in Psychiatry JITENDER JAKHAR, DEBANJAN BANERJEE, NAND KUMAR	538
50	Optimising Patient Care in Psychiatry: Psychosocial Rehabilitation DURVA SAIL, CHITRITA SENGUPTA CHAKI, AVINASH DE SOUSA	545
51	Optimising Patient Care in Psychiatry – Impact of the COVID-19 Pandemic KARISHMA RUPANI, SUSHMA SONAVANE, AVINASH DE SOUSA	557
	Index	568

Contributors

Yash Acchapalia
Medical Researcher
Lokmanya Tilak Municipal Medical College
Mumbai

Shilpa Adarkar
Associate Professor
Department of Psychiatry
Seth G.S. Medical College and
K.E.M. Hospital
Mumbai, India

Shruti Agarwal
Resident Doctor
Department of Psychiatry
Jawaharlal Nehru Medical College
Wardha, Maharashtra
India

Elvina Akhmetova
Department for Alcohol Dependence
  Treatment
V.M. Bekhterev National Medical Research
  Center for Psychiatry and Neurology
Ministry of Health of the Russian
  Federation, Saint Petersburg, Russian
  Federation
Department of Psychiatry and Addiction
  Medicine with a Course of the Institute
  for Continued Professional Education
Bashkir State Medical University
Ministry of Health of the Russian
  Federation, Ufa, Russian Federation

Mike Akroyd
Consultant Psychiatrist
Clinical Director & Clinical Teaching
  Fellow
Derbyshire Healthcare NHS Foundation
  Trust

Janet Allison
Clinical Educationalist
Post-Graduate Researcher in Psychiatry
Doctorate Student
Anglia-Ruskin University, UK

Shabbir Amanullah
Adjunct Professor
University of Toronto and Western Ontario,
  Canada

Azat Asadullin
Department of Psychiatry and Addiction
  Medicine with a Course of the
  Institute for Continued Professional
  Education
Bashkir State Medical University
Ministry of Health of the Russian
  Federation, Ufa, Russian Federation
Centre for Personalized Psychiatry and
  Neurology
V.M. Bekhterev National Medical Research
  Center for Psychiatry and Neurology
Ministry of Health of the Russian
  Federation, Saint Petersburg, Russian
  Federation

CONTRIBUTORS • xi

Suvarna Badhe
Independent Researcher
Mumbai, India

Debanjan Banerjee
Senior Resident
National Institute of Mental Health and
 Neurosciences (NIMHANS)
Bengaluru, India

Aniket Bansod
Assistant Clinical Director
Forensic Mental Health and Alcohol,
 Tobacco and Other Drug Service
Senior Staff Specialist
Prison Mental Health Service
Cairns and Hinterland Hospital and Health
 Service, Cairns, QLD

Aniruddh P. Behere
Helen Devos Children's Hospital
Assistant Professor
Department of Pediatrics and Human
 Development
Michigan State University College of Human
 Medicine, Grand Rapids MI, USA

Prakash B. Behere
Former Vice Chancellor
D.Y. Patil University, Kolhapur (MS)
Director Professor
Department of Psychiatry
Jawaharlal Nehru Medical College
Director – School of Advanced Studies,
 DMIMS
Sawangi, Wardha
Maharashtra, India

Anuja Bendre
Resident Doctor
Department of Psychiatry
Lokmanya Tilak Municipal Medical College
Mumba, India

Sarmishtha Bhattacharyya
Consultant Psychiatrist
Clinical Lead
North Wales, BCUHB
Visiting Professor
University of Chester, UK

Colin Brewer
Retired Psychiatrist
Formerly Medical Director
The Stapleford Clinic, London
Director of the Community Alcoholism
 Treatment Service
Westminster Hospital, London, UK

Chitrita Sengupta Chaki
Independent Researcher
Consultant Psychologist
Kolkata, India

Debolina Chowdhury
Resident Doctor
Department of Psychiatry
Jawaharlal Nehru Medical College
Wardha, Maharashtra
India

Paul Cumming
International Centre for Education and
 Research in Neuropsychiatry
Samara State Medical University
Samara, Russia
Department of Nuclear Medicine
Inselpital, Bern University
Bern, Switzerland
School of Psychology and Counselling,
 Queensland University of Technology,
 Brisbane, Australia

Anweshak Das
Consultant Psychiatrist
Psychiatric Clinic
Guwahati
Assam, India

Jayashree Das
Consultant Clinical Psychologist
Psychiatric Clinic
Guwahati
Assam, India

Riteeka Deshpande
Ex – Assistant Professor
Department of Psychiatry
Lokmanya Tilak Municipal Medical
 College
Mumbai, India

Avinash De Sousa
Consultant Psychiatrist
Research Associate
Department of Psychiatry
Lokmanya Tilak Municipal Medical College
Founder Trustee – Desousa Foundation
Mumbai, India

Richard M. Duffy
The Rotunda Hospital
Parnell Square
Dublin, Ireland

Cheryl Forchuk
Lawson Health Research Institute
University of Toronto
University of Windsor
Wayne State University
Western University
Canada

Konstantinos N. Fountoulakis
3rd Department of Psychiatry
Division of Neurosciences
School of Medicine
Aristotle University of Thessaloniki
Greece

Abhishek Ghosh
Assistant Professor
Department of Psychiatry
Post Graduate Institute of Medical
    Education and Research
Chandigarh, India

Sandeep Grover
Professor,
Department of Psychiatry
Post Graduate Institute of Medical
    Education & Research
Chandigarh, India

Gautam Gulati
Graduate Entry Medical School
University of Limerick
Ireland

Boniface Harerimana
College of Medicine and Health Sciences,
    University of Rwanda
King's College, London
Lawson Health Research Institute
Neuro-psychiatric Hospital Caraes Ndera,
    Referral Hospital for Mental Health care
    in Rwanda, Western University

Lata Hemchand
Senior Consultant Psychologist
Richmond Fellowship Society
Bangalore, India

Jitender Jakhar
Senior Resident
Govind Ballabh Pant Institute of
    Postgraduate Medical Education and
    Research (MAMC), New Delhi, India

S. Kalyanasundaram
Honorary Advisor
Richmond Fellowship Society
Bangalore, India

Pooja Kapri
Resident Doctor
Department of Psychiatry
Lokmanya Tilak Municipal Medical College
Mumbai, India

Sagar Karia
Assistant Professor
Department of Psychiatry
Lokmanya Tilak Municipal Medical
    College
Mumbai, India

Olga Karpenko
Mental-health Clinic No 1
Named after N.A. Alexeev
Moscow, Russian Federation

Brendan D. Kelly
Department of Psychiatry
Trinity College Dublin
Trinity Centre for Health Sciences
Tallaght University Hospital
Dublin, Ireland

Prerna Khar
Consultant Psychiatrist
Mindtemple Clinic and Rotary Service
    Centre
Mumbai, India

Svetlana Kopishinskaia
Department of Neurology, Neurosurgery and Neurorehabilitation
Kirov State Medical University
Russian Federation
International Centre for Education and Research in Neuropsychiatry
Samara State Medical University
Samara, Russia

Mariia Korotysh
LTD "Genome"
Nizhny Novgorod
Russian Federation

George Kostyuk
Mental-health Clinic No 1
Named after N.A. Alexeev
Moscow, Russian Federation

Evgeny Krupitsky
Department for Alcohol Dependence Treatment
V.M. Bekhterev National Medical Research Center for Psychiatry and Neurology
Ministry of Health of the Russian Federation, Saint Petersburg, Russian Federation
Clinical Pharmacology Laboratory for Addictive Disorders
Institute of Pharmacology n.a. A.V. Valdman, Pavlov First St. Petersburg State Medical University
Ministry of Health of the Russian Federation, Saint Petersburg, Russian Federation

Nand Kumar
Professor
Department of Psychiatry
All India Institute of Medical Sciences (AIIMS)
New Delhi, India

Marat Kurmyshev
Mental-health Clinic No 1
Named after N.A. Alexeev
Moscow, Russian Federation

Paul S. Links
Professor
Psychiatry & Behavioural Neurosciences
Faculty of Health Sciences
McMaster University
Canada

Pragya Lodha
Clinical Psychologist & Researcher
Desousa Foundation
Mumbai, India

Elvin Lukose
Assistant Professor
Department of Psychiatry
Seth G.S. Medical College and K.E.M. Hospital
Mumbai, India

Tanya Malik
Department of Clinical and Counselling Psychology
Teachers College
Columbia University, USA

Shivananda Manohar
Assistant Professor
Department of Psychiatry
JSS Medical College & Hospital
JSS Academy of Higher Education and Research, Mysore
India

Shorouq Motwani
Senior Medical Officer
Department of Psychiatry
Lokmanya Tilak Municipal Medical College, Mumbai, India

Akshata Mulmule
Staff Specialist
Mental Health Inpatient Unit
Cairns and Hinterland Hospital and Health Service
Cairns, QLD

Nikita Nalawade
Consultant Psychiatrist
Private Practice and Researcher
Mumbai, India

Regina F. Nasyrova
V. M. Bekhterev National Medical Research Centre for Psychiatry and Neurology
Saint-Petersburg, Russian Federation

Nikolay G. Neznanov
V. M. Bekhterev National Medical Research Centre for Psychiatry and Neurology
Saint-Petersburg, Russian Federation

Swateja Nimkar
Associate Professor
University of Southern Indiana
USA

Urveesha Nirjar
Department of Clinical and Counselling Psychology
Teachers College
Columbia University, USA

Vinyas Nisarga
Assistant Professor
Department of Psychiatry
K.J. Somaiya Medical College, Hospital and Research, Centre
Mumbai, India

Tarek Okasha
Okasha Institute of Psychiatry
Faculty of Medicine
Ain Shams University
Cairo, Egypt

Heena Merchant Pandit
Associate Professor
Department of Psychiatry
Lokmanya Tilak Municipal Medical College
Mumbai, India

Swaroopa Lunge Patil
Resident Doctor
Department of Psychiatry
Jawaharlal Nehru Medical College
Wardha, Maharashtra
India

Prajakta Patkar
Assistant Professor
Department of Psychiatry
B.Y.L. Nair Hospital and T.N. Medical College
Mumbai, India

Sayuri Perera
Senior Lecturer in Psychiatry
Faculty of Medicine
University of Peradeniya
Honorary Consultant Psychiatrist
Teaching Hospital, Peradeniya
Sri Lanka

Aathira J. Prakash
Department of Psychiatry
King George's Medical University
Lucknow, India

Ajay Prakash
Forensic Psychiatrist
Southwest Centre for Forensic Mental Health Care – St. Joseph's Health Care London
London, Ontario, Canada
Assistant Professor
The University of Western Ontario
Canada

Arun Prakash
Medical Director
Southwest Centre for Forensic Mental Health Care – St. Joseph's Health Care London
Adjunct Professor
The University of Western Ontario, London
Canada

Jason Quinn
Forensic Psychiatrist
Southwest Centre for Forensic Mental Health Care – St. Joseph's Health Care London
London, Ontario, Canada
Assistant Professor
The University of Western Ontario
Canada

Shazia Farheen Qureshi
Consultant Psychiatrist
Mental Health Hospital, Taif
Kingdom of Saudi Arabia

Suman S. Rao
Resident Doctor

Department of Psychiatry
JSS Medical College & Hospital
JSS Academy of Higher Education and
    Research, Mysore
India

T.S. Sathyanarayana Rao
Professor and Head
Department of Psychiatry
JSS Medical College & Hospital
JSS Academy of Higher Education and
    Research, Mysore
India

Salmi Razali
Department of Psychiatry
Faculty of Medicine
Sg Buloh Selangor Campus
Universiti Teknologi MARA
Malaysia

Parijat Roy
Specialist Medical Officer
Department of Psychiatry
Lokmanya Tilak Municipal Medical College
Mumbai, India

Karishma Rupani
Assistant Professor
Department of Psychiatry
Seth G.S. Medical College and
    K.E.M. Hospital
Mumbai, India

Swapnajeet Sahoo
Assistant Professor
Department of Psychiatry
Post Graduate Institute of Medical
    Education & Research
Chandigarh, India

Durva Sail
Specialist Medical Officer
Department of Psychiatry
Lokmanya Tilak Municipal Medical College
Mumbai, India

Victor Savilov
Mental-health Clinic No 1
Named after N.A. Alexeev
Moscow, Russian Federation

Jared Scott
Forensic Outreach Ambulatory Team,
    Facilitator
Southwest Centre for Forensic Mental
    Health Care – St. Joseph's Health Care
    London
London, Ontario, Canada
Member of the Faculty of Graduate Studies
The University of Western Ontario
Canada

Mary V. Seeman
Professor Emerita
Department of Psychiatry
University of Toronto
Toronto
Ontario, Canada

Swar Shah
Graduate Entry Medicine Student
Royal College of Surgeons in Ireland
Dublin, Ireland

Mikhail Sherman
Department of Neurology, Neurosurgery
    and Neurorehabilitation
Kirov State Medical University
Russian Federation

Shiva K. Shivakumar
Associate Professor
Northern Ontario School of Medicine
Health Sciences North, Sudbury
Ontario, Canada

Natalia A. Shnayder
V. M. Bekhterev National Medical Research
    Centre for Psychiatry and Neurology
Saint-Petersburg, Russian Federation
V. F. Voino-Yasenetsky Krasnoyarsk State
    Medical University
Krasnoyarsk, Russian Federation

Amresh Shrivastava
Professor Emeritus
Department of Psychiatry

University of Western Ontario
Ontario, London, Canada

Prathiksha Shukla
Deputy Rehab Manager
Richmond Fellowship Society
Bangalore, India

Javed Ather Siddiqui
Consultant Psychiatrist
Mental Health Hospital, Taif
Kingdom of Saudi Arabia

Deshwinder S. Sidhu
Social and Rehabilitation Psychiatry
Phoenix Care Centre, Grangegorman
North Circular Road
Dublin, Ireland

Daria Smirnova
International Centre for Education and Research in Neuropsychiatry
Department of Psychiatry, Narcology, Psychotherapy and Clinical Psychology, Samara State Medical University
Samara, Russia

Sushma Sonavane
Professor and Head
Department of Psychiatry
B.Y.L. Nair Charitable Hospital and T.N. Medical College
Mumbai, India

Sergey Svetozarskii
FBIHC "Volga District Medical Center", Nizhny Novgorod
Russian Federation

Gustavo E. Tafet
Department of Psychiatry and Neurosciences
Maimonides University
Buenos Aires, Argentina
International Foundation for the Development of Neurosciences

Catrin Thomas
Psychiatry Higher Trainee
Betsi Cadwaladr University Health
North Wales

Adarsh Tripathi
Department of Psychiatry
King George's Medical University
Lucknow, India

Efi Tsomaka
Psychiatry Department
General Hospital for Chest Diseases
Sotiria, Athens
Greece

Dina Tukhvatullina
Barts and The London School of Medicine and Dentistry
Institute of Population Health Sciences
Queen Mary University of London
London, United Kingdom

Ivan Velichko
Department of Neurology and Neurosurgery, Kuban State Medical University
Krasnodar, Russian Federation

Eric H. Wainwright
Department of Psychiatry and Neurosciences
Maimonides University
Buenos Aires, Argentina
International Foundation for the Development of Neurosciences
Universidad Católica Argentina
Buenos Aires British Hospital
Hospital Braulio A. Moyano

Richa Yadav
Assistant Professor
Department of Psychiatry and Behavioural Sciences
OU College of Medicine, Oklahoma City, Oklahoma, USA

Chee Kok Yoon
Consultant Neuropsychiatrist
NEURON
Department of Psychiatry & Mental Health
Kuala Lumpur Hospital
Kuala Lumpur, Malaysia

Optimizing Patient Care in Psychiatry – Preface

Amresh Shrivastava[1]
Avinash De Sousa[2]
Nilesh Shah[3]

There are potent evidence-based medical, psychological, and psychosocial treatments for patients who suffer from mental illness and have varying mental health needs. There are, however, marked differences in the approaches that people have towards mental illness, the methods of treatment they advise, and the drugs that they prescribe. Marked differences in psychotherapeutic and family psychoeducation approaches also exist that vary from psychiatrist to psychiatrist. There is a need for a standard approach to many psychiatric disorders and their management, but a hurdle in this regard are the marked variations in symptomatology and clinical presentations that a patient may present with. What do we mean by optimization in psychiatric care? We mean that psychiatric care must be standard and non-varying across centres and yet at the same time must be the best that can be provided to the patient irrespective of environment.

Most doctors and healthcare workers need to be aware of the standard of care available and the best practices that are possible. There is a need for optimization in various areas due to a wide variety of treatments available. The current volume is aimed at case managers of patients, and the book shall provide them with an overview of the optimized management of various psychiatric conditions and also has some general chapters on concepts that are needed for optimization. There is a need to optimize psychopharmacological care as well, and some chapters look at various facets of this. The authors who have contributed chapters are from various countries all over the world and add diversity and completeness to the volume. Optimization of psychiatric care is a distant dream, and the book aims at achieving it. It is a good read for both case managers and doctors and shall provide a holistic perspective to optimizing patient care in psychiatry.

Notes

1. Professor Emeritus, Department of Psychiatry, Western University & Scientist – Mental Health, Lawson Health Research Institute, Canada.
2. Research Associate, Department of Psychiatry, Lokmanya Tilak Municipal Medical College and Founder Trustee and Consultant Psychiatrist, Desousa Foundation, Mumbai.
3. Professor and Head, Department of Psychiatry, Lokmanya Tilak Municipal Medical College, Mumbai.

Section 1
Concept and Scope of Optimization of Patient Care in Psychiatry

1
Educational Strategies to Optimise Patient Care in Psychiatry

Janet Allison and Mike Akroyd

Introduction	3
What Do Healthcare Professionals Need to Know?	4
Addressing the 'How'	4
Learning Objectives – Defining the Desired Learning	5
Pedagogical Strategies – The 'Best Tools for the Job'	5
Models of Learning, Pedagogical Strategies and Teaching Methods	6
Instructivism	6
Social Cognitivism	6
Situated Learning	7
Social Constructivism	8
Transfer of Learning Into Practice	10
Summary of the Design Process	10
An Example From Practice	11
Context	11
Overall Aim of Teaching Intervention	11
Learning Objectives	11
Pedagogical Strategies and Teaching Methods	11
Conclusion	15

INTRODUCTION

Education to optimise patient care in psychiatry is a far more complex process than simply teaching facts about diagnoses or memorising lists of questions. In addition to accurate knowledge, a healthcare professional needs skills in order to elicit relevant information and compassion to show understanding of presenting difficulties. It is only through the combination of such knowledge, skills and positive attitudes that professionals can work out the best way to help. Knowledge, skills and attitudes are equally important, and each needs to be addressed in the educational context. However, how these three elements are taught can have a significant impact on whether that learning is acquired at a deep or superficial level and on whether the learning will later transfer into clinical practice. We argue that knowledge, skills and attitudes cannot be taught in the same way and that each requires a specific pedagogical or teaching and learning strategy.

We will therefore explore the core pedagogical strategies utilised in teaching psychiatric assessment and the learning theories from which they arise. We will address the necessity of alignment between clinical learning needs, educational learning objectives and the pedagogical strategies and teaching methods used. In the educational context, we propose that there is no 'one size fits all' approach, but in order to maximise learning, educators need to identify and apply the 'right tool for the job'.

To illustrate this process, we present an example of how different pedagogical approaches can be combined in a community healthcare setting in order to teach the assessment and management of a patient experiencing low mood with suicidal ideation.

WHAT DO HEALTHCARE PROFESSIONALS NEED TO KNOW?

Education in psychiatric assessment and management is important to enable community-based healthcare professionals to address the mental health needs of their population effectively. There are a number of psychiatric screening or assessment tools widely available, with a general focus on content or knowledge, as in 'what' needs to be assessed – the psychiatric symptoms, where the identification of a certain number of features indicates a particular diagnosis or differential diagnoses and suggests a possible treatment plan. These commonly take the form of checklists such as the Beck Depression Inventory (Beck et al., 1996) or Brief Psychiatric Rating Scale (BPRS) (Ventura et al., 1993). Tools such as the mhGAP assessment tool (WHO, 2016), now available as an application for mobile devices or app (WHO, 2017), offer an easy-access means for assessing what might be happening more broadly in a patient's mental health and can suggest treatment options. As with other checklist-based systems, the mhGAP very much focuses on the content to be covered – *what* to ask, with minimal instruction on *how* to ask it or the communication skills required to optimise assessment.

However, it can be argued that *how* you ask the questions in mental health will have a significant bearing on the accuracy and utility of that assessment. If a patient feels able to 'open up', that is, to be honest about their symptoms and experiences, and then feels listened to and understood, research shows us that their level of concordance with suggested management strategies will increase (Stewart, 1995; Fallowfield et al., 2003), meaning any treatment or advice offered has a higher chance of being effective. Similarly, medical curricula worldwide state that practitioners should not only have the knowledge of a given condition (the *what*) but also the skills and attitudes required to assess and treat (the *how*) (World Psychiatry Association (WPA), 2017a; Medical Council of India, (MCI), 2018; General Medical Council, (GMC), 2020), thus explicitly recognising that knowledge alone is insufficient for effective patient care.

Therefore it would seem that whilst including knowledge of diagnostic facts, optimum mental healthcare education also needs to address the skills and attitudes underlying assessment and treatment – the *how* as well as the *what*. And as the mhGAP implies (2016), it is the *how* that is often harder to learn and where education needs to focus.

ADDRESSING THE 'HOW'

How a mental health-related consultation is undertaken differs across cultures, with variability in patient expectation, as well as in the hierarchical relationship between healthcare professionals and patients. Stigma about mental illness is more universal, as is reticence when talking about struggling to cope. Enabling people to talk about their mental health is a skill that can not only lead to more accurate diagnosis and hence more effective management planning but also to the subjective patient experience of compassion as one human reaches out to another, seeking to understand and help. Expressions of compassion can be different in different cultures, with some more verbal or explicit than others. Demonstration of a willingness to understand is nevertheless a key element in enabling disclosure of mental distress, opening channels for help to be received and thereby optimising the potential effectiveness of any care subsequently provided.

However, *how* a consultation is undertaken is not as straightforward as considering *what* should be covered and includes elements such as how to communicate clearly, how to control an interview, how to connect with a patient and also the underlying attitudes and values that inform how these skills are applied. If a healthcare professional is actively trying to understand the experiences of the patient in front of them, that will be experienced by the patient. If the professional does not believe in the validity of anxiety symptoms or feels their professional skills would be better spent on physical problems, that too will be felt, with a resultant impact upon the outcomes of the interaction. To explore such attitudes and their impact is an important part of the educational process and comes under the heading of *how* an interview is undertaken, as well as the more behavioural mechanics.

Providing education about *how* a mental health consultation is best undertaken in addition to *what* content needs to be covered will have a significant impact on mental health assessment practice and so significantly add to the overall aim of optimising psychiatric patient care. The *what* and the *how*, however, require different pedagogical strategies. The first point of devising an educational intervention, therefore, is to decide the priorities of what needs to be learned, or the learning objectives, and then to work out the best pedagogical strategy to enable that learning to occur – the 'best tool for the job'.

LEARNING OBJECTIVES – DEFINING THE DESIRED LEARNING

Learning objectives specify the intended learning that teachers expect participants to have achieved by the end of a teaching session or learning intervention. According to the aims of adult learning as defined by Knowles (1980), such learning objectives need to be viewed as relevant and practically applicable for the learners and also connect to previous knowledge and experience. When adult learners see how new learning connects to their previous experiences plus the relevance of the teaching for their current clinical practice, then motivation to engage and learn greatly increase (Merriam, 2001; Kahu, 2013).

To structure the learning objectives, Bloom's taxonomy (1956) offers a tool that contains a progression through knowledge, skill and affective or attitudinal engagement, with all three elements requiring consideration. The learning objectives each need to contain a verb in order to describe the anticipated learning behaviour – or how the learning will be achieved. When considering anticipated learning for undertaking a psychiatric assessment, objectives need to relate to knowledge acquisition, or *what* needs to be assessed, and also to the skills and attitudes that need to be practiced and explored, or *how* the assessment needs to be undertaken. When describing objectives, it is usual to begin with simpler verbs: such as to identify, to remember, to practice, and to work sequentially towards more complex processes: such as to evaluate, to conceptualise, to synthesise. Such verbs need to be matched to both the identified learning needs and the level of ability of the group.

If the learning objectives are clear and specifically connect to what the learners need to know, this will help to structure the teaching session and to provide a clear measure to gauge whether the expected learning has been achieved.

PEDAGOGICAL STRATEGIES – THE 'BEST TOOLS FOR THE JOB'

In educational theory, the concept of 'constructive alignment' describes the creation of a connection between what needs to be learned, or the content, and the optimum way for that learning to occur – the teaching methods, that is, the 'best tools for the job'. In some contexts, how learning is assessed is also significant and also needs to align. There are a range of pedagogical strategies, each used in different medical education contexts depending on *what* is to be learned and *how* the learning will occur. Choice of pedagogical strategy is also informed by the beliefs that the teachers hold about how learning takes place or their epistemological position.

Each strategy or approach has strengths and drawbacks, with some significantly more suitable to teach some content than others (Verduin et al., 2013). It is not a 'one size fits all' scenario. Then there are different methods or tools to address different objectives within each approach. Knowledge of a range of the pedagogical strategies and the various teaching methods that they contain will enable a healthcare educator to choose the most appropriate method for each given learning objective and so greatly increase the likelihood of that learning taking place.

We will now consider some of the common models of learning and related pedagogical strategies that could enable community healthcare professionals to learn not only *what* to look for when assessing someone presenting with possible mental ill health but also *how* to do it, including how different teaching methods, learning activities or tools can be optimised in order to address different learning objectives. We will then present a case study looking at a pedagogical strategy incorporating different teaching methods to learn both *what* and *how* to assess in someone presenting with low mood and suicidal ideation in a community healthcare setting.

MODELS OF LEARNING, PEDAGOGICAL STRATEGIES AND TEACHING METHODS

Instructivism

Instructivism has been the traditional learning methodology in medical education for many years and involves transmission of knowledge from those who know more to those who need to acquire it. It is fact focused and delivered through lectures, the reading of textbooks, or knowledge-focused e-learning. Once facts have been taught and memorised, learning is generally assessed in an exam, often consisting of multiple-choice questions. The main learning outcome from a student perspective is to have memorised the prescribed knowledge, most commonly to pass an assessment (McLeod et al., 2009). Strengths of this approach include its efficiency in the delivery of knowledge to a large number of people simultaneously and its ability to provide basic facts that underpin medical practice.

However, one key criticism of instructivism is that it creates passive learners who only achieve superficial levels of learning (McLachlan, 2006). Being able to remember information can be seen as more important than the ability to process that information or to understand its application in a clinical scenario. It has also been criticised as a potential means to power, with those who write the curriculum deciding what the 'objective truth' that should therefore be 'transmitted' is, with the passive recipients having little or no opportunity to consider alternatives, so enabling the dominant organisational discourse to perpetuate (Freire, 1996). This can create a static learning environment, not open to challenge or change, where the same facts are passed on to each generation, and progress of the educational system is therefore minimal.

Medical curricula across the world now state that an instructivist approach should not be the sole methodology in medical education but should instead be supplemented and enhanced by more interactive methods of learning (Verduin et al., 2013; World Federation of Medical Educators (WFME), 2015; WPA, 2017a). Teaching methodologies have been changing in the United Kingdom since the 1980s, when more social cognitivist and constructivist methodologies were introduced, such as problem-based learning and skill-based simulation. However, despite such innovations, the instructivist teaching model remains the mainstay of medical education worldwide.

Social Cognitivism

Social cognitivism focuses not on knowledge transmission but on information processing (Bandura, 2001). It considers how to integrate different streams of knowledge and process them to conceptualise and arrive at sound conclusions. The knowledge is important, but it is the processing or assimilation of that knowledge that is key in this approach. This is a necessary skill in healthcare, where, for example, during a patient assessment, different biological, psychological and social (bio-psycho-social) information will be presented and clinical reasoning or formulation will be needed in order to reach differential diagnoses and to construct subsequent management plans. Social cognitivism teaches the cognitive skills required to undertake that process.

Learning based in social cognitivism commonly occurs in a small group setting, where the tutor presents a problem or a case that needs research and exploration in order for solutions to emerge. The tutor acts as more of a designer and a guide than as a teacher, as the aim is that learners engage in self-directed learning. The most common learning strategies are problem-based learning (Barrows, 1996) or case-based learning, both of which start with a particular issue to be explored, with individuals in a group taking on specific tasks of discovery, then working together to create a solution which is then shared with the wider group. Working with a patient with 'lived experience' could also be considered social cognitivism, where learners can have the opportunity to hear a patient's story in a small group setting and can be guided to collaboratively integrate their previous knowledge with the real-life experiences of a patient in order to understand a more personal and holistic picture of a theoretical diagnosis.

Social cognitivist learning has been well integrated across many medical schools in the United Kingdom and is named as an option in medical curricula worldwide. However, this too has limitations, and some have questioned whether methods such as problem-based learning are as universally applicable as others suggest (Thirunavukarasu and Thirunavukarasu, 2009). As students discovering their own learning rather than being instructed, it could be argued that learning may be incomplete, lack sufficient depth or even leave learners with unchecked inaccurate deductions (Thirunavukarasu and Thirunavukarasu, 2009). Any learning that occurs could also remain theoretical, with transfer of learning to practice proposed to occur at some unspecified time in the future and far from guaranteed. The tutor in this type of teaching mainly has a design role, which is time consuming. It also requires skill and experience in order to create the correct level of challenge, plus sufficient activities for a small group such that all participants can contribute at a similar level and achieve the learning required.

Situated Learning

Situated learning happens in situ, such as in a healthcare setting, and involves the learner observing and modelling the practice of those with more experience, also known as an apprentice model. This connects with the "see one, do one, teach one" approach: vicarious learning by observation, followed by practice and then the teaching of that practice to others. A learner would commence their learning on the periphery of what has been named a 'community of practice' (Wenger, 1998), such as a clinic or department, and gradually work their way towards a more central role as expertise accumulates. It is claimed that learning in this way integrates knowledge, skills and attitudes because in practice all three elements work cohesively and are not separated out as they can be in a classroom (Lave and Wenger, 1991; Nicolini et al., 2016). The tutor role is taken on by a more senior practitioner, who demonstrates and explains their personal and professional expertise. As the learner progresses to the 'doing' phase, the tutor provides feedback on the learner's performance. Lave and Wenger (1991) explain how this way of working is beneficial in gaining professional identity, as it is not only applied knowledge and skill that is demonstrated but also professional values in practice.

To learn in such an environment, however, requires a 'good enough' role model, who can not only demonstrate skill as a clinician but also has the time and motivation to explain their own practice, to observe the learner and to provide proactive feedback on performance, with clear direction on how to progress. In a clinical environment, there may be limited time for teaching due to the pressure of clinical caseloads. There may also be gaps in learning, as the methodology is dependent upon the arrival of the range of patient presentations required to cover the intended learning, meaning if a patient with a certain condition is not present, the learning will not occur, potentially creating a 'hit and miss' approach to curriculum design.

Social Constructivism

Constructivism comes from the ontological position that there is no external positivist reality waiting to be discovered or transmitted but that knowledge is constructed by each of us individually as we experience and interpret the world around us. Social constructivism enables these interpretations to be co-constructed with others through a process of accommodation, working in a social or small group context guided by a tutor who facilitates the process, acting as a 'more knowledgeable other' (Vygotsky, 1978) or 'midwife' (Jones, 2005) to learning. Constructivism requires an experiential or practice element on which to reflect and conceptualise, as "learning is formed and re-formed through experience" rather than remaining theoretical. Like social cognitivism, social constructivism enables a measure of cognitive processing but has the added component of experimentation as ideas are not only conceptualised theoretically but can also be put into practice and reflected upon further, in relation to learning from previous experimentation. As such, a cycle of construction of collective learning occurs: an active process of 'working things out together', facilitated by someone with greater knowledge and experience, who understands the cumulative learning process.

The application and experimentation phase of learning can be undertaken in clinical practice, with regular re-groupings. One example of this would be group supervision, where participants can be supported to reflect retrospectively upon clinical experiences and prospectively plan how they might change practice based on those reflections with consideration of alternative approaches. Social constructivism can also be used in a classroom setting through an activity such as experiential simulation (Fanning and Gaba, 2007; Dave, 2012). Classroom-based simulation involves experimentation with how to undertake challenging tasks in a safe practice environment, such as undertaking a mental state examination, managing disinhibition or breaking bad news. It utilises the concept of 'playing' in a virtual world: a safe space in which to experiment (Schon, 1987), where in addition to 'playing' with different skills and reflecting on the impact, the group with the facilitator can identify individual attitudinal reactions within the simulation and explore why those reactions may be occurring. This enables learning about the skills required for the task, as well as exploration of the attitudes and feelings that inevitably inform practice.

The use of constructivist learning strategies is not necessarily simple, requiring skilful facilitation and at times design in order to create an educationally challenging yet safe space for learning to occur. The tutor should have an awareness of the group's learning needs and should be facilitating progression into the next stage of learning at all times, a progression that Vygotsky refers to as moving into a learner's 'zone of proximal development' (1978). As this is an approach that primarily considers skills and attitudes, there may be need for prior learning of appropriate knowledge before the session can commence, which may include more instructivist methods. There is no guarantee that all participants would have completed such preparatory activities. There is also the need of a second tutor in the group taking the part of a simulated patient, able not only to act but also to interpret their own reactions to the skills and attitudes of the learners in the consultation. This has potential cost implications which need to be weighed against the benefits of learning in this methodology.

For a summary of the common models of learning and related pedagogical strategies, please see Table 1.1.

EDUCATIONAL STRATEGIES TO OPTIMISE CARE • 9

Table 1.1 Summary of common models of learning and related pedagogical strategies.

Models of learning	Pedagogical strategies	Learning objectives	Role of teacher	Positives	Potential drawbacks	Proponents
Instructivism. Transmission model.	Lectures.	To acquire knowledge. To memorise facts.	To impart knowledge or direct reading.	Provides knowledge which can then be applied. Cost effective.	Superficial learning of facts. Can be politically motivated – what is valid knowledge?	Jones (2007) Carpenter (2006)
Social cognitivism.	Small group discussion. Problem-based, case-based learning.	To process information. To enable conceptual thinking.	To design self-directed learning activities. To facilitate the process.	Enables knowledge to be applied theoretically. Promotes processing/assimilation skills needed for clinical decision making.	Requires prior knowledge. Remains theoretical.	Bruner (1986) Barrows (1996)
Situated learning. Communities of Practice.	Observation	To gain skills and professional values.	To model skills and values.	Combines the learning of knowledge, skills and attitudes.	Requires a 'good' role model who can teach. May be incomplete – 'hit and miss'.	
Social constructivism. Experiential learning.	Experiential simulation.	To apply knowledge. To explore attitudes and values.	To facilitate. To be a 'midwife' to learning.	Applies knowledge.	Requires prior knowledge. Requires a simulated patient – potential financial implications.	Vygotsky (1978) Diekmann (2009)

TRANSFER OF LEARNING INTO PRACTICE

If education is to have any impact on optimising patient care, learning needs to leave the classroom and transfer into clinical practice. The content of learning that needs to be transferred is driven by the learning objectives. If the learning objective is that knowledge be transmitted, this can be assessed easily by the use of a knowledge test, for example, through multiple-choice questions or a viva. Transfer of this knowledge into practice could be measured by assessing the accuracy of patients' diagnoses and management plans. However, it has been identified that knowledge alone does not promote patient engagement or concordance with management plans, (Zimmermann and Del Piccolo, 2007; Cushing and Metcalfe, 2007) and as such, the memorising of facts alone is unlikely to have any significant impact in the ongoing optimisation of patient care. The measurement of learning *how* an assessment has been undertaken and the skills and attitudes displayed is more complex. Skills such as communication or structuring an interview are largely behavioural and, as such, observable. Research shows us that, if taught well, these skills can transfer from the classroom to practice *and* be sustained after several months (Fallowfield et al., 2003). Attitudes, however, drive *how* an assessment is undertaken, *what* is valued in a patient history and *what* is addressed in management. Learning of professional attitudes is much more difficult to assess, as changes in conceptual understanding always precede a change in performance, and such internal changes in concepts are not directly observable (Glaserfeld, 1997). However, it could also be argued that once one has explored or reflected on new insights and has been empowered to act differently, it is hard to remain as you were, as: "the rehearsal stimulates the practice of the act in reality" (Boal, 2000: 120) both in attitudes and subsequent actions. Likewise, learning related to alternative attitudinal constructs, once conceptualised, leads to thoughts that are more difficult to deconstruct. Evidence suggests that knowledge built in this way is associated with deeper levels of learning and therefore has a much higher likelihood of transfer into practice (Moon, 2004; Mann et al., 2007). Ways to assess such transfer of attitudinal change include reflection, supervision and group discussion, possibly through a community of practice, in reality or online.

SUMMARY OF THE DESIGN PROCESS

When designing pedagogical strategies to optimise patient care, the factors that we have discussed that need to be in place are:

1. The overall aim of the educational intervention.
2. The learning objectives – what the learner needs to know, using a taxonomy such as Bloom's (1956).
3. The pedagogical strategies to address the learning objectives, including the need for constructive alignment.
4. The most appropriate teaching methods in line with each pedagogical strategy – the learning activities that will be used to address the different learning elements and how those activities will be facilitated.
5. How any learning will be transferred into practice.

We will now consider how this process can be applied in practice, considering how to enable a group of healthcare workers in a community setting to assess and manage a patient presenting with moderate low mood and suicidal ideation.

AN EXAMPLE FROM PRACTICE

Context

A group of healthcare practitioners working in a primary care community setting – the first point of contact for the patient experiencing low mood with suicidal ideation.

Overall Aim of Teaching Intervention

The overall aim of the teaching session is to enable more effective assessment of a patient presenting with low mood and suicidal ideation and negotiate an appropriate management plan. Depression is the most common presentation of mental illness worldwide (WHO, 2013), contributing 4.3% to the global burden of disease (WHO, 2013) and being the third most leading cause of 'years lived with disability' (YLD) worldwide, behind low back pain and headache (The Lancet, 2017). In some developing countries, it is estimated that only 12–15% of people with depression receive treatment (Murthy, 2017), creating a treatment gap of 85%. It is estimated that 15–20% of patients with depression end their life by suicide (WHO, 2001), which has its own impact upon the mental wellbeing (including risk of further suicide) in the families of those affected. Low mood with suicidal ideation is extremely common in all countries of the world and is frequently managed by non-psychiatrists. To address this subject in a teaching session should create a resonance of relevance for all healthcare workers in a healthcare setting, and all should have some baseline experience and knowledge upon which to build.

Learning Objectives

The learning objectives for this educational intervention are:

1. To *be aware* of the knowledge required when assessing a patient with low mood and suicidal ideation and the appropriate management options, with particular emphasis on risk.
2. To *identify* the challenges in assessing a patient who presents with depression and suicidal ideation, from a patient, professional and organisational perspective.
3. To *experiment* with different communication skills that explore the symptomatology, risk and management of a 'patient' with low mood and suicidal ideation.
4. To *appraise* the impact of different communication skills upon the consultation and conceptualise alternatives.
5. To *explore* the effect on the professional of talking with a patient about low mood and suicide and how pre-existing value systems and attitudes can impact the conversation and subsequent decisions made.
6. To *reflect* on anticipated and actual changes to healthcare practice in this context following the training.

Pedagogical Strategies and Teaching Methods

1. Learning Objective 1 – to be aware of the knowledge required to undertake an appropriate assessment of low mood and suicidal ideation, including risk, and to decide an appropriate management plan. As certain elements of key knowledge are central, an instructivist pedagogical strategy would be optimal to address this outcome. Given that this is a highly relevant subject to healthcare practice and that participants are

likely to have a degree of motivation to learn – (a key principle of adult learning as described by Knowles [1980]), participants would be asked to read about the core symptoms of depression, the associated risks and the potential management options prior to the session. The mhGAP Intervention Guide, as published by the World Health Organisation (WHO, 2016), would be a useful tool in this context, as it aims at how to assess and manage mental, neurological and substance use disorders in non-specialised health settings, with specific sections on depression, self-harm and suicide. A shorter version is available as a smartphone application (app) (WHO, 2017). In the classroom context, participants can be asked to share what they have learned and, based on their prior reading, create a consensus of key symptoms, risks and management options.

2. Learning Objective 2 – to identify how and why assessing and treating low mood and suicidal risk is challenging in practice. This again reinforces the relevance of the subject for participants and gives credence to prior learning and experience (Knowles, 1980). As this learning uses group discussion to explore and analyse different perceptions of a challenge or problem, it is rooted in a social cognitivist pedagogy. Learning is optimised if the group is divided into smaller sub-sections of three to four people, allowing opportunity for greater active discussion about prior knowledge and experience (Mills and Alexander, 2013). Discussion points from the small groups are then shared with the larger group, and an overall picture of the challenges in practice for professionals, patients and organisations is created. As this educational intervention aims not only to teach knowledge and skills but also attitudes and professional values, it is important to explore the challenges brought by healthcare professionals' personal perceptions about mental illness and how these may impact both the accuracy and depth of assessment and the subjective experience of compassion for those being assessed. This is particularly important to explore, as if the patient feels judged or not understood, the level of concordance with management will decrease (Cushing and Metcalfe, 2007).

As well as establishing common ground of understanding for participants, this discussion also enables the facilitator to identify the participants' 'zone of proximal development' (Vygotsky, 1978), or what they need to learn next based on their current knowledge and experience. This awareness will inform how the facilitator can help participants move into their neighbouring 'zone', building on their current level of 'knowing' and hence making learning easier. This is a precursor to social constructivist learning and fits well with the learning objectives that follow.

3. Learning objectives 3, 4 and 5 – to experiment with different communication skills in experiential simulation when assessing a patient with low mood and suicidal ideation, including the resultant impact upon the patient, the process and the professional. As this approach is one of experimentation in a group setting, alongside reflection, conceptualisation and re-experimentation, it uses the pedagogical strategy of social constructivism.

In a teaching context, simulation can be described as a re-enactment of a reality-based situation in a safe environment, where skills can be practiced and reflected upon, and conceptual thinking can be honed (McNaughton et al., 2008). In psychiatry this commonly involves a psychiatric interview or management of a challenging situation, either as an individual or as part of a team. Simulation can be used in a variety of ways, and such differences in application allow for it to be aligned with all the pedagogical strategies. In the context of social constructivism, simulation can be used not only as a place to rehearse skills and reflect upon impact but also as a means for a group to collectively conceptualise alternatives and continually experiment in Kolb's ongoing learning cycle (1994). It must be noted that the impact of the interview is felt not only by the patient but also by the professional involved. Asking about symptoms of low mood and suicidal ideation is not easy and can create anxiety and raise unconscious bias in anyone having to talk in depth about such challenging subjects. Simulation methodology is increasingly being seen as applicable to exploring the human relations at the heart of mental healthcare (Nestel et al., 2018), as it allows a facilitator to draw out any emotional or attitudinal difficulties and enables the group to consider how such professional challenges can be addressed.

The experiential simulation being used in this context is inspired by forum theatre, created by Augusto Boal (2000) with roots in the pedagogy of Freire (Dwyer, 2004). Forum theatre involves the presentation of a scenario based in real experiences where the conclusion is not perceived as ideal. In experiential simulation, this could be the presentation of a patient brought to a healthcare centre by their family with symptoms of being withdrawn, with poor sleep, weight loss, no enjoyment, not working and feeling hopeless, with repetitive ideas of suicide. In forum theatre, the audience or group offers suggestions of how to approach the scenario, which are then tried out or experimented with, and the group discusses the effectiveness of these approaches, conceptualises alternatives and continues to experiment in this cycle until a satisfactory conclusion is reached. Twomey-Fosnot describes how social constructivism often uses symbolic representations such as storytelling, film and theatre that enable us to "go beyond the immediacy of the concrete . . . to encounter multiple perspectives that generate new possibilities, to become conscious of our actions on the world in order to gain new knowledge with which to act" (2005: 30). This form of experiential simulation enables that process.

Experiential simulation requires a facilitator who, in terms of social constructivism, acts as the 'more knowledgeable other' (Vygotsky, 1978) or 'midwife to learning' (Jones, 2005). The facilitator does not provide the answers or promote one correct way to perform the interview but instead prompts participants to collectively construct meaning or 'work it out for themselves'. It is this element of needing to process learning, not just receive information, that creates the deeper levels of learning that have been shown to have a measurable effect upon practice (Mann et al., 2007; Moon, 2004). The skill in such facilitation is in enabling a group to reach its *own* conclusions, ensuring that they remain in line with accepted practice and in resisting of temptation to simply provide the 'correct answer'. Experiential simulation also requires a second tutor to simulate or take the role of a patient: that is, a simulated patient. Where possible, it is preferable to use a trained actor, although this has obvious cost implications. It needs someone who can be representative of real patients in similar situations, who can see and feel from the patient's point of view, reacting to the interviewer and their skills and attitudes as a real patient would and able to articulate that reaction; it is far more than simply 'saying the words'.

For this methodology to work, the participants need to 'buy in' to the scenario as if it were real. This is known as the 'as if' concept (Vaihinger, 1927), which is aligned with simulation fidelity (Hamstra et al., 2014). How the methodology is presented by the facilitator and how accurately the simulated patient represents the patient are key elements to promoting fidelity and thus 'buy-in'.

The scenario for the simulated patient needs to cover the content of everything a healthcare professional could ask and how to deliver that information in alignment with the diagnosis. It is necessary to cover such information as:

1. Symptoms to be examined in a mental state examination, including how they are experienced, for example, that there is difficulty in concentration or processing information,

including in this interview; experiences of guilt or hopelessness, so reducing eye contact and manifesting in negative content about self in the simulation.
2. Physical presentation related to low mood – such as wearing unkempt clothes, dirty hair, slouched posture, slowed gait, reduced eye contact, slowed speech.
3. History – chronology of significant recent events and symptoms; social background including work, family, finances, interests and the *impact* of low mood in these areas.
4. Previous experiences of similar symptoms and help received.
5. Suicidal ideation – detail in relation to method, frequency of thought, intent, preparations and protective factors.
6. How the 'patient' feels about seeing the healthcare professional and how this is demonstrated. What will help them trust and connect with the professional and what will not.

THE SIMULATION FORMAT

1. The scenario or patient story is presented to the group in brief, such as the limited information that could be included in a referral letter. If, as is commonly the case in some settings, there is no referral mechanism, then no such information is given to the group, and the participant meets the simulated patient with no prior knowledge, as they would in real life. Ideas are sought from the group as to how to approach an assessment, and feelings and thoughts approaching the assessment are shared. One group member takes the interview chair, or 'hot seat', and is advised they are the mouthpiece for the group and that they can stop any time they struggle.
2. The simulated patient enters the group, and the participant begins the interview, as instructed in the group discussion. The simulated patient responds in line with the scenario.
3. After a few minutes, the participant or facilitator stops the scenario; the 'patient' remains in the room and in role, not speaking unless spoken to. The facilitator leads group discussion, reflecting on *what* has been discovered, including symptoms from the 'patient' story in alignment with earlier learning of knowledge, and *how* it was found out or what skills were used with what impact. The simulated patient can be asked by the facilitator how they experienced the interview so far, responding in role. The group are encouraged to conceptualise about where the interview could go next, both in terms of symptoms or history – the *what*, or skills that could be tried – the *how*.
4. The scenario restarts, with experimentation with some of the alternative approaches. This could resume at the point that the interview stopped or perhaps 'rewind' to an earlier point in order to try an alternative, using a different participant as mouthpiece for the group.
5. The process is repeated until sufficient information is elicited to determine the severity of low mood and the level of risk associated with the suicidal ideation. Discussion can then take place about management options. The simulated patient is asked what management options would create the greatest level of concordance and why that might be, drawing out the principle that if the patient feels their situation is understood, concordance increases.
6. The group summarises both what needs to be covered and the skills that enabled both disclosure and concordance. An action plan for this type of assessment is created in small groups and discussed in the large group, aiming at an acceptable consensus in line with local practice.
7. Revisiting of attitudes to a patient with depression and suicidal ideation – exploration of if attitudes have changed and why that might be.

8. Learning outcome 6 – to reflect upon anticipated and actual changes to participants' practice in this context. In order for learning to occur at a deeper level than simple transfer of factual knowledge, and to encourage integration of learning into practice, reflection on one's own work is necessary, for example, through use of a reflective diary (Moon, 2004). Ideally this would be supported in a situated learning pedagogy by having one's assessments being observed, with feedback provided about *how* the learned skills are being applied. In situations where this is not possible, alternatives may include the use of online communities, where individuals can discuss progress and challenges and support each other to apply the learning taken from the classroom (Mann et al., 2007). It would also be optimal for the group to meet again with the facilitator some weeks later to discuss progress in the transfer of learning to the workplace, as even with the constraints of time, evidence suggests that knowledge which is socially constructed is embedded at a deeper level for the learner and therefore has a much higher likelihood of transfer (Moon, 2004).

CONCLUSION

When considering education to optimise patient care, it is important to begin with what the healthcare professionals need to learn relevant to their daily clinical practice – the learning objectives. Once identified, a range of pedagogical strategies should be considered in order to identify the optimum way for the learning objectives to be achieved – the 'best tools for the job'. Once the combination of necessary pedagogical strategies is known, appropriate teaching methods can be aligned so that, working in combination, they can equip healthcare professionals with the knowledge, skills and professional attitudes required, so that each may confidently undertake accurate and compassionate assessments and achieve subsequent concordance with ongoing management plans. Hence the optimum psychiatric care has a higher chance of being secured for the many patients currently not receiving the help that they need.

References

Bandura, A., (2001). Social cognitive theory: An agentic perspective. *Annual Review of Psychology.* 52: 1–26.
Barrows, H.S., (1996). Problem-based learning in medicine and beyond: A brief overview. *New Directions for Teaching and Learning.* 68: 3–12.
Beck, A.T., Steer, R.A., Brown, G.K. (1996). *Manual for the Beck Depression Inventory-II*. San Antonio, TX: Psychological Corporation.
Bloom, B.S., (1956). *Taxonomy of Educational Objectives: The Classification of Educational Goals. Handbook 1, Cognitive Domain*. New York, NY: McKay.
Boal, A. (2000). *Theatre of the Oppressed*. London: Pluto Press.
Bruner, J., (1986). *Actual Minds, Possible Worlds*. Cambridge, MA: Harvard University Press.
Carpenter, J., (2006). Effective teaching methods for large classes. *Journal of Family and Consumer Sciences Education.* 24: 13–23.
Cook, V., Daly, C., Newman, M., (Editors) (2012). *Work-Based Learning in Clinical Settings – Insights from a Socio-Cultural Perspective*. London: Radcliffe Publishing.
Cushing, A., Metcalfe, R. (2007). Optimizing medicines management: From compliance to concordance. *Therapeutics and Clinical Risk Management*, 3(6): 1047–1058.
Dave, S., (2012). Simulation on psychiatric teaching. *Advances in Psychiatric Teaching*, 18: 292–298.
Dieckmann, P., (Editor) (2009). *Using Simulations for Education, Training and Research*. Lengerich: Pabst Science Publishers.
Dwyer, P., (2004). Making bodies talk in forum theatre. *Research in Drama Education: The Journal of Applied Theatre and Performance.* 9(2): 199–210.

Fallowfield, L., Jenkins, V., Farewell, V., Solis-Trapala, I., (2003). Enduring impact of communication skills training: Results of a 12-month follow-up. *British Journal of Cancer*, 89: 1445–1449.
Fanning, R., Gaba, D., (2007). The role of debriefing in simulation-based learning. *Simulation in Healthcare: The Journal of the Society for Simulation in Healthcare*, 2(2): 115–125.
Freire, P., (1996). *Pedagogy of the Oppressed*. Toronto, CA: Penguin Books.
General Medical Council – UK (GMC), (2020). *Outcomes for Graduates*. GMC UK. www.gmc-uk.org/education/standards-guidance-and-curricula/standards-and-outcomes/outcomes-for-graduates/outcomes-for-graduates/structure-and-overarching-outcome. Accessed 21st May 2020.
Glaserfeld, E.V., (1997). *Radical Constructivism—Way of Knowing and Learning*. London: The Falmer Press.
Hamstra, S.J., Brydges, R., Hatala, R., Zendejas, B., Cook, D.A., (2014). Reconsidering fidelity in simulation-based training. *Academic Medicine*. 89(3).
Jones, G.G., (2005). *Gatekeepers, Midwives and Fellow-Travellers: The Craft and Artistry of Adult Educators*. London: Mary Ward Centre.
Jones, S.E., (2007). Reflections on the lecture: Outmoded medium or instrument of inspiration? *Journal of Further and Higher Education*, 31(4): 397–406.
Kahu, E., (2013). Framing student engagement in higher education. *Studies in Higher Education* 38(5): 758–773.
Knowles, M.S., (1980). *The Modern Practice of Adult Education: From Pedagogy to Androgogy* (2nd ed.). New York: Cambridge Books.
The Lancet, (2018). Global, regional, and national incidence, prevalence, and years lived with disability for 354 diseases and injuries for 195 countries and territories, 1990–2017: A systematic analysis for the Global Burden of Disease Study 2017. *The Lancet*. 392: 1789–1858.
Lave, J., Wenger, E., (1991). *Situated Learning: Legitimate Peripheral Participation*. Cambridge: Cambridge University Press.
Mann, K., Gordon, J., Macleod, A., (2007) Reflection and reflective practice in health professions education: a systematic review. *Advance in Health Science Education*. 14: 595–621.
McLachlan, J. C. (2006). The relationship between assessment and learning [Editorial]. *Medical Education*. 40(8): 716–777.
McLeod, P., Steinert, Y., Chalk, C., Cruess, R., Cruess, S., Meterissian, S., Razack, S., Snell, L. (2009). Which pedagogical principles should clinical teachers know? Teachers and education experts disagree: Disagreement on important pedagogical principles. *Medical Teacher*. 31(4): e117–e124.
McNaughton, N., Ravitz, P., Wadell, A., Hodges, B.D., (2008). Psychiatric education and simulation: A review of the literature. *The Canadian Journal of Psychiatry*. 53(2): 85–93.
Medical Council of India (MCI), (2018). *Competency Based Undergraduate Curriculum for the Indian Medical Graduate 2018* (Vol. 1). Delhi, India, p. 14.
Merriam, S.B., (2001). Androgogy and self-directed learning: Pillars of adult learning theory. *New Directions for Adult and Continuing Education*, 89, Spring.
Mills, D., Alexander, P., (2013). *Small Group Teaching: A Toolkit for Learning*. UK: The Higher Education Academy.
Moon, J. A., (2004). *A Handbook of Reflective and Experiential Learning—Theory and Practice*. London: Routledge Falmer.
Murthy, R.S., (2017). National mental health survey of India 2015–2016. *Indian Journal of Psychiatry*, 59(1): 21–26.
Nestel, D., McNaughton, N., Smith, C., Schlegel, C., Tierney, T., (2018). Values and value in simulated participant methodology: A global perspective on contemporary practices. *Medical Teacher*. DOI: 10.1080/0142159X.2018.1472755
Nicolini, D., Scarbrough, H., Gracheva, J., (2016). Communities of practice and situated learning in healthcare. In *Oxford Handbook of Health Care Management* (ed. Ferlie, E., Montgomert, K.). Oxford: Oxford University Press.
Schon, D., (1987). *Educating the Reflective Practitioner*. San Francisco, CA: Jossey-Bass Ltd.
Stewart, M.A., (1995). Effective physician-patient communication and health outcomes: A review. *Canadian Medical Association Journal*. 152(9).
Thirunavukarasu, M., Thirunavukarasu, P., (2009). Retrospective introspection. *Indian Journal of Psychiatry*. 51(2): 85–87.
Twomey Fosnot, C., (2005). *Constructivism: Theory, Perspectives and Practice*. UK: Teachers' College Press.
Vaihinger, H., (1927). *The Philosophy of the As-If System of the Theoretical, Pragmatic, and Religious Fictions of Mankind Based on an Idealistic Positivism*. Aalen: Scientia.

Ventura, J., Lukoff, D., Nuechterlein, K. H., Liberman, R. P., Green, M., Shaner, A., (1993). Appendix 1: Brief Psychiatric Rating Scale (BPRS) expanded version (4.0) scales, anchor points and administration manual. *International Journal of Methods in Psychiatric*. 3: 227–244.

Verduin, M.L., Boland, R.J., Guthrie, T.M., (2013). New directions in medical education related to psychiatry. *International Review of Psychiatry*. 25(3): 338–346.

Vygotsky, L., (1978). *Mind in Society: Development of Higher Psychological Processes*. Cambridge, MA: Harvard University Press.

Wenger, E., (1998). *Communities of Practice. Learning Meaning and Identity*. Cambridge: Cambridge University Press.

World Federation of Medical Educators (WFME), (2015). *Basic Medical Education WFME Global Standards 2015*. WFME, p. 18.

World Health Organisation (WHO), (2001). *World Health Report, 2001-Mental Health – New Understanding, New Hope*. WHO, Geneva.

World Health Organisation (WHO), (2008). *mhGAP Mental Health Gap Action Programme–Scaling Up Care for Mental, Neurological, and Substance Use Disorders*. WHO.

World Health Organisation (WHO), (2013). *Mental Health Action Plan, 2013–2020*. WHO, Geneva.

World Health Organisation (WHO), (2016). *mhGAP Intervention Guide for Mental, Neurological and Substance Use Disorders in Non-Specialized Health Settings V2*. WHO, Geneva.

World Health Organisation (WHO), (2017). *mhGAP App*. www.who.int/mental_health/mhgap/e_mhgap/en/. Accessed 17th May 2020.

World Psychiatry Association (WPA), (2017a). WPA Action Plan–2017–2020. *World Psychiatry*, 16(3).

World Psychiatry Association (WPA), (2017b). *WPA Recommendations: Principles and Priorities for a Framework for Training Psychiatrists*, pp. 15–27. https://3ba346de-fde6-473f-b1da-536498661f9c.filesusr.com/ugd/e172f3_9e614f64a8ee4675b8b3dedbc6488686.pdf. Accessed 21st May 2020.

Zimmermann, C., Del Piccolo, L., (2007). Cues and concerns by patients in medical consultations: A literature review. *Psychological Bulletin*. 133(3): 438–463.

2
Optimising Patient Care in Psychiatry – Focus on Quality of Life

Sandeep Grover and Swapnajeet Sahoo

Introduction	18
Defining QoL	19
Measurement of QoL	20
Research on QoL in Major Psychiatric Disorders	22
Strategies to Improve QoL	28
Conclusions	28

INTRODUCTION

Medicine has always been traditionally focused on the objective clinical or biological outcomes to determine improvement in patients suffering from various illnesses. However, the patient's personal viewpoint of illness and social perspectives is equally important for the overall holistic management of the patient's health condition. In this regard, researchers have tried to capture these attributes by using different outcome measures, and the concept of "quality of life" (QoL) is one such outcome.

The concept of QoL was introduced about 45 years ago in 1975 in medical indexes, mainly in the field of oncology, since oncologists were often questioned about their viewpoint on whether to add years to life or life to years.[1] With the improvement in understanding of the concept, QoL is now regarded as an important patient-reported outcome measure.[2] Over the years, the concept of QoL has moved beyond the boundaries of mortality and symptomatic improvement, and now it also encompasses the patient's experience with illness, that is, how one feels to live with illness, how satisfied one is with his/her treatment and so on. QoL is now regarded as an important outcome measure to evaluate the effectiveness of therapeutic interventions in any chronic illnesses. The concept of QoL has broadened to a great extent now, and it gives due weight to the concerns of the patients and regards them as human beings and not just as 'cases', as every individual has different aspects of his/her life which are not directly connected to disease.[3] In addition to physical functioning, QoL includes psychological functioning and well-being (emotional and mental), social functioning (interpersonal relationships and community participation), perception of health status and overall satisfaction with life.[4–6]

With regard to mental disorders, the concept of QoL has a much wider scope.[7] QoL received significant attention among patients with mental disorders soon after the beginning of the deinstitutionalisation movement in the 1960s. Further, with the emergence of the concept of recovery, more emphasis was given to the personal perspectives of the patients' lives, along with implementation of community psychiatric services.

DEFINING QOL

Various researchers have tried to define QoL differently. While some have proposed it is the perception and reaction to health problems and other components of one's life,[4] others regard it as the difference between an individual's expectations and actual achievements.[8] A panel of experts and researchers at the World Health Organization (WHO) developed an unifying and transcultural definition of QoL as

> the individual's perception of his or her position in life, within the cultural context and value system he or she lives in, and in relation to his or her goals, expectations, parameters and social relations. It is a broad ranging concept affected in a complex way by the person's physical health, psychological state, level of independence, social relationships and their relationship to salient features of their environment.[9]

This definition takes into account the subjective nature of QoL along with the earlier experiences of the subject in his/her cultural background. WHO also defined different domains and facets included under the domain of QoL (Table 2.1).[9] Although the WHO definition of QoL is widely used, there is no universally accepted definition of QoL. However, for all practical purposes, in simpler words, QoL is the degree of well-being as perceived by the individual or a group of people or one's own evaluation of the impact of illness on one's life spheres.

Apart from the different domains of QoL, the main dimensions of QoL are adaptive functioning (personal self-care and social roles) and life satisfaction or subjective feeling of well-being. Social support has also been regarded as a dimension of QoL by some authors.[10]

Table 2.1 WHO QoL domains [9].

Domain	Facets
Physical	• Pain and discomfort
	• Energy and fatigue
	• Sexual activity
	• Sleep and rest
	• Sensory function
Psychological	• Positive feelings
	• Thinking, learning, memory and concentration
	• Self-esteem
	• Bodily image and appearance
	• Negative feelings
Level of independence	• Mobility
	• Activities of daily living
	• Dependence on medicinal substances and medical aids
	• Dependence on non-medicinal substances (alcohol, tobacco, drugs)
	• Communication capacity
	• Work capacity

(Continued)

Table 2.1 (Continued)

Domain	Facets
Social relationships	• Personal relationships
	• Practical social support
	• Activities as provider/supporter
Environment	• Freedom, physical safety and security
	• Home environment
	• Work satisfaction
	• Financial resources
	• Health and social care: accessibility and quality
	• Opportunities for acquiring new information and skills
	• Participation in and opportunities for recreation/leisure activities
	• Physical environment: (pollution/noise/traffic/climate)
	• Transport
Spirituality/religion/personal beliefs	• Feeling life to be meaningful, how much one's personal beliefs give strength to face difficulties and understand difficulties in life, faith in God, opportunities for religious activities
Overall QoL and general health beliefs	• Rating overall QoL, satisfaction with one's own QoL, satisfaction with one's life and health

More recently, QoL has been termed health-related QoL (HRQoL) and has been regarded as one of the core components of patient-reported outcome measures (PROs). Patients have been considered the most valid reporters of their suffering and coping with illness. Therefore, HRQoL assessment provides an additional viewpoint to the overall assessment of patient's self perception of his/her symptoms and treatment-related problems/side effects along with physical, social and mental well-being.[11,12] Further, the ambit of QoL has broadened for persons with mental illnesses, and occupational function, life satisfaction, treatment tolerability and adherence have been added to the assessment of HRQoL.[13] Despite the use of several definitions of QoL in psychiatry, there is a lack of a conceptual model of QoL in psychiatry, resulting in overlap of other outcome measures.[11]

MEASUREMENT OF QOL

As QoL is a complex multi-dimensional construct which is often very difficult to assess clinically, researchers have developed various instruments to measure QoL. Evidence suggests that two approaches have been adopted to understand the concept of QoL and its subsequent measurement. These are (a) assessing QoL through the assessment of general life satisfaction with ongoing circumstances and (b) assessing QoL as a health-related outcome measure which involves assessing disease experience and one's functioning in his/her different life domains.[14] However, there are several issues pertaining to the assessment of QoL. Some of these issues are discussed in the following section.

1. **Subjective vs objective assessment of QoL:** Most QoL measurement instruments rely on subjective assessment (mostly by using self-rated scales or clinician interview-based scales/questionnaires designed to pick up the patient's viewpoint). Subjective assessment is the ideal way of assessing QoL, as it takes into account the person's well-being and satisfaction with life along with his/her perception of his/her daily functioning in all aspects. However, some researchers point out that solely focusing upon the subjective perspective of patients could be misleading, as it is prone to distortion due to altered psychological states (for example, in patients with depression).[15,16] It is suggested that subjective reporting of QoL can be coloured by "psychopathological fallacies", that is, affective conditions (affective fallacy – a depressed person would rate his well-being and functioning worse, and a manic patient would rate his well-being and functioning as excellent and more favourable than their significant others),[17] cognitive errors/negative cognitive schema (cognitive fallacy) or reality distortion/delusions/hallucinations (reality distortion fallacy). All these fallacies are difficult to correct and may lead to wrong inferences in assessment of subjective QoL. Further, perceived and internalised stigma in patients suffering from severe mental illness can also colour the subjective evaluation of QoL.[18] Hence, it is usually recommended to control for the presence of psychopathological symptoms to avoid spurious rating of QoL. In view of the limitations of the subjective evaluation of QoL, some researchers suggest incorporation of objective evidence from other sources to quantify QoL. Accordingly, it is suggested that while evaluating QoL in patients with psychiatric disorders, necessary information must be collected from caregivers and key informants, too. Accordingly, some QoL instruments have 'patient version', 'carer version' and 'professional version' so as to take into account the actual QoL of the patient from different perspectives (for example, Wisconsin Quality of Life).[19,20] However, others are of the view that taking information from family members and medical staff would be more for 'objective' assessment of QoL and patients' perspectives are not taken into account; hence, the evaluation might not be genuine. Despite all these arguments, caregiver information has been considered vital and valuable to understand others' perception of the patient.[21] Further, assessment of QoL solely from the patient can be unreliable in subjects with intellectual disability and severe cognitive impairment due to severe mental illness or head trauma.[22] In summary, though the subjective assessment of QoL is better than objective assessment, the assessment measure needs to be acknowledged, with the possible fallacies it can account for.
2. **Role of contextual factors in QoL evaluation in patients with psychiatric disorders:** QoL assessment in patients with psychiatric disorders is difficult when one looks into the role of various contextual factors which can affect the appropriate assessment of QoL. It was proposed that QoL is the gap between one's expectations and achievements.[8] However, this statement about QoL might not be applicable to patients with psychiatric disorders, as it is often seen that most patients with chronic psychiatric illnesses lower their expectations as an adaptation to their psychological process/illness and report themselves well satisfied with their current living standards and life conditions. In other words, the gap between expectations and achievements in these patients appears to be quite narrow, and such satisfaction with limited expectations may be regarded as inadequate by healthy individuals.[16] Further, one's will to achieve in different spheres of life also depends largely on the opportunities available in the environment. Therefore, a genuine assessment of QoL should try to include the real-time available environmental factors (both social and material) related to the subject. These can also be assessed by assessing the actual 'needs' and 'unmet needs' of the subject, the concept of which is very closely linked with QoL and subjective well-being, as it has

been suggested that to improve one's QoL, fulfilment of one's needs is essential.[23] Therefore, issues related to housing/supported housing, social support, occupational facilities, financial requirements and so on in patients with psychiatric disorders (with limited cognitive and social skills) are relevant contextual factors which need a detailed assessment to provide an accurate estimate of QoL for a subject with mental illness. Some of the available instruments of QoL have taken into account these aspects, and in some cases, more appropriate assessment instruments for patients' needs such as the Camberwell Assessment of Needs (CAN) have been developed.

3. **Impact of time on QoL assessment:** It has been reported that QoL does not remain constant over a period of time in patients undergoing treatment for chronic psychiatric disorders. Some researchers evaluated patients with depression during depression and after attaining remission and found that patients tend to rate their social adjustment negatively during the acute illness phase.[24] Therefore, it has been suggested that health-related QoL is a changing construct.[25] Further, the various domains of QoL (i.e., social support, living conditions, occupation, etc.) tend to vary from time to time, leading to different interpretations. Duration of illness has a significant impact on the assessment of QoL. Therefore, it should be kept in mind that definite changes in the QoL after any pharmacological/non-pharmacological intervention over a short period of time would signify subjective well-being (symptomatic improvement in functioning), and more long-term improvement in QoL would suggest additional factors responsible for its improvement (supported rehabilitation plans, disability benefits, etc.).

4. **Generic scales vs disorder-specific scales:** Currently there are several generic scales and some disorder-specific scales (Table 2.2) developed to measure QoL. Disorder-specific scales have the advantage of being able to assess additional issues particularly relevant to the disorder such as chronicity of illness and daily activities, support in doing self-care and so on. Further, any improvement in a particular domain with the use of any medication/non-pharmacological measure would be able to mark the change in the domain previously measured by the disorder-specific scale. However, there are several limitations of disorder-specific scales, and researchers have advised using them to provide complementary data and in general advocate the use of generic scales of QoL while assessing QoL as an outcome measure.[3,7,26]

RESEARCH ON QOL IN MAJOR PSYCHIATRIC DISORDERS

QoL has been widely researched in almost every psychiatric disorder. While it is relevant to understand QoL in patients with various psychiatric disorders, the research on QoL is very heterogeneous; that is, it has been linked with effectiveness of medications or non-pharmacological intervention strategies. On the other hand, it has also been evaluated as a correlate of other psychosocial variables (such as assessment of needs, social support, symptomatology), various treatment settings (primary care vs hospital setting) and so on. Accordingly, it is important to understand that QoL is not only a multi-dimensional construct, but its assessment and interpretation also depend on the context of measurement.

Studies evaluating quality of life can be broadly divided into four groups. First, studies that have compared QoL of patients with various psychiatric disorders and healthy controls in general suggest that the QoL of patients with any type of psychiatric disorder is inferior to that of the healthy controls.[10,35] Second, studies which have compared the QoL of patients with different psychiatric disorders suggest the QoL of patients with more severe mental disorders is more impaired than those with common mental disorders. Third, studies which have evaluated the efficacy/effectiveness of various interventions in general suggest

Table 2.2 Commonly used instruments to assess QoL.

Instrument	Clinician/self-administered	No. of items	Time taken	Remarks
Generic scales				
Quality of Life Interview (QOLI)	Structured interview	158 (long version) 78 (brief version)	45 mins (long version) 16 mins (short version)	Usually used to assess QoL in patients with Severe Mental Illness (SMI)
Wisconsin Quality of Life Index (W-QLI)	Self-rated	• 42 items – client version • 68 items – provider version • 28 items – family member version	• 25 mins • 15 mins • 10 mins	QoL in patients with SMI
Medical Outcomes Study Short Form – 36 items (SF-36)	Self- or clinician-administered	36	20 mins	Measures health-related QoL – includes general health perceptions, general mental health and physical health
Quality of Life Enjoyment & Satisfaction Questionnaire (Q-LES-Q)	Self-administered	60	15 mins	Measures degree of enjoyment and satisfaction in daily life functioning
Quality of Life Index (QLI)	Self-report	35	variable	Measures satisfaction in different domains of life
Quality of Life Inventory (QOLI)	Self-administered	16	5–10 mins	Measures overall satisfaction
Psychosocial Adjustment to Illness Scale, interview version (PAIS), and Self-Report Version (PAIS-SR)	Self-administered	46	variable	Measures overall adjustment to present or past medical conditions

(Continued)

Table 2.2 (Continued)

Spitzer Quality of Life Index (Spitzer QL-Index)	Clinician-rated	5	5–10 mins	Measures overall QoL in patients with chronic illness
World Health Organization's Quality of Life Instrument (WHOQOL)	Self-administered	100 (long version) 26 items (short version)	25 mins (long version) 5 mins (short version)	Measures QoL in 5 broad domains (Table 2.1)
The EuroQoL five-dimension (EQ-5D)	Three types – self, interviewer and proxy	Available in electronic and paper form; 15 items grouped under five dimensions	5 mins	Allows for the calculation of quality-adjusted life years by adopting preference-based index scores derived from it. One of the most frequently used scales; validated in many languages and disease states[27] Has five dimensions – mobility, self-care, usual activities, pain/discomfort and anxiety/depression
Disorder-specific scales				
Quality of Life Scale (QLS) (used for schizophrenia)	Semi-structured interview	21	45 mins	Can be used for assessment of QoL in patients with schizophrenia
The Lancashire Quality of Life Profile (LQoLP) (used for schizophrenia and other psychosis)	Self-administered (with assistance from clinicians in severely ill patients)	58	20–30 mins	Can be used for assessment of QoL in patients with schizophrenia and other psychoses; nine life domains – living situation, family, social relationships, leisure activities, work/education, finances, personal safety, health and religion; offers both objective QoL indicators and a subjective QoL estimate[28]
Quality of Life in Depression Scale (QLDS)	Self-administered	34	5–10 mins	Used for assessment of QoL for patients with depressive disorders

Quality of life in Bipolar Disorder (QoL-BD)	Self-rated	Brief version – 12 Full version – 56	10–20 mins	Measures QoL more specifically and reliably in patients with BD. Has 14 factors – physical, sleep, cognitive, mood, leisure, social, finances, household, spirituality, self-esteem, identity, independence, work and education.[29] It has been translated and validated in more than ten languages[30]
Quality of Life in Alzheimer's Disease Self-Rating scale (QoL-AD-SR)	Two versions: self-rated and proxy-rated	13	Depends on the severity of illness – mildly to moderately impaired AD subjects	Measures the patient's QoL from both the patient's and caregiver's perspective. Provides both patient's and caregiver's appraisal of the patient's physical condition, mood, interpersonal relationships, ability to participate in meaningful activities, financial situations and an overall assessment of self as a whole and life quality as a whole[31]
The Smoking Cessation QoL (SCQoL) Questionnaire	Self-rated Likert scale	51; 13 categories	10 mins	Assesses change in well-being and functioning associated with smoking cessation; has smoking cessation-specific component: social interactions, self-control, sleep, cognitive functioning, anxiety[32]
AL QoL (alcohol-related QoL)	Self-rated Likert scale	9	5 mins	Items have been derived from SF-36 generic scale; has good specificity for subjects with alcohol dependence and had good clinical utility – complement to motivational counselling[33]
The Injection Drug User QoL Scale (IDUQoL)	Self-rated Likert scale	22	10 mins	Evaluates health and non-health-related aspects of injected drug users, with an emphasis on individual circumstances and environmental factors;; looks into the physical, social, psychological, occupational and geographical reality of substance users[34]

beneficial effects of various interventions. Finally, studies have evaluated QoL as a correlate of various psychosocial variables, and these suggest that the QoL of patients with various disorders is associated with variables like unmet needs, social support, insight, medication adherence, neurocognitive functioning and so on.

In the following section, an attempt is made to summarise the findings with respect to some of the specific psychiatric disorders.

QoL in patients with intellectual disability (ID): Very few studies have looked into the QoL aspects of patients with ID. Available studies have mostly used generic QoL scales or Schalok and Keith's QoL questionnaire to assess QoL in subjects with ID and have reported low QoL in subjects with ID as compared to healthy controls. Among subjects with ID, studies have reported better QoL in those subjects who have functional ability and supported open employment.[36] Further, community-based interventions have been found to be more beneficial in improving QoL in subjects with ID than campus-based activities/inpatient stays.[37] Most of the studies do suggest developing more rehabilitation facilities in the form of supported residential facilities and opening employment for better outcome.

QoL in patients with dementia (PwD): Although many studies have evaluated QoL of PwD, there are conflicting data with respect to QoL of PwD, mainly because of the use of different measures and methodological issues.[38] Recent systematic review and meta-analysis on studies related to QoL research in PwD suggest that both qualitative studies and cross-sectional self-rated studies involving PwD are available, and many studies have used the disease-specific QoL scale, the QoL Alzheimer's Disease Scale.[38] Most studies have reported having greater social engagement, positive relationships within family and caregivers, having a degree of control over their lives and having religious beliefs/spirituality are moderately associated with better QoL,[39–41] and the presence of depression and neuropsychiatric symptoms are associated with poorer QoL.[38] Further, greater severity of dementia, pain, anxiety, unmet needs, living alone and greater carer burden/stress are associated with poor QoL. With regard to type of rating scale used, studies which have used self-rated QoL have found better QoL than staff-rated QoL scales.[42,43] These findings stress the fact that efforts to improve QoL in PwD should focus on relationships, social engagement, addressing poor physical and mental health and everyday functioning.

QoL in patients with schizophrenia/psychotic disorders: Many studies have evaluated the QoL in patients with schizophrenia/psychosis. Most of these studies have either used generic scales to measure QoL such as the Medical Outcomes Study Short Form Health Survey, WHO-QOL/WHOQOL-BREF or Quality of Life Index for Mental Health or disease-specific scales for schizophrenia such as Lancashire Quality of Life Profile, Lehman Quality of Life Interview and Quality of Life Scale. Almost all studies which have compared QoL of patients with schizophrenia with healthy controls have found QoL to be significantly poor in patients with schizophrenia.[44] Studies which used the most commonly used generic scale – WHOQOL/WHOQOL-BREF – have found QoL to be significantly low in the domains of physical health, psychological health, social relationships and environment.[44] Studies which have compared patients with first-episode schizophrenia and chronic schizophrenia suggest that patients with first-episode schizophrenia have reported poorer subjective QoL than those with chronic illness.[45,46] With regard to the predictors of QoL, the majority of studies have found higher levels of psychopathology, side effects of medications, loneliness, unemployment, affective symptoms and poor physical health to be associated with poorer QoL.[47,48] A few studies have also found an association between higher levels of negative symptoms with poor subjective QoL.[49–51] Studies which have compared QoL of patients with schizophrenia and BD have come up with conflicting results, with some studies reporting low subjective QoL for patients with schizophrenia,[52] while others have reported poor QoL in subjects with BD.[53] Studies have also compared QoL in patients with schizophrenia with patients with BD and reported poorer QoL in the former.[52] Some studies have also focused upon the spiritual aspects or spiritual domain of QoL in patients with residual schizophrenia/those in remission, have reported the spirituality domain to explain about one-third variance of the level of independence domain of QoL and have suggested that spirituality and religiosity have a significant influence on overall QoL and also are associated with adaptive and active coping.[54,55] In summary, it can be said that for a satisfactory QoL in patients with schizophrenia, along with symptom resolution, social network, community participation and family support, having good adaptive religious coping skills and spirituality can be beneficial.[56–58]

QoL in patients with bipolar disorder: Available literature on QoL research in BD subjects is variable due to the inclusion of heterogeneous group of patients during different phases of illness. However, overall, it has been reported that BD subjects, even in the euthymic phase, have significantly poorer QoL when compared with healthy controls. It is further noted that longer the period of euthymia, better the QoL.[59] Usually, generic scales such as WHOQOL-BREF, Short Form Health Survey, QoL Enjoyment and Satisfaction Questionnaire and a depression-specific scale – Quality of Life in Depression Scale – have been used for assessing QoL. More recently, a specific QoL-BD scale was developed to look into the more specific QoL aspects in subjects with BD.[29] Studies which have tried to evaluate the clinical correlates of QoL in subjects with BD report a higher number of previous depressive episodes to be more strongly associated with poor QoL than the number of previous manic episodes.[60,61] Other clinical correlates reported to be associated with poor QoL include younger age of onset.[62] Studies which have evaluated QoL as an outcome of various interventions suggest that olanzapine[63,64] and lithium prophylaxis[52] are associated with better QoL outcomes. Similarly, studies which have evaluated the impact of psychoeducational intervention for a period of 3 months among patients receiving lithium suggest that psychoeducation leads to improvement in QoL.[65]

QoL in patients with depressive disorders: Most of the studies which have evaluated QoL among patients with depression have relied upon generic scales like the Short Form Health Survey and QoL Enjoyment and Satisfaction Questionnaire, and some studies have used a depression-specific scale (Quality of Life In Depression Scale) to assess QoL. Studies have evaluated the relationship of severity of symptoms and QoL and reported it to be an independent variable which adversely affects QoL,[66] and QoL is uniquely associated with measures of functioning.[67,68] Studies evaluating the impact of various interventions, such as venlafaxine, duloxetine, bupropion, escitalopram, cognitive therapy and so on suggest that these interventions lead to improvement in QoL.[69–74]

QoL in patients with anxiety disorders: The QoL domain is less researched in patients with various anxiety disorders when compared with other psychiatric disorders. Studies which have evaluated QoL among patients with anxiety disorders have mostly relied on generic scales to assess QoL such as SF-36, QoL inventory, Life Satisfaction Index, Satisfaction with Life Scale and QoL Enjoyment and Satisfaction Questionnaire. Available literature suggests that across all anxiety disorders, compared to healthy controls, patients with anxiety disorder have poorer QoL.[75] Overall, the impact of anxiety disorders on the QoL affect multiple domains and has been found to be independent of symptom severity, demographic variables and co-morbid conditions.[75] Among the various variables, poor QoL among patients with panic disorder is associated with marital and financial problems,[76] whereas among patients with social phobia, poor QoL is associated with a moderate level of impairment in areas of education and relationships due to social anxiety and avoidance.[77] Poor QoL among patients with obsessive-compulsive disorder is associated with role limitation.[78]

QoL in subjects with substance abuse disorders: QoL research in substance use disorders has yielded inconclusive results due to several methodological issues.[79] Although earlier studies relied upon Short Form-36, Lancashire QoL Profile and QoL Index and Euro-QoL, recent studies have used specific questionnaires developed to capture more key components of QoL in patients with substance dependence such as QoL Scale for Drug Addicts, the Smoking Cessation QoL Questionnaire, AL QoL and the Injection Drug User QoL Scale. In general, it is suggested that persons with substance use disorders have poor QoL compared to non-users. Available studies on QoL of patients with alcohol dependence indicate QoL improves with brief intervention programs and detoxification management by general practitioners.[80–82] In subjects with opioid dependence disorder, a higher severity of opioid dependence is associated with poorer QoL, irrespective of the presence of comorbid psychiatric disorders, and QoL of patients with opioid dependence improves with buprenorphine/methadone maintenance therapy.[83–85] Studies involving patients with nicotine dependence suggest that smokers have low QoL and heavy smokers experience a decrease in QoL while attempting to quit smoking.[86,87]

QoL research in caregivers of patients with psychiatric disorders: Caregivers play an important role in management of patients with various psychiatric disorders. Hence, understanding the caregiver's QoL is an important outcome variable for various mental disorders. Available literature undoubtedly suggests that mental disorders, especially severe mental disorders, are associated with significant caregiver burden.[88,89] Data also suggest that most caregivers suffer from poor psychological well-being, and some also suffer from clinical depression and anxiety disorders when compared to the general population.[90,91] Overall, studies have reported poor QoL in caregivers of patients with psychiatric disorders more than in patients with severe mental illnesses. Some of the factors identified to be associated with QoL of caregivers of persons with mental disorders are caregiver satisfaction with health of patient; environment; and some caregivers' variables such as their education status, psychological well-being and having spiritual well-being.[92,93] Some factors which have been consistently found to be associated with low QoL of caregivers include presence of depressive symptoms among the caregivers,[94] being a young caregiver, having patients with chronic illness, low education level and experiencing more caregiving burden.[95] Accordingly, any effort to improve QoL of caregivers must take these variables into account, and suitable interventions need to be designed.

STRATEGIES TO IMPROVE QOL

Some strategies to improve QoL in patients with psychiatric disorders include providing basic facilities to lead a satisfactory and dignified life. These can include provision of community residential programs, occupational rehabilitation strategies, emphasising patient empowerment and self-help groups and promotion of positive mental health.[16] Activities focusing on psychoeducational programs, psychotherapeutic group programs and increasing community awareness about psychiatric illnesses help in reducing public and perceived stigma about mental illness and also indirectly help in improving QoL. Family and carer burden assessment and planning strategies to alleviate it can further improve the QoL of the patients.

CONCLUSIONS

QoL is a complex multidimensional construct which should be regarded as an important and reliable outcome measure in assessing conditions of patients suffering from mental disorders in routine practice so as to provide complete and holistic care. Several generic and disease-specific QoL instruments are available which can be used to assess QoL as well as to plan interventions. It is necessary to focus on improving QoL in patients with psychiatric disorders as a public health policy and develop national-level strategies for mental health promotion.

References

1. Soni MK, Cella D. Quality of life and symptom measures in oncology: An overview. *Am J Manag Care* 2002;8(18 Suppl):S560–S573.
2. Schwartz CE, Sprangers MAG. An introduction to quality of life assessment in oncology: The value of measuring patient-reported outcomes. *Am J Manag Care* 2002;8(18 Suppl):S550–S559.
3. Orley J, Saxena S, Herrman H. Quality of life and mental illness: Reflections from the perspective of the WHOQOL. *Br J Psychiatry* 1998;172:291–293.
4. Gill TM, Feinstein AR. A critical appraisal of the quality of quality-of-life measurements. *JAMA* 1994;272(8):619–626.
5. Higginson IJ, Carr AJ. Measuring quality of life: Using quality of life measures in the clinical setting. *BMJ* 2001;322(7297):1297–1300.
6. McKenna S, Whalley D. Can quality of life scales tell us when patients begin to feel the benefits of antidepressants? *Eur Psychiatry* 1998;13(3):146–153.
7. Berlim MT, Fleck MPA. "Quality of life": A brand new concept for research and practice in psychiatry. *Braz J Psychiatry* 2003;25(4):249–252.
8. Calman KC. Quality of life in cancer patients: An hypothesis. *J Med Ethics* 1984;10(3):124–127.
9. The WHOQOL Group. The World Health Organization Quality of Life Assessment (WHOQOL): Development and general psychometric properties. *Soc Sci Med* 1998;46(12):1569–1585.
10. Katschnig H. How useful is the concept of quality of life in psychiatry? *Curr Opin Psychiatry* 1997;10(5):337–345.
11. Awad AG, Voruganti LNP. Measuring quality of life in patients with schizophrenia: An update. *Pharmacoeconomics* 2012;30(3):183–195.
12. Reininghaus U, Priebe S. Measuring patient-reported outcomes in psychosis: Conceptual and methodological review. *Br J Psychiatry* 2012;201(4):262–267.
13. Revicki DA, Kleinman L, Cella D. A history of health-related quality of life outcomes in psychiatry. *Dialogues Clin Neurosci* 2014;16(2):127–135.
14. Kaasa S, Loge JH. Quality of life in palliative care: Principles and practice. *Palliat Med* 2003;17(1):11–20.
15. Atkinson MJ, Caldwell L. The differential effects of mood on patients' ratings of life quality and satisfaction with their care. *J Affect Disord* 1997;44(2–3):169–175.
16. Katschnig H. Quality of life in mental disorders: Challenges for research and clinical practice. *World Psychiatry* 2006;5(3):139–145.
17. Schwarz N, Clore GL. Mood, misattribution, and judgments of well-being: Informative and directive functions of affective states. *J Personal Soc Psychol* 1983;45(3):513–523.
18. Pukrop R, Schlaak V, Möller-Leimkühler AM, Albus M, Czernik A, Klosterkötter J, et al. Reliability and validity of quality of life assessed by the short-form 36 and the modular system for quality of life in patients with schizophrenia and patients with depression. *Psychiatry Res* 2003;119(1–2):63–79.
19. Diamond R, Becker M. The Wisconsin quality of life index: A multidimensional model for measuring quality of life. *J Clin Psychiatry* 1999;60(Suppl 3):29–31.
20. Sainfort F, Becker M, Diamond R. Judgments of quality of life of individuals with severe mental disorders: Patient self-report versus provider perspectives. *Am J Psychiatry* 1996;153(4):497–502.
21. Bullinger M, Quitmann J. Quality of life as patient-reported outcomes: Principles of assessment. *Dialogues Clin Neurosci* 2014;16(2):137–145.
22. Bertelli M, Brown I. Quality of life for people with intellectual disabilities. *Curr Opin Psychiatry* 2006;19(5):508–513.
23. Tay L, Diener E. Needs and subjective well-being around the world. *J Pers Soc Psychol* 2011;101(2):354–365.
24. Morgado A, Smith M, Lecrubier Y, Widlöcher D. Depressed subjects unwittingly overreport poor social adjustment which they reappraise when recovered. *J Nerv Ment Dis* 1991;179(10):614–619.
25. Bernhard J, Lowy A, Mathys N, Herrmann R, Hürny C. Health related quality of life: A changing construct? *Qual Life Res* 2004;13(7):1187–1197.
26. Skevington SM. Advancing cross-cultural research on quality of life: Observations drawn from the WHOQOL development. *Qual Life Res* [Internet] 2002 [cited 2020 Mar 5];11(2):135–144. https://doi.org/10.1023/A:1015013312456

27. Rabin R, Gudex C, Selai C, Herdman M. From translation to version management: A history and review of methods for the cultural adaptation of the EuroQoL five-dimensional questionnaire. *Value Health* 2014;17(1):70–76.
28. van Nieuwenhuizen CH, Schene AH, Koeter MWJ, Huxley PJ. The Lancashire quality of life profile: Modification and psychometric evaluation. *Soc Psychiatry Psychiatr Epidemiol* 2001;36(1):36–44.
29. Michalak EE, Murray G, Collaborative RESearch Team to Study Psychosocial Issues in Bipolar Disorder (CREST.BD). Development of the QoL.BD: A disorder-specific scale to assess quality of life in bipolar disorder. *Bipolar Disord* 2010;12(7):727–740.
30. Xiao L, Gao Y, Zhang L, Chen P, Sun X, Tang S. Validity and reliability of the "Brief version of Quality of Life in Bipolar Disorder" (Bref QoL.BD) among Chinese bipolar patients. *J Affect Dis* 2016;193:66–72.
31. Logsdon RG, Gibbons LE, McCurry SM, Teri L. Quality of life in Alzheimer's disease: Patient and caregiver reports. *J Ment Health Aging* 1999;5(1):21–32.
32. Olufade AO, Shaw JW, Foster SA, Leischow SJ, Hays RD, Coons SJ. Development of the smoking cessation quality of life questionnaire. *Clin Ther* 1999;21(12):2113–2130.
33. Malet L, Llorca P-M, Beringuier B, Lehert P, Falissard B. ALQOL 9 for measuring quality of life in alcohol dependence. *Alcohol Alcohol* 2006;41(2):181–187.
34. Hubley AM, Russell LB, Palepu A. Injection Drug Use Quality of Life scale (IDUQOL): A validation study. *Health Qual Life Outcomes* 2005;3:43.
35. Connell J, Brazier J, O'Cathain A, Lloyd-Jones M, Paisley S. Quality of life of people with mental health problems: A synthesis of qualitative research. *Health Qual Life Outcomes* 2012;10(1):138.
36. Kober R, Eggleton IRC. The effect of different types of employment on quality of life. *J Intellect Disabil Res* 2005;49(Pt 10):756–760.
37. Hartnett E, Gallagher P, Kiernan G, Poulsen C, Gilligan E, Reynolds M. Day service programmes for people with a severe intellectual disability and quality of life: Parent and staff perspectives. *J Intellect Disabil* 2008;12(2):153–172.
38. Martyr A, Nelis SM, Quinn C, Wu Y-T, Lamont RA, Henderson C, et al. Living well with dementia: A systematic review and correlational meta-analysis of factors associated with quality of life, well-being and life satisfaction in people with dementia. *Psychol Med* 2018;48(13):2130–2139.
39. Cahill S, Diaz-Ponce AM. "I hate having nobody here. I'd like to know where they all are": Can qualitative research detect differences in quality of life among nursing home residents with different levels of cognitive impairment? *Aging Ment Health* 2011;15(5):562–572.
40. Moyle W, O'Dwyer S. Quality of life in people living with dementia in nursing homes. *Curr Opin Psychiatry* 2012;25(6):480–484.
41. Moyle W, Venturto L, Griffiths S, Grimbeek P, McAllister M, Oxlade D, et al. Factors influencing quality of life for people with dementia: A qualitative perspective. *Aging Ment Health* 2011;15(8):970–977.
42. Nakanishi K, Hanihara T, Mutai H, Nakaaki S. Evaluating the quality of life of people with dementia in residential care facilities. *Dement Geriatr Cogn Disord* 2011;32(1).
43. Gräske J, Fischer T, Kuhlmey A, Wolf-Ostermann K. Quality of life in dementia care–differences in quality of life measurements performed by residents with dementia and by nursing staff. *Aging Ment Health* 2012;16(7):819–827.
44. Dong M, Lu L, Zhang L, Zhang Y-S, Ng CH, Ungvari GS, et al. Quality of life in schizophrenia: A meta-analysis of comparative studies. *Psychiatr Q* 2019;90(3):519–532.
45. Sim K, Mahendran R, Siris SG, Heckers S, Chong SA. Subjective quality of life in first episode schizophrenia spectrum disorders with comorbid depression. *Psychiatry Res* 2004;129(2):141–147.
46. Priebe S, Roeder-Wanner UU, Kaiser W. Quality of life in first-admitted schizophrenia patients: A follow-up study. *Psychol Med* 2000;30(1):225–230.
47. Skantze K, Malm U, Dencker SJ, May PR, Corrigan P. Comparison of quality of life with standard of living in schizophrenic out-patients. *Br J Psychiatry* 1992;161:797–801.
48. Bengtsson-Tops A, Hansson L. Clinical and social needs of schizophrenic outpatients living in the community: The relationship between needs and subjective quality of life. *Soc Psychiatry Psychiatr Epidemiol* 1999;34(10):513–518.
49. Neil AL, Carr VJ, Mackinnon A, Foley DL, Morgan VA. Health-related quality of life in people living with psychotic illness and factors associated with its variation. *Value in Health* 2018;21(8):1002–1009.
50. Packer S, Husted J, Cohen S, Tomlinson G. Psychopathology and quality of life in schizophrenia. *J Psychiatry Neurosci* 1997;22(4):231–234.

51. Ho B-C, Nopoulos P, Flaum M, Arndt S, Andreasen NC. Two-year outcome in first-episode schizophrenia: Predictive value of symptoms for quality of life. *AJP* 1998;155(9):1196–1201.
52. Chand PK, Mattoo SK, Sharan P. Quality of life and its correlates in patients with bipolar disorder stabilized on lithium prophylaxis. *Psychiatry Clin Neurosci* 2004;58(3):311–318.
53. Atkinson M, Zibin S, Chuang H. Characterizing quality of life among patients with chronic mental illness: A critical examination of the self-report methodology. *Am J Psychiatry* 1997;154(1):99–105.
54. Shah R, Kulhara P, Grover S, Kumar S, Malhotra R, Tyagi S. Contribution of spirituality to quality of life in patients with residual schizophrenia. *Psychiatry Res* 2011;190(2–3):200–205.
55. Shah R, Kulhara P, Grover S, Kumar S, Malhotra R, Tyagi S. Relationship between spirituality/religiousness and coping in patients with residual schizophrenia. *Qual Life Res* 2011;20(7):1053–1060.
56. Vitorino LM, Lucchetti G, Leão FC, Vallada H, Peres MFP. The association between spirituality and religiousness and mental health. *Scientific Reports* 2018;8(1):1–9.
57. Smith S, Suto MJ. Religious and/or spiritual practices: Extending spiritual freedom to people with schizophrenia. *Can J Occup Ther* 2012;79(2):77–85.
58. Hasanah CI, Razali MS. Quality of life: An assessment of the state of psychosocial rehabilitation of patients with schizophrenia in the community. *J R Soc Promot Health* 2002;122(4):251–255.
59. Pascual-Sánchez A, Jenaro C, Montes-Rodríguez JM. Quality of life in euthymic bipolar patients: A systematic review and meta-analysis. *J Affect Disord* 2019;255:105–115.
60. MacQueen GM, Young LT, Robb JC, Marriott M, Cooke RG, Joffe RT. Effect of number of episodes on wellbeing and functioning of patients with bipolar disorder. *Acta Psychiatr Scand* 2000;101(5):374–381.
61. Ozer S, Uluşahin A, Batur S, Kabakçi E, Saka MC. Outcome measures of interepisode bipolar patients in a Turkish sample. *Soc Psychiatry Psychiatr Epidemiol* 2002;37(1):31–37.
62. Perlis RH, Miyahara S, Marangell LB, Wisniewski SR, Ostacher M, DelBello MP, et al. Long-term implications of early onset in bipolar disorder: Data from the first 1000 participants in the systematic treatment enhancement program for bipolar disorder (STEP-BD). *Biol Psychiatry* 2004;55(9):875–881.
63. Namjoshi MA, Rajamannar G, Jacobs T, Sanger TM, Risser R, Tohen MF, et al. Economic, clinical, and quality-of-life outcomes associated with olanzapine treatment in mania: Results from a randomized controlled trial. *J Affect Disord* 2002;69(1–3):109–118.
64. Shi L, Namjoshi MA, Swindle R, Yu X, Risser R, Baker RW, et al. Effects of olanzapine alone and olanzapine/fluoxetine combination on health-related quality of life in patients with bipolar depression: Secondary analyses of a double-blind, placebo-controlled, randomized clinical trial. *Clin Ther* 2004;26(1):125–134.
65. Doğan S, Sabanciogullari S. The effects of patient education in lithium therapy on quality of life and compliance. *Arch Psychiatr Nurs* 2003;17(6):270–275.
66. Gao K, Su M, Sweet J, Calabrese JR. Correlation between depression/anxiety symptom severity and quality of life in patients with major depressive disorder or bipolar disorder. *J Affect Disord* 2019;244:9–15.
67. IsHak WW, Greenberg JM, Balayan K, Kapitanski N, Jeffrey J, Fathy H, et al. Quality of life: The ultimate outcome measure of interventions in major depressive disorder. *Harv Rev Psychiatry* 2011;19(5):229–239.
68. IsHak WW, Mirocha J, James D, Tobia G, Vilhauer J, Fakhry H, et al. Quality of life in major depressive disorder before/after multiple steps of treatment and one-year follow-up. *Acta Psychiatr Scand* 2015;131(1):51–60.
69. Jha MK, Minhajuddin A, Thase ME, Jarrett RB. Improvement in self-reported quality of life with cognitive therapy for recurrent major depressive disorder. *J Affect Disord* 2014;167:37–43.
70. Hudson JI, Perahia DG, Gilaberte I, Wang F, Watkin JG, Detke MJ. Duloxetine in the treatment of major depressive disorder: An open-label study. *BMC Psychiatry* 2007;7:43.
71. Dunner DL, Kwong WJ, Houser TL, Richard NE, Donahue RMJ, Khan ZM. Improved health-related quality of life and reduced productivity loss after treatment with bupropion sustained release: A study in patients with major depression. *Prim Care Companion J Clin Psychiatry* 2001;3(1):10–16.
72. Cervera-Enguix S, Soutullo CA, Landecho I, Murillo-Jelsbak R. Quality of life in 833 outpatients with major depression treated with open-label venlafaxine extended release: An observational 24-week study. *Int J Psychiatry Clin Pract* 2003;7(3):193–197.
73. Hofmann SG, Curtiss J, Carpenter JK, Kind S. Effect of treatments for depression on quality of life: A meta-analysis. *Cogn Behav Ther* 2017;46(4):265–286.

74. Demyttenaere K, Hemels MEH, Hudry J, Annemans L. A cost-effectiveness model of escitalopram, citalopram, and venlafaxine as first-line treatment for major depressive disorder in Belgium. *Clin Ther* 2005;27(1):111–124.
75. Olatunji BO, Cisler JM, Tolin DF. Quality of life in the anxiety disorders: A meta-analytic review. *Clin Psychol Rev* 2007;27(5):572–581.
76. Weissman MM. Panic disorder: Impact on quality of life. *J Clin Psychiatry* 1991;52(Suppl.):6–8; discussion 9.
77. Schneier FR, Heckelman LR, Garfinkel R, Campeas R, Fallon BA, Gitow A, et al. Functional impairment in social phobia. *J Clin Psychiatry* 1994;55(8):322–331.
78. Hollander E, Kwon JH, Stein DJ, Broatch J, Rowland CT, Himelein CA. Obsessive-compulsive and spectrum disorders: Overview and quality of life issues. *J Clin Psychiatr* 1996 [cited 2020 Mar 6];57(Suppl. 8):3–6.
79. Zubaran C, Foresti K. Quality of life and substance use: concepts and recent tendencies. *Curr Opin Psychiatry* 2009;22(3):281–286.
80. Malet L, Reynaud M, Llorca P-M, Chakroun N, Blanc O, Falissard B. Outcomes from primary care management of alcohol dependence in France. *J Subst Abuse Treat* 2009;36(4):457–462.
81. Foster JH, Powell JE, Marshall EJ, Peters TJ. Quality of life in alcohol-dependent subjects–a review. *Qual Life Res* 1999;8(3):255–261.
82. Pal HR, Yadav D, Mehta S, Mohan I. A comparison of brief intervention versus simple advice for alcohol use disorders in a North India community-based sample followed for 3 months. *Alcohol Alcohol* 2007;42(4):328–332.
83. Maremmani I, Pani PP, Pacini M, Perugi G. Substance use and quality of life over 12 months among buprenorphine maintenance-treated and methadone maintenance-treated heroin-addicted patients. *J Subst Abuse Treat* 2007;33(1):91–98.
84. Astals M, Domingo-Salvany A, Buenaventura CC, Tato J, Vazquez JM, Martín-Santos R, et al. Impact of substance dependence and dual diagnosis on the quality of life of heroin users seeking treatment. *Subst Use Misuse* 2008;43(5):612–632.
85. Ponizovsky AM, Grinshpoon A. Quality of life among heroin users on buprenorphine versus methadone maintenance. *Am J Drug Alcohol Abuse* 2007;33(5):631–642.
86. Erickson SR, Thomas LA, Blitz SG, Pontius LR. Smoking cessation: A pilot study of the effects on health-related quality of life and perceived work performance one week into the attempt. *Ann Pharmacother* 2004;38(11):1805–1810.
87. Schmitz N, Kruse J, Kugler J. Smoking and its association with disability in chronic conditions: Results from the Canadian community and health survey 2.1. *Nicotine Tob Res* 2007;9(9):959–964.
88. Del-Pino-Casado R, Espinosa-Medina A, López-Martínez C, Orgeta V. Sense of coherence, burden and mental health in caregiving: A systematic review and meta-analysis. *J Affect Disord* 2019;242:14–21.
89. Schulze B, Rössler W. Caregiver burden in mental illness: Review of measurement, findings and interventions in 2004–2005. *Current Opinion in Psychiatry* [Internet] 2005 [cited 2020 Mar 6];18(6):684–691. https://journals.lww.com/co-psychiatry/Fulltext/2005/11000/Caregiver_burden_in_mental_illness__review_of.17.aspx
90. Basheer S, Anurag K, Garg R, Kumar R, Vashisht S. Quality of life of caregivers of mentally ill patients in a tertiary care hospital. *Industrial Psychiatry J* 2015;24(2):144.
91. Sales E. Family burden and quality of life. *Qual Life Res* 2003;12(Suppl. 1):33–41.
92. Ndikuno C, Namutebi M, Kuteesa J, Mukunya D, Olwit C. Quality of life of caregivers of patients diagnosed with severe mental illness at the national referral hospitals in Uganda. *BMC Psychiatry* 2016;16.
93. Kate N, Grover S, Kulhara P, Nehra R. Relationship of quality of life with coping and burden in primary caregivers of patients with schizophrenia. *Int J Soc Psychiatry* 2014;60(2):107–116.
94. Jeyagurunathan A, Sagayadevan V, Abdin E, Zhang Y, Chang S, Shafie S, et al. Psychological status and quality of life among primary caregivers of individuals with mental illness: A hospital based study. *Health Qual Life Outcomes* 2017;15(1):106.
95. Wong DFK, Lam AYK, Chan SK, Chan SF. Quality of life of caregivers with relatives suffering from mental illness in Hong Kong: Roles of caregiver characteristics, caregiving burdens, and satisfaction with psychiatric services. *Health Qual Life Outcomes* 2012;10:15.

3

Optimising Patient Care in Psychiatry With Sound Mental Health Legislation

Brendan D. Kelly, Gautam Gulati and Richard M. Duffy

Introduction	33
Mental Health Legislation Focused on Traditional Themes: Ireland	35
Mental Health Legislation Focused on Broader Themes: India	37
Conclusions	39
Acknowledgements	40

INTRODUCTION

Mental health law forms a key component of mental healthcare in virtually every country in the world. Different jurisdictions have, however, developed different approaches to the purpose, nature, extent and implementation of legislation in this area. This chapter examines two of these different approaches using Ireland and India as examples and relates legislation in these countries to the positions outlined by the World Health Organisation (WHO) and United Nations (UN). The purpose of these comparisons is to highlight key issues shaping approaches to mental health legislation as a central element of mental healthcare in different countries around the world. The final section of the chapter presents conclusions and suggested directions for future work in this field.

To begin, it is necessary to pose some fundamental questions about the purpose of mental health legislation in the first place. Why does mental health legislation exist? Is it necessary? Could mental health services function without legislation? Why does mental health legislation continue to exist despite clear evidence of the misuse of such legislation in the past? Can mental health legislation be adapted to the societies and human rights standards of the twenty-first century? If so, how?

The first reason for the persistence of mental health legislation is an historical one. In virtually all countries for which there is recorded history, there has been long-standing recognition of both the existence of mental illness and the need for treatment (Scull, 1993). While certain aspects of societal responses to the mentally ill have varied between jurisdictions, recent centuries have seen clear evidence of both the emergence of community-based mental healthcare and continued provision for the involuntary treatment of a minority of people with severe mental disorders who pose a significant risk to themselves or others (Scull, 2015).

As a result of these developments, mental health legislation was introduced in order to govern such practices in a more accountable way and move involuntary care out of the private sphere, often in private homes and unregulated facilities during the nineteenth century,

DOI: 10.4324/9780429030260-4

and into the public sphere, starting initially with government-operated asylums with inspection systems. These developments were at their most intense during the nineteenth century, which saw the establishment of large networks of mental hospitals across many countries (Shorter, 1997). For the most part, these institutions went into decline during the latter part of the twentieth century as ideas about "community care" became more prominent. Despite these changes, treatment without consent has continued, and there is, as a result, a continued need for laws to govern it.

The second reason for the existence of mental health legislation is that the evolution of mental healthcare along the lines outlined previously led to a clear need to protect the rights of the mentally ill, especially when they were confined in institutions (Kelly, 2016a). In other words, just as it was deemed important to provide care without consent to the seriously mentally ill, it was soon recognised as equally important that the mentally ill not experience disproportionate denial of rights while such care was being provided.

Today, it is clear that mental health legislation still serves a number of key purposes. These include not only the provision of care to people who are unable to provide consent and the protection of such persons from unjustified denial of rights during care but also the need to achieve social justice for the mentally ill more broadly (Gostin et al., 2010). This third reason for existence of mental health law – achieving social justice – reflects a more expansive view of the role of mental health legislation and often involves such laws reaching into new and unfamiliar areas, such as social care, housing policy, general health services and politics more broadly.

Today, there is still a clear and urgent need to reach into these areas in order to achieve meaningful justice for the mentally ill. People with mental illness, especially those with enduring illnesses such as schizophrenia, are at increased risk of poor access to healthcare, homelessness, imprisonment and social exclusion (Kelly, 2005). The negative effects of these social, economic and societal factors, along with the social stigma of mental illness, constitute a form of "structural violence" that amplifies the effects of mental illness in the lives of sufferers. As a result of these over-arching social and economic factors, many people with severe mental illness are systematically excluded from full participation in civic and social life and are constrained to live lives that are shaped, in large part, by stigma, isolation, homelessness and denial of rights. This is a global scandal.

Addressing these gross inequities and injustices requires a careful combination of psychiatric care, general health services, social support, reform of the criminal justice system, economic assistance, family support and political empowerment of the mentally ill and their families. There is a clear role for mental health legislation in this process, combatting the discrimination and social injustice still experienced by the mentally ill around the world (Callard et al., 2012). More broadly, the WHO (2017) argues that there is a substantial and compelling role for law in achieving the "right to health" for all, not just people with mental illness (Wolff, 2012). Clearly, achieving these rights for the mentally ill is particularly important, now more than ever.

Against this background, this chapter looks at two different approaches to mental health legislation in order to identify lessons about how such legislation can best help optimise patient care and achieve meaningful justice for the mentally ill. More specifically, this chapter uses two contrasting examples of mental health law in order to explore this topic. The first example is Ireland, which is a typical example of a jurisdiction in which mental health legislation focuses almost exclusively on two areas of traditional concern in mental health law: regulations governing treatment without consent and ways to ensure that high standards are maintained in mental health facilities. This traditional approach to mental health law is also seen in New Zealand's Mental Health (Compulsory Assessment and Treatment) Act, 1992, and England and Wales's Mental Health Act, 1983 (amended in 2007).

The second example is India, where new mental health legislation addresses the same areas as Ireland's legislation but also seeks to ensure equitable access to services, enhanced social care for the mentally ill, support for families and the protection and promotion of a broader range of rights. Other countries have enacted similar legislation in recent years, such as Ghana's Mental Health Act, 2012, and Peru's Mental Health Law 29889.

This chapter compares Ireland's rather narrow, focused approach with the much broader approach of India; relates the legislation in these two countries to the views of the WHO and UN; and, in the final section, presents conclusions and suggests directions for future work.

MENTAL HEALTH LEGISLATION FOCUSED ON TRADITIONAL THEMES: IRELAND

Ireland's Mental Health Act, 2001, was fully implemented in November 2006. The legislation aims, in its own words,

> to provide for the involuntary admission to approved centres of persons suffering from mental disorders, to provide for the independent review of the involuntary admission of such persons and, for those purposes, to provide for the establishment of a Mental Health Commission and the appointment of Mental Health Commission Tribunals and an Inspector of Mental Health Services.
>
> (Preamble)

From the outset, then, the clear, stated purpose of the Irish legislation is to govern involuntary mental healthcare and create an updated inspection system for mental health facilities (Kelly, 2016b). In relation to the former, the legislation states that "a person may be involuntarily admitted to an approved centre . . . on the grounds that he or she is suffering from a mental disorder" (Section 8(1)), but not "by reason only of the fact that the person (a) is suffering from a personality disorder, (b) is socially deviant, or (c) is addicted to drugs or intoxicants" (Section 8(2)).

"Mental disorder" is defined in the legislation as

> mental illness, severe dementia or significant intellectual disability where (a) because of the illness, disability or dementia, there is a serious likelihood of the person concerned causing immediate and serious harm to himself or herself or to other persons, or (b) (i) because of the severity of the illness, disability or dementia, the judgment of the person concerned is so impaired that failure to admit the person to an approved centre would be likely to lead to a serious deterioration in his or her condition or would prevent the administration of appropriate treatment that could be given only by such admission, and (ii) the reception, detention and treatment of the person concerned in an approved centre would be likely to benefit or alleviate the condition of that person to a material extent.
>
> (Section 3(1))

More detailed definitions are provided for the terms "mental illness", "severe dementia" and "significant intellectual disability" (Section 3(2)).

The 2001 Act outlines a three-step involuntary admission process that involves (a) an "application" for involuntary admission (e.g., by a family member or police officer), (b) a "recommendation" made by a general practitioner or other doctor and (c) an "admission order" made by a consultant psychiatrist in an "approved centre" (inpatient psychiatry unit). The involuntary patient receives free legal aid and a free independent psychiatric examination. The involuntary admission order or renewal order is subject to review by an independent mental health tribunal within 21 days of the order being made.

There is a different process for the involuntary retention of a person who already is a voluntary inpatient in a psychiatry unit but expresses a desire to leave. If such a person fulfils criteria for "mental disorder" (Section 3(1)), they can be retained in the inpatient facility by a nurse or doctor for up to 24 hours. Within this period, the patient is assessed by two consultant psychiatrists, and a decision is made about whether or not the patient's status should be changed from voluntary to involuntary. Such a decision is also subject to review by a mental health tribunal within 21 days of the involuntary order being made.

Ireland's Mental Health Act, 2001 also deals with other areas of involuntary treatment. It makes provisions for the administration of medication (Section 60), electro-convulsive therapy (ECT) (Section 59) and seclusion and restraint (Section 69).

This, then, is the first focus of Ireland's mental health legislation: regulating involuntary care and reviews of involuntary admission decisions by mental health tribunals. The second focus of the legislation is the creation and maintenance of a new and updated system of inspection for mental health facilities. The 2001 Act specifies that the principal functions of Ireland's Inspector of Mental Health Services are "to visit and inspect every approved centre at least once in each year" and "to visit and inspect any other premises where mental health services are being provided as he or she thinks appropriate" (Section 51(1)). The inspector writes an annual report which is published each year on the website of the Mental Health Commission (www.mhcirl.ie).

In these two areas – involuntary care and assuring standards of care – Ireland's mental health legislation meets the great majority of relevant human rights standards outlined by the WHO in its *Resource Book on Mental Health, Human Rights and Legislation* (2005). Areas of low compliance with these standards relate to promoting rights (which impacts other areas within the legislation, such as information management), treatment of voluntary patients (especially non-protesting, incapacitated patients), the protection of vulnerable groups and emergency treatment (Kelly, 2011). The WHO *Resource Book* also emphasizes the protection of social rights, such as rights to housing, employment and social security. These are not considered under 'mental health law' in Ireland. While protections from discrimination exist in these areas, people with mental illness do not get the level of consideration that their specific needs require.

The reason the Irish legislation does not score highly in some of these areas relates chiefly to the fact that the legislation does not seek to address many of them, opting instead to focus almost exclusively on involuntary care and inspections. The legislation has, for example, very few provisions relating to voluntary patients. It defines a "voluntary patient" as "a person receiving care and treatment in an approved centre who is not the subject of an admission order or a renewal order" (Section 2(1)), but it provides very little further information about the management of voluntary patients or any other issues pertaining to them.

This is not necessarily a flaw in the legislative provisions of the 2001 Act, but rather a reflection of the limited scope of the legislation, which is strongly focused on regulating involuntary care and the functions of the Inspector of Mental Health Services. There is some evidence that this rather narrow focus is useful: Ireland now has a highly functional system of mental health tribunals to protect patients' rights and Ireland's rate of involuntary care is low by international standards, being less than half of the rate in neighbouring England (Gilhooley and Kelly, 2018).

There are, however, also significant limitations with this focused approach, with the result that the Irish legislation does not meet WHO requirements in many important areas, chiefly relating to broader protections of rights (Kelly, 2011). As a result, some of the key areas in need of attention in Ireland's mental health legislation include measures to protect and promote the rights of voluntary patients; issues relating to competence, capacity and consent (which will be partly addressed in the new Assisted Decision-Making (Capacity) Act, 2015); and the extent to which Ireland wishes to protect the economic and social rights of the mentally ill through mental health legislation rather than general legislation or social policy.

These matters are currently unresolved in Ireland. In seeking to address them, Irish legislators could usefully look to recent developments in India for possible lessons about a more ambitious, extended view of the role of mental legislation in protecting and promoting the rights of the mentally ill and their families.

MENTAL HEALTH LEGISLATION FOCUSED ON BROADER THEMES: INDIA

On 29 May 2018, new mental health legislation commenced in India, titled the Mental Healthcare Act, 2017. The new legislation sought explicitly to comply with the UN Convention on the Rights of Persons with Disabilities (CRPD) (UN, 2006) and therefore covered both (a) areas traditionally addressed in mental health legislation, such as treatment without consent and oversight of standards, and (b) the broader areas that are often neglected in such laws, such as broader protections of rights. India's legislation is undoubtedly the most interesting and potentially educational development in mental health law in several decades, and it merits close attention as a result.

In the first instance, India's new act, like similar legislation in other jurisdictions, includes new definitions of certain key terms (such as "mental illness" and "mental health establishment"); an updated consideration of "capacity" in relation to mental healthcare; "advance directives" to permit people with mental illness to direct future care; changes in the roles of family and "nominated representatives" (who need not be family members); revised procedures for admission (both with and without patient consent); new "Mental Health Review Boards" to review admissions and other matters; new rules governing treatment, restraint and research; and the establishment of various governmental authorities to oversee services (Duffy and Kelly, 2019). There is also *de facto* decriminalization of suicide, which has been widely welcomed.

Most dramatically, however, the new Indian legislation steps well beyond the confines of traditional mental health law and grants a legally binding right to mental healthcare to the entire population of India. This is a very expansive right impacting many aspects of the lives and experiences of people with mental illness and their families. The granting of this right is a notably dramatic development for mental health law in India or, indeed, anywhere.

More specifically, India's 2017 Act states that "every person shall have a right to access mental healthcare and treatment from mental health services run or funded by the appropriate Government" (Section 18(1)). The legislation goes on to specify the inclusive nature of this right:

> The right to access mental healthcare and treatment shall mean mental health services of affordable cost, of good quality, available in sufficient quantity, accessible geographically, without discrimination on the basis of gender, sex, sexual orientation, religion, culture, caste, social or political beliefs, class, disability or any other basis and provided in a manner that is acceptable to persons with mental illness and their families and care-givers.
>
> (Section 18(2))

As a result of this provision, all of the 1.3 billion people in India, amounting to one-sixth of the planet's population, have been granted a fully justiciable, legal right to mental healthcare. The legislation is quite specific about what this involves, stating that "the appropriate

Government shall make sufficient provision as may be necessary, for a range of services required by persons with mental illness" (Section 18(3)), including:

(a) Provision of acute mental healthcare services such as outpatient and inpatient services;
(b) Provision of half-way homes, sheltered accommodation, supported accommodation as may be prescribed;
(c) Provision for mental health services to support family of person with mental illness or home-based rehabilitation;
(d) Hospital and community-based rehabilitation establishments and services as may be prescribed;
(e) Provision for child mental health services and old age mental health services.

(Section 18(4))

This provision of a right to mental healthcare overcomes a highly problematic and common injustice. Jurisdictions that allow involuntary treatment without providing a right to mental healthcare can facilitate individuals oscillating between being "well and untreated" and being "unwell and treated involuntarily". An individual's mental health might be in decline, but they might have no way of accessing care until they reach the threshold for involuntary treatment. Often this occurs when they present a risk to themselves or others. As a result, a right to *voluntary* treatment for mental health conditions is vital to optimising mental healthcare.

Using mental health legislation to grant rights in this way is broadly consistent with the approaches of both the UN CRPD (UN, 2006) and the *WHO Resource Book on Mental Health, Human Rights and Legislation* (2005). As a result, India's new act meets 96 (55%) of the 175 relevant WHO human rights standards (Duffy and Kelly, 2017). When other relevant Indian legislation is taken into account, some 118 (67%) of the WHO standards are now addressed in Indian law – an outcome that compares very favourably with many other jurisdictions (Kelly, 2011).

Despite the clear vision and ambition of India's approach, however, there are significant issues which still need to be resolved with the legislation. The first issue is that there are still some important areas of low concordance with WHO standards, relating chiefly to the rights of families and carers, competence and guardianship, non-protesting patients and involuntary treatment in the community. These areas require further attention, possibly in regulations or further rules. In addition, certain provisions, such as the act's ban on ECT without muscle relaxants and anaesthesia, have proven controversial among psychiatrists in India (Andrade et al., 2012; Duffy et al., 2019). It is to be hoped that these issues can be resolved during the course of implementation across the country.

The second issue with India's new legislation is, perhaps, more fundamental, and it concerns whether the rights outlined in the new Indian legislation can truly be achieved in practice. Even prior to this legislation, it was clear that Indian mental health services are significantly under-resourced. In 2016, the *National Mental Health Survey of India, 2015–16* reported a "treatment gap" of approximately 85% for common mental disorders and 74% for severe mental disorders, including such conditions as psychosis (75%) and bipolar affective disorder (70%) (Gururaj et al., 2016).

This situation is largely attributable to the facts that less than 1% of the Indian health budget is allocated to mental healthcare (Patel et al., 2016), and there is a long-standing shortage of human resources (Jiloha, 2015). India has just 0.3 psychiatrists per 100,000 population, compared to 2.2 in China and 10.5 in the United States (WHO, 2019). There is a similar paucity of nurses, with just 0.8 mental health nurses per 100,000 people in India compared to 5.4 in China and 4.3 in the United States. These are profound resource problems that will be difficult to remedy quickly, even though India's new legislation clearly requires steps to be taken in this direction as a matter of urgency.

Against this background, it is clear that closing the treatment gaps in India's mental health services presents a substantial challenge to full implementation of the new legislation, even before the act's additional rights, such as rights to accommodation, can be achieved. Other key challenges with the new legislation include resourcing the new structures outlined in the act, the appropriateness of apparently increasingly legalized approaches to care (especially the consequences of potentially lengthy judicial proceedings) and the possible negative effects of specific aspects of the legislation that could result in barriers to care (e.g., revised licensing requirements for general hospital psychiatry units) (Duffy and Kelly, 2019).

Notwithstanding these challenges, India's new legislation clearly offers substantial potential benefits to India and, by example, to other countries that wish to align their mental health laws with the CRPD. At the same time, however, India's 2017 act also stands in stark contrast with more traditional mental health legislation, such as that in Ireland, which does not grant legally binding rights to mental healthcare and is far more circumspect in its ambitions.

Interestingly, both India and Ireland have stopped short of embracing some of the most recent guiding principles proposed for mental health legislation. One interpretation of the CRPD, for example, proposes removing all involuntary treatment from mental healthcare. These ideas have been most clearly articulated by the UN Committee on the Rights of Persons with Disabilities (2014) and the WHO's QualityRights initiative (WHO, 2012). This emphasis on a particular interpretation of autonomy as the key ethical principle in mental healthcare has proven controversial, on the basis that it might, paradoxically, curtail certain rights of persons with mental illness (Appelbaum, 2019; Raveesh et al., 2019).

Such dramatic proposals for reform of mental health legislation pose many difficult questions that currently remain unanswered. While the pragmatic realisation of entirely voluntary mental healthcare is still being debated, however, India appears to have struck a difficult balance by enacting broad-based mental health law that seeks to provide greater autonomy to patients and provide care to all. Its Mental Healthcare Act, 2017, includes many of the elements of traditional legislation but attempts to minimise conceive practices and facilitate individual choice were possible.

The final section of this chapter examines the extent to which each of these different approaches in Ireland and India effectively use mental health legislation to help optimise patient care.

CONCLUSIONS

Mental health legislation forms an important element of patient care in psychiatry. Regardless of the contrasting approaches in countries such as Ireland and India, virtually all jurisdictions recognise a need for dedicated mental health legislation that both facilitates delivery of care to people who lack the decision-making capacity to consent and helps protect and promote the rights of the mentally ill and their families.

There are, however, undeniable differences between jurisdictions. In Ireland, as we have seen, mental health legislation focuses on areas of traditional concern in mental health law, chiefly treatment without consent and ensuring standards in mental health facilities. This is a very narrow, focused vision of the role of mental health law.

In other jurisdictions, such as India, mental health legislation addresses these areas of traditional concern but also seeks to ensure equitable access to services, enhanced social care for the mentally ill, support for families and the protection and promotion of a broader range of rights. This is an approach that is explicitly informed by the UN CRPD, which was not published when Ireland's Mental Health Act, 2001, was developed.

In broad terms, both the WHO and UN provide strong support for India's more expansive vision of the role of law in protecting the right to mental health. This is, perhaps, a more modern approach to mental health legislation, compared to Ireland, and it is an approach that is likely to gain traction in other countries, following the ambitious example set by India's legislators.

It is important, however, that the approach to mental health legislation in any jurisdiction takes careful account of the history, traditions and pre-existing legislative structures in that jurisdiction, as well as the specific needs of the population in question. One size does not fit all. In the case of India, while many aspects of the 2017 act have been welcomed, important questions have been raised about the extent to which rights-based legislation can achieve its stated goals.

Raveesh and colleagues (2019), for example, note that the UN CRPD is a major milestone but also note, among other observations, that the concept of vulnerability is not addressed, that mental illness is not necessarily associated with disability, that empirical research on certain aspects of the UN CRPD is scarce and that more evidence is needed in this area. They also note that the UN CRPD has the potential to undermine certain rights if, for example, the insanity defence were to be abolished. In addition, rights are not always the only, or even the best, way to distribute scarce resources or meet all human needs; other methods include political (rather than judicial) allocation of public resources, myriad forms of exchange, community relations, charitable activities and various other local arrangements (Osiatyński, 2009).

These compelling arguments point to some of the potential limitations of relying exclusively or even very heavily on the UN CRPD in shaping approaches to mental health legislation. Clearly there is a balance to be reached between the narrow focus of legislation in countries such as Ireland and the expansive ambition displayed in India's 2017 act. While it is important that legislation have ambition and vision, it is also important that legislation work on the ground; that at least some of its goals are achievable; and that ideas about human rights do not inadvertently result in legislation becoming irrelevant, stakeholders becoming disenchanted and patients being paradoxically neglected as a result of legislation intended to assist them.

India's ambitious step forward into rights-based mental health law merits close attention over the years to come. Future research could usefully examine the extent of implementation across the country, the benefits of the new legislation, any paradoxical negative effects and any lessons that are potentially transferrable to other jurisdictions. The new Indian legislation presents a once-in-a-generation opportunity to gain an understanding of the extent to which such legislation can truly impact mental health services and improve the position of the mentally ill and their families.

Ultimately, optimising patient care and protecting rights are the twin goals of all mental health legislation, which needs to form an embedded part of health and social services if it is to achieve its goals. The optimal approach probably lies somewhere between the approach in Ireland and that in India, but further work is needed to identify precisely what that optimal approach involves.

ACKNOWLEDGEMENTS

The authors are very grateful to everyone who assisted them with their research work in India and to the editors of this volume for inviting this chapter.

References

Andrade C, Shah N, Tharyan P, Reddy MS, Thirunavukarasu M, Kallivayalil RA, Nagpal R, Bohra NK, Sharma A, Mohandas E. Position statement and guidelines on unmodified electroconvulsive therapy. *Indian Journal of Psychiatry* 2012; 54: 119–133.

Appelbaum PS. Saving the UN convention on the rights of persons with disabilities–from itself. *World Psychiatry* 2019; 18: 1–2.

Callard F, Sartorius N, Arboleda-Flórez J, Bartlett P, Helmchen H, Stuart H, Taborda J, Thornicroft G. *Mental Illness, Discrimination and the Law: Fighting for Social Justice*. Chichester: Wiley-Blackwell, 2012.

Duffy RM, Gulati G, Paralikar V, Kasar N, Goyal N, De Sousa A, Kelly BD. A focus group study of Indian psychiatrists' views on electroconvulsive therapy under India's Mental Healthcare Act 2017: "the ground reality is different". *Indian Journal of Psychological Medicine* 2019; 41: 507–515.

Duffy RM, Kelly BD. Concordance of the Indian Mental Healthcare Act 2017 with the World Health Organization's checklist on mental health legislation. *International Journal of Mental Health Systems* 2017; 11: 48.

Duffy RM, Kelly BD. India's mental healthcare act, 2017: Content, context, controversy. *International Journal of Law and Psychiatry* 2019; 62: 169–178.

Gilhooley J, Kelly BD. Return of the asylum. *British Journal of Psychiatry* 2018; 212: 69–70.

Gostin L, Bartlett P, Fennell P, McHale J, Mackay R. Preface. In L. Gostin, P. Bartlett, P. Fennell, J. McHale and R. Mackay (Eds.), *Principles of Mental Health Law and Policy* (pp. v–viii). Oxford: Oxford University Press, 2010.

Gururaj G, Varghese M, Benegal V, Rao GN, Pathak K, Singh LK, Mehta RY, Ram D, Shibukumar TM, Kokane A, Lenin Singh RK, Chavan BS, Sharma P, Ramasubramanian C, Dalal PK, Saha PK, Deuri SP, Giri AK, Kavishvar AB, Sinha VK, Thavody J, Chatterji R, Akoijam BS, Das S, Kashyap A, Ragavan VS, Singh SK, Misra R, NMHS collaborators group. *National Mental Health Survey of India, 2015–16: Prevalence, Patterns and Outcomes (NIMHANS Publication No. 129)*. Bengaluru: National Institute of Mental Health and Neuro Sciences, 2016.

Jiloha RC. The Mental Health Act of India. In S. Malhotra and S. Chakrabarti (Eds.), *Developments in Psychiatry in India: Clinical, Research and Policy Perspectives* (pp. 611–622). New Delhi: Springer, 2015.

Kelly BD. Structural violence and schizophrenia. *Social Science and Medicine* 2005; 61: 721–730.

Kelly BD. Mental health legislation and human rights in England, Wales and the Republic of Ireland. *International Journal of Law and Psychiatry* 2011; 34: 439–454.

Kelly BD. *Hearing Voices: The History of Psychiatry in Ireland*. Dublin: Irish Academic Press, 2016a.

Kelly BD. *Mental Illness, Human Rights and the Law*. London: RCPsych Publications, 2016b.

Osiatyński W. *Human Rights and Their Limits*. Cambridge: Cambridge University Press, 2009.

Patel V, Xiao S, Chen H, Hanna F, Jotheeswaran AT, Luo D, Parikh R, Sharma E, Usmani S, Yu Y, Druss BG, Saxena S. The magnitude of and health system responses to the mental health treatment gap in adults in India and China. *Lancet* 2016; 388: 3074–3084.

Raveesh BN, Gowda GS, Gowda M. How right is right-based mental health law? *Indian Journal of Psychiatry* 2019; 61: S640–S644.

Scull A. *The Most Solitary of Afflictions: Madness and Society in Britain, 1700–1900*. New Haven and London: Yale University Press, 1993.

Scull A. *Madness in Civilization: A Cultural History of Insanity, From the Bible to Freud, From the Madhouse to Modern Medicine*. London: Thames and Hudson Ltd., 2015.

Shorter E. *A History of Psychiatry: From the Era of the Asylum to the Age of Prozac*. New York: John Wiley and Sons, 1997.

United Nations. *Convention on the Rights of Persons with Disabilities*. New York: United Nations, 2006.

United Nations Committee on the Rights of Persons with Disabilities. *General Comment No. 1: Article 12: Equal Recognition Before the Law*. New York: United Nations, 2014.

Wolff J. *The Human Right to Health*. New York and London: W.W. Norton and Company, 2012.

World Health Organisation. *WHO Resource Book on Mental Health, Human Rights and Legislation*. Geneva: World Health Organization, 2005.

World Health Organization. *WHO QualityRights Tool Kit Assessing and Improving Quality and Human Rights in Mental Health and Social Care Facilities*. Geneva: World Health Organization, 2012.

World Health Organization. *Advancing the Right to Health: The Vital Role of Law*. Geneva: World Health Organization, 2017.

World Health Organization. *Global Health Observatory Data Repository: Human Resources Data by Country*. Geneva: World Health Organization, 2019. http://apps.who.int/gho/data/node.main.MHHR?lang=en. Accessed 9 April 2020.

4
Improving Patient Outcomes by Integration of Public Health and Mental Health

Swateja Nimkar

Introduction	42
Fighting the Stigma	43
Health Promotion and Disease Prevention in Mental Health	44
Use of mHealth and Tele-Psychiatry	45
Examples of Public Health-Mental Health Integration	45
Mental Health First Aid	45
Suicide Prevention Programs	46
Wellness Recovery Action Plan	46
Substance Abuse Education Programming	46
Pandemics and Mental Health	47
Future Trends	47

INTRODUCTION

Mental illnesses contribute significantly to the public health burden across the globe. In the 2017 World Health Organization (WHO) Mental Health Atlas, the Comprehensive Mental Health Action Plan 2013–2020 was discussed, which aimed at developing mental health leadership and policy that is effective in providing mental healthcare as an integral part of public health (WHO, 2018). The action plan called upon psychiatrists, the leaders of mental health, to "pave the way" for a community health approach in mental health using principles of public health and recognizing the biopsychosocial model that is at the foundation of all mental health disorders (Saxena, Funk, & Chisholm, 2014, p. 108). It is evident from the plan and its outcomes that evidence-based research and the principles of public health are paramount for mental health. This chapter discusses the immensely crucial role played by mental health in achieving public health.

Efforts for prevention and control are necessary in the field of mental health given the alarming rate at which mental illnesses are rising around the world. WHO reports that 25% of individuals in the world will develop a psychiatric illness or a behavioral disorder at some point during their lifetime and have consistently formed more than 14% of age-standardized years lived with disabilities for an appalling three decades (Global Burden of Diseases, 2017). Based on these statistics reported at the global level, there is a demonstrable need for increased mental health personnel and other resources. Collaboration of public health with psychiatric service providers can enhance management of care and allow seamless integration of the mental health system into mainstream healthcare.

FIGHTING THE STIGMA

To fight the stigma associated with mental illnesses is no less challenging than fighting the illness itself. Vigo, Thornicroft, and Atun (2016) argue that the public health estimates of the global burden of mental illnesses are underestimated due to various reasons related to diagnosis, changing definitions of psychiatric disorders, and insufficient attention given to this category of diseases. In a 2007 *Lancet* series on global mental health, more than 70% of young individuals and adults who need professional mental health services do not receive them due to the stigma associated with seeking mental healthcare. A decade later, the statistics have changed enough to reflect the changing attitudes and landscape when it comes to mental healthcare (Frankish, Boyce, & Horton, 2018). According to Corbiere et al. (2012, p. 1), "stigma is a complex term defined as a visible or invisible attribute, deeply discrediting, that disqualifies its bearer from full social acceptance, often resulting in several forms of discrimination". In the twenty-first century, stigma has assumed a slightly different meaning, even though the derogatory outcomes of stigmatizing behavior remain the same. Today, stigma manifests mainly in the form of social disapproval, often accompanied by perceived fear and discrimination (Corbiere et al., 2012).

Health care professionals have a very important role to play in reducing the stigma toward mental illnesses. A study conducted among Indian physicians showed the quality of undergraduate training in medicine and exposure to psychiatric patients is a significant determinant of stigmatizing attitudes expressed by the healthcare provider toward patients suffering from mental illnesses (Chandramouleeswaran et al., 2017). Furthermore, a detailed review conducted on several other studies have shown that healthcare providers' negative attitudes towards individuals suffering from serious mental illnesses have an adverse effect on clinician decision making, and can potentially alter the treatment outcomes in an unfavorable manner Stone et al., 2019; Henderson, Evans-Lacko, & Thornicroft, 2013). Some of the specifics that should be focused on in the sensitivity trainings of healthcare workers are use of the empowering language, debunking of myths, discouraging labeling and stereotyping, encouraging support groups for patients, increasing compassion and free speech, and finally, discussing mental health in the same manner as one would physical health.

Mental disorders can in themselves bring about a certain level of disconnect from roles and responsibilities in society. We all have daily tasks in which we engage in order to maintain a level of balance within our own lives in order to maintain autonomy within society. In individuals with mental health disorders, this everyday functioning is affected, which ultimately spirals into a disruption in their relationships, professional roles, and social status. It is not enough that individuals suffering from mental illnesses may be misunderstood, bullied, or even ostracized, but even worse is the fact that those seeking treatment and their families are severely stigmatized. Among all the barriers to psychiatric treatment in the western countries such as the United States, stigma and discrimination against people diagnosed with mental illnesses still unfortunately not only lead to significant delays in receiving treatment and add to non-compliance but also cause patients to avoid seeking mental health services altogether (Yilmaz & Okanli, 2015; Henderson et al., 2013).

Cultural factors can impact people's attitudes toward mental health. So, it is important that the family and close friends of sufferers accept mental illnesses as health conditions that need medical attention, just like physiological diseases. The use of tele-psychiatry and mobile health apps (discussed in detail in the section "Use of mHealth and Tele-Psychiatry") can help reduce the stigmatizing experiences of patients, as doctor's visits can be held discreetly from the patient's home setting. However, such a use of technology may not be feasible in all circumstances. A long-term and rather permanent solution would be a change in attitudes and perspectives toward mental health through pervasive education of clinicians and communities and a paradigm shift in the focus on mental health *promotion* and not only on treating the illness.

HEALTH PROMOTION AND DISEASE PREVENTION IN MENTAL HEALTH

> The science of psychology has been far more successful on the negative than on the positive side; it has revealed to us much about man's shortcomings, his illnesses, his sins, but little about his potentialities, his virtues, his achievable aspirations, or his full psychological height. It is as if psychology had voluntarily restricted itself to only half its rightful jurisdiction, and that the darker, meaner half.
> (Abraham Maslow, as cited in *Gross, 2018*, p. 243)

Although the terminology is often used interchangeably, health promotion and disease prevention are two distinct and important areas in public health that resonate very closely with the mental health system. There is a notable difference between mental health promotion and mental illness prevention. This difference is related to the community health goals or clinical outcomes generated by the interventions used in each of them. According to WHO (2016), health promotion is the phenomenon of enabling people to increase control over their personal health through policy-making, health literacy, and healthy environment. It has a positive connotation to it. In the world of mental health, health promotion goes hand in hand with positive psychology or, simply put, the *pursuit of happiness and contentment.*

Although concepts of mental well-being and the importance of positivity have been around in the western countries for over five decades, they are recently starting to fill the gap in the literature with evidence-based programs such as SAFECARE, Triple P, and so on focusing on interventions based on positive psychology and preventive educational programs such as mindfulness (Marsenich, 2020). Wellness and contentment are some of the most widely studied and acknowledged concepts of positive psychology in India, often tied to cultural and spiritual aspects of health and regarded as quintessential in an individual's overall spectrum of well-being. However, their application in clinical practice is limited (Shukla, 2016).

Mental health promotion aims to develop and maintain a positive mental health status and enable individuals to achieve their fullest psychological potential. By creating conducive social and environmental conditions, mental health promotion can increase the quality of life for not only individuals but also families and communities. However, mental illness prevention and mental health promotion are not exclusive to each other but rather two intertwined, yet distinct components of our mental health system (Saxena, Jane-Llopis, & Hosman, 2006). Practical applications of disease prevention and health promotion may include similar programming strategies, plans, and activities, but they are aimed at producing "different but complementary outcomes".

Disease prevention is the process of minimizing the onset and public health burden of disease. Prevention by using various levels of prevention strategies. These levels are broadly categorized into primary, secondary, and tertiary levels. The outcomes at the primary level focuses on preventing the disease. The rapidly emerging personal and community needs for positive psychology and emotional wellness have built a significant target audience for primary prevention mental health programs in healthy individuals. At the secondary level, the interventions focus on screening, early identification, and controlling disease. Finally, the prevention strategies at the tertiary level aim to reduce complications arising from diseases. In mental health, primary prevention would include substance use education with the aim of continued abstinence and prolonging the onset of substance use as long as possible. Depression and anxiety screenings are among the most commonly used screening exams used in mental health, even in low- and middle-income countries (Gemma-Claire, Grace, & De Silva, 2016). Suicide prevention, on the other hand, is an example of tertiary prevention, where the goal is to prevent the complication of existing and potentially co-morbid psychiatric illnesses that can potentially lead to suicidal ideation, plan, or action.

USE OF MHEALTH AND TELE-PSYCHIATRY

There exists a considerable amount of literature supporting the conclusion that technology has had a huge impact on individual health as well as the healthcare system. However, there is a need to assess and implement technology in the mentally ill population, especially knowing that a majority of this population owns at least one technology device that has the potential to promote individual health.

According to Pfefferbaum and North (2020), the use of tele-medicine in the field of psychiatry, also known as tele-psychiatry, has seen a tremendous surge during the out-of-ordinary times of this pandemic. According to Nimkar (2016a), there is mounting evidence for the effectiveness of self-assessments conducted using mobile health (also known as mHealth) applications such as screenings and other interventions such as global positioning system (GPS) tracking for dementia care and smartphone applications (apps) for home-based care. Mobile apps have been designed for medication reminders, allowing for improved medication compliance, a verifiable need in psychiatry (Nimkar, 2016b). The literature undeniably points to the fact that the field of telepsychiatry has a vast scope to incorporate mHealth in the areas of prevention, screening, and treatment, more so in regions affected by shortage of mental healthcare providers. Additionally, the idea and use of remote social services and virtual counseling centers and support groups needs to promulgate in all strata of society.

EXAMPLES OF PUBLIC HEALTH-MENTAL HEALTH INTEGRATION

The majority of mental health programs conducted in community settings are designed and implemented through the lens of public health. The approaches of prevention and early identification are at the core of these programs. Inarguably, these programs contribute to creating awareness about mental health, push the need to seek professional help in high-risk situations, and contribute to narrowing the gap between physical and mental health needs when it comes to increasing accessibility of mental health services. The following select programs provide a brief overview of the availability and types of the integrated public health-mental health programs around the world.

Mental Health First Aid

Mental Health First Aid is a widely implemented and evidence-based mental health literacy program that aims at increasing awareness, reducing stigma, and preventing mental illnesses in high-risk as well as average-risk populations, addressing both crisis and non-crisis situations (Hung, Lam, & Chow, 2019). It has been shown to "expand psychological support in ways that enhance dignity and respect for all" (Douglas, p. 494).

It uses the gatekeeper training approach to educate public about the knowledge and skills required to intervene and prevent distressing feelings and suicidal thoughts (Ziedonis et al., 2016). In a mixed-methods feasibility trial of the Mental Health First Aid program, it was found that the program can increase acceptance of mental illnesses by reducing stigma and help develop culturally relevant strategies to identify and respond to mental health crisis situations in a community-based setting (Crooks et al., 2018).

Suicide Prevention Programs

Suicide is the most dreaded and irreversible outcome of any mental health condition.

Due to issues of medication non-adherence in mentally ill patients, as well as the variation in persistence of suicidal thoughts, it is extremely difficult to predict the effect of antidepressants on those at risk for suicide. Statistics show that one in five patients with clinically diagnosed major depressive disorder receiving antidepressant treatment for at least 12 weeks experienced suicidal ideation even while they were on antidepressant treatment (Madsen et al., 2019). This substantiates the need for effective public health programming that can prevent or control the very complex phenomenon of suicide. Suicide prevention programs aim to intervene at earlier stages of the mental illness such that suicidal ideations or intent could be identified well before the attempt takes place. These programs are planned to nurture peer support, self-awareness, and understanding using underlying principles of public health promotion and disease prevention.

The SEYLE study employed a randomized controlled trial to assess the effectiveness of a three-pronged approach to suicide prevention, an awareness program, a screening program, and a gate-keeping program for education and early intervention among at-risk adolescents from 11 countries in Europe, Asia, and the Middle East (Wasserman et al., 2015).

Wellness Recovery Action Plan

Wellness Recovery Action Plan (WRAP) is an example of a privately run, evidence-based program that promotes mental well-being using innovative strategies. According to the Copeland Center (2020, para 1), the creators of WRAP, this program is a personalized wellness and recovery system that can "help individuals to monitor uncomfortable and distressing feelings and behaviors and, through planned responses, reduce, modify, or eliminate those feelings". It is one of the peer-led, evidence-based programs recognized by the United States Substance Abuse and Mental Health Services Administration (SAMHSA) that promotes individual wellness through peer support groups led by individuals who themselves have been patients of the mental health system. Additionally, WRAP is one of the few mental health promotion programs that offers electronic wellness plans and a confidential and safe set of self-management tools.

Substance Abuse Education Programming

Substance use disorders affect millions of people worldwide, often leading to problems such as distorted personal and professional relationships, overdose, poor quality of life, increased violence, motor vehicle accidents, and other co-morbid health conditions. Approximately 80% of individuals suffering from a substance use disorder and living in low- and middle-income countries do not have regular access to professional care and treatment, because of which at least half of these cases go undiagnosed and untreated (Erskine et al., 2018; WHO, 2010). Structured public health programs can help create awareness and improve the accessibility of professional care and treatment options as observed in case of opioid and alcohol abuse disorders (WHO, 2010). Thus, once again, it is evident that psychiatry and public health categorically overlap in the areas of prevention, control, and treatment for substance abuse as well.

PANDEMICS AND MENTAL HEALTH

Pandemics are a form of public health emergencies that affect people worldwide and trigger a wide variety of psychological reactions. In the last hundred years, the world has witnessed multiple pandemics, such as the H1N1 pandemic in 2009, the H3N2 pandemic that occurred in 1968, H2N2 from the 1950s, or a century-old pandemic of H1N1 influenza, also known as the Spanish flu, that occurred in 1918 toward the end of the First World War. Pandemics can certainly add to the mental health burden of the affected communities. Individual reactions to pandemics may cover a wide spectrum of negativity, and people experience damaging feelings and emotions such as fear, distress, sadness, anger, helplessness, and hopelessness.

One of the most dreaded patient outcomes in psychiatry is suicide, and prevention of suicide is an important goal in treatment plans. Challenges such as isolation, anxiety, and newly emerging stressors due to an unprecedented environment add to the suicide risk and the overall mental health burden of communities during pandemics. The most recent one, the coronavirus (COVID-19) pandemic, significantly exacerbated the mental health of communities affected by it. In addition to the concerns of the infection itself, communities were also dealing with shortages of personal protective equipment; individuals experiencing isolation due to home confinement; and anxiety related to healthcare, continuity in education, and financial insecurity (Pfefferbaum & North, 2020).

The first case of suicide occurred in India on February 12, 2020, barely 13 days after the first case of COVID-19 was confirmed in the country (Goyal et al., 2020). It was later discovered that the victim committed suicide by hanging himself on a tree after learning from his physician that he had contracted an unknown viral illness, all because of the fear and panic he suffered induced by COVID-19. Based on this case, Goyal and his team (2020) have advised a more responsible use of social media to circulate information related to newly emerging diseases, especially those that have the potential to turn into pandemics. According to Panigrahi and colleagues (2021), 151 COVID-19–related suicide cases have been reported in India, with male gender, age 25 to 60 years, and urban non-metro location being strong risk factors.

The COVID-19 pandemic has been rampantly spreading in waves all over the world. In the first half of the pandemic, multiple cases were observed primarily ranging between the ages of 19 and 65 (Thakur & Jain, 2020). Identifying suicidal predictors or risk factors associated with suicides that are also related to pandemics, such as fear of social isolation, economic recession, stress, and discrimination is of the utmost importance in preventing suicidal ideations and plans (Thakur & Jain, 2020). The mental healthcare system and faith-based organizations are both capable of providing much-needed support networks during the difficult times experienced by individuals during a pandemic. Therefore, psychosocial services such as community clinics, crisis care teams, psychiatric services for medication management, in-patient facilities, faith-based counseling, and social workers at the grassroots levels, all of whom play a critical role in fighting the mental health pandemic in its various stages.

FUTURE TRENDS

History is witness to the fact that there are several challenges for the public health systems across the globe pertaining to mental health. These challenges mainly relate to early identification of risk factors, reducing stigma, and compliance problems associated with mental health disorders. The collateral damage resulting from these challenges is the skewed utilization and limited effectiveness of treatment, which tends to exacerbate mental health disparities and restrict access to services for individuals predominantly belonging to populations that are disproportionately affected.

Going forward, evidence-based public health programs can be used to identify needs and risk factors related to mental health and also to increase the awareness of and accessibility to psychiatric services. The use of telepsychiatry and other virtual services in mental health needs to be explored to establish evidence of effectiveness in various parts of the world, as psychiatric services backed by technology can have a far-reaching, positive impact on stigma and global shortages in mental healthcare.

The public health approach allows mental healthcare workers to implement interventions on large groups of people and sometimes entire communities and populations, unlike clinical fields, where clinicians usually work on one patient at a time. Public health strategies certainly cannot and should not replace clinical interventions but need to be incorporated to increase resourcefulness, have broader reach, and complement psychiatric medicine to prevent and control mental illnesses.

References

Chandramouleeswaran, S., Rajaleelan, W., & Edwin, N. C., et al. (2017). Stigma and attitudes toward patients with psychiatric illness among postgraduate Indian physicians. *Indian Journal of Psychological Medicine, 39*(6), 746.

Copeland Center for Wellness and Recovery (2020). *What is WRAP®?* Retrieved from https://copeland-center.com/wellness-recovery-action-plan-wrap

Corbiere, M., Samson, E., Villotti, P., & Pelletier, J. (2012). Strategies to fight stigma toward people with mental disorders: Perspectives from different stakeholders. *Scientific World Journal, 2012*, 516358.

Crooks, C., Lapp, A., Auger, M., van der Woerd, K., Snowshoe, A., Rogers, B. J., Tsuruda, S., & Caron, C. (2018). A feasibility trial of mental health first aid first nations: Acceptability, cultural adaptation, and preliminary outcomes. *American Journal of Community Psychology, 61*, 459–471. https://doi.org/10.1002/ajcp.12241

Erskine, H. E., Moffitt, T. E., Copeland, W. E., Costello, E. J., Ferrari, A. J., Patton, G., Degenhardt, L., Vos, T., Whiteford, A. J., & Scott, J. G. (2018). A heavy burden on young minds: The global burden of mental and substance use disorders in children and youth. *Psychological Medicine, 45*(7), 1551–1563.

Frankish, H., Boyce, N., & Horton R. (2018). Mental health for all: A global goal. *The Lancet, 392*(10157): 1493–1494. http://doi.org/10.1016/S0140-6736(18)32271-2

GBD 2017 Disease and Injury Incidence and Prevalence Collaborators (2018). Global, regional, and national incidence, prevalence, and years lived with disability for 354 diseases and injuries for 195 countries and territories, 1990–2017: A systematic analysis for the global burden of disease study 2017. *The Lancet, 392*(10159), 1789–1858. https://doi.org/10.1016/S0140-6736(18)32279-7

Gemma-Claire, A., Grace, R., & De Silva, M. J. (2016). Validated screening tools for common mental disorders in low and middle income countries: A systematic review, *PLoS One, 11*(6), e0156939.

Goyal, K., Chauhan, P., Chhikara, K., Gupta, P., & Singh, M. P. (2020). Fear of COVID 2019: First suicidal case in India! *Asian Journal of Psychiatry, 49*, 101989. https://doi.org/10.1016/j.ajp.2020.101989

Gross, R. (2018). *Psychology in its historical context: Theories and debates.* Abingdon, UK: Routledge.

Henderson, C., Evans-Lacko, S., & Thornicroft, G. (2013). Mental illness stigma, help seeking, and public health programs. *American Journal of Public Health, 103*, 777–780. https://doi.org/10.2105/AJPH.2012. 301056.

Hung, M. S. Y., Lam, S. K. K., & Chow, M. C. M. (2019). Nursing students' experiences of mental health first aid training: A qualitative descriptive study. *Collegian, 26*(5), 534–540. https://doiorg.ezproxy.umuc.edu/10.1016/j.colegn.2019.02.006

Madsen, T., et al. (2019). Trajectories of suicidal ideation during 12 weeks of escitalopram or nortriptyline antidepressant treatment among 811 patients with major depressive disorder. *Journal of Clinical Psychiatry, 80*(4), 18m12575. https://doi.org/10.4088/JCP.18m12575

Marsenich (2020). *Using evidence-based programs to meet the mental health needs of California children and youth.* Retrieved from www.cibhs.org/sites/main/files/fileattachments/ebp children_youth_070811.pdf

Nimkar, S. (2016a). Promoting individual health using information technology: Trends in the US health system. *Health Education Journal, 75*(6), 744–752. https://doi.org/10.1177/0017896916632790

Nimkar, S. (2016b, September). Medication compliance in patients with mental health problems. [Guest Editorial]. *Indian Journal of Mental Health*, 237–239.

Panigrahi, M., Pattnaik, J. I., Padhy, S. K., Menon, V., Patra, S., Rina, K., Padhy, S. S., & Patro, B. (2021). COVID-19 and suicides in India: A pilot study of reports in the media and scientific literature. *Asian Journal of Psychiatry, 57*, 102560.

Pfefferbaum, B., & North, C. S. (2020). Mental health and the Covid-19 pandemic. *The New England Journal of Medicine: Perspectives*. https://doi.org/10.1056/NEJMp2008017

Saxena, S., Funk, M., & Chisholm, D. (2014). WHO's mental health action plan 2013–2020: What can psychiatrists do to facilitate its implementation? *World Psychiatry, 13*(2), 107–109. https://doi.org/10.1002/wps.20141

Saxena, S., Jane-Llopis, E., & Hosman, C. (2006). Prevention of mental and behavioural disorders: implications for policy and practice. *World Psychiatry, 5*(1), 5–14. www.ncbi.nlm.nih.gov/pmc/articles/PMC1472261/

Shukla, P. (2016). Positive psychology, Indian psychology, and spirituality. *Dev Sanskriti: Interdisciplinary International Journal, 7*, 12–26.

Stone, E. M., Chen, L. N., Daumit, G. L., et al. (2019). General medical clinicians' attitudes toward people with serious mental illness: A scoping review. *Journal of Behavioral Health Services and Research, 46*, 656–679.

Thakur, V., & Jain, A. (2020). COVID 2019-suicides: A global psychological pandemic. *Brain Behavior & Immunity* [Epub ahead of print]. https://doi.org/10.1016/j.bbi.2020.04.062

Vigo, D., Thornicroft, G., & Atun, R. (2016). Estimating the true global burden of mental illness. *The Lancet: Psychiatry, 3*(2), 171–178. https://doi.org/10.1016/S2215-0366(15)00505-2

Wasserman, D., et al. (2015). School-based suicide prevention programmes: The SEYLE cluster-randomised, controlled trial. *Lancet, 385*(9977), 1536–1544.

World Health Organization (2010). *mhGAP intervention guide for mental, neurological and substance use disorders in non-specialized health settings*. Geneva: World Health Organization. Retrieved from www.who.int/mental_health/publications/mhGAP_intervention_guide/en

World Health Organization (2016, August 20). *What is health promotion?* Retrieved from www.who.int/news-room/q-a-detail/what-is-health-promotion2016

World Health Organization (2018, June 6). *Mental health: Massive scale-up of resources needed if global targets are to be met*. Retrieved from www.who.int/mental_health/evidence/atlas/atlas_2017_web_note/en/

Yilmaz, E., & Okanli, A. (2015). The effect of internalized stigma on the adherence to treatment in patients with schizophrenia. *Archives of Psychiatric Nursing, 29*, 297–301. https://doi.org/10.1016/j.apnu.2015.05.006

Ziedonis, D., Larkin, C., & Appasani, R. (2016). Dignity in mental health practice & research: Time to unite on innovation, outreach & education. *Indian Journal of Medicine and Research, 144*(4), 491–495. https://doi.org/10.4103/0971-5916.200885

5
Building Resilience at a Community and Family Level for Care in Psychiatry

Yash Acchapalia and Avinash De Sousa

The Concept of Resilience	50
The Psychobiology of Resilience	51
Hypothalamus-Pituitary-Adrenal Axis	*51*
Noradrenergic System	*51*
Serotonergic and Dopaminergic Systems	*51*
Neuropeptide Y	*52*
Brain-Derived Neurotrophic Factor	*52*
The Molecular Genetics of Resilience	52
Epigenetic Mechanisms of Resilience	*52*
Transcriptional Mechanisms of Resilience	*52*
Neural Circuitry of Resilience	53
Neural Circuitry of Fear	*53*
Neural Circuitry of Reward	*53*
Neural Circuitry of Emotion Regulation	*54*
Additional Relevant Neural Circuits	*54*
Factors Determining Resilience	54
Personal Factors	*54*
Biological Factors	*54*
Environmental Factors	*55*
Interaction Between Personal, Biological and Environmental Factors	*55*
Indicators of Resilience	55
Resilience and Schizophrenia	56
Resilience and Rehospitalization	56
Resilience-Based Interventions	57
Conclusion	57

THE CONCEPT OF RESILIENCE

Human beings have the potential to endure and persevere against adverse conditions as an inherent survival instinct. This conviction and capacity to sustain even in difficult situations despite all odds is what is commonly referred to as 'resilience'. There are multiple definitions of the term resilience[1]. Resilience is a term used to describe the unique characteristics that allow a person to confront external or internal hardships and to overcome periods of suffering. A number of psychiatric disorders have been linked to the levels of resilience in subjects[2][3].

It is a construct that plays a role in resolving stress and safeguarding one's psychobiological homeostasis[4]. A high level of resilience works as a protective element, while a lower level of resilience increases the susceptibility to develop a psychiatric disorder[5]. Resilience is a dynamic and multidimensional abstraction which expresses psychological flexibility[2].

Resilience is now emerging as an imperative approach in preventive psychiatry, with resilience-promoting interventions being deliberated in various preventive mental health community programmes[7]. Resilience is now gaining attention as one of the predictors of sound mental health and as something to be developed in individuals to better combat mental illnesses[8].

THE PSYCHOBIOLOGY OF RESILIENCE

The physiological response of the body to any kind of stress is controlled by a number of hormones, neurotransmitters, neuropeptides and other body chemicals. The function, balance and interaction of these factors bring about the inter-individual variability resilience.

Hypothalamus-Pituitary-Adrenal Axis

The hypothalamus releases corticotropin-releasing hormone (CRH) in response to stress, which activates the hypothalamus-pituitary-adrenal (HPA) axis and releases cortisol. Short-term actions of cortisol are protective and promote adaptation; however, continuous exposure to abnormally high levels of cortisol can be harmful, leading to hypertension, immunosuppression, cardiovascular disease, and so on[9]. Excessive cortisol is associated with complex structural effects in the amygdala and hippocampus, including atrophic effects in certain types of neurons[10][11] Thus, low levels of CRH release and adaptive changes in CRH receptor activity might promote resilience. DHEA is also released in response to stress and has antiglucocorticoid effects in the brain. It has additional central effects, particularly on the GABA (γ-aminobutyric acid)-ergic system, which could also play a part in resilience[12]. Resilience is associated with the capacity to curb unnecessary increases in CRH and cortisol through an refined negative feedback system, involving optimal function and balance of glucocorticoid and mineralocorticoid receptors[13][14].

Noradrenergic System

The locus coeruleus in the brainstem releases noradrenaline during periods of stress, which, if remaining unchecked, is associated with anxiety disorders and cardiovascular problems[15][16]. This suggests that decreased responsiveness of the locus coeruleus noradrenergic system could promote resilience.

Serotonergic and Dopaminergic Systems

Acute stress is associated with a rise in serotonin turnover in several areas of the cortex, which modulates neural responses to stress, with both anxiogenic and anxiolytic effects depending on the receptor subtype and brain region involved. Serotonin function is also closely linked to mood regulation. Dopamine signalling aids fear extinction, but its part in resilience per se is ambiguous.

Neuropeptide Y

Neuropeptide Y (NPY) is thought to have anxiolytic-like effects and to enhance cognition under stressful conditions. NPY also negates the anxiogenic effects of CRH in the amygdala, the hypothalamus, the hippocampus and the locus coeruleus. Resilience might play a role in maintaining a harmony between NPY and CRH levels during stress[17]. Moreover, intra-amygdala NPY administration promotes resilient responses to stress, in the form of reduced anxiety-like behaviours[18].

Brain-Derived Neurotrophic Factor

Brain-derived neurotrophic factor (BDNF) levels in the hippocampus are reduced by stress, which can be reversed by chronic antidepressant treatment[19]. But chronic stress increases BDNF, causing prodepression-like effects[20][21].

THE MOLECULAR GENETICS OF RESILIENCE

The degree of adaptability of neurochemical stress response systems to new adverse exposures is determined by complex interactions between one's genetic make-up and history of exposure to environmental stressors.

Polymorphisms and haplotypes of the CRH type 1 receptor gene, functional variants of the brain mineralocorticoid and glucocorticoid receptor (GR) genes and genetic variations in FKBP5 gene have strong influences on the HPA axis and therefore in the development of resilience[22].

The most-researched gene-environment interaction involves naturally occurring variations in the promoter of the human serotonin transporter gene (5-HTTLPR)[23].

Polymorphisms found in the gene that codes for COMT (Val158Met) play a significant role in resilience[24].

A recent study showed higher amygdala reactivity to threat-related facial expressions in people with a low-expression diplotype of the gene that encodes NPY[25].

An single nucleotide polymorphisms (G196A, Val66Met) in the gene that encodes BDNF significantly blunts BDNF's intracellular trafficking and activity-dependent release[26].

Epigenetic Mechanisms of Resilience

Epigenetics refers to stable non-heritable changes in chromatin structure causing long-lasting modifications in gene expression and that are not associated with changes in DNA sequence[27]. Epigenetic changes that occur at the time of brain development are an additional means by which behavioural variability is established in individuals, preparing them for a host of possible environmental stresses[30]. Various research on behavioural changes during stages of early and adulthood due to epigenetic modifications carried out in animal models suggests that drugs that influence DNA methylation and related epigenetic mechanisms might promote resilience[28][29].

Transcriptional Mechanisms of Resilience

One series of studies which focuses on the ventral tegmental area (VTA)-nucleus accumbens reward circuit is a social defeat stress model[21] in which resilience, among a population of inbred mice, is linked to the absence of many of the changes in gene expression that are seen in the VTA-nucleus accumbens of vulnerable mice and also with the induction of distinct changes in gene expression that occur in resilient mice only[30]. Chronic defeat stress in resilient mice increases expression of several K+ channel subunits in VTA dopamine neurons, which prevents the stress-induced increase in VTA excitability and the consequent release of BDNF onto the nucleus accumbens. The transcriptional regulation of multiple additional genes in the VTA and nucleus accumbens of resilient mice now contribute to new directions in understanding the molecular basis of resilience along with developing new treatments for depression and other stress-related disorders. Similar studies among inbred mice suggest the use of substance P antagonists (neurokinin 1 receptor antagonists) as a way to promote resilience in humans[32].

NEURAL CIRCUITRY OF RESILIENCE

A plethora of imaging studies of the human brain, along with research among animal models, are beginning to delineate the brain circuits that intercede distinct aspects of mood and emotion under normal circumstances and in distinct pathological conditions that are indicative of low resilience. Several limbic regions in the forebrain have been recognized which are highly interlinked and function as a series of integrated parallel circuits that regulate emotional states and thus resilience.

Neural Circuitry of Fear

Recent designs of the patho-physiology of PTSD, an example of diminished resilience on exposure to a traumatic stressor, involve abnormal fear learning and an underlying dysfunction in the neural circuitry of fear, comprising the amygdala, the hippocampus and the ventromedial prefrontal cortex (PFC)[33][34]. Preliminary findings suggest that managing patients with PTSD using cognitive behaviour therapy might have favourable effects by reducing amygdala activation and increasing rostral anterior cingulate cortex activation during fear processing[35]. The amygdala and hippocampus-dependent fear conditioning in animals have been related to lasting potentiation and synaptic plasticity. Accordingly, the N-methyl-D-aspartate (NMDA) glutamate receptor blockade in the amygdala impedes cue-associated fear conditioning, while the NMDA receptor blockade in the hippocampus blocks context-dependent fear conditioning[36]. Administration of D-cycloserine, a partial agonist of NMDA receptors, can augment extinction of fear conditioning in patients with PTSD undergoing prolonged exposure therapy[37]. The β-adrenergic receptor blockade in the amygdala can also block cue-dependent fear conditioning, and β-adrenergic antagonists have been tested in patients exposed to trauma, with mixed results[16][39]. Further, activation of GRs in the hippocampus and perhaps in the amygdala regulates fear conditioning and its extinction, which suggests the potential use of glucocorticoids in the treatment of trauma[40].

Neural Circuitry of Reward

In recent fMRI studies among patients of PTSD and major depressive disorder, evidence of reward system dysfunction was found, with decrease in strial activation during performance of reward-related tasks[41][42][43]. Several novel studies have found that Val158met COMT polymorphisms are somewhat accountable for inter-individual variations in neural responses to reward anticipation in healthy individuals[44]. Animal studies have greatly increased our knowledge of the brain's reward circuitry and its possible significance for resilience. The mesolimbic dopamine system is the best-established reward circuit. It involves dopaminergic neurons of the VTA and their innervation of the nucleus accumbens and many other forebrain limbic regions. The trait optimism, which is linked to resilience, might relate to reward circuit function. Optimism bias, which is the propensity to expect future events to be positive, was associated with higher activation in the amygdala and the rostral anterior cingulate cortex (ACC) and therefore influence individual resilience[45].

Neural Circuitry of Emotion Regulation

Studies of individuals with psychiatric disorders suggest that they have abnormalities in their emotion regulation systems[46][47]. A greater capacity for emotion regulation has also been related to stress resilience. Studies in mood and anxiety disorders have led to identification of abnormalities in amygdala, hippocampus, subgenual ACC and PFC function[48]. Additionally, individual differences in cortico-limbic connectivity point towards genetic predisposition to inflexible emotion processing in certain individuals[49].

Cognitive reappraisal is one mechanism of emotion regulation that has received particular attention. Recent fMRI studies have shown decreased amygdala activation and increased activation in lateral and medial PFC regions during reappraisal, which is associated with reappraisal success[50][51]. It has thus been speculated that the PFC regulates the intensity of emotional responses by fine-tuning the activation of the amygdala.

Incorporation of reappraisal in day-to-day activities has also been linked to greater PFC and lower amygdala activation to negative stimuli. This points towards the notion that there might be a central mechanism through which reappraisal could promote successful coping and reduce the risk of mood disorder onset[52].

Additional Relevant Neural Circuits

A few other neuronal circuits that are suggested to play an important role in the development of resilience, either directly or indirectly, include the mirror neuron system[53] and the role of oxytocin in promoting social attachment[54][55].

FACTORS DETERMINING RESILIENCE

Personal Factors

Personality attributes such as self-esteem, mindfulness, receptivity, extraversion, cognitive appraisal and optimism all ultimately contribute to the development of resilience.

The findings of pioneering investigators indicate that cognitive flexibility, positive self-concepts, intellectual functioning, emotional regulation and coping mechanisms, are also very much associated with resilience[56]. Demographic factors such as age, sex, gender, race and ethnicity, social relationships and population characteristics are variably related to resilience. Some factors that positively affect resilience may be life stage specific, while others may operate across the lifespan.

Biological Factors

Recent research in biological factors of resilience indicates that harsh early environments can adversely affect the developing brain structure, function and neurobiological systems[57][67]. These include changes in brain size, receptor sensitivity, neural networks and neurotransmitter metabolism[59]. These changes can affect the capacity to mitigate negative emotions and thereby affect resilience to stress and adversities. An EEG study compared between maltreated and nonmaltreated children aged 6 to 12 years found significant interaction in patterns of EEG activity between resilience, maltreatment status and gender[60]. There is strong evidence to prove that supportive, sensitive early caregivers in infancy and childhood can increase resilience and reduce the effects of unhealthy environments and that there may be specific sensitive periods of life where interventions to modify resilience may work best[61]. Exposure to stressful events in early childhood and adolescence has persistently shown to produce chronic amendments in the HPA axis, which increases susceptibility to mood and anxiety disorders[62]. Studies of healthy people exposed to childhood maltreatment have identified numerous biological variables where personality, cortisol and dehydroepiandrosterone were independent contributors to resilience[63].

Environmental Factors

Relationships with immediate family, peers and other social support form the microenvironment level are directly proportionately related to resilience. Non-abusive parents with healthy parenting, non-broken and stable family structure; secure attachment to mother; family stability; and absence of maternal depression or substance abuse are associated with fewer behavioural problems and better psychological well-being. On a macrosystemic level, community factors such as good schooling and education, community services, sports and athletics and artistic opportunities, cultural diversity, spirituality and religion and lack of exposure to violence contribute to resilience[64][65].

Interaction Between Personal, Biological and Environmental Factors

Susceptibility and vulnerability to the development of mental disorders are known to be related to genetic predisposition in combination with the person's life experiences and environments. Social experiences can lead to substantial and enduring changes in gene expression that can in turn affect behaviour in a person and be transmitted to the next generation[66]. Genetic variations may interact protectively against both acute and chronic environmental stressors and have a protective function for some maltreated children[67][68]. These include polymorphisms of monoamine oxidase A (MAOA),[69] the serotonin transporter gene[70] and genes that regulate the HPA axis[75]. Resilience arises from a complex interaction of forces at various levels, consolidating a person's genetic heritage, environment-gene reactions, life experiences, social interactions and cultural setting[72].

INDICATORS OF RESILIENCE

In addition to the diverse definitions, the measurements used affect assessments of resilience. Studies on children and adolescents concentrates on developmental domains, including behavioural, emotional and educational functioning, thus making this the quantification and qualification of resilience complex. Competence in one domain does not ensure competence in another[73]. Children who show high resilience are comparable to the average population in domains of academic performance, interpersonal relationships, behavioural problems, emotional regulation and social competence. Some indicators of a lack of resilience include symptoms of mental disorders such as depression or anxiety, academic performance, substance abuse, social skills and delinquency. Domains which can be assessed in adults include employment, criminal behaviour, substance abuse and homelessness[74]. Using cut-off scores or standard deviations on standardized psychopathological measurement tools for depression, anxiety and PTSD is a common means of measuring resilience in the population[75] More recently, researchers have developed specific scales to measure resilience, such as the Connor-Davidson Resilience Scale[76] or the Resilience Scale for Adults[77].

RESILIENCE AND SCHIZOPHRENIA

Schizophrenia encompasses a wide spectrum of symptoms where a number of aetiological factors and pathophysiological mechanisms come into play. It has a profound impact on the person's life and may lead to several adversities[78]. Resilience is an important factor contributing to recovery in individuals with schizophrenia, with evidence that it increases the probability for long-term recovery[79].

A Norwegian study was done on patients fully recovered from schizophrenia who were followed up for a period of 15 years. Seventeen subjects were interviewed with semi-structured interviews and the Connor-Davidson Resilience Scale (CD-RISC) to assess resilience. The results show that approximately 50% of the participants maintained full recovery. No neuroleptic medication had been used by these subjects for about 17 years.

The prospect of being cured of schizophrenia instilled optimism and hope in patients and helped reduce stigma about the disease, showing that people with schizophrenia do not have to live a life of disability[80]. Optimism and willpower instilled in the recovered individuals in this study were reflected in their high scores on the resilience scale[81].

Another study was done on transcultural attributes in internalized stigma, self-esteem and hopelessness to measure resilience among patients of schizophrenia between Austria and Japan. Among the Japanese subjects, marked lower resilience and self-esteem scores as well as higher scores of hopelessness were observed. Both Austrian and Japanese patients observed significantly lower degrees of resilience, self-esteem and hope compared to healthy control subjects. The conclusion drawn was that patients of schizophrenia from Japanese and Western Europe may have different needs to achieve recovery[81]. Resilience has been proven much lower among ultrahigh-risk individuals who progress to full-blown psychosis compared to those who do not[83]. Patients meeting the full diagnostic criteria for schizophrenia were studied for resilience as the capacity to cope with and to gain insight into the illness, and resilience was shown to have a favourable effect on the course of the illness[84].

The parent-infant relationship is an important preventative intervention to identify very early risk and resilience factors[85]. Another study explored resilience and its correlation among the offspring of parents with schizophrenia. The findings showed that a majority of the offspring reported medium resilience[86].

Henderson and Cock studied a qualitative approach to study how ten patients experienced recovery after a first episode of psychosis. Based on unstructured interviews, two styles of resilience were identified. One was "tenacity," requiring effort over a period of time, and another was "rebounding," springing back to normal life almost immediately. Internal and environmental resources, including self-pacing and support from others, were described as mechanisms of "harnessing resilience"[87].

RESILIENCE AND REHOSPITALIZATION

Patients are often hospitalized for very specific common causes: (1) those related to individual patient characteristics such as personality traits, treatment acceptance and attitude, stigma and discrimination, resilience and coping ability; (2) illness-related causes such as early onset of illness, prolonged duration of untreated illness, severe psychopathology and treatment resistance, comorbidities and suicide attempts; (3) treatment-related causes such as delayed intervention, poor access to care, inadequate treatment, side effects and lack of specialized treatments; and (4) systemic factors such as lack of human resources, modern treatment facilities, training and competency of professional staff. Resilience is one important factor to consider that can prevent rehospitalization by promoting positive treatment outcome and preventing relapses[71][82].

RESILIENCE-BASED INTERVENTIONS

Studies to determine the effectiveness of resilience enhancement in a younger population have been done in Russia, which offered 94 participants who were taken hostage in a 2004 school tragedy combined recreational sport and psychosocial rehabilitation. The results indicated a significant mean increase in resilience at follow-up assessment and higher self-reported improvement in resilience processes for participants who experienced more traumatic events. Therefore, mentalization and cognitive training can help modify and enhance resilience[88].

Another study examined the effect of mindfulness training on resilience mechanisms in active-duty marines preparing for deployment. Mechanisms related to stress recovery could be modified in healthy individuals prior to stress exposure, as shown in this study[89].

Resilience programs can be developed to increase treatment efficacy and improve outcome for patients suffering from multiple mental health conditions as well as physical disorders[6].

Those who experience childhood adversities seem to demonstrate a certain level of post-traumatic growth, and this unique inter-individual resilience is significant for responding to adversities faced in adulthood. Resilience is now being thought of as a paradigm to be incorporated into nursing and medical curricula, corporate wellness training and mental health rehabilitation programmes. It is also an important part of emotional intelligence interventions for frontline workers that may increase coping resources and enhance social skills, which may benefit their long-term occupational health[31].

An emerging role of resilience enhancement training with at-risk children and adolescents and resilience enhancement interventions at a school level for the prevention of development of psychopathology in childhood and adolescence may help in the prevention of adult psychopathology.[38]

Resilience also has a pivotal role to play in trauma and natural disasters[58].

CONCLUSION

Resilience is an active, dynamic, unique trait with interpersonal variability which determines an individual's capacity for successful adaptation to both acute trauma or chronic adversities. It is not just the absence of psychopathology. It is said to have both genetic and acquired influences in a person's lifetime. There is a complex interaction between one's genetic, epigenetic, biological, environmental and personal factors which keeps this trait ever changing and dynamic. The functional capacity of the brain structures, including neurotransmitter metabolism and neuronal plasticity, mediate resilience. An individual's level of resilience is better if they have a greater adaptive functioning of fear, reward, emotion regulation or social-behaviour circuits which in turn helps them to better face fears, experience positive emotions, increase their ability to search for positive ways to reframe stressful events and derive benefit from supportive relationships. It has an extremely vital role in the prevention and determining the course of disease and treatment for a vast number of common mental health disorders such as depression, PTSD, ADHD, schizophrenia, substance abuse and so on. The role of psychopharmacological treatments in the enhancement of resilience is still in question. A few quantitative methods for assessment of resilience have been developed, but its being such a complex entity makes this extremely difficult. There is a dire need for establishment of mental health programs at community and school levels as well as for rehabilitation of people who have suffered from mental health diseases. Much more research into this field is warranted to get a better understanding of the vital role of resilience at all levels of not only mental but also physical health and medicine.

References

1. De Sousa A, Shrivastava A. Resilience among people who face natural disaster. *Journal of Psychiatrists' Association of Nepal.* 2015;4(1):1–4.
2. Fletcher D, Sarkar M. Psychological resilience. *European Psychologist.* 2013 Apr 8.
3. Black K, Lobo M. A conceptual review of family resilience factors. *Journal of Family Nursing.* 2008 Feb;14(1):33–55.
4. Bonanno GA. Loss, trauma, and human resilience: Have we underestimated the human capacity to thrive after extremely aversive events? *American Psychologist.* 2004 Jan;59(1):20.
5. Tusaie K, Dyer J. Resilience: A historical review of the construct. *Holistic Nursing Practice.* 2004 Jan 1;18(1):3–10.
6. Jha AP, Morrison AB, Parker SC, Stanley EA. Practice is protective: Mindfulness training promotes cognitive resilience in high-stress cohorts. *Mindfulness.* 2017 Feb;8(1):46–58.
7. Leve LD, Harold GT, Chamberlain P, Landsverk JA, Fisher PA, Vostanis P. Practitioner review: Children in foster care—Vulnerabilities and evidence-based interventions that promote resilience processes. *Journal of Child Psychology and Psychiatry.* 2012 Dec;53(12):1197–1211.
8. Almedom AM. Resilience, hardiness, sense of coherence, and posttraumatic growth: All paths leading to "light at the end of the tunnel"? *Journal of Loss and Trauma.* 2005 Apr 20;10(3):253–265.
9. Karlamangla AS, Singer BH, McEwen BS, Rowe JW, Seeman TE. Allostatic load as a predictor of functional decline: MacArthur studies of successful aging. *Journal of Clinical Epidemiology.* 2002 Jul 1;55(7):696–710.
10. McEwen BS, Milner TA. Hippocampal formation: Shedding light on the influence of sex and stress on the brain. *Brain Research Reviews.* 2007 Oct 1;55(2):343–355.
11. Brown ES, Woolston DJ, Frol AB. Amygdala volume in patients receiving chronic corticosteroid therapy. *Biological Psychiatry.* 2008 Apr 1;63(7):705–709.
12. Dubrovsky BO. Steroids, neuroactive steroids and neurosteroids in psychopathology. *Progress in Neuro-Psychopharmacology and Biological Psychiatry.* 2005 Feb 1;29(2):169–192.
13. Southwick SM, Vythilingam M, Charney DS. The psychobiology of depression and resilience to stress: Implications for prevention and treatment. *Annual Reviews in Clinical Psychology.* 2005 Apr 27;1:255–291.
14. Carver CS. You want to measure coping but your protocol's too long: Consider the brief cope. *International Journal of Behavioral Medicine.* 1997 Mar;4(1):92–100.
15. Charney DS. Neuroanatomical circuits modulating fear and anxiety behaviors. *Acta Psychiatrica Scandinavica.* 2003 Sep;108:38–50.
16. McGaugh JL. The amygdala modulates the consolidation of memories of emotionally arousing experiences. *Annual Reviews in Neuroscience.* 2004 Jul 21;27:1–28.
17. Sajdyk TJ, Shekhar A, Gehlert DR. Interactions between NPY and CRF in the amygdala to regulate emotionality. *Neuropeptides.* 2004 Aug 1;38(4):225–234.
18. Sajdyk TJ, Johnson PL, Leitermann RJ, Fitz SD, Dietrich A, Morin M, Gehlert DR, Urban JH, Shekhar A. Neuropeptide Y in the amygdala induces long-term resilience to stress-induced reductions in social responses but not hypothalamic–adrenal–pituitary axis activity or hyperthermia. *Journal of Neuroscience.* 2008 Jan 23;28(4):893–903.
19. Duman RS, Monteggia LM. A neurotrophic model for stress-related mood disorders. *Biological Psychiatry.* 2006 Jun 15;59(12):1116–1127.
20. Eisch AJ, Bolaños CA, De Wit J, Simonak RD, Pudiak CM, Barrot M, Verhaagen J, Nestler EJ. Brain-derived neurotrophic factor in the ventral midbrain–nucleus accumbens pathway: A role in depression. *Biological Psychiatry.* 2003 Nov 15;54(10):994–1005.
21. Berton O, McClung CA, DiLeone RJ, Krishnan V, Renthal W, Russo SJ, Graham D, Tsankova NM, Bolanos CA, Rios M, Monteggia LM. Essential role of BDNF in the mesolimbic dopamine pathway in social defeat stress. *Science.* 2006 Feb 10;311(5762):864–868.
22. Bradley RG, Binder EB, Epstein MP, Tang Y, Nair HP, Liu W, Gillespie CF, Berg T, Evces M, Newport DJ, Stowe ZN. Influence of child abuse on adult depression: Moderation by the corticotropin-releasing hormone receptor gene. *Archives of General Psychiatry.* 2008 Feb 1;65(2):190–200.

23. Kendler KS, Kuhn JW, Vittum J, Prescott CA, Riley B. The interaction of stressful life events and a serotonin transporter polymorphism in the prediction of episodes of major depression: a replication. *Archives of General Psychiatry.* 2005 May 1;62(5):529–535.
24. Heinz A, Smolka MN. The effects of catechol O-methyltransferase genotype on brain activation elicited by affective stimuli and cognitive tasks. *Reviews in the Neurosciences.* 2006 Jun 1;17(3):359–368.
25. Zhou Z, Zhu G, Hariri AR, Enoch MA, Scott D, Sinha R, Virkkunen M, Mash DC, Lipsky RH, Hu XZ, Hodgkinson CA. Genetic variation in human NPY expression affects stress response and emotion. *Nature.* 2008 Apr;452(7190):997–1001.
26. Chen ZY, Jing D, Bath KG, Ieraci A, Khan T, Siao CJ, Herrera DG, Toth M, Yang C, McEwen BS, Hempstead BL. Genetic variant BDNF (Val66Met) polymorphism alters anxiety-related behavior. *Science.* 2006 Oct 6;314(5796):140–143.
27. Tsankova N, Renthal W, Kumar A, Nestler EJ. Epigenetic regulation in psychiatric disorders. *Nature Reviews Neuroscience.* 2007 May;8(5):355–367.
28. Meaney MJ, Szyf M. Environmental programming of stress responses through DNA methylation: Life at the interface between a dynamic environment and a fixed genome. *Dialogues in Clinical Neuroscience.* 2005 Jun;7(2):103.
29. Weaver IC, Cervoni N, Champagne FA, D'Alessio AC, Sharma S, Seckl JR, Dymov S, Szyf M, Meaney MJ. Epigenetic programming by maternal behavior. *Nature Neuroscience.* 2004 Aug;7(8):847–854.
30. Krishnan V, Han MH, Graham DL, Berton O, Renthal W, Russo SJ, LaPlant Q, Graham A, Lutter M, Lagace DC, Ghose S. Molecular adaptations underlying susceptibility and resistance to social defeat in brain reward regions. *Cell.* 2007 Oct 19;131(2):391–404.
31. Brennan EJ. Towards resilience and wellbeing in nurses. *British Journal of Nursing.* 2017 Jan 12;26(1):43–47.
32. Berton O, Covington III HE, Ebner K, Tsankova NM, Carle TL, Ulery P, Bhonsle A, Barrot M, Krishnan V, Singewald GM, Singewald N. Induction of ΔFosB in the periaqueductal gray by stress promotes active coping responses. *Neuron.* 2007 Jul 19;55(2):289–300.
33. Rauch SL, Shin LM, Phelps EA. Neurocircuitry models of posttraumatic stress disorder and extinction: Human neuroimaging research—Past, present, and future. *Biological Psychiatry.* 2006 Aug 15;60(4):376–382.
34. Yehuda R, LeDoux J. Response variation following trauma: A translational neuroscience approach to understanding PTSD. *Neuron.* 2007 Oct 4;56(1):19–32.
35. Felmingham K, Kemp A, Williams L, Das P, Hughes G, Peduto A, Bryant R. Changes in anterior cingulate and amygdala after cognitive behavior therapy of posttraumatic stress disorder. *Psychological Science.* 2007 Feb;18(2):127–129.
36. Davis M, Myers KM. The role of glutamate and gamma-aminobutyric acid in fear extinction: Clinical implications for exposure therapy. *Biological Psychiatry.* 2002 Nov 15;52(10):998–1007.
37. Davis M, Ressler K, Rothbaum BO, Richardson R. Effects of D-cycloserine on extinction: Translation from preclinical to clinical work. *Biological Psychiatry.* 2006 Aug 15;60(4):369–375.
38. Prince-Embury S, Saklofske DH, editors. *Resilience in children, adolescents, and adults: Translating research into practice.* Springer Science & Business Media; 2012 Nov 6.
39. Stein MB, Kerridge C, Dimsdale JE, Hoyt DB. Pharmacotherapy to prevent PTSD: Results from a randomized controlled proof-of-concept trial in physically injured patients. *Journal of Traumatic Stress: Official Publication of the International Society for Traumatic Stress Studies.* 2007 Dec;20(6):923–932.
40. Cai WH, Blundell J, Han J, Greene RW, Powell CM. Postreactivation glucocorticoids impair recall of established fear memory. *Journal of Neuroscience.* 2006 Sep 13;26(37):9560–9566.
41. Gibbons RD, Brown CH, Hur K, Marcus SM, Bhaumik DK, Erkens JA, Herings RM, Mann JJ. Early evidence on the effects of regulators' suicidality warnings on SSRI prescriptions and suicide in children and adolescents. *American Journal of Psychiatry.* 2007 Sep;164(9):1356–1363.
42. Sailer U, Robinson S, Fischmeister FP, König D, Oppenauer C, Lueger-Schuster B, Moser E, Kryspin-Exner I, Bauer H. Altered reward processing in the nucleus accumbens and mesial prefrontal cortex of patients with posttraumatic stress disorder. *Neuropsychologia.* 2008 Sep 1;46(11):2836–2844.
43. Drevets WC, Price JL, Furey ML. Brain structural and functional abnormalities in mood disorders: Implications for neurocircuitry models of depression. *Brain Structure and Function.* 2008 Sep 1;213(1–2):93–118.
44. Schmack K, Schlagenhauf F, Sterzer P, Wrase J, Beck A, Dembler T, Kalus P, Puls I, Sander T, Heinz A, Gallinat J. Catechol-O-methyltransferase Val158met genotype influences neural processing of reward anticipation. *Neuroimage.* 2008 Oct 1;42(4):1631–1638.

45. Sharot T, Riccardi AM, Raio CM, Phelps EA. Neural mechanisms mediating optimism bias. *Nature*. 2007 Nov;450(7166):102–105.
46. Masten AS, Coatsworth JD. The development of competence in favorable and unfavorable environments: Lessons from research on successful children. *American Psychologist*. 1998 Feb;53(2):205.
47. Johnstone T, Van Reekum CM, Urry HL, Kalin NH, Davidson RJ. Failure to regulate: Counterproductive recruitment of top-down prefrontal-subcortical circuitry in major depression. *Journal of Neuroscience*. 2007 Aug 15;27(33):8877–8884.
48. Ressler KJ, Mayberg HS. Targeting abnormal neural circuits in mood and anxiety disorders: From the laboratory to the clinic. *Nature Neuroscience*. 2007 Sep;10(9):1116–1124.
49. Drabant EM, Hariri AR, Meyer-Lindenberg A, Munoz KE, Mattay VS, Kolachana BS, Egan MF, Weinberger DR. Catechol O-methyltransferase val158met genotype and neural mechanisms related to affective arousal and regulation. *Archives of General Psychiatry*. 2006 Dec 1;63(12):1396–1406.
50. Goldin PR, McRae K, Ramel W, Gross JJ. The neural bases of emotion regulation: Reappraisal and suppression of negative emotion. *Biological psychiatry*. 2008 Mar 15;63(6):577–586.
51. Ochsner KN, Ray RD, Cooper JC, Robertson ER, Chopra S, Gabrieli JD, Gross JJ. For better or for worse: Neural systems supporting the cognitive down-and up-regulation of negative emotion. *Neuroimage*. 2004 Oct 1;23(2):483–499.
52. Drabant EM, McRae K, Manuck SB, Hariri AR, Gross JJ. Individual differences in typical reappraisal use predict amygdala and prefrontal responses. *Biological Psychiatry*. 2009 Mar 1;65(5):367–373.
53. Schulte-Rüther M, Markowitsch HJ, Fink GR, Piefke M. Mirror neuron and theory of mind mechanisms involved in face-to-face interactions: A functional magnetic resonance imaging approach to empathy. *Journal of Cognitive Neuroscience*. 2007 Aug;19(8):1354–1372.
54. Kosfeld M, Heinrichs M, Zak PJ, Fischbacher U, Fehr E. Oxytocin increases trust in humans. *Nature*. 2005 Jun;435(7042):673–676.
55. Kirsch P, Esslinger C, Chen Q, Mier D, Lis S, Siddhanti S, Gruppe H, Mattay VS, Gallhofer B, Meyer-Lindenberg A. Oxytocin modulates neural circuitry for social cognition and fear in humans. *Journal of Neuroscience*. 2005 Dec 7;25(49):11489–11493.
56. Joseph S, Linley PA. Growth following adversity: Theoretical perspectives and implications for clinical practice. *Clinical Psychology Review*. 2006 Dec 1;26(8):1041–1053.
57. Luthar SS, Brown PJ. Maximizing resilience through diverse levels of inquiry: Prevailing paradigms, possibilities, and priorities for the future. *Development and Psychopathology*. 2007;19(3):931.
58. Shah R. Protecting children in a situation of ongoing conflict: Is resilience sufficient as the end product? *International Journal of Disaster Risk Reduction*. 2015 Dec 1;14:179–185.
59. Curtis WJ, Nelson CA. Toward building a better brain: Neurobehavioral outcomes, mechanisms, and processes of environmental enrichment. *Resilience and Vulnerability: Adaptation in the Context of Childhood Adversities*. 2003:463–488.
60. Curtis WJ, Cicchetti D. Emotion and resilience: A multilevel investigation of hemispheric electroencephalogram asymmetry and emotion regulation in maltreated and nonmaltreated children. *Development and Psychopathology*. 2007 Jun;19(3):811–840.
61. Gunnar MR, Fisher PA. Bringing basic research on early experience and stress neurobiology to bear on preventive interventions for neglected and maltreated children. *Development and Psychopathology*. 2006 Sep;18(3):651–677.
62. Gladstone GL, Parker GB, Mitchell PB, Malhi GS, Wilhelm K, Austin MP. Implications of childhood trauma for depressed women: An analysis of pathways from childhood sexual abuse to deliberate self-harm and revictimization. *American Journal of Psychiatry*. 2004 Aug 1;161(8):1417–1425.
63. Cicchetti D, Rogosch FA. Personality, adrenal steroid hormones, and resilience in maltreated children: A multi-level perspective. *Development and Psychopathology*. 2007;19(3):787.
64. Luthar SS, Cicchetti D, Becker B. The construct of resilience: A critical evaluation and guidelines for future work. *Child Development*. 2000 May;71(3):543–562.
65. Luthar SS, Cicchetti D. The construct of resilience: Implications for interventions and social policies. *Development and Psychopathology*. 2000;12(4):857.
66. Parent C, Zhang TY, Caldji C, Bagot R, Champagne FA, Pruessner J, Meaney MJ. Maternal care and individual differences in defensive responses. *Current Directions in Psychological Science*. 2005 Oct;14(5):229–233.
67. Cicchetti D, Curtis WJ. Multilevel perspectives on pathways to resilient functioning. *Development and Psychopathology*. 2007 Jun;19(3):627–629.
68. Moffitt TE, Caspi A, Rutter M. Measured gene-environment interactions in psychopathology: Concepts, research strategies, and implications for research, intervention, and public understanding of genetics. *Perspectives on Psychological Science*. 2006 Mar;1(1):5–27.

69. Youdim MB, Edmondson D, Tipton KF. The therapeutic potential of monoamine oxidase inhibitors. *Nature Reviews Neuroscience*. 2006 Apr;7(4):295–309.
70. Kaufman J, Yang BZ, Douglas-Palumberi H, Grasso D, Lipschitz D, Houshyar S, Krystal JH, Gelernter J. Brain-derived neurotrophic factor–5-HTTLPR gene interactions and environmental modifiers of depression in children. *Biological Psychiatry*. 2006 Apr 15;59(8):673–680.
71. Davydow DS, Ribe AR, Pedersen HS, Fenger-Grøn M, Cerimele JM, Vedsted P, Vestergaard M. Serious mental illness and risk for hospitalizations and rehospitalizations for ambulatory care-sensitive conditions in Denmark. *Medical Care*. 2016 Jan 1;54(1):90–97.
72. Davydov DM, Stewart R, Ritchie K, Chaudieu I. Resilience and mental health. *Clinical Psychology Review*. 2010 Jul 1;30(5):479–495.
73. Walsh WA, Dawson J, Mattingly MJ. How are we measuring resilience following childhood maltreatment? Is the research adequate and consistent? What is the impact on research, practice, and policy? *Trauma, Violence, & Abuse*. 2010 Jan;11(1):27–41.
74. Daigneault I, Hébert M, Tourigny M. Personal and interpersonal characteristics related to resilient developmental pathways of sexually abused adolescents. *Child and Adolescent Psychiatric Clinics of North America*. 2007 Apr 1;16(2):415–434.
75. Gillespie CF, Phifer J, Bradley B, Ressler KJ. Risk and resilience: Genetic and environmental influences on development of the stress response. *Depression and Anxiety*. 2009 Nov;26(11):984–992.
76. Friborg O, Hjemdal O, Rosenvinge JH, Martinussen M, Aslaksen PM, Flaten MA. Resilience as a moderator of pain and stress. *Journal of Psychosomatic Research*. 2006 Aug 1;61(2):213–219.
77. Friborg O, Hjemdal O, Rosenvinge JH, Martinussen M. A new rating scale for adult resilience: What are the central protective resources behind healthy adjustment? *International Journal of Methods in Psychiatric Research*. 2003 Jun;12(2):65–76.
78. Insel TR. Rethinking schizophrenia. *Nature*. 2010 Nov;468(7321):187–193.
79. Ridgway P. Restorying psychiatric disability: Learning from first person recovery narratives. *Psychiatric Rehabilitation Journal*. 2001;24(4):335.
80. Torgalsbøen AK. Sustaining full recovery in schizophrenia after 15 years: Does resilience matter? *Clinical Schizophrenia & Related Psychoses*. 2012 Jan 1;5(4):193–200.
81. Hofer A, Mizuno Y, Frajo-Apor B, Kemmler G, Suzuki T, Pardeller S, Welte AS, Sondermann C, Mimura M, Wartelsteiner F, Fleischhacker WW. Resilience, internalized stigma, self-esteem, and hopelessness among people with schizophrenia: Cultural comparison in Austria and Japan. *Schizophrenia Research*. 2016 Mar 1;171(1–3):86–91.
82. Marom S, Munitz H, Jones PB, Weizman A, Hermesh H. Expressed emotion: Relevance to rehospitalization in schizophrenia over 7 years. *Schizophrenia Bulletin*. 2005 Jan 1;31(3):751–758.
83. Kim KR, Song YY, Park JY, Lee EH, Lee M, Lee SY, Kang JI, Lee E, Yoo SW, An SK, Kwon JS. The relationship between psychosocial functioning and resilience and negative symptoms in individuals at ultra-high risk for psychosis. *Australian & New Zealand Journal of Psychiatry*. 2013 Aug;47(8):762–771.
84. Reddy SK, Thirthalli J, Channaveerachari NK, Reddy KN, Ramareddy RN, Rawat VS, Narayana M, Ramkrishna J, Gangadhar BN. Factors influencing access to psychiatric treatment in persons with schizophrenia: A qualitative study in a rural community. *Indian Journal of Psychiatry*. 2014 Jan;56(1):54.
85. Beeghly M, Tronick E. Early resilience in the context of parent–infant relationships: A social developmental perspective. *Current Problems in Pediatric and Adolescent Health Care*. 2011 Aug 1;41(7):197–201.
86. Herbert HS, Manjula M, Philip M. Growing up with a parent having schizophrenia: Experiences and resilience in the offsprings. *Indian Journal of Psychological Medicine*. 2013 Apr;35(2):148.
87. Henderson AR, Cock A. The responses of young people to their experiences of first-episode psychosis: Harnessing resilience. *Community Mental Health Journal*. 2015 Apr;51(3):322–328.
88. Makhnach AV. Resilience in Russian youth. *International Journal of Adolescence and Youth*. 2016 Apr 2;21(2):195–214.
89. Johnson DC, Thom NJ, Stanley EA, Haase L, Simmons AN, Shih PA, Thompson WK, Potterat EG, Minor TR, Paulus MP. Modifying resilience mechanisms in at-risk individuals: A controlled study of mindfulness training in Marines preparing for deployment. *American Journal of Psychiatry*. 2014 Aug;171(8):844–853.

Section 2
Specific Strategies for Management

6

Comprehensive Management of Violence Against Women
Putting WHO Recommendations Into Practice

Salmi Razali, Dina Tukhvatullina, Daria Smirnova

Introduction	65
Type of Violence	66
Contributing Factors to Violence	67
Distal Factors	67
Proximal Factors	68
Individual Factors	68
Consequences of Violence Against Women	70
Strategies and Intervention – Integrated Socioecological Framework	70
Distal-Level Intervention	70
Proximal-Level Intervention	73
Individual-Level Interventions	74
Conclusions	74

ABBREVIATIONS

   ADHD – Attention Deficit and Hyperactivity Disorder
   CDC – Centers for Disease Control and Prevention
   IPV – Intimate Partner Violence
   GWH – Gender, Women, Health
   PTSD – Post-traumatic Stress Disorder
   UN – United Nations
   VAW – Violence Against Women
   WHO – World Health Organisation

INTRODUCTION

Violence against women (VAW) is a form of abuse and aggression against human rights, not merely posing a physical threat but causing psychological harm to women and girls by denying their equality, rejecting their demands for dignity and self-worth, violating their security and restricting their right to enjoy fundamental freedoms. This pervasive violence results in immense psychological consequences to survivors of violence and likewise to their children, family and friends as well as significant others residing at every level of the socioecological system. Mental health professionals are positioned to play significant roles in addressing these damaging behaviours.

DOI: 10.4324/9780429030260-8

VAW was defined by the United Nations in the New York Declaration on the Elimination of Violence Against Women (1993) as

> any act of gender-based violence that results in, or is likely to result in, physical, sexual, or mental harm or suffering to women, including threats of such acts, coercion or arbitrary deprivation of liberty, whether occurring in public or private life.

Global data from the World Health Organisation (WHO) indicates that almost one in every three women has been in an abusive relationship and may have experienced physical and/or sexual violence committed by their intimate partner. The prevalence of this problem varies between regions, ranging from estimates of 23% in high-income countries to 38% in the South-East Asia region (Stake, Ahmed, Tol et al., 2020). Moreover, an increased level of domestic violence against women, female professionals at their workplaces in the health sector (e.g., frontline workers), financial difficulties in females as compared to males and the associated growth of depression and anxiety symptoms rates among women have been registered during the COVID-19 pandemic worldwide (Thibaut & van Wijngaarden-Cremers, 2020).

TYPE OF VIOLENCE

Violence, abuse and victimisation can come in many forms, including physical, sexual, psychological, economic and sociocultural violence. The term physical violence may be easy to understand, but sexual, psychological, economic and social violence are sometimes in need of further clarification. While sexual violence can be hard to distinguish from sexual harassment, both may have detrimental consequences for the survivors (Harris, McFarlane, & Wieskamp, 2020). In certain parts of the world, marital rape is condoned in the name of culture, honour and power (Gul & Schuster, 2020; Sheehy, 2020). Being less overt than sexual violence, psychological abuse is difficult to detect and disclose. It can come in the public form of verbal aggression (such as yelling, swearing) but also in emotional manipulation, intimidation, control, degrading, pervasive criticism, humiliation, threatening behaviour and forced isolation from others (Capezza, D'Intino, Flynn, & Arriaga, 2017). Economic violence or financial abuse is another form of VAW, which involves acts aimed at controlling, exploiting or interfering with women's economic resources, including property and gainful employment (Postmus, Hoge, Breckenridge, Sharp-Jeffs, & Chung, 2020). Sociocultural violence is a variant of VAW; a girl or woman is harmed as a result of social, cultural, religion or traditional practices, such as honour killing or genital mutilation.

The 2002 World Report on Violence and Health by the WHO classified violence into three groups: (i) self-directed violence, (ii) interpersonal violence and (iii) collective violence. Self-directed violence includes suicidal behaviour and self-abuse, such as self-mutilation. Interpersonal violence can be divided into family and interpersonal violence (such as child abuse, intimate partner violence and elder abuse) and community violence (such as youth violence and violence in institutional settings such as schools and the workplace). The third type is collective violence, which can be divided into social, political and economic violence, such as what occurs during terrorist acts, war, conflict and economic fragmentation or segmentation.

Collective violence was also described by Johan Galtung (1969) as "indirect violence or structural violence". This consists of systematic harm or violence inflicted by a group of people or state operators that denies equal distribution of resources and encourages social disparity and marginalisation of some group or of an individual. Most forms of self-directed, interpersonal and collective or structural violence are interconnected in a common "web of violence" (Hamby & Grych, 2012; Hamby et al., 2018; Renvoize, 1978). In this era of the internet, the rise of cyberviolence brings a covert and complex aspect to the landscape of abuse and aggression (Backe, Lilleston, & McCleary-Sills, 2018; Peterson & Densley, 2017). VAW does not stand alone but is entwined within the "web of violence" and structures of polyvictimisation.

The survivors of the "web of violence" may include most women and girls, children, the elderly, people with disabilities and transgender people. The survivor may not be an isolated figure but a victim of family or community violence. The co-occurrence of several types of violence, which results in polyvictimisation, is not uncommon. A survivor can experience different types of direct victimisation (such as bullying, assault, sexual victimisation, child abuse and infanticide) or indirect victimisation (such as domestic violence, economic deprivation and gender disparity). A recent review of 59 publications on polyvictimisation reported an overall co-occurrence of polyvictimisation in a family of about 10% among the general population and 36.% among the clinical population (Chan, Chen, & Chen, 2019). In low- and lower-income countries, the co-occurrence rates were as high as 77% (Le, Holton, Romero, & Fisher, 2018). Since VAW is such a complex matter, understanding the intricate relationship of VAW with various types of non-gendered violence is crucial to overcome present challenges, inform early preventive measures and deliver effective interventions to the target population (Colombini, Dockerty, & Mayhew, 2017; Hamby et al., 2018).

CONTRIBUTING FACTORS TO VIOLENCE

No single contributing factor can entirely explain violence perpetrated against women. The intercalation of various factors can directly or indirectly predispose towards, precipitate or perpetuate VAW, and these factors can be simplified according to the socioecological model. The framework proposed by Urie Bronfenbrenner (1992) and applied by the WHO (2010) and several respective centres summarises the interaction of factors contributing to VAW (Terry, 2014). It explains the interaction between personal or individual factors with proximal factors (such as spousal, family, workmate, workplace superior) and more distal factors (such as community, legal, cultural and political influences) (Heise, 1998; Razali, Kirkman, & Fisher, 2020a)

Distal Factors

Chief among the distal factors contributing to VAW are economic factors such as poverty or financial difficulties and economic dependence of women upon men (Buller et al., 2018; Hess & Del Rosario, 2018). Also, women the world over are more likely to have informal domestic work than formal employment. They will consequently have less access to cash and credit and own minimal property. Even in the United States, women only gained the right to have a bank account within living memory (Legal Information Institute, n.d.). The persistence of economic insecurity limits a women's opportunities to have a better life and creates a hurdle for seeking help and obtaining agency and empowerment (Buller et al., 2018; Hess & Del Rosario, 2018).

The second fundamental distal element in the genesis of VAW consists of sociocultural factors, including gender disparity and gender-specific socialisation such as cultural bias in sex roles, inherent patriarchal belief and practice and marriage customs such as dowry and teenage or consanguineous marriage (Semahegn et al., 2019; Willie & Kershaw, 2019). A not uncommon factor is the culture of victim-blaming and stigmatisation, from nonprofessional service providers (such as healthcare workers, law enforcement personnel, spiritual advisors, traditional healers, community leaders and legal officers), and secondary victimisation perpetuates further VAW, in particular domestic violence (Ivert, Merlo, & Gracia, 2018; Kruahiran, Boonyasiriwat, & Maneesri, 2020).

Acting in concert with socioeconomic factors are legal factors. Discriminatory legal provisions against women such as disfavoured legal status regarding divorce, child custody, maintenance and inheritance are imposing hurdles to women's empowerment (Walklate, Fitz-Gibbon, & McCulloch, 2018). The absence of provisions for welfare and legal rights of vulnerable women (especially domestic helpers, immigrants, refugees and asylum-seekers) may increase a woman's vulnerability to abuse and aggression (Gangoli, 2020; Jennings, Powers, & Perez, 2021). Moreover, inadequate understanding and low levels of legal literacy present a great challenge to deterring and curbing VAW (Gangoli, 2020; Walklate et al., 2018).

Politics is another crucial distal factor for VAW. Indeed, war and civil conflicts expose women and girls to a violent environment (Bronson, 2021; Quenivet, 2020). Also, underrepresentation of women in power structure and politics, and the perpetuation of genderbased agendas by the media, undermine the recognition of VAW. If women remain without political power, abuse and aggression in domestic milieu are too often perceived as a private matter, outside the control of the government and authorities (Krook, 2020).

Proximal Factors

Most perpetrators of VAW are the intimate partner (intimate partner violence; IPV) or someone in the survivor's milieu such as employer or workmate, whereas violence from strangers is a relatively minor component of VAW. Theorisation to explain how those perpetrators continue to inflict violence has evolved from the concept of "battered women syndrome" and "cycle of violence" first proposed in the 1850s to the struggle for "power and control" introduced by the Duluth Domestic Abuse Intervention Programme in the 1980s (Barner & Carney, 2011; Bohall, Bautista, & Musson, 2016) (refer to Figure 6.1). The former theory posits cyclic phases of tension building, explosion and a reset to the initial honeymoon phase that results in trapping the survivor within the violent environment. The later "power and control" model later explained further that the perpetrator uses intimidation, male privilege, economic control, psychological abuse, hostage-taking of children, social isolation, denial, blaming, threats and various other tactics to assert control (Barner & Carney, 2011; Bohall et al., 2016). Nowadays, the widespread access to information technology and the internet connection have extended conflict beyond the wheel of power and control through devices such as mobile phones and social media (Havard & Lefevre, 2020). Furthermore, other crucial proximal factors include alcohol and other substance abuse among the perpetrators of VAW (Abramsky et al., 2011; Cafferky, Mendez, Anderson, & Stith, 2018). Moreover, at the proximal level, friends, neighbourhood and community play essential roles in the genesis of VAW. A negative social environment characterised by social disorder and community violence and aspects of the physical environment such as access to alcohol and population density are contributing factors for VAW (Voith, 2019).

Individual Factors

Self-agency can be described as "the individual's perception that an action is the consequence of his/her own intention" (Nahab et al., 2011), the "voluntaristic theory of action," on "how apparently free actions lead individuals to (often) unconsciously reproduce their social-structural milieu" (Hitlin & Elder Jr, 2007). A poor support system, gender inequality, inadequate financial resources and structural disparity may limit survivors of VAW in their choices and attainment of empowerment and self-agency, leading to poor help-seeking, self-blaming and

MANAGEMENT OF VIOLENCE AGAINST WOMEN • 69

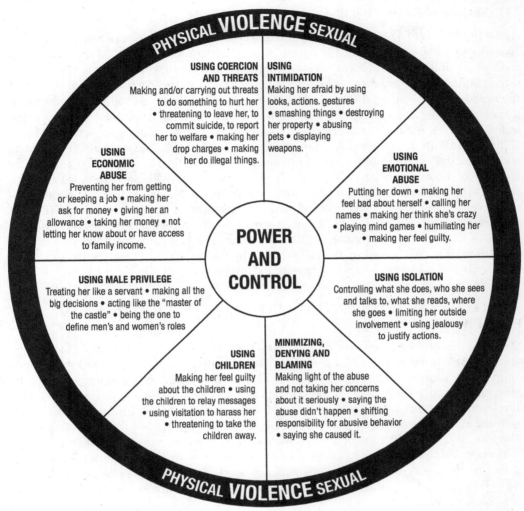

Figure 6.1 The wheel of power control.

Source: The Wheel of Power Control, Domestic Abuse Intervention Programs, Home of the Duluth Model; retrieved from www.theduluthmodel.org/wheels/

a failure to free oneself from the cycle of violence (Grose, Roof, Semenza, Leroux, & Yount, 2019; Mandal, Muralidharan, & Pappa, 2017; Razali, Fisher, & Kirkman, 2019). Moreover, according to the multination study by WHO, other possible contributing factors include young age, cohabitation, having experienced childhood abuse and growing up in a violent environment, while the attainment of secondary education, high socioeconomic status and formal marriage provide a certain protection (Abramsky et al., 2011; Cafferky et al., 2018; Graham-Kevan & Bates, 2020). For the perpetrator, critical predisposing factors are having outside sexual partners, as well as alcohol or substance abuse (Abramsky et al., 2011; Cafferky et al., 2018; Graham-Kevan & Bates, 2020). Additional traits of perpetrations include psychopathologies such as borderline and antisocial personality traits or disorders (Green & Browne, 2020) and mental illness such as adult ADHD manifesting with substance abuse, impulsivity and aggressive behaviour (Buitelaar, Posthumus, & Buitelaar, 2020).

CONSEQUENCES OF VIOLENCE AGAINST WOMEN

As for the genesis of VAW, the self-perpetuating consequences of violence result in a multi-layered impact to each level of the socioecological system. Certainly, VAW has direct and indirect encumbrances, such as the cost of materials and labour for the implementation of intervention and services such medical and mental healthcare, property damage and loss and the need for social and legal services. Included among these costs are reduced productivity, loss of wages and less tangible psychological costs arising from pain and suffering. At the individual level, physical consequences of VAW include physical injuries; permanent disability; and death due to homicide, infanticide and neonaticide. The psychological impacts include mental illness, poor quality of life, suicide, poor mother-baby bonding and attachment. VAW sometimes occurs along with filicide-suicide, infanticide and neonaticide (Razali et al., 2019; Razali et al., 2020a; Razali, Kirkman, & Fisher, 2020b). Among the sexual consequences are unintended pregnancies; sexually transmitted infections including HIV and miscarriages; and low birth weight babies, with epigenetic consequences. Given the diverse nature of VAW, which is often intercalated within the web of violence and polyvictimisation, those damaging effects are experienced not only by the survivors but also by their children and family and bring a risk of transgenerational propagation.

STRATEGIES AND INTERVENTION – INTEGRATED SOCIOECOLOGICAL FRAMEWORK

Many countries have ratified the Convention on the Elimination of All Forms of Discrimination against Women (CEDAW), the Beijing World Conference on Women and the Millennium Declaration of the September 2000 Millennium Summit, thus committing to make progress in gender equity and equality. In concert with efforts towards progress in gender development, a multi-layered socioecological framework has served as a foundation for management and interventions of VAW violence (CDC, 2020; Terry, 2014; World Health Organization, 2002). The planning and implementation of the interventions must be informed by the opinions and information arising from various levels in the ecological systems if the unmet needs of survivors, perpetrators and secondary victims such as children and family are to be addressed. These efforts also require top-down collaborative management of various stakeholders.

Distal-Level Intervention

Global and International Level

At the international level, the stakeholders include international organisations such as the United Nations agency, the WHO, the World Bank and regional development banks. The United Nations through its women's division functions to support inter-governmental bodies in formulating policies, preparing global standards and norms and assisting with suitable technical and financial support to encourage effective partnerships between various stakeholders and with civil society and to ensure regular monitoring (VAWNet, 2020). Also, the World Bank provides financial and technical assistance for poorly resourced countries. In terms of health, the Gender, Women and Health (GWH) of the WHO gathers data, develops norms and standards for mainstreaming gender equality in health policies and programmes, strengthens health capacity and engages in advocacy on gender inequality (VAWNet, 2020; WHO, 2021). Various initiatives have been and continue to be planned and implemented to address VAW effectively. Examples of such initiatives include the Spotlight Initiative and the UNiTE campaign of the United Nations (2020).

Sociocultural Transformation

The 1993 Vienna Human Rights Conference defined VAW as a violation of human rights which was rooted in unequal patriarchal relations. Hence, the sociocultural beliefs, values and norms that directly or indirectly condone VAW must be transformed. To achieve this goal, it is crucial to transform societal and community gender norms to eradicate subordination of women to men and to extirpate gender disparity and violent behaviours perpetrated against women and girls. Promoting gender equality does not mean elevating women to a higher level than men but rather entails simply giving equality of rights and opportunities. This allows women to progress hand in hand with men while embracing the acceptable sociocultural values and religious beliefs that place men and women at an equal level. Furthermore, stakeholders must be aware of the stigmatisation, victim-blaming attitudes and negative perceptions towards VAW survivors, which could hamper their emancipation in basic areas in life, such as education and health. Progress in these areas is needed to ensure that women (especially vulnerable and marginalised women) are safe from discrimination and oppression. To reduce VAW, every level of society must treat women with respect and dignity.

Structural Interventions

Gender inequities should be addressed at multiple socioecological levels aiming to eliminate VAW in key areas, to rectify inequitable gender norms in economic, education, health, legal and politics (Bourey, Williams, Bernstein, & Stephenson, 2015). For example, a practical strategy should include empowering women with instruments such as microfinance, economic self-reliance, financial literacy, job and skills training, attaining positions in managerial and decision-making posts and general participation in the labour force (Buvinić & O'Donnell, 2019; Hahn & Postmus, 2014). In terms of health, women and girls should be well informed about their rights regarding mental health, fertility, reproductive health and sexuality (Grose et al., 2019; Mandal et al., 2017; Najmabadi & Sharifi, 2019). Moreover, in terms of legislation, reform in policies and legislation in every aspect of the law, including torts, reproductive rights, criminal law, employment law, civil rights, international human rights and especially family law is crucial to ensure women's equality and freedom from VAW. Women and girls must be treated equally in terms of entitlement for full citizenship, social equality, work opportunity, economic independence and health status (Laing, 2017). Moreover, networking, community mobilisation, the creation of awareness and web-based dissemination of information and media coverage on the impact of violence on communities are key factors in mitigating against VAW (Dragiewicz et al., 2018; Johnson, 2019).

Service Enhancement

Lack of proper policies and guidelines, lack of or inaccessible facilities, poor collaboration among multidisciplinary teams and negative attitudes of service providers as well as secondary victimisation should be tackled immediately to enhance the services required to eradicate VAW. A collaborative approach is needed so that multiple stakeholders can work together synergistically work to develop a multi-stranded response. Stakeholders from diverse disciplines, which include government agencies, non-governmental organisations, private parties and volunteers, should collaborate to address any challenges and loopholes in providing effective management of programs directed against VAW. Examples of such a multidisciplinary approach are presented in Table 6.1.

In the era of information technology, web-based interventions may add to the traditional face-to-face interventions offered to VAW survivors (Anderson et al., 2019). In the future, the

Table 6.1 Multidisciplinary approaches to prevent violence against women.

Service Provider		Some Examples of the Scope of Services
Health services	Emergency Psychiatrist, psychologist, counsellor	• One-stop crisis centre • Early detection, treatment and care for mental illness (postpartum psychiatric disorders, major mental illness), substance abuse • Early detection, treatment and care for adolescents with behavioural problems, adolescent pregnancy, ex-nuptial pregnancy • Early detection, treatment and care for survivors of violence (domestic violence, sexual assault, rape, incest) • Treatment care for family and children of survivors of violence • Rehabilitation for offenders
	Obstetrician and gynaecologist	• Treatment and care for unintended and adolescent pregnancies • Services for sex and fertility management (contraception, abortion) • Care for victims of violence (domestic violence, sexual assault, rape, incest)
	Paediatrician	• Treatment and care for child abuse, neglect and abandonment • Treatment and care for adolescent pregnancy
	Primary carer	• Necessary treatment and care for the above
Education	Teacher, counsellor	• Comprehensive sexuality education promoting gender equality, sexuality and reproductive rights, mental health and implications of violence against women • School-based gender equality, reproductive and mental health promotion
Religious body	Counsellor, faith leader	• Comprehensive sexuality education integrating the cultural and spiritual approach
Social department	Counsellor, social worker	• Care for victims of violence (domestic violence, sexual assault, rape, incest) • Care for children, young people, women, and families at risk of violence, mental illness, substance abuse • Care for single mothers and their children

Service Provider		Some Examples of the Scope of Services
Other agencies, departments	Registration	• Non-discriminatory registration for immigrant, single mothers, other vulnerable women and their children
	Finance	• Financial support for families with children who are vulnerable and disadvantaged by poverty and dysfunction
	Enforcement	• Enforcement for perpetrators of violence against women (domestic violence, sexual assault, rape, incest) and children (abuse, neglect, abandonment, filicide)
	National Anti-Drug Agency	• Comprehensive care not only for drug abusers but also their families, who are at risk of violence, mental illness, and substance abuse
	Immigration	• Care for immigrant children, young people, women and families, including those experiencing violence
NGOs	Counsellor, activist	• Care for children, young people, women, families at risk of violence, mental illness, substance abuse
		• Shelters for unmarried mothers and their children
Private sector	Factories, hotels, and so on	• Promote organisational-level reproductive and mental health

use of blockchain-based solutions integrating multidisciplinary service providers and other stakeholders (such as social welfare departments, healthcare services, law and enforcement and non-governmental organisations) may be the way forward to prevent and manage VAW.

Proximal-Level Intervention

Children and Family

The web of violence and polyvictimisation that occurs in VAW requires service providers to be comprehensive in managing any particular case (Hamby & Grych, 2012; Hamby et al., 2018; Johnson, 2019; Le et al., 2018). The damage inflicted by intimate partner violence not merely targets the survivor (most often women) but also extends to their children, family and other significant others. Hence, addressing VAW should include planning and providing interventions for the survivors of VAW and also the people surrounding them. For example, early detection and intervention of child abuse in cases of IPV should be made a compulsory aspect of routine casework by primary healthcare and child welfare agencies (Turner et al., 2017). Equally important is the co-occurrence of elder abuse, which calls for a holistic approach in managing VAW (Ramsey-Klawsnik, 2017). Most often, an effective intervention calls for separation from the offenders from their victims, but in cases where separation is impossible, a "whole family intervention" based on family system therapy may be helpful (Stanley & Humphreys, 2017).

Perpetrators

Managing VAW at the proximal level is not complete without provisions for the prevention, early detection and rehabilitation of the perpetrator (Graham-Kevan & Bates, 2020; Karakurt, Koç, Çetinsaya, Ayluçtarhan, & Bolen, 2019). Intervention should not focus exclusively on educating the offenders but should include the targeting criminogenic factors such as managing alcohol or substance abuse; treating the perpetrators' emotional dysregulation and mental illness; and supporting them to overcome the underlying poverty, financial insecurity and unemployment (Graham-Kevan & Bates, 2020; Karakurt et al., 2019). The Duluth model is a foundation for instilling insight into the consequences of inequality in gender roles with respect to power and control (Pence & Paymar, 1993). Other essential psychological elements include focusing on therapy for offenders to bring them improved skills in communication, coping, impulse control and conflict resolution, as well as anger management, self-awareness, meditation and relaxation exercises, all aiming to change pro-violent/irrational thought patterns (Bates, Graham-Kevan, Bolam, & Thornton, 2017).

Individual-Level Interventions

Informed by previous research on VAW, we can state that promoting empowerment and improving literacy and knowledge about violence prevention, mental health and reproductive health and sexuality among women and girls are essential factors in preventing VAW (Buvinić & O'Donnell, 2019; Grose et al., 2019; Mandal et al., 2017). Furthermore, women and girls should be provided with counselling to enhance their basic psychological autonomy through acquiring problem-solving and assertiveness skills, learning help-seeking behaviours for self-efficacy and stress management. Possessing these skills may help women and girls at risk to deal with a violent environment and stress and increase their agency in preventing VAW (Brecklin & Ullman, 2005; Gotcă et al., 2019; Karmakar, Arora, & Franky). Helpful interventions for survivors will recognise their trauma and life experiences and instil in them an insight into the impacts of the cycle of violence and the wheel of power and control (Ferrari et al., 2018). Well-known consequences of VAW are post-traumatic disorders (PTSD), depression, anxiety, stress-related disease and substance abuse, and managing these mental illnesses is a priority (Dillon, Hussain, Loxton, & Rahman, 2013). While it is vital to provide medications and supportive therapy for anxiety, depression and PTSD, it is insufficient to focus solely on treating psychiatric consequences of VAW; there is no resolution without addressing the violent behaviours of the offender (Ferrari et al., 2018). Extra caution must be exercised in context when couple's and family therapy may place the victim at increased risk from further VAW. Furthermore, shelters or temporary housing interventions must be available to ensure the immediate safety and security of a survivor (Klein, Chesworth, Howland-Myers, Rizo, & Macy, 2019).

CONCLUSIONS

Addressing the complex issues necessary for the prevention of VAW and for effective responses to VAW calls for a multidisciplinary approach to achieve the programme's goals. In order to achieve long-term change, it is essential to adopt and implement comprehensive management in every level of the socioecological framework. The holistic management of VAW is thus a multilevel endeavour, calling for early detection, interventions and care at the individual level while also targeting proximal factors (spousal, family, workmate, neighbourhood) and distal factors (legal, economic, sociocultural, media and political). Taking into account the adjustment of measures to the current COVID-19 pandemic period conditions also seems very important worldwide. The goals of primary prevention not allowing VAW to occur in the first place – and secondary prevention in developing national plans and policies should be tailored to the national context, as strategies effective for high-income countries might not work in low-resource settings (WHO, 2017). As mental health professionals, it is crucial for the involved psychiatrist, psychologist or counsellor to be well informed about how VAW arises in the web of violence and the risk that survivors may suffer from polyvictimisation. Furthermore, VAW is often hidden and often masked by a diagnosis of mental illness. Hence, it is inadequate to consider only the phenomenology and psychopathology manifested by survivors with mental illness. Obtaining a holistic and in-depth history of social, family and marital factors and the survivor's relationships with significant others is crucial for effective case management of VAW.

References

Abramsky, T., Watts, C. H., Garcia-Moreno, C., Devries, K., Kiss, L., Ellsberg, M., . . . Heise, L. (2011). What factors are associated with recent intimate partner violence? Findings from the WHO multicountry study on women's health and domestic violence. *BMC Public Health*, *11*(1), 109.

Anderson, E. J., McClelland, J., Krause, C. M., Krause, K. C., Garcia, D. O., & Koss, M. P. (2019). Web-based and mHealth interventions for intimate partner violence prevention: A systematic review protocol. *BMJ Open*, *9*(8), e029880.

Backe, E. L., Lilleston, P., & McCleary-Sills, J. (2018). Networked individuals, gendered violence: A literature review of cyberviolence. *Violence and Gender*, *5*(3), 135–146.

Barner, J. R., & Carney, M. M. (2011). Interventions for intimate partner violence: A historical review. *Journal of Family Violence*, *26*(3), 235–244.

Bates, E. A., Graham-Kevan, N., Bolam, L. T., & Thornton, A. J. (2017). A review of domestic violence perpetrator programs in the United Kingdom. *Partner Abuse*, *8*(1), 3–46.

Bohall, G., Bautista, M.-J., & Musson, S. (2016). Intimate partner violence and the Duluth model: An examination of the model and recommendations for future research and practice. *Journal of Family Violence*, *31*(8), 1029–1033.

Bourey, C., Williams, W., Bernstein, E. E., & Stephenson, R. (2015). Systematic review of structural interventions for intimate partner violence in low-and middle-income countries: Organizing evidence for prevention. *BMC Public Health*, *15*(1), 1165.

Brecklin, L. R., & Ullman, S. E. (2005). Self-defence or assertiveness training and women's responses to sexual attacks. *Journal of Interpersonal Violence*, *20*(6), 738–762.

Bronfenbrenner, U. (1992). *Ecological systems theory*: Jessica Kingsley Publishers.

Bronson, J. (2021). Intimate partner violence, firearm violence, and human rights in the United States. In *Why we are losing the war on gun violence in the United States* (pp. 49–61): Springer.

Buitelaar, N. J., Posthumus, J. A., & Buitelaar, J. K. (2020). ADHD in childhood and/or adulthood as a risk factor for domestic violence or intimate partner violence: A systematic review. *Journal of Attention Disorders*, *24*(9), 1203–1214.

Buller, A. M., Peterman, A., Ranganathan, M., Bleile, A., Hidrobo, M., & Heise, L. (2018). A mixed-method review of cash transfers and intimate partner violence in low-and middle-income countries. *The World Bank Research Observer*, *33*(2), 218–258.

Buvinić, M., & O'Donnell, M. (2019). Gender matters in economic empowerment interventions: A research review. *The World Bank Research Observer*, *34*(2), 309–346.

Cafferky, B. M., Mendez, M., Anderson, J. R., & Stith, S. M. (2018). Substance use and intimate partner violence: A meta-analytic review. *Psychology of Violence*, *8*(1), 110.

Capezza, N. M., D'Intino, L. A., Flynn, M. A., & Arriaga, X. B. (2017). Perceptions of psychological abuse: The role of perpetrator gender, victim's response, and sexism. *Journal of Interpersonal Violence*, 0886260517741215.

CDC. (2020). *Centres for disease control and prevention; the social-ecological model: A framework for prevention*. Retrieved from www.cdc.gov/violenceprevention/publichealthissue/social-ecologicalmodel.html.

Chan, K. L., Chen, Q., & Chen, M. (2019). Prevalence and correlates of the co-occurrence of family violence: A meta-analysis on family polyvictimization. *Trauma, Violence, & Abuse*, 1524838019841601.

Colombini, M., Dockerty, C., & Mayhew, S. H. (2017). Barriers and facilitators to integrating health service responses to intimate partner violence in low-and middle-income countries: A comparative health systems and service analysis. *Studies in Family Planning, 48*(2), 179–200.

Dillon, G., Hussain, R., Loxton, D., & Rahman, S. (2013). Mental and physical health and intimate partner violence against women: A review of the literature. *International Journal of Family Medicine, 2013*.

Dragiewicz, M., Burgess, J., Matamoros-Fernández, A., Salter, M., Suzor, N. P., Woodlock, D., & Harris, B. (2018). Technology facilitated coercive control: Domestic violence and the competing roles of digital media platforms. *Feminist Media Studies, 18*(4), 609–625.

Ferrari, G., Feder, G., Agnew-Davies, R., Bailey, J. E., Hollinghurst, S., Howard, L., . . . Peters, T. J. (2018). Psychological advocacy towards healing (PATH): A randomized controlled trial of psychological intervention in a domestic violence service setting. *PloS One, 13*(11), e0205485.

Galtung, J. (1969). Violence, peace, and peace research. *Journal of Peace Research, 6*(3), 167–191.

Gangoli, G. (2020). Gender-based violence, law, justice and health: Some reflections. *Public Health Ethics, 13*(1), 29–33.

Gotcă, I., Ioan, B. G., Cărăușu, E. M., Dascălu, C. G., Anton-Păduraru, D. T., Antohe, I., & Mocanu, V. (2019). The effect of assertiveness training on the self-esteem, violence and stress response in adolescents. *Acta Medica Marisiensis, 65*.

Graham-Kevan, N., & Bates, E. A. (2020). Intimate partner violence perpetrator programmes: Ideology or evidence-based practice? In *The Wiley handbook of what works in violence risk management: Theory, research and practice* (pp. 437–449): John Wiley and Sons, UK.

Green, K., & Browne, K. (2020). Personality disorder traits, trauma, and risk in perpetrators of domestic violence. *International Journal of Offender Therapy and Comparative Criminology, 64*(2–3), 147–166.

Grose, R. G., Roof, K. A., Semenza, D. C., Leroux, X., & Yount, K. M. (2019). Mental health, empowerment, and violence against young women in lower-income countries: A review of reviews. *Aggression and Violent Behavior, 46*, 25–36.

Gul, P., & Schuster, I. (2020). Judgments of marital rape as a function of honor culture, masculine reputation threat, and observer gender: A cross-cultural comparison between Turkey, Germany, and the UK. *Aggressive Behavior, 46*(4), 341–353.

Hahn, S. A., & Postmus, J. L. (2014). Economic empowerment of impoverished IPV survivors: A review of best practice literature and implications for policy. *Trauma, Violence, & Abuse, 15*(2), 79–93.

Hamby, S., & Grych, J. (2012). *The web of violence: Exploring connections among different forms of interpersonal violence and abuse*: Springer.

Hamby, S., Taylor, E., Jones, L., Mitchell, K. J., Turner, H. A., & Newlin, C. (2018). From poly-victimization to poly-strengths: Understanding the web of violence can transform research on youth violence and illuminate the path to prevention and resilience. *Journal of Interpersonal Violence, 33*(5), 719–739.

Harris, K. L., McFarlane, M., & Wieskamp, V. (2020). The promise and peril of agency as motion: A feminist new materialist approach to sexual violence and sexual harassment. *Organization, 27*(5), 660–679.

Havard, T. E., & Lefevre, M. (2020). Beyond the power and control wheel: How abusive men manipulate mobile phone technologies to facilitate coercive control. *Journal of Gender-Based Violence, 4*(2), 223–239.

Heise, L. L. (1998). Violence against women: An integrated, ecological framework. *Violence Against Women, 4*(3), 262–290.

Hess, C., & Del Rosario, A. (2018). *Dreams deferred: A survey on the impact of intimate partner violence on survivors' education, careers, and economic security*: Institute for Women's Policy Research. Retrieved from https://iwpr. org/wpcontent/uploads/2020/09/C475_IWPRReportDreamsDeferred. Pdf

Hitlin, S., & Elder Jr, G. H. (2007). Time, self, and the curiously abstract concept of agency. *Sociological Theory, 25*(2), 170–191.

Ivert, A.-K., Merlo, J., & Gracia, E. (2018). Country of residence, gender equality and victim blaming attitudes about partner violence: a multilevel analysis in EU. *The European Journal of Public Health, 28*(3), 559–564.

Jennings, W. G., Powers, R. A., & Perez, N. M. (2021). A review of the effects of the violence against women act on law enforcement. *Violence Against Women, 27*(1), 69–83.

Johnson, E. (2019). Evaluation of web-based my voice, my choice for decreasing sexual violence victimization in college women. *Psychology*. Corpus ID: 201684925.

Karakurt, G., Koç, E., Çetinsaya, E. E., Ayluçtarhan, Z., & Bolen, S. (2019). Meta-analysis and systematic review for the treatment of perpetrators of intimate partner violence. *Neuroscience & Biobehavioral Reviews, 105*, 220–230.

Karmakar, N., Arora, S., & Franky, S. Effectiveness of assertiveness training programme on knowledge and attitude of adolescent girls regarding prevention of sexual abuse. *Journal of Nursing and Science Practice 2020, 10*(2), 57–61.

Klein, L., Chesworth, B. R., Howland-Myers, J. R., Rizo, C. F., & Macy, R. J. (2019). Housing interventions for intimate partner violence survivors: A systematic review. *Trauma, Violence, & Abuse*, 1524838019836284.

Krook, M. L. (2020). Violence against women in politics. In *How gender can transform the social sciences* (pp. 57–64): Springer.

Kruahiran, P., Boonyasiriwat, W., & Maneesri, K. (2020). Thai police officers' attitudes toward intimate partner violence and victim blaming: The influence of sexism and female gender roles. *Journal of Interpersonal Violence*, 0886260520969405.

Laing, L. (2017). Secondary victimization: Domestic violence survivors navigating the family law system. *Violence Against Women, 23*(11), 1314–1335.

Le, M. T., Holton, S., Romero, L., & Fisher, J. (2018). Polyvictimization among children and adolescents in low-and lower-middle-income countries: A systematic review and meta-analysis. *Trauma, Violence, & Abuse, 19*(3), 323–342.

Legal Information Institute (n.d.). *15 U.S. Code § 1691 – Scope of prohibition*. [Online]. LII/Legal Information Institute. Retrieved from www.law.cornell.edu/uscode/text/15/1691 [Accessed: 24 January 2021].

Mandal, M., Muralidharan, A., & Pappa, S. (2017). A review of measures of women's empowerment and related gender constructs in family planning and maternal health program evaluations in low-and middle-income countries. *BMC Pregnancy and Childbirth, 17*(2), 342.

Nahab, F. B., Kundu, P., Gallea, C., Kakareka, J., Pursley, R., Pohida, T., . . . Hallett, M. (2011). The neural processes underlying self-agency. *Cerebral Cortex, 21*(1), 48–55.

Najmabadi, K. M., & Sharifi, F. (2019). Sexual education and women empowerment in health: A review of the literature. *International Journal of Women's Health and Reproduction Sciences, 7*(2), 150–155.

Pence, E., & Paymar, M. (1993). *Education groups for men who batter*: Springer Pub. Co.

Peterson, J., & Densley, J. (2017). Cyber violence: What do we know and where do we go from here? *Aggression and Violent Behaviour, 34*, 193–200.

Postmus, J. L., Hoge, G. L., Breckenridge, J., Sharp-Jeffs, N., & Chung, D. (2020). Economic abuse as an invisible form of domestic violence: A multicountry review. *Trauma, Violence, & Abuse, 21*(2), 261–283.

Quenivet, N. (2020). Violence against women in armed conflict: An overview. In W. Nortje & N. Quenivet (Eds.), *Child soldiers and the defence of duress under international criminal law*: Palgrave Macmillan.

Ramsey-Klawsnik, H. (2017). Older adults affected by polyvictimization: A review of early research. *Journal of Elder Abuse & Neglect, 29*(5), 299–312.

Razali, S., Fisher, J., & Kirkman, M. (2019). "Nobody came to help": Interviews with women convicted of filicide in Malaysia. *Archives of Women's Mental Health, 22*(1), 151–158.

Razali, S., Kirkman, M., & Fisher, J. (2020a). *In Wong, Gina and George Parnham, JD; Infanticide and filicide: Foundations in maternal mental health forensics*: American Psychiatric Pub.

Razali, S., Kirkman, M., & Fisher, J. (2020b). Why women commit filicide: Opinions of health, social work, education and policy professionals in Malaysia. *Child Abuse Review, 29*(1), 73–84.

Renvoize, J. (1978). *Web of violence: A study of family violence*: Routledge & Kegan Paul.

Semahegn, A., Torpey, K., Manu, A., Assefa, N., Tesfaye, G., & Ankomah, A. (2019). Are interventions focused on gender-norms effective in preventing domestic violence against women in low and lower-middle-income countries? A systematic review and meta-analysis. *Reproductive Health, 16*(1), 93.

Sheehy, E. (2020). The right to say no: Marital rape and law reform in Canada, Ghana, Kenya and Malawi ed. by Melanie Randall, Jennifer Koshan, and Patricia Nyaundi. *Canadian Journal of Women and the Law, 32*(1), 231–236.

Stake, S., Ahmed, S., Tol, W., Ahmed, S., et al. (2020) Prevalence, associated factors, and disclosure of intimate partner violence among mothers in rural Bangladesh. *Journal of Health, Population and Nutrition*, [Online] 39(1). doi:10.1186/s41043-020-00223-w [Accessed: 24 January 2021].

Stanley, N., & Humphreys, C. (2017). Identifying the key components of a whole family intervention for families experiencing domestic violence and abuse. *Journal of Gender-Based Violence, 1*(1), 99–115.

Terry, M. S. (2014). Applying the social-ecological model to violence against women with disabilities. *Journal of Women's Health Care, 3*(6), 193. doi:10.4172/2167-0420.1000193

Thibaut, F., & van Wijngaarden-Cremers, P. J. M. (2020) Women's mental health in the time of Covid-19 pandemic. *Front. Glob. Women's Health, 1,* 588372. doi:10.3389/fgwh.2020.588372

Turner, W., Hester, M., Broad, J., Szilassy, E., Feder, G., Drinkwater, J., . . . Stanley, N. (2017). Interventions to improve the response of professionals to children exposed to domestic violence and abuse: A systematic review. *Child Abuse Review, 26*(1), 19–39.

United Nations. (2020). *Spotlight initiative.* Retrieved from www.spotlightinitiative.org/.

VAWNet. (2020). *Websites on international initiatives to end violence against women.* Retrieved from https://vawnet.org/sc/websites-international-initiatives-end-violence-against-women.

Voith, L. A. (2019). Understanding the relation between neighborhoods and intimate partner violence: An integrative review. *Trauma, Violence, & Abuse, 20*(3), 385–397.

Walklate, S., Fitz-Gibbon, K., & McCulloch, J. (2018). Is more law the answer? Seeking justice for victims of intimate partner violence through the reform of legal categories. *Criminology & Criminal Justice, 18*(1), 115–131.

WHO. (2021). *World health organization, gender, equity and human rights.* Retrieved from www.who.int/teams/gender-equity-and-human-rights/about.

Willie, T. C., & Kershaw, T. S. (2019). An ecological analysis of gender inequality and intimate partner violence in the United States. *Preventive Medicine, 118,* 257–263.

World Health Organization. (2002). *World report on violence and health.* 1–360.

World Health Organization. (2010). *Preventing intimate partner and sexual violence against women; taking actions and generating evidence.* Retrieved from www.who.int/violence_injury_prevention/publications/violence/9789241564007_eng.pdf.

World Health Organization (2017) *Violence against women.* [Online]. Who.int. Retrieved from www.who.int/news-room/fact-sheets/detail/violence-against-women [Accessed: 21 January 2021].

7

Mental Health Access to the Unreached Using Mobile Mental Health

Prakash B. Behere, Swaroopa Lunge Patil, Debolina Chowdhury, Aniruddh P. Behere and Richa Yadav

Introduction	79
Role of Primary Health Care	79
Mental Health Policies, Plans and Laws	80
Role of Mobile Phones in Mental Health	80
Awareness Regarding Mental Health Problems	81

INTRODUCTION

The problems of availability and accessibility of mental health services faced in rural areas are high, and the impact of mental health disorders in these areas is great. Furthermore, the acceptance of these services by the rural population acts as a barrier to the full utilization of the available services[1]. Various factors contribute to this, such as transportation difficulties to use these services, shortage of mental health professionals in these areas[2], stigma regarding mental health due to strongly held traditional beliefs and the lack of understanding of mental illnesses in general[3].

According to the 2011 Census of the total population of India, 68.84% of the Indian population is rural. This includes mostly people with lower income, poor education and limited employment. According to data from the National Mental Health Survey completed in 2016, mental health disorders are high in such households[4]. This can be attributed to their blind faith in supernatural beliefs, which results in a negative attitude towards mental health[5]. A longer time to seek the appropriate treatment is seen because faith healers are the primary help sought rather than medical help[6].

Ironically, even the urban population of India does not adequately make use of mental health services. The reasons for this may be low perceived need for treatment more due to attitudinal barriers rather than structural barriers,[7] which further causes the rate of treatment dropout to be higher in severe mental illness[8].

ROLE OF PRIMARY HEALTH CARE

Primary healthcare is essentially healthcare made universally accessible to individuals and families by means acceptable to them, through their full participation and at a cost that the communities and country can afford, thus making it the mainstay of country's health system and a major contributor to the social and economic development of the country[9]. It should focus on brief psychotherapeutic interventions and community-based rehabilitation

DOI: 10.4324/9780429030260-9

programs for people with disability due to chronic mental health disorders and implement more mental health policies[10].

Integrating mental healthcare with primary healthcare will ensure that people have easy access to these services with assurance that these services are rendered to people at affordable prices and in a way acceptable to them. Primary healthcare services ensure continuity of care rather than mere consultation and poor drug adherence, thus taking care of the main barriers of mental health services[11]. On this basis, many mental health disorders can be managed effectively. Depression can be substantially managed with low-cost anti-depressants and psychological interventions. Anti-psychotics may be made available at cost-effective basis suited for populations of all types. Psychopharmacological management of patients with alcohol dependence has already successfully been executed[12].

Primary care physicians (PCPs) can play an important role in this. There has been an increasing trend of patients being prescribed psychiatric medications by PCPs[13]. Such trends thus indicate that these PCPs play the role of primary psychiatric care physicians (PPCPs) to many patients. In addition, safer psychotropic medications with fewer side effects can put the PCPs at ease prescribing them. The tendency of society with regard to psychiatric disorders has been changing, and society is now visualizing these disorders as medical problems which need medical attention. This has expanded the role of primary healthcare to providing additional psychiatric care. With the advent of electronic media, with an important role of advertising media in this, people have greater access to knowledge about psychiatric disorders, leading to the development of a positive attitude for seeking medical help for psychiatric disorders. This in turn motivates physicians in a positive way for providing relief of psychiatric ailments to patients[14].

MENTAL HEALTH POLICIES, PLANS AND LAWS

By enforcing proper mental health laws and keeping legislative watch over the implementation of these laws, the integration of mental healthcare with primary healthcare can be reinforced[15]. A commitment at higher level of authority and proper policy drafting by our government can make this successful.

More primary health workers should be armed with proper skill training to identify mental health disorders in the population, to provide primary aid to them, to give the required referral to specific mental health centres when required and to create awareness among people by giving them psychoeducation about various mental health disorders and the role of family members towards such patients[16]. To support this, a strong referral system should exist between primary and secondary healthcare centres, and the availability of trained mental health specialists at secondary healthcare centres is essential[17].

Regarding policy, strong primary healthcare delivery can be potentiated through mental health policies ant the integration of mental health into the primary healthcare system. These mental health policies can form an outline of specific objectives that can lead to integrating of mental health, whereas the specific strategies and activities required to do so can be done by implementing mental health plans[11].

ROLE OF MOBILE PHONES IN MENTAL HEALTH

Besides making calls, mobile phones can be used as a treatment aid in mental health problems, as consultations and primary counselling can be done through mobile phones. Over a period of time, these electronic gadgets are found among all strata of society, and thus a wider population can be covered in this way. In a study conducted by Sood et al., it was found that most psychiatry patients have a positive attitude toward using a mobile phone as an aid in treatment[18]. The findings in a study by Ainsworth et al. were that mobile phones can be used effectively in assessment of patients with schizophrenia[19]. Primary healthcare workers can also be trained in optimizing the use of these devices and thus play an important role in rendering mental health services to the population. Telepsychiatry using these electronic gadgets can work as a link between primary and secondary healthcare centres.

Mobile phone technologies should be integrated with clinic-based services to bridge the gap between services and users. This will help to provide psychosocial interventions to the population in need. Easy-to-use and affordable mobile technologies can be used in increasing awareness about mental illnesses in the population. Caregiver groups can be formed on social networking sites to increase awareness among them in a simpler, convenient way[20]. Mobile phones can also be used to conduct surveys regarding mental health disorders, as done in a study in Kashmir to collect data on the prevalence of depression, anxiety and post-traumatic stress disorder[21]. Additionally, there exists a scarcity of mental health professionals in military services; hence, telepsychiatry can be a useful tool in aiding mental health problems in the defence sector of our country[22].

A study done by Fortney et al. showed that off-site telepsychiatry collaborative care was more cost effective than on-site practice-based collaborative care interventions. Such telepsychiatry collaborative care can have fruitful outcomes in rural areas[23].

Telepsychiatry has potential and is a great solution for the problem of people being under-diagnosed with mental illness and the scarcity of trained health professionals at the root levels of a healthcare setting[24]. With the proper implementation of telepsychiatry at affordable prices and the wider availability of increasingly secure technologies, this mode of service can be useful for both patients and mental health professionals[25].

AWARENESS REGARDING MENTAL HEALTH PROBLEMS

The main barrier to help seeking in people with mental health problems is the stigma regarding them. Other barriers in improvement of mental health services are the lack of availability of health professionals trained in mental healthcare and prevailing public health priorities and their influence on the funding of these services, thus making it challenging to cater to mental healthcare needs in a primary health setup[26].

Large-scale mental health awareness programs can be undertaken for the masses. These awareness programs can result in a positive attitude of people about psychiatric disorders and thus can bring about a favourable change in their views about mental illness[27]. Anti-stigma campaigns should be undertaken to increase awareness among people and develop a positive attitude in them regarding mental healthcare. This is supported by findings of study conducted by Henderson et al. in which conducting an anti-stigma awareness program increased comfort among people in coming forward with their mental health problems and also positively influenced their treatment-seeking behaviour[28]. Plans and policies should be implemented for the enforcement of such awareness programs on a large scale for the public.

Thus, by integrating primary healthcare with mental healthcare supplemented by mental health policies and laws, access to the unreached in the community can be achieved with the help of mental health awareness programs and technology. This can change the scenario of mental health disorders in a positive way.

References

1. Human J, Wasem C. Rural mental health in America. *Am Psychol*. 1991;46(3):232–239.
2. Bird DC, Dempsey P, Hartley D. *Addressing mental health workforce needs in underserved rural areas: Accomplishments and challenges*. Muskie School; 2001.

3. Letvak S. The importance of social support for rural mental health. *Issues Ment Health Nurs*. 2002 May;23(3):249–261.
4. Murthy RS. National mental health survey of India 2015–2016. *Indian J Psychiatry*. 2017;59(1):21–26.
5. Kermode M, Bowen K, Arole S, Pathare S, Jorm AF. Attitudes to people with mental disorders: A mental health literacy survey in a rural area of Maharashtra, India. *Soc Psychiatry Psychiatr Epidemiol*. 2009 Dec;44(12):1087–1096.
6. Lahariya C, Singhal S, Gupta S, Mishra A. Pathway of care among psychiatric patients attending a mental health institution in central India. *Indian J Psychiatry*. 2010 Oct 1;52(4):333.
7. Sareen J, Jagdeo A, Cox BJ, Clara I, ten Have M, Belik S-L, et al. Perceived barriers to mental health service utilization in the United States, Ontario, and the Netherlands. *Psychiatr Serv Wash DC*. 2007 Mar;58(3):357–364.
8. Drapalski AL, Milford J, Goldberg RW, Brown CH, Dixon LB. Perceived barriers to medical care and mental health care among veterans with serious mental illness. *Psychiatr Serv Wash DC*. 2008 Aug;59(8):921–924.
9. Primary health care: International conference on primary health care, Alma-Ata, USSR, 6–12 September 1978. *Nurs J India*. 1979 Nov;70(11):285–295.
10. Ventevogel P. Integration of mental health into primary healthcare in low-income countries: Avoiding medicalization. *Int Rev Psychiatry Abingdon Engl*. 2014 Dec;26(6):669–679.
11. Funk M, Saraceno B, Drew N, Faydi E. Integrating mental health into primary healthcare. *Ment Health Fam Med*. 2008 Mar;5(1):5–8.
12. Patel V, Araya R, Chatterjee S, Chisholm D, Cohen A, Silva MD, et al. Treatment and prevention of mental disorders in low-income and middle-income countries. *The Lancet*. 2007 Sep 15;370(9591):991–1005.
13. Olfson M, Marcus SC, Druss B, Elinson L, Tanielian T, Pincus HA. National trends in the outpatient treatment of depression. *JAMA*. 2002 Jan 9;287(2):203–209.
14. Abed Faghri NM, Boisvert CM, Faghri S. Understanding the expanding role of primary care physicians (PCPs) to primary psychiatric care physicians (PPCPs): Enhancing the assessment and treatment of psychiatric conditions. *Ment Health Fam Med*. 2010 Mar;7(1):17–25.
15. Funk M, Drew N, Saraceno B, De Almeida J, Agossou T, Wang X, et al. A framework for mental health policy, legislation and service development: Addressing needs and improving services. *Harv Health Policy Rev*. 2005a;6:57–69.
16. Bhalla P, editor. *Human resources and training in mental health*. Geneva: World Health Organization; 2005. 123 p. (Mental health policy and service guidance package).
17. Funk M, Saraceno B, Pathare S, World Health Organization, editors. *Organization of services for mental health*. Geneva: World Health Organization; 2003. 74 p. (Mental health policy and service guidance package).
18. Sood M, Chadda RK, Deb KS, Bhad R, Mahapatra A, Verma R, et al. Scope of mobile phones in mental health care in low resource settings. *J Mob Technol Med*. 2016 Jul 31;5(2):33–37.
19. Ainsworth J, Palmier-Claus JE, Machin M, Barrowclough C, Dunn G, Rogers A, et al. A comparison of two delivery modalities of a mobile phone-based assessment for serious mental illness: Native smartphone application vs text-messaging only implementations. *J Med Internet Res*. 2013 Apr 5;15(4):e60.
20. Sood M, Chadda RK, Singh P. Mobile health (mHealth) in mental health: Scope and applications in low-resource settings. *Nat Medi J India*. 2016;29(6):3.
21. Papadimitriou N, Housen T, Ara S. Use of mobile technologies in data collection for a mental health survey in Kashmir, India: A pilot study. *Meĩdecins Sans FrontieÃres*. 2015.
22. Grady BJ. A comparative cost analysis of an integrated military telemental health-care service. *Telemed J E-Health Off J Am Telemed Assoc*. 2002;8(3):293–300.
23. Pyne JM, Fortney JC, Mouden S, Lu L, Hudson TJ, Mittal D. Cost-effectiveness of on-site versus off-site collaborative care for depression in rural FQHCs. *Psychiatr Serv Wash DC*. 2015 May 1;66(5):491–499.
24. Malhotra S, Chakrabarti S, Shah R. Telepsychiatry: Promise, potential, and challenges. *Indian J Psychiatry*. 2013 Jan;55(1):3–11.
25. Behere PB, Mansharamani HD, Kumar K. Telepsychiatry: Reaching the unreached. *Indian J Med Res*. 2017 Feb 1;146(2):150.
26. Saraceno B, van Ommeren M, Batniji R, Cohen A, Gureje O, Mahoney J, et al. Barriers to improvement of mental health services in low-income and middle-income countries. *Lancet Lond Engl*. 2007 Sep 1;370(9593):1164–1174.

27. Pinfold V, Stuart H, Thornicroft G, Arboleda J. Working with young people: The impact of mental health awareness programmes in schools in the UK and Canada. *World Psychiatry*. 2005;4(supplement):48–52.
28. Henderson C, Robinson E, Evans-Lacko S, Thornicroft G. Relationships between anti-stigma programme awareness, disclosure comfort and intended help-seeking regarding a mental health problem. *Br J Psychiatry J Ment Sci*. 2017 Nov;211(5):316–322.

8
Optimising Patient Care When Working With Children of Patients With Mental Illness

Sandeep Grover and Abhishek Ghosh

Introduction	84
Risks and Resilience of Children of Parents With Mental Illness	84
Effect of Maternal Depression on Children	86
Outcomes and Their Predictors in Children of Parents With Mental Illness	86
Intervention Programs for Children of Parents With Mental Illness COPMI	86
Interventions for Parents With Mental Illness	87
Interventions for Children	87
Interventions for Professionals	88
Intervention for the Community	88
A Combined and Integrated Intervention Program	88
Conclusion	88

INTRODUCTION

The advent and growth of de-institutionalisation and community-based care have resulted in greater exposure of children to parental mental illness. Although the change was much anticipated, the challenges associated with this change were not anticipated. Surveys from across the globe have shown 6–30% of patients with mental illness have identified themselves as parents (Parker et al., 2008; Howe et al., 2009). Standard psychiatric care so far has concentrated on patients, and little attention is given to their young offspring. This is despite the fact that there has been increased vulnerability to emotional and behavioural problems in the offspring because of the adverse genetic, familial, and broader social-environmental influences. A few countries have already initiated prevention programs directed to the children of parents with mental illness (COPMI) at a national level (Doesum & Hosman, 2009; Solantaus & Toikka, 2006).

RISKS AND RESILIENCE OF CHILDREN OF PARENTS WITH MENTAL ILLNESS

There are five identified risk factors for COPMI: the genetic transmission of risk, risk due to prenatal adverse influences, maladaptive parent-child interactions, stressful family environment, and social influences from outside the family (Doesum & Hosman, 2009). The dynamic cycle of familial mental illness, based on the model of stress vulnerability, succinctly describes the interactions between parental mental illness, the family's and society's reaction, and the effect on the offspring (Murphy et al., 2014). The dynamic cycle posits that the diagnosis of mental illness brings about a changing self-concept and reduces the self-worth of parents with mental illness. These changes in the self might occur as a result of the social construction of mental illness and the social stigma (Murphy et al., 2014). Children suffer from emotional distress because of their strained relationship with the parents, worry and uncertainty during the time of parental hospitalisation, and limited understanding of mental illness. The parents might be physically available but emotionally distant. Studies have described unrecognised and protracted grief among COPMI (Mordoch & Hall, 2002). The episodic nature of various mental illnesses exacerbates these grief reactions. Children also feel the courtesy stigma, typically described as fear of being contaminated by parental illness (Corrigan & Miller, 2004). The child's reaction determines the next course of the family dynamic cycle. The child might react with emotional distancing and further withdrawal from their parents, which could result in parental disenfranchisement. This would add to parental distress and trigger mental illness because of "stress vulnerability" (Murphy et al., 2014). However, studies have also focused on the positive coping and resilience of children with parents with mental illness. With support from others in the family and information about mental illness, the child might use problem-solving coping to deal with parental mental illness and the associated emotional distress (Polkki et al., 2004). Positive coping might terminate the dynamic family cycle. Figure 8.1 illustrates the risk-resilience model for COPMI.

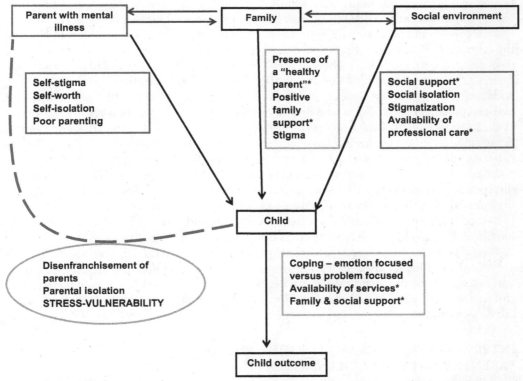

Figure 8.1 Illustrating the risk and protective factors* for children of parents with mental illness and the interactions between these factors to determine the mental health outcome of COPMI.

EFFECT OF MATERNAL DEPRESSION ON CHILDREN

Given the magnitude of disability resulting from major depressive illness and the common occurrence of depression in the peri-natal period, the effect of maternal depression on children require special discussion.

To begin with, maternal depression affects the mother-infant interaction by either excessive intrusiveness or withdrawal. Intrusive mothers manifest hostile affect, whereas withdrawn mothers are disengaged. Impaired interaction results in poor attachment between the infant and mother.

Maternal depression affects the children throughout their life course.

In addition to the immediate effect, maternal depression has been shown to have long-term effects. In a longitudinal study from the United States, more than 150 offspring of depressed mothers were followed up for 20 years. Maternal depression was shown to increase the odds of anxiety disorders, major depression, and substance dependence by nearly three times. Social impairment was also greater in those offspring with maternal depression. The risk of medical disorders and mortality showed an emerging trend (Weismann et al., 2006). The findings are not very different from low- and middle-income countries. A large birth-cohort study with 10-year follow-up from South Africa showed that the children whose mothers had postnatal depression were more likely to have psychological difficulties at the age of 10 years (Verkuijl et al., 2014).

OUTCOMES AND THEIR PREDICTORS IN CHILDREN OF PARENTS WITH MENTAL ILLNESS

Parental mental illness affects children in more than one way. COPMI were observed to lag behind in academics, communication, and social functioning compared to their counterparts with "normal" parents. COPMI were more likely to take up age-inappropriate roles to take care of their parents and other siblings, resulting in conflicts with appropriate activities and attending schools. A wide range of parental mental illness, from psychosis to depression to eating disorders, has been found to be associated with an equally wide spectra of mental illness in children. COPMI are vulnerable to both externalising (conduct, oppositional defiant disorders) and internalising disorders (anxiety, depressive disorder) (Reupert et al., 2012). The association between parental mental illness, and disorder in the children is largely non-specific (Keshavan et al., 2008; Weissman et al., 2006). A comparison between the effect of maternal and paternal depression has shown the former has a greater effect on emotional problems, but the effect on behavioural problems of the children is equivalent (Ramchandani & Psychogiou, 2009).

In addition to an increased vulnerability to psychiatric disorders, COPMI are also predisposed to several maladaptive traits and cognitive styles. Children of mothers with eating disorders showed higher restraint, shape concern, and weight concern (Stein et al., 2006). Increased impulsivity, difficulty in affect modulation, and internalised negative self-image have been seen in children whose mothers have borderline personality disorders.

Overall, the diagnosis, severity, chronicity, and current psychopathology of the parents are found to influence their parenting competencies and therefore the effect on children. Parents' age, academic qualifications, and economic status are said to mediate the effect on children. Nevertheless, maternal mental health seems to exert an independent effect (Mensah & Kieman, 2010).

INTERVENTION PROGRAMS FOR CHILDREN OF PARENTS WITH MENTAL ILLNESS COPMI

Programs intended to address the needs of COPMI have been established in the United States, United Kingdom, Australia, Netherlands, and other Scandinavian countries (Fraser et al., 2006; Solantaus et al., 2012). Such programs are aimed at improving mental health outcome of children, enhancing quality of family life, and reducing the expensive psychiatric treatment needs of parents. However, finding the most effective means is often challenging because of the presence of the multitude of potential risk factors and the wide range of adverse outcomes. The interventions programs are typically directed to parents with mental illness, children of parents with mental illness, professionals, and the community. There are several critical reviews of program effectiveness (Fraser et al., 2006; Schrank et al., 2015; Doesum & Hosman, 2009).

Interventions for Parents With Mental Illness

In their systematic review Schrank and colleagues (2015) identified 14 articles on the nature and effectiveness of parent-based interventions. Four types of service delivery models could be observed: home-based, a component of a complex community-based program, routine inpatient-based, and online interventions. The services were largely psycho-education oriented and provided by peer educators or treatment providers. The common components of psycho-education were parenting skills (especially to deal with behavioural problems in the children and to improve the quality of parent-child interaction) and on the impact of mental illness of parents on their children. Web-based programs are largely supplemented by face-to-face meetings (Doesum & Hosman, 2009). Practical and social support was only covered in the inpatient-based and complex community-based programs. The evidence of effectiveness of these interventions was mixed. Nevertheless, preliminary evidence suggested positive outcomes in terms of improvement in self-rated parenting skills and parent-rated child outcome measures (Schrank et al., 2015).

Among other special interventions not discussed in the review by Schrank and colleagues (2015), Knowledge of positive parenting (KOPP) mother-baby intervention is worth a mention. It is an early intervention meant to improve the quality of interaction between mother and baby and help the growth of a secure attachment. Mother and infant together during their interaction are videotaped in the natural environment and feedback based on this is provided by a trained home visitor. The standard number of sessions is 8–10. In a randomised clinical trial, significant improvement was seen in the quality of interaction of the mother-infant dyad. Infants in the intervention group had greater attachment security and higher emotional competence.

KOOP mother-baby intervention is resource intensive and applicable only to infants. A less resource-intensive program, which can be applied to a wide age range, is the "let's talk about children" discussion. The aim of this treatment is to support parents to identify their children's strengths and difficulties, to inform parents of ways to help their children with mental health problems, and to guide to additional mental health services (if required). The efficacy of the intervention is yet to be established in a controlled trial.

Interventions for Children

Intervention in COPMI depends on the age of the children. Nevertheless, the common goals are providing practical support and scientific information to enhance competencies to reduce emotional distress and burden (Doesum & Hosman, 2009). The interventions are largely group based, although online interventions have also been tried. The web-based programs are psycho-educative in nature, whereas the group-based programs aim at skill building, learning problem solving, drawing support from others and the treatment providers, and also dissemination of information on parents' disorders. Open educational meetings for information dissemination and providing tips to tackle daily life stress in the family are mainly targeted to adolescents and young adults (Doesum & Hosman, 2009). Local activity days for children (8–16 years) is a program in Netherlands, which runs during the school holidays with active co-operation from mental health centres and addiction clinics (Doesum & Hosman, 2009).

Interventions for Professionals

All professional staff expected to deal with patients with mental illness are trained to raise awareness of the risk to children, talk to children and their families, detect problems in an early stage, and offer help whenever required. This is done either by an educational approach through periodic workshops, lectures, and conferences or by ensuring integrated care of children and parents with mental illness across the mental healthcare facilities. A specific program developed for professionals is the basic care management (BCM) program. This is a theory-driven program focusing on support for children yet to show any specific signs of mental illness in a patient's family. The intervention includes three elements: 1) the structured screening and monitoring of risk and protective factors and parenting skills and the assessment of early signs of child behavioural problems; 2) tailored to the risk and protective factors identified, organising and coordinating supportive services for these families; and 3) evaluation of the implementation of the services. Parenting skill improvement with the BCM was established in a randomised controlled trial from the Netherlands, but the intervention was costlier than control (Wansink et al., 2016).

Intervention for the Community

The interventions focused on the community aim to address public stigma and discrimination, break through the social isolation of the family with mental illness, and improve social and community support for the family (and children) with mental illness. Routine and periodic activities are done either in the community or in schools. Families with mental illness and volunteer workers from the community and mental health service establishments come together for this kind of intervention program. Intervention for the context and community has not been studied in a clinical trial.

A Combined and Integrated Intervention Program

Preventive family intervention (PFI), originating in the United States is a family-based service integrated with all levels of care, primary, mental health, and substance abuse services. This service is said to be manualised, user-friendly, flexible, and easily adaptable. PFI has been shown to be effective in clinical trials to improve communication and understanding of parental mental illness in the family (Fraser et al., 2006).

Figure 8.2 illustrates and summarises the domains and types of intervention for COPMI.

There are several barriers in implementation of the aforementioned intervention programs even in relatively resource-rich countries. Future challenges are using the already strained resources for those who are in real need of care – a stepped care approach. This would require development and validation of structured screening tools for cost-effective risk assessment. To ensure continuity of care, long-term cooperation is required between the youth and adult care services.

CONCLUSION

Children of parents with mental illness are inherently a high-risk population, not only because of genetic factors but also because of several family-environmental-social factors. COMPI are at higher risk for both mental illnesses and other non-specific emotional and behavioural

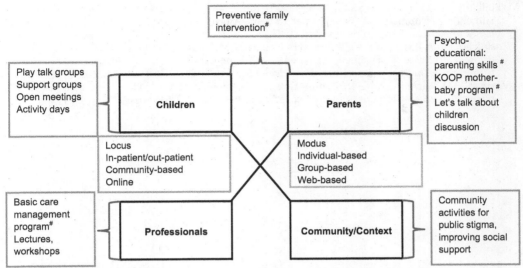

Figure 8.2 Illustrating the interventions for children of parents with mental illness.
suggests intervention with evidence of efficacy from at least one randomised controlled trial

problems. Early screening and identification of such problems is one of the key measures for COPMI. Interventions for COPMI are directed to the parents, the children, the professionals, and the context/community. Most research has been done on parental interventions. However, the evidence is also emerging for interventions for children and professionals.

References

Corrigan PW, Miller FE. Shame, blame, and contamination: A review of the impact of mental illness stigma on family members. *Journal of Mental Health*. 2004;13(6):537–548.
Fraser C, James EL, Anderson K, Lloyd D, Judd F. Intervention programs for children of parents with a mental illness: A critical review. *International Journal of Mental Health Promotion*. 2006;8(1):9–20.
Howe D, Batchelor S, Bochynska K. Estimating consumer parenthood within mental health services: A census approach. *Australian e-Journal for the Advancement of Mental Health*. 2009;8(3):231–241.
Keshavan M, Montrose DM, Rajarethinam R, Diwadkar V, Prasad K, Sweeney JA. Psychopathology among offspring of parents with schizophrenia: Relationship to premorbid impairments. *Schizophrenia Research*. 2008;103(1–3):114–120.
Mordoch E, Hall WA. Children living with a parent who has a mental illness: A critical analysis of the literature and research implications. *Archives of Psychiatric Nursing*. 2002;16(5):208–216.
Murphy G, Peters K, Wilkes L, Jackson D. A dynamic cycle of familial mental illness. *Issues in Mental Health Nursing*. 2014;35(12):948–953.
Parker G, Beresford B, Clarke S, Gridley K, Pitman R, Spiers G, Light K. *Research reviews on prevalence, detection and interventions in parental mental health and child welfare: Summary report*. York: Social Policy Research Unit, University of York. 2008.
Ramchandani P, Psychogiou L. Paternal psychiatric disorders and children's psychosocial development. *The Lancet*. 2009;374(9690):646–653.
Schrank B, Moran K, Borghi C, Priebe S. How to support patients with severe mental illness in their parenting role with children aged over 1 year? A systematic review of interventions. *Social Psychiatry and Psychiatric Epidemiology*. 2015;50(12):1765–1783.
Solantaus T, Toikka S. The effective family programme: Preventative services for the children of mentally ill parents in Finland. *International Journal of Mental Health Promotion*. 2006;8(3):37–44.
Stein A, Woolley H, Cooper S, Winterbottom J, Fairburn CG, Cortina-Borja M. Eating habits and attitudes among 10-year-old children of mothers with eating disorders: Longitudinal study. *The British Journal of Psychiatry*. 2006;189(4):324–329.

Verkuijl NE, Richter L, Norris SA, Stein A, Avan B, Ramchandani PG. Postnatal depressive symptoms and child psychological development at 10 years: A prospective study of longitudinal data from the South African birth to twenty cohort. *The Lancet Psychiatry*. 2014;1(6):454–460.

Wansink HJ, Drost RM, Paulus AT, Ruwaard D, Hosman CM, Janssens JM, Evers SM. Cost-effectiveness of preventive case management for parents with a mental illness: A randomized controlled trial from three economic perspectives. *BMC Health Services Research*. 2016;16(1):228.

Weissman MM, Wickramaratne P, Nomura Y, Warner V, Pilowsky D, Verdeli H. Offspring of depressed parents: 20 years later. *American Journal of Psychiatry*. 2006;163(6):1001–1008.

9
Forensic Risk Assessment and Management of Community Case Managed Clients

Aniket Bansod and Akshata Mulmule

Case Management and Risks	91
Prevalence of Mental Illnesses and Associated Risks	92
Forensic Patients	92
Risk Prediction vs Prevention	93
Risk Assessments	93
First Generation or Unstructured Clinical Judgement	93
Second Generation: Actuarial Methods	93
Structured Professional Judgement	94
Three-Tiered Risk Framework Used in Queensland, Australia	95
Special Mention: Firearms	96
Newer Developments	96
Management of Risks	96
Duty to Disclose	97
Developing a Safety Culture	97
Implications of Better Risk Management	97

CASE MANAGEMENT AND RISKS

Mental illnesses, particularly severe mental illnesses, have a long history of management in institutions. However, with deinstitutionalisation that happened in the 1960s and 1970s, most of these patients with major mental illnesses are now being managed in the community. Case management is one of the most popular types of aftercare provided to patients post-discharge from hospitals. There are several models of management that have had variable success in achieving the goals set, like preventing repeated hospitalisations and managing the risks in the community. Of these models, standard case management, assertive community treatment (ACT) and intensive case management (ICM) are popular models. These models consist of management of the mental illness and provision of rehabilitation and social support needs of the patients for an indefinite period by multidisciplinary teams, with each member carrying varying case loads. (Dieterich et al., 2017). Many services have capacity to operate all these models of care within their service for clients with differing needs. ICM, though the most effective, is however the most resource-intensive model, while standard management, on the other hand, has pitfalls but serves the purpose when client needs are not too complex. In any of these models, however, the role of the case manager is undertaking assessments; monitoring mental state and risks; planning care; advocacy; and linking the consumer with disability, rehabilitation and support services, including NGOs. (Intagliata, 1982). Risk assessment and management forms an integral part of a case manager's role when they are dealing with these clients. Moreover, most community management teams have to manage involuntary patients and patients with forensic history and/or risks. Thus, knowing the basics of risk assessment and management becomes vital for any case manager to be effective in their role while managing these clients.

PREVALENCE OF MENTAL ILLNESSES AND ASSOCIATED RISKS

The WHO has defined violence as "the intentional use of physical force or power, threatened or actual, against oneself, another person, or against a group or community, that either results in or has a high likelihood of resulting in injury, death, psychological harm, maldevelopment or deprivation" (World Health Organization, 2002). Violence is commonly associated with mental illnesses, particularly psychoses. In a study by Wallace et al. (2004), they found that the rate of violent offending in schizophrenia was about 8%. However, there is a high rate of other psychiatric diagnoses in patients with schizophrenia which influences and increases these risks significantly. Wallace et al. (2004) found that the rate of violence increased to 26% when patients with schizophrenia had a co-morbid substance abuse diagnosis. Similar observations about patients discharged from a hospital with a diagnosis of a major mental disorder alone and with co-morbid substance use disorder have been made, which suggests a significant impact of co-morbid diagnoses on the risk of violence (Steadman et al., 1998). Nonetheless, in public perception, mental illnesses are closely associated with violence, which may be the result of the tendency to combine the concept of mental illnesses with dangerousness. This is also fuelled by sensationalist media coverage of incidents involving mentally ill offenders (Varshney, Mahapatra, Krishnan, Gupta, & Deb, 2016). Hence, violence risk assessment and management both form not only an important part of a mental health clinician's duties but are also societal expectations from them. The public is unlikely to accept excuses by mental health services when failures occur and a person in the community is seriously harmed, no matter how legitimate they may be.

FORENSIC PATIENTS

Forensic patients are patients who are given this particular status by the legal system, that is, the courts, and in some jurisdictions the mental health courts, when these patients have committed an indictable offense and are found to be of unsound mind, that is, not guilty due to their mental illness and/or unfit to stand a trial. The court must make a forensic order if it believes that is necessary to protect the safety of the community, including risk of serious harm to other persons or property. Forensic orders are not only made for offenders who have serious mental illness but also for people with intellectual disabilities who are perpetrators of serious offenses and are found to be of unsound mind or unfit due to an intellectual disability.

These patients form a special group of clientele who require a careful focus on their risks and are subject to periodic reviews under tribunals and various risk management committees set up by the service to manage these clients. A clinician plays a vital role in liaising with various agencies involved in the clinical governance of these patients and provides mental state and risk updates to the various layers of clinical governance starting with a multidisciplinary team, specialist forensic services, clinical directors and sometimes the executives or the boards. They are also responsible for presenting risk assessments to tribunals at their hearings, either periodically or as requested by clients or their legal representation. These patients often not only require specialist forensic risk assessments apart from the clinician or case manager–driven assessments but this is also sometimes mandated by the courts. However, the role of the case manager in managing the risks of these clients remains vital.

RISK PREDICTION VS PREVENTION

Violence has been regarded as a behavioural manifestation of a complex mental illness in a portion of patients. There are studies based on prisoners that have established an empirical relationship between serious mental illness and violence (Mullen, Burgess, Wallace, Palmer, & Ruschena, 2000; Swanson, Holzer, Ganju, & Jono, 1990; Wallace et al., 2004). Hence its assessment and management in patients with such complex mental illnesses is understandably expected out of a mental health clinician (Mullen, 2006).

Risk assessment is the process of identifying empirical and clinically derived risk factors. Risk management is a process of ameliorating this propensity through multidisciplinary intervention, addressing the identified risk factors that moderate the interaction between mental illness and violent behaviour (Mullen, 2006). Monahan's review of studies involving risk assessment using unstructured clinical judgement lead to the conclusion that no one can predict who shall or shall not be violent using these methods. However, his work led to the development of improved assessment procedures (Monahan, 1981). It has been proven that using structured approaches for assessment that have an empirical basis are not only more reliable compared to unstructured clinical judgement alone but also provide stronger predictive validity (Aegisdottir et al., 2006; Hanson & Morton-Bourgon, 2009; Mossman, 2000)

There is a debate amongst experts about mental health clinicians engaging in risk assessments based on statistical observations that risks cannot be predicted (Large, Ryan, Singh, Paton, & Nielssen, 2011; Ryan, Nielssen, Paton, & Large, 2010). However, the primary goal of violence risk assessment is the prevention rather than the prediction of violence (Allnutt et al., 2013). It is important to note that violence risk management is done by developing strategies for managing risk factors, which relate to propensity (Allnutt et al., 2013)

RISK ASSESSMENTS

Bonta (1996) has outlined three generations of risk assessment tools that identify the level of risk for violent (and sexual) offenders.

First Generation or Unstructured Clinical Judgement

In the 1970s, mental health clinicians used the term "dangerousness" to predict violence in forensic patients. This was based on the clinician's observations, assessments and verbal reports from the patients. There are strengths to this method, including less resource intensiveness, speed, flexibility and no need to rely on or be bound by any particular framework. This method, however, has been deemed ineffective in predicting rates of violence, and these methods are no longer considered an acceptable method to assess risks (Heilbrun, Ogloff, & Picarello, 1999).

Second Generation: Actuarial Methods

The actuarial assessment is an objective evaluation of factors empirically related to recidivism and reoffending (Grove & Meehl, 1996). These were developed as it was realised that unstructured clinical or professional judgements have a poor predictive value compared to more structured measures. These methods are based on an explicit method of combining the available information and then linking this to a probability figure based on empirically derived relative frequencies. These methods categorise risks into levels like low, medium and high risk.

The positives of these methods are their usefulness for a large size of offenders like in correctional centres, where an estimate of whether a prisoner would reoffend is the basis of custodial management. However, on the other hand these measures fail to address the reasons for the behaviours they are predicting and are unable to handle individual patterns well.

The Violence Risk Appraisal Guide (VRAG) is a 12-item test developed by Harris, Rice and Quinsey in 1993 that assesses the risk for general violence. VRAG scores range from −26 to +38. Each VRAG score is associated with a particular percentile so that the violence risk of an individual assessee is evaluated according to his or her standing relative to a large sample of violent offenders. Although requiring resources and expertise, the VRAG is the most accurate and empirically supported actuarial method for assessing the risk of violent recidivism in forensic populations.

Static-99 is the most common actuarial risk measure used due to availability of extensive research data on its reliability and validity to assess risk of sexual violence and recidivism. It is easy to conduct, only requiring a file review to ascertain the risk scores in various historical or static risk factors like age, relationships and previous offending. Static-99 has ten items and produces estimates of future risk based on a number of risk factors present in any one individual. Use of Static-99 and its updated version, Static-99R, require training on manual updates before using it in practice.

However, it has also been argued that due to the low predictive accuracy of actuarial methods, their use in making high-stakes decisions should be avoided. Moreover, their reliance on static risk factors while failing to consider dynamic risk factors is considered a shortcoming when it comes to their predictive accuracies. Despite these shortcomings, these are commonly used in the criminal justice system rather than in the mental health system for risk assessment and management. However, clinicians should remain familiar with these, as they will frequently be liaising with criminal justice agencies while managing high-risk consumers.

Structured Professional Judgement

Structured professional judgement is a widely used approach for risk assessments and considered the most "state of the art," transparent and evidence based of the three approaches to risk assessment.

It is used mostly by specialist forensic services and provides an in-depth assessment of the risks considering a detailed review of the presence of a number of empirically identified risk factors. These not only help identify risk factors and the relevance of these factors to the individual but also help guide treatment and management strategies tailored to the individual. However, the limitation of using this approach is that it is time consuming and requires clinicians to be trained specifically to use these tools.

The Historical, Clinical Risk Management-20 (HCR-20) is the most widely used structured professional judgement tool used worldwide. This has been validated in studies throughout the world and by most standards required of a risk assessment tool in a variety of settings, including forensic psychiatric, correctional centre and civil psychiatric and both inpatient and outpatient settings. It consists of 20 items from the historical, clinical and risk domains, which are scored for presence and relevance to the individual. Scoring is based on a manual provided when a clinician is trained in its use and needs to be strictly adhered to in order to maintain validity and standards. The HCR-20 as a tool can, for research purposes, produce numerical scores by totalling its 20 items, producing total scores in the range 0–40. This "actuarial" approach is not advocated in clinical practice (nor do the authors of the

HCR-20 advocate this approach), because it is a "tick box" approach and ignores other clinical factors (Allnutt et al., 2013).

The Risk for Sexual Violence Protocol (RSVP) is a tool used to assess and develop management strategies for individuals with sexual violence risks. Another example of a structured professional judgement tool is the Spousal Assault Risk Assessment (SARA), which is designed to assess the risk of spousal violence.

The clinician must have regard to the clinical, personal and social context of a patient that will help in defining the intervention needed.

Risk formulation is an important aspect of these assessments, where rather than allocating a patient to the low, medium or high risk categories, clinicians attempt to formulate and understand their risks. It involves the description of the potential nature of violence, motives, patterns, victims and factors that can potentially precipitate and perpetuate violence. Also, there is merit in identifying protective factors.

THREE-TIERED RISK FRAMEWORK USED IN QUEENSLAND, AUSTRALIA

Risk assessment, if done in the most comprehensive way, not only requires a huge amount of time and resources but also requires experienced and trained staff. Most services are short on both these valuable resources. A novel way to tackle this is to develop a tiered system for risk assessment. This has been successfully implemented in mental health services across the Australian state of Queensland and provides Queensland Health mental health services with a systematic approach for the identification, assessment and management of consumers who may pose a risk of violence towards others. This system supports a structured and standardised approach to risk assessment and management through the provision of a three-tiered approach, principles of good practice, clinical tools to underpin clinical expertise, training and a quality assurance cycle for continuous improvement (Health, 2019).

This risk framework proposes that all individuals who are consumers of the service should have a risk assessment done by the primary clinician. This is through a locally developed risk screening tool, which is based on empirically identified static and dynamic risk factors and also focusses on identifying protective factors which can mitigate the risks. It is recommended that this risk screen be conducted for all consumers every three months and to align with their care reviews in a multidisciplinary meeting.

When this screening identifies elevated risk factors, a multidisciplinary discussion should happen to mitigate immediate risks, if any. This discussion, however, then triggers evaluation whether a Tier 2 assessment is warranted. Important considerations here include recent violent behaviour, history of serious violent behaviour or a history of a group of concerns that may require a closer look at the risks. For this, a tool called Violence Risk Assessment and Management (VRAM) has been introduced, and training, supervision and online resources have been developed for it. The responsibilities for these Tier 2 assessments lie with the senior clinicians in the team or with the consultant psychiatrist. Risk management strategies are then developed as a part of the multidisciplinary team, and where possible, the consumer, families, primary health network, NGOs and any other support are included in the risk management plans. Local police and ambulance personnel may also be a part of this or may be informed to tailor a response to these clients in high-risk situations.

If required after this Tier 2 assessment, in cases where risks are deemed to be elevated to such a level with that a referral to the specialist forensic mental health services is required to manage these risks. The specialist services make use of structured professional judgement tools like the HCR-20 to assess the risk and develop a risk management plan in conjunction with the referring team and where possible involving the consumer, families, primary health network, NGOs and any other support in the process. Specialist forensic services work in close liaison with the local police and ambulance services, and they are involved in making any risk management strategies for these consumers with elevated risks.

SPECIAL MENTION: FIREARMS

Mental health clinicians are often called upon to assess violence risk where firearms are involved. Although access to firearms is closely linked to the risks and has implications for client and community safety, most clinicians are not trained about discussing firearms with clients while conducting risk assessments. Also, knowledge about firearm legislation can help clinicians identify risk management strategies around this. Clinicians should make themselves familiar with these and seek supervision from specialist services around such assessments (Barnhorst & Kagawa, 2018).

NEWER DEVELOPMENTS

A Swiss study (Arborelius, Fors, Svensson, Sygel, & Kristiansson, 2013) on the use of computer simulation systems for risk assessment for mentally unwell violent offenders has shown that this was not only more acceptable to the offenders but also helped to identify their responses to particular simulated circumstances while not relying only on their verbal abilities and may more effectively assess their emotional reactions, making it superior to the standard question-and-answer approaches. This style of risk assessment may provide a useful complement to the more traditional modes of assessing risks in the near future.

No risk assessment approach is perfect, and clinicians should be aware of the limitations and benefits of the different approaches.

MANAGEMENT OF RISKS

Risk management aims to reduce the likelihood of violence or any such risk behaviours while safely managing the clinical condition of the client, planning care and thus achieving the best possible outcome for the consumer, service and community. This risk management is best informed by risk assessment and a proportionate response to the identified risk factors. Where possible, the consumer, family, support, NGOs, carers, primary health professionals and, if they are willing to participate, victims should be included in developing risk management strategies.

For major mental illnesses and associated risks, it is recommended to focus on some of the common domains to address the risks, but these should be tailored to the individual. Treatment recommendations should be focused upon, including treatment of substance use disorders, as often optimum treatment of the symptoms of the illness is one of the most effective strategies to prevent the client from re-offending or engaging in violence. Treatment not only includes pharmacological but also non-pharmacological interventions like psychotherapy, psychoeducation to family members and carers, preparing relapse prevention plans with the consumer and involving the police and ambulance officers in these plans.

Monitoring clients closely can be an effective risk management strategy. Regular risk assessment and updating risk management plans should be recommended, and moreover any major change in risk factors should prompt a risk review.

Supervision and control, if able to be exercised per the local legislation, can prove an effective strategy to manage risks. Restrictions on client movement to certain places or beyond certain times could be imposed. Subjecting the client to urine drug and alcohol screens could also be possible depending upon the local legislation. Removing or limiting access to weapons like guns should be considered, if relevant.

Victim safety and planning is a vital aspect of risk management. Structured professional judgements can outline a few potential victims that may be at higher risk. There may be previous victims with whom clients still have contact like family members or intimate partners. Victims should be protected, under most legislations, by restraining orders, ordered by the court or requested by the victims themselves. Victims who are unable to avoid being with the client due to virtue of the relationship or living arrangements should be psycho-educated about the illness and any early warning signs and should be included to contribute to developing any relapse prevention and risk management strategies.

DUTY TO DISCLOSE

Clinicians are bound by the duty to protect the wider community, particularly if there is a risk to a specific identified person. Confidentiality can be breached to protect third parties in certain circumstances. Professional codes of ethics allow clinicians to disclose confidential information like serious concern about risk of violence to a named person.

DEVELOPING A SAFETY CULTURE

It is important for services to develop a safety culture which learns from adverse events and builds good practice. For this, services need to lead and support staff, integrate risk management activity, promote reporting of incidents into risk management systems, involve consumers and consumer representatives in various governance projects, regularly share learning from adverse incidents, develop good practice and develop and implement timely solutions to prevent further harm.

It is important that staff receive regular training in risk assessment and that regular refreshers be conducted for trained staff. Peer support is also vital in managing day-to-day challenges, and staff should be supported where they wish to access this. Personal safety is paramount, and occupational violence prevention and self-defence workshops should be offered to all clinicians, with regular refreshers for these.

It is common for staff working in high acute and constant high-risk situations to feel burnout. Recognising and managing staff burnout is vital in maintaining the quality of the risk assessment and in turn its management. Staff should be supported to take regular time off, and secondments and upskilling should be encouraged where possible. Confidential helplines for employee assistance should be available if staff wish to access support. Employers should cover their staff with indemnity insurance, especially while working in high-risk situations.

IMPLICATIONS OF BETTER RISK MANAGEMENT

Having a robust risk management strategy for individuals with elevated risks and the necessary resources to manage these clients can have a great impact on service delivery and patient flow within the service. Patients with elevated risks can present repeatedly to the hospital, requiring use of precious and already pressured acute and emergency services, if not managed and supported well. These presentations themselves can lead to escalation of risks, particularly to staff working in these environments.

Intensive case management and, as a consequence, intensive risk management and support for clients are known to reduce the rate of hospitalisation and prevent overuse of hospital beds by these clients.

Having effective risk management strategies is not only important for the service but also for the community at large. It protects the larger community from any potential risks through these clients. Managing risks effectively can lead to reduced rates of violence and re-offending and thus reduce the rates of incarceration.

One aware and trained clinician can be the difference between a client's journey being steady and recovery bound versus ending up in a revolving door. Thus, risk-aware and competent clinicians are an asset to any service.

References

Aegisdottir, S., White, M., Spengler, P., Maugherman, A., Anderson, L., Cook, R., . . . Rush, J. (2006). The meta-analysis of clinical judgment project: Fifty-six years of accumulated research on clinical versus statistical prediction. *The Counseling Psychologist, 34*, 341–382. doi:10.1177/0011 000005285875

Allnutt, S. H., Ogloff, J. R., Adams, J., O'Driscoll, C., Daffern, M., Carroll, A., . . . Chaplow, D. (2013). Managing aggression and violence: The clinician's role in contemporary mental health care. *Aust N Z J Psychiatry, 47*(8), 728–736. doi:10.1177/0004867413484368

Arborelius, L., Fors, U., Svensson, A. K., Sygel, K., & Kristiansson, M. (2013). A new interactive computer simulation system for violence risk assessment of mentally disordered violent offenders. *Crim Behav Ment Health, 23*(1), 30–40. doi:10.1002/cbm.1849

Barnhorst, A., & Kagawa, R. M. C. (2018). Access to firearms: When and how do mental health clients become prohibited from owning guns? *Psychol Serv, 15*(4), 379–385. doi:10.1037/ser0000185

Bonta, J. (1996). *Risk-Needs Assessment and Treatment*. London, UK: Sage Publications, Inc.

Dieterich, M., Irving, C. B., Bergman, H., Khokhar, M. A., Park, B., & Marshall, M. (2017). Intensive case management for severe mental illness. *Cochrane Database of Systematic Reviews, 1*. doi:10.1002/14651858.CD007906.pub3

Grove, W. M., & Meehl, P. E. (1996). Comparative efficiency of informal (subjective, impressionistic) and formal (mechanical, algorithmic) prediction procedures: The clinical–statistical controversy. *Psychology, Public Policy, and Law, 2*, 293–323. doi:10.1037/1076-8971.2.2.293

Hanson, R. K., & Morton-Bourgon, K. E. (2009). The accuracy of recidivism risk assessments for sexual offenders: A meta-analysis of 118 prediction studies. *Psychol Assess, 21*(1), 1–21. doi:10.1037/a0014421

Harris, G. T., Rice, M. E., & Quinsey, V. L. (Producer). (1993). Violent recidivism of mentally disordered offenders: The development of a statistical prediction instrument. *Criminal Justice and Behavior, 20*(4), 315–335. doi:10.1177/0093854893020004001

Health, Q. (2019). *Violence Risk Assessment and Management Framework – Mental Health Services*. Retrieved from www.health.qld.gov.au/research-reports/reports/departmental/annual-report/case-study-1

Heilbrun, K., Ogloff, J. R., & Picarello, K. (1999). Dangerous offender statutes in the United States and Canada: Implications for risk assessment. *Int J Law Psychiatry, 22*(3–4), 393–415. doi:10.1016/s0160-2527(99)00017-5

Intagliata, J. (1982). Improving the quality of community care for the chronically mentally disabled: The role of case management. *Schizophrenia Bulletin, 8*(4), 655–674. doi:10.1093/schbul/8.4.655

Large, M. M., Ryan, C. J., Singh, S. P., Paton, M. B., & Nielssen, O. B. (2011). The predictive value of risk categorization in schizophrenia. *Harv Rev Psychiatry, 19*(1), 25–33. doi:10.3109/10673229.2 011.549770

Monahan, J. (1981). *Predicting Violent Behavior: An Assessment of Clinical Techniques* (Vol. 114). New York: United States of America: Sage Publications, Inc.

Mossman, D. (2000). Evaluating violence risk "by the book": A review of HCR-20: Assessing risk for violence, version 2 and the manual for the sexual violence risk 20. *Behavioral Sciences & the Law, 18*, 781–789. doi:10.1002/bsl.418

Mullen, P. E. (2006). Schizophrenia and violence: From correlations to preventive strategies. *Advances in Psychiatric Treatment, 12*(4), 239–248. doi:10.1192/apt.12.4.239

Mullen, P. E., Burgess, P., Wallace, C., Palmer, S., & Ruschena, D. (2000). Community care and criminal offending in schizophrenia. *Lancet, 355*(9204), 614–617. doi:10.1016/s0140-6736(99)05082-5

Organization, W. H. (2002). *The World Health Report 2002: Reducing Risks, Promoting Healthy Life*. Geneva, Switzerland: World Health Organization.

Ryan, C., Nielssen, O., Paton, M., & Large, M. (2010). Clinical decisions in psychiatry should not be based on risk assessment. *Australas Psychiatry, 18*(5), 398–403. doi:10.3109/10398562.2010. 507816

Steadman, H. J., Mulvey, E. P., Monahan, J., Robbins, P. C., Appelbaum, P. S., Grisso, T., . . . Silver, E. (1998). Violence by people discharged from acute psychiatric inpatient facilities and by others in the same neighborhoods. *Arch Gen Psychiatry, 55*(5), 393–401. doi:10.1001/archpsyc.55.5.393

Swanson, J. W., Holzer, C. E., 3rd, Ganju, V. K., & Jono, R. T. (1990). Violence and psychiatric disorder in the community: Evidence from the epidemiologic catchment area surveys. *Hosp Community Psychiatry, 41*(7), 761–770. doi:10.1176/ps.41.7.761

Varshney, M., Mahapatra, A., Krishnan, V., Gupta, R., & Deb, K. S. (2016). Violence and mental illness: What is the true story? *Journal of Epidemiology and Community Health, 70*(3), 223. doi:10.1136/jech-2015-205546

Wallace, C., Mullen, P. E., & Burgess, P. (2004). Criminal offending in schizophrenia over a 25-year period marked by deinstitutionalization and increasing prevalence of comorbid substance use disorders. *Am J Psychiatry, 161*(4), 716–727. doi:10.1176/appi.ajp.161.4.716

10
Optimizing Patient Care in Sexual Dysfunction in Severe Mental Illness

Shivananda Manohar, Suman S. Rao, T.S. Sathyanarayana Rao

The Sexual Response Cycle	101
Neurobiology of Sexual Response Cycle	101
Neurotransmitters	*101*
Hormones	*101*
Sexual Dysfunction	102
Sexual Functioning in Mental Illness	102
Sexual Dysfunction in Schizophrenia Patients	*102*
Impact of Depression on Sexual Functioning	103
Sexual Response Cycle in Depression	103
Sexual Functioning in Bipolar Disorders	*105*
Sexual Functioning in Anxiety and Personality Disorders	*105*
Sexual Functioning in Cognitive Impairment	*106*
Conclusion	106

The definition of sexuality by the World Health Organization in 2006 states:

> Sexuality is a central aspect of being human throughout life and encompasses sex, gender identities and roles, sexual orientation, eroticism, pleasure, intimacy and reproduction. Sexuality is experienced and expressed in thoughts, fantasies, desires, beliefs, attitudes, values, behaviors, practices, roles and relationships. While sexuality can include all of these dimensions, not all of them are always experienced or expressed. Sexuality is influenced by the interaction of biological, psychological, social, economic, political, cultural, ethical, legal, historical and religious and spiritual factors.

The multidimensional concept of sexuality is constructed socially and shaped by sexual and gender norms and inequalities. Various dimensions of sexuality include intimacy, sensuality, sexual practices and behavior, gender identity and sexual orientation and reproductive and sexual health. Sensuality refers to the fulfillment of bodily appetite, especially sexual, with free indulgence in carnal pleasures. There is the possibility of a strong feeling of deep affection in every possible human interaction.[1] Love is dedication and total submission of self to the beloved.[2] Three components of love was described by Sternberg: passion, intimacy and commitment.[3] Intimacy may not always culminate in sex, and it's very much possible for two friends to be truly intimate without any sexual connection. Romance, physical attraction and sexual commitment are driven by passion. The decision to love and maintain for the long term is determined by commitment.[4]

Sexuality is one of the key components of the physical, intellectual and psychosocial wellbeing of an individual. Patient-centered approaches are used to define 'normal' or 'healthy' sexuality. When an individual presents with problems with the physical and emotional aspects of sexual functioning, it is considered a sexual problem. Disruption in any phase of the sexual response cycle is considered sexual dysfunction.

THE SEXUAL RESPONSE CYCLE

One of the simplest models of the sexual response cycle is given by Robinson and Kaplan, the DEOR model. The desire phase is represented as D, which is the desire to have sex and includes sexual drive and fantasies. The excitement phase begins with physiological and psychological stimulation. During the excitement phase in men, there will be testicular enlargement and penile tumescence. In women, the excitement phase is characterized by vaginal lubrication, clitoral engorgement, thickening of labia majora, enlargement of breast size and erection of the nipple. An increase in blood pressure, respiratory rate and heart rate happens in both sexes during the excitement phase. Sexual pleasure peaks during the orgasm phase, and contraction of perineal muscles happen both in men and women. Inevitably, ejaculation happens in men, and contraction of the lower third of the uterus and vagina characterizes the orgasm phase in women. Disengorgement of blood from the genitals characterizes the resolution phase, which may last up to six hours. There will be a general sense of wellbeing during the resolution phase.[5,6]

NEUROBIOLOGY OF SEXUAL RESPONSE CYCLE

Various endocrine factors, along with neurotransmitters and neuropeptides, regulate the sexual response cycle. Serotonin, norepinephrine, dopamine and nitric oxide are a few neurotransmitters that impact sexual functioning. Testosterone influences all phases of the sexual response cycle through its action on the hypothalamus, limbic system and cortex. Opiate receptors and enkephalins in the amygdala motivate pleasure-seeking behavior.[7,8,9]

The brainstem, through its influence on the spinal cord, exerts inhibitory as well as excitatory influence on the sexual response cycle. The sympathetic nervous system involving T10–L2 is implicated in emission, while the parasympathetic system involving S2–S4 is implicated in ejection.[10]

Neurotransmitters

Dopamine plays an important role in the sexual response cycle. Activation of the median preoptic nucleus of the hypothalamus and nucleus accumbens is implicated in sexual motivation. Serotonin has an inhibitory role in all phases of the sexual response cycle. With regard to norepinephrine, decreased activity at alpha receptors and increased activity at beta receptors is required for erection. Gamma-aminobutyric acid also plays a role in erection.[11–18]

Hormones

Testosterone influences libido in both men and women. Lifestyle and stress level also influence testosterone level. Progesterone, estrogen and testosterone promote sexual desire. Oxytocin has positive influence on sexual activity in both sexes and promotes orgasm. Arousal is inhibited by prolactin.[19–21]

SEXUAL DYSFUNCTION

Sexual dysfunction is usually classified based on which phase of the sexual response cycle is affected. Desire phase disorders include hypoactive sexual desire disorder, which is seen in both men and women. It is characterized by persistently low desire or fantasies concerning sexual activity. Excitement phase disorders in male include erectile dysfunction and premature ejaculation. Erectile dysfunction is characterized by persistent complete or partial failure to maintain an erection throughout the a sexual act. Premature ejaculation is the most common sexual dysfunction in men, characterized by ejaculation with minimal sexual stimulation – before the individual wishes to. Female sexual arousal disorder is characterized by persistent complete or partial failure to maintain lubrication throughout the completion of a sexual act. To make a diagnosis, it should be present on at least 20–30% of occasions. Orgasm disorders include inhibited male and female orgasm. Female orgasm disorder is characterized by lack of orgasm after an adequate sexual excitement phase, while male orgasm disorder is characterized by absence or delay in ejaculation despite an adequate sexual excitement phase.[22]

SEXUAL FUNCTIONING IN MENTAL ILLNESS

The prevalence of sexual dysfunction in mental illness is very high. The disease process by itself as well as the medication used in treatment both contribute to the increased prevalence of sexual dysfunction.

Sexual Dysfunction in Schizophrenia Patients

Negative symptoms of schizophrenia like avolition, blunted affect and anhedonia significantly impair sexual functioning. Recurrent psychotic episodes also impact self-esteem and the ability to establish relationships. Studies suggest that the prevalence of sexual dysfunction is around 82% in men and 96% in women suffering from schizophrenia[23] Historically, sexual problems have been implicated in the origin of delusions, but not much literature is available about sexual dysfunctions in delusional disorder. The usefulness of PDE5 inhibitors in sexual dysfunction in delusional disorders has been reported. The available literature on sexual functioning and schizophrenia focus more on male sexual problems. Aizen et al. found a higher prevalence of sexual dysfunction in both untreated and treated male patients. Untreated patients had desire and excitement problems, while treatment with antipsychotics worsened erection and orgasm.[24] A study focusing on sexual functioning in female schizophrenia patients found 70% prevalence. Among them, all reported desire disorders; 92% reported arousal problems, while 48% reported poor lubrication.[25] More than 75% reported impaired orgasm, around 70% reported poor satisfaction and more than 35% reported pain during intercourse.[25]

Earlier studies comparing first-generation antipsychotics found the prevalence of sexual dysfunction was greater in patients receiving thioridazine when compared to other first-generation antipsychotics.[26]

The use of dopamine agonists to treat typical antipsychotic-induced sexual dysfunction did not bring desirable changes. Use of Levodopa caused exacerbation of psychotic symptoms, while apomorphine caused severe nausea.[27] A six week open-label study using Amanatidine, a dopamine reuptake inhibitor, showed some statistical improvement in sexual functioning.[28] Use of low doses of selegline, which is a selective monoaminooxidase B inhibitor, did not show any effect on improving sexual functioning.[29]

Newer atypical antipsychotics that have stronger 5HT2A receptor affinity compared to D2 receptors carry a lower risk of increasing prolactin levels. Second-generation antipsychotics are associated with lower risk of prolactin elevation and a lesser effect on peripheral cholinergic receptors and alpha1 adrenergic receptors.[30]

Studies comparing second- and first-generation antipsychotics in terms of sexual functioning have shown mixed results. A study done by Hummer et al. could not find any difference between haloperidol and clozapine. A study done by Aisenberg et al. found people receiving clozapine had better orgasm, enjoyment of sex and sexual satisfaction.[31]

Another prospective study was done using a sample size of 570 patients, in which patients were evaluated on sexual functioning at baseline and at 3 and 6 months after starting antipsychotics. The study sample consisted of three groups, the first group receiving olanzapine, the second receiving risperidone and the third receiving first-generation antipsychotics. At baseline, 37% of the participants reported sexual dysfunction. After treatment, the group receiving olanzapine reported significantly lower sexual dysfunction when compared to risperidone and first-generation antipsychotics.[32]

Another study done by Dossenbach et al. using a larger sample of 3,828 comparing sexual dysfunction in patients receiving olanzapine, risperidone, quetiapine and haloperidol found the group receiving olanzapine and quetiapine had less sexual dysfunction compared to the group receiving haloperidol and risperidone.[33]

There is accumulation of data regarding the use of sildenafil in treating sexual dysfunction in male patients with schizophrenia. A study done on a small sample of schizophrenia and delusional disorder patients suffering from erectile dysfunction found people receiving sildenafil had better frequency and duration of erection as well as sexual satisfaction when compared to placebo.[33]

In summary, sexual dysfunction is more prevalent in schizophrenia, both as part of the illness as well as psychotropically induced. Lack of recognition would lead to non-compliance and recurrence of psychotic symptoms. Reducing psychotropics to the minimal effective dose as well as using atypical medication like olanzapine, quetiapine and ziprasidone would cause less sexual dysfunction, which in turn improves quality of life.

IMPACT OF DEPRESSION ON SEXUAL FUNCTIONING

The estimated prevalence of sexual dysfunction in people suffering from depression is around 70–80% in various studies.

SEXUAL RESPONSE CYCLE IN DEPRESSION

Depression negatively affects all phases of the sexual response cycle. Studies done on males about the impact of depression on sexual functioning showed 40% of men had sexual interest problems, while 20% had difficulty in ejaculation or reaching orgasm. FMRI studies done on women suffering from depression showed decreased activation of certain areas of the brain when presented with sexually stimulating visual images. These areas included the middle occipital gyrus, middle temporal gyrus, inferior frontal gyrus, insula, hypothalamus, septal area, anterior cingulate gyrus, parahippocampal gyrus, thalamus and amygdala.[34]

A study that compared sexual functioning in unipolar and bipolar depression with a sample size of 132 found 72% with unipolar depression and 77% with bipolar depression had sexual dysfunction. This study also found that in some patients, loss of desire may be the presenting complaint; some people revealed sexual dysfunction on enquiry, and sexual dysfunction predated the onset of illness in others.[35]

Studies comparing sexual functioning in depressed individuals with controls found that desire disorders are more common than arousal and orgasm disorders. A comparative study found that desire disorders were more common in depressed individuals, while erectile, ejaculatory and orgasmic disorders did not differ from controls.[36] A Zurich study found that sexual dysfunctions were twice as common in depressive disorders, which included major depression, dysthymia and recurrent brief depressive disorders, when compared to controls. This study included an age group from 28–35 years and may not be applicable for older adults. The Zurich study also compared sexual functioning in treated and untreated patients. Treatment included antidepressants, benzodiazepines or psychotherapy. Sixty-two percent of individuals who received treatment had sexual dysfunction, which was higher than untreated patients (45%).[37]

A cross-sectional study done in the United Kingdom and France with a sample size of 502 found that selective serotonin reuptake/serotonin norepinephrine reuptake inhibitor-induced sexual dysfunction was around 26.6% in France and 39.2% in United Kingdom.[38] Sexual dysfunction in patients receiving antidepressants ranged from 25.8% to 80.3% according to a MET analysis. According to this study, antidepressants causing sexual dysfunction in descending order were sertraline, venlafaxine, citalopram, paroxetine, fluoxetine, imipramine, phenelzine, duloxetine, escitalopram and fluvoxamine. Bupropion, mirtazapine and nefazodone were associated with lesser sexual dysfunction.[39]

All SSRIs have been reported to cause absent or delayed orgasm/ejaculation and, in some instances, a reduction in libido and arousal. A study that evaluated sexual dysfunction in patients taking paroxetine, fluoxetine or sertraline using a valid questionnaire reported treatment of emergent sexual dysfunction in 60% of men. Delayed orgasm (35%) was the most common dysfunction, followed by inability to reach orgasm and requirement of greater stimulation to maintain erection each in 30% of subjects and diminished intensity of orgasm (24%) in about one-fourth of the subjects.[40] Other studies have also shown that SSRIs predominantly impair orgasm. Studies comparing different SSRIs and their impact on sexual functioning have had mixed results. Among SSRIs, paroxetine is more likely to cause sexual dysfunction, while fluvoxamine has a modest advantage. There is some evidence that paroxetine may be more likely than other SSRIs to cause sexual dysfunction and that fluvoxamine may have some modest advantage. Studies evaluating the effects of SSRIs on ejaculation in men with premature ejaculation found greater delays in ejaculation in men taking paroxetine and the least delay in those receiving fluvoxamine.[41] Though there is some evidence that the noradrenergic effect may mitigate serotonin's influence on sexual function, studies evaluating the sexual effects of SNRIs have been inconsistent. Studies comparing duloxetine with paroxetine or escitalopram found treatment of emergent sexual dysfunction was significantly lower. After 12 weeks of treatment, the difference was not maintained, suggesting that duloxetine has only a short-term advantage over SSRIs.[42] Earlier studies found that sexual side effects by venlafaxine were significantly lower in women when compared to men. Further studies could not replicate the same findings and found that venlafaxine was associated with decreased desire and delayed orgasm.[43] Initial studies that relied on spontaneous self reports about desvenlafaxine, which is an active metabolite of venlafaxine, found fewer sexual adverse effects in women compared to men. Later a meta-analysis done by Clayton et al. revealed around 7% of men receiving desvenlafaxine had erectile dysfunction, and 1% of women had anorgasmia. Another SNRI with predominant norepinephrine reuptake inhibition, milnacipran, has been claimed to have fewer sexual side effects.[44,45]

Mirtazapine has agonistic action on post-synaptic 5HT1A receptors and antagonistic action on 5HT2A receptors. As it antagonizes 5HT2A receptors, serotonin-mediated sexual adverse events are minimized. An outpatient study which systematically assessed sexual functioning in depressed individuals found mirtazapine enhances sexual functioning in both men and women. In patients who had remitted from depression with treatment with SSRIs and had sexual dysfunction, when switched to mirtazapine, 50% of individuals had no sexual dysfunction at the end of 8 weeks.[46]

Mirtazapine stimulates noradrenergic and serotonergic activity by its agonist effects on postsynaptic 5-HT1A receptors and concurrent antagonist effects on 5-HT2 and 5-HT3 receptors. The 5-HT2 blockade mechanism is thought to prevent serotonin-mediated adverse effects on sexual function. On the basis of this, it is claimed that in comparison to SSRIs and venlafaxine, mirtazapine is significantly less likely to produce sexual dysfunction. In fact, a systematic assessment of sexual function among depressed outpatients found that mirtazapine may enhance functioning of some of the phases in both men and women. Ozmenler et al. also reported that when remitted patients with SSRI-induced sexual dysfunction were switched to mirtazapine, approximately half of them reported no sexual dysfunction at the end of the 8-week treatment. Preliminary evidence suggests that mirtazapine improves duloxetine-induced sexual dysfunction. Studies comparing mirtazapine to serotonergic antidepressants with respect to sexual side effects have come up with inconsistent results.[46,47]

Sexual Functioning in Bipolar Disorders

Sexual functioning can be impaired in bipolar disorder as a direct consequence of the illness. Though there are reports of hypersexuality as well as high-risk sexual behavior in manic or hypomanic states, overall, people with bipolar disorder report sexual dissatisfaction. One study reports up to 40% of individuals with bipolar disorder have hypersexuality as an interepisodic trait.[48,49] Comparative studies with schizophrenia show that people with bipolar disorder have more stable sexual partners and more intense sexual relationships.[50,51] The literature suggests that in comparison with unipolar patients, bipolar patients are less sexually active.[52] Studies comparing men and women with bipolar disorder show that men tend to have more partners as well a high tendency to have sex with strangers.[53] Bipolar disorder impacts all phases of the sexual response cycle, which in turn can lead to feelings of worthlessness as well as suicidal ideas.[54] Youths with bipolar disorder with comorbid post-traumatic stress disorder have higher chances of sexual aggression, so proper identification and treatment is essential.[55]

Even the drugs used in bipolar disorder can cause sexual dysfunction.[56] Lithium, which is one of the major drug used for bipolar disorder, causes impairment in sexual functioning.[57] Literature suggests that lithium causes decreased libido, erectile dysfunction and reduction in sexual satisfaction.[58] When compared with antipsychotics, lithium has fewer sexual side effects.[59,60,61] Another mood stabilizer, valproate, which is an antiepileptic, actually increases testosterone and also dehydroepiandrosterone.[62] There are reports of valproate causing erectile dysfunction in men and menstrual irregularity in women.[63] Carbamazepine, which is a antiepileptic mood stabilizer, decreases progesterone, estrogen and testosterone. It increases serum hormone binding globulin (SHBG), which in turn decreases bioactive testosterone.[64] Carbamazepine is also reported to decrease sexual desire and cause erectile dysfunction.[65]

Sexual Functioning in Anxiety and Personality Disorders

Anxiety disorders have been associated with higher prevalence of sexual dysfunction. Men suffering from social phobia also have higher chances of having premature ejaculation, impaired sexual enjoyment and sexual satisfaction.[66] Woman suffering from anxiety disorders have impairment in all phases of the sexual response cycle.[67] Up to 80% of individuals with post-traumatic stress disorder report sexual dysfunction.[68] Patients suffering from eating disorders also have sexual inadequacies. Fear of intimacy and decreased sexual interest are seen in patients with anorexia nervosa.[69]

Personality disorders, specifically borderline personality disorder, is associated with higher sexual assertiveness, sexual avoidance, promiscuity, sexual dissatisfaction and sexual preoccupation.[70]

Patients suffering from Alzheimer's and related dementia have a multitude of sexual problems, which include sexual apathy, sexually inappropriate behavior, decreased sexual desire and inappropriate sexual behavior, causing disrupted marital relationships.[71]

Adolescents with mental retardation have a higher chance of non-consensual sexual abuse, which may include fondling, exposure to sexual material, exhibitionism, oral sex or sexual intercourse.

Sexual Functioning in Cognitive Impairment

An older study done in an elderly population without any impairment showed 33% of the population were involved in sexual activity, while 40% reported that they still had sexual interest. An Indian study found that only 27.4% of individuals above 60 years were sexually active. It progressively dropped as age advanced, and after 75 years none were sexually active.[72] There are varied findings regarding the association between sexuality and cognitive functioning. A study done among menopausal women did not show any association between sexual functioning and cognitive decline.[73] An Italian study showed subjects who continued sexual interest or activity had better cognitive functioning. Another study that found a prevalence of minimal cognitive impairment in the range of 3–20% found that only one-third of cognitively impaired individuals had sexual activity when compared to 62.3% of the healthy cognitive group. This study revealed minimal cognitive impairment significantly impaired sexual functioning. The factors that contributed to sexual decline in these individuals included organic, relational and comorbid medical conditions. Organic changes included vasculopathy, neuropathy, decrease in sex hormones and erectile dysfunction. Relationship factors include bereavement and role transition from caregivers to care receivers. Comorbid medical conditions include diabetes, hypertension and depression. Use of prescribed medications like anticholinergics, antidepressants, antipsychotics and others can cause impotence and impaired ejaculation.[74]

CONCLUSION

Sexuality involves the whole experience of a person's sense of self, a person's ability to form relationships with others and feeling about themselves. Sexuality has a significant impact on quality of life. People of all ages and abilities are involved in sexual intimacy as a means of connecting with partners and also to enhance a sense of wellbeing. Life-threatening illness often precludes discussion on sexual health; even after recovery, practitioners persistently fail to acknowledge sexual dysfunction. This is due to a lack of knowledge about sexual dysfunction and treatment among healthcare professionals. The first step in treating sexual dysfunction is becoming aware of its association with almost every diseased organ system. Patients willingly discuss sexual problems if the healthcare professional broaches the topic. By identifying and treating sexual dysfunction, practitioners will not only help to enhance patients' quality of life but also make complicated treatment more bearable.

References

1. Hornby AS, Crowther J. (Eds.) *Oxford advanced learner's dictionary of current English*, Fifth Edition, Oxford University Press, Oxford, 1996, pp. 699–700.
2. Chandwani A. *Kama Sutra elixir of love*. Brijbasi Art Press Ltd., Delhi, India, 2006, pp. 43–66.

3. Sternberg R. A triangular theory of love. *Psychological Review* 1986;93: 119–135.
4. Stanway A. *The art of sexual intimacy A guide for lovers*. Headline Book Publishing, London, UK, 1993, pp. 6–17, 32–51, 72–138.
5. Kaplan H. *Disorders of sexual desire*. Simon and Schuster, New York, 1979.
6. Robinson P. *The modernization of sex*. Cornell University Press, Ithaca, NY, 1976.
7. Georgiadis J, Holstege G. Human brain activation during stimulation of the penis. *Journal of Comparative Neurology* 2005;493:33–38.
8. Hamann S, Herman R, Nolan C, Wallen K. Men and women differ in amygdala response to visual sexual stimuli. *Nature Neuroscience* 2004;7(4):325–326.
9. Zimmer C. The brain: Where does sex live in the brain? From top to bottom. *Discover Magazine*, October 2009 Issue.
10. Rowland D, McMahon CG, Abdo C, Cheh J, Jannini E, Waldinger MD, Ahn TY. Disorders of orgasm and ejaculation in men. *The Journal of Sexual Medicine* April 2010;7(2):1668–1686.
11. Rao TSS, Rao VS, Guptha AR, Raman R, Urs O, Basavaraju M, Pande S. A study on desire disorders in women. *Indian Journal of Psychiatry* 2003;45(supplement):86.
12. Sadock BJ, Sadock VA. Human sexuality. In: *Kaplan & Sadock's synopsis of psychiatry: Behavioral sciences/clinical psychiatry*, Tenth Edition. Lippincott Williams & Wilkins, New York, NY, 2007;21:680–717.
13. McMahon CG, Abdo C, Incrocci L, et al. Disorders of orgasm and ejaculation in men. *J Sex Med* 2004;1:58–65.
14. Graf H, Walter M, Metzger CD, et al. Antidepressant-related sexual dysfunction-perspectives from neuroimaging. *Pharmacol Biochem Behav* 2014;121:138–145.
15. Stahl SM. The psychopharmacology of sex, part 2: Effects of drugs and disease on the 3 phases of human sexual response. *J Clin Psychiatry* 2001;62(3):147–148.
16. Stahl SM. The psychopharmacology of sex, Part 1: Neurotransmitters and the 3 phases of the human sexual response. *J Clin Psychiatry* 2001;62(2):80–81.
17. Just MJ. The influence of atypical antipsychotic drugs on sexual function. *Neuropsychiatr Dis Treat* 15;11:1655–1661.
18. Meston CM, Frohlich PF. The neurobiology of sexual function. *Arch Gen Psychiatry* Nov 2000;57(11):1012–1030.
19. Corona G, Isidori AM, Aversa A, Burnett AL, Maggi M. Endocrinologic control of men's sexual desire and arousal/erection. *J Sex Med* Mar 2016;13(3):317–337.
20. Davis SR, Worsley R, Miller KK, Parish SJ, Santoro N. Androgens and female sexual function and dysfunction-findings from the fourth international consultation of sexual medicine. *J Sex Med* Feb 2016;13(2):168–178
21. Worsley R, Santoro N, Miller KK, Parish SJ, Davis SR. Hormones and female sexual dysfunction: Beyond estrogens and androgens-findings from the fourth international consultation on sexual medicine. *J Sex Med* 2016;13(3):283–290.
22. Gregoire A. (1999) ABC of sexual health: Assessing and managing male sexual problems. *BMJ* 1999;318(3):15–317.
23. Macdonald S1, Halliday J, MacEwan T, Sharkey V, Farrington S, Wall S, McCreadie RG. Nithsdale schizophrenia surveys 24: Sexual dysfunction: Case-control study. *Br J Psychiatry* Jan 2003;182:50–56
24. Aizenberg, D, Zemishlany, Z, Dorfman-Etrog, P, Weizman, A. Sexual dysfunction in male schizophrenic patients. *The Journal of Clinical Psychiatry* Apr 1995;56(4):137–141.
25. Simiyon M, Chandra PS, Desai G. Sexual dysfunction among women with schizophrenia: A cross sectional study from India. *Asian J Psychiatr* Dec 2016;24:93–98.
26. Kotin J, Wilbert DE, Verburg D, Soldinger SM. Thioridazine and sexual dysfunction. *Am J Psychiatry* Jan 1976;133(1):82–85.
27. Schiavi RC, Segraves RT. The biology of sexual function. *Psychiatr Clin North Am* Mar 1995;18(1):7–23.
28. Valevski A, Modai I, Zbarski E, Zemishlany Z, Weizman A. Effect of amantadine on sexual dysfunction in neuroleptic-treated male schizophrenic patients. *Clin Neuropharmacol* Nov–Dec 1998;21(6):355–357.
29. Berry MD, Juorio AV, Paterson IA. Possible mechanisms of action of (-)deprenyl and other MAO-B inhibitors in some neurologic and psychiatric disorders. *Prog Neurobiol* Oct 1994;44(2):141–161.
30. Cutler AJ. Sexual dysfunction and antipsychotic treatment. *Psychoneuroendocrinology* Jan 2003;28(Suppl. 1):69–82.

31. Hummer M, Kemmler G, Kurz M, Kurzthaler I, Oberbauer H, Fleischhacker W. Sexual disturbances during clozapine and haloperidol treatment for schizophrenia. *Am J Psychiatry* Apr 1999;156(4):631–633.
32. Tran PV, Hamilton SH, Kuntz AJ, Potvin JH, Andersen SW, Beasley C Jr, Tollefson GD. Double-blind comparison of olanzapine versus risperidone in the treatment of schizophrenia and other psychotic disorders. *J Clin Psychopharmacol* Oct 1997;17(5):407–418.
33. Dossenbach M, Dyachkova Y, Pirildar S, et al. Effects of atypical and typical antipsychotic treatments on sexual function in patients with schizophrenia: 12-month results from the Intercontinental Schizophrenia Outpatient Health Outcomes (IC-SOHO) study. *European Psychiatry: The Journal of the Association of European Psychiatrists* 2006;21(4):251–258.
34. Yang JC, Park K, Eun SJ, et al. Assessment of cerebrocortical areas associated with sexual arousal in depressive women using functional MR imaging. *J SexMed* 2008;5(3):602–609.
35. Schreiner-Engel, P, Schiavi RC. Lifetime psychopathology in individuals with low sexual desire. *Journal of Nervous and Mental Disease* 1986;174:646–651.
36. Mathew RJ, Weinman ML. Sexual dysfunctions in depression. *Archives of Sexual Behavior* 1982;11:323–325.
37. Ernst C, Foldenyi M, Angst J. The Zurich study: XXI. Sexual dysfunctions and disturbances in young adults. *European Archives of Psychiatry and Clinical Neuroscience* 1993;243:179–188.
38. Williams VS, Baldwin DS, Hogue SL, Fehnel SE, Hollis KA, Edin HM. Estimating the prevalence and impact of antidepressant-induced sexual dysfunction in 2 European countries: A cross-sectional patient survey. *J Clin Psychiatry* 2006;67:204–210.
39. Clayton AH, Pradko JF, Croft HA, Montano CB, Leadbetter RA, Bolden-Watson C, et al. Prevalence of sexual dysfunction among newer antidepressants. *J Clin Psychiatry* 2002;63:357–366.
40. Jacobsen FM. Fluoxetine-induced sexual dysfunction & an open trial of yohimbine. *J Clin Psychiatry* 1992;53:119–122.
41. Waldinger MD, Hengeveld MW, Zwinderman AH, Olivier B. Effect of SSRI antidepressants on ejaculation: A double blind, randomized, placebo-controlled study with fluoxetine, fluvoxamine, paroxetine, and sertraline. *J Clin Psychopharmacol* 1998;18:274–281.
42. Clayton A, Kornstein S, Prakash A, Mallinckrodt C, Wohlreich M. Changes in sexual functioning associated with duloxetine, escitalopram, and placebo in the treatment of patients with major depressive disorder. *J Sex Med* 2007;4:917–929.
43. Thase ME, Clayton AH, Haight BR, Thompson AH, Modell JG, Johnston JA. A double-blind comparison between bupropion XL and venlafaxine XR: Sexual functioning, antidepressant efficacy, and tolerability. *J Clin Psychopharmacol* 2006;26:482–488.
44. Liebowitz MR, Manley AL, Padmanabhan SK, Ganguly R, Tummala R, Tourian KA. Efficacy, safety, and tolerability of desvenlafaxine 50 mg/day and 100 mg/day in outpatients with major depressive disorder. *Curr Med Res Opin* 2008;24:1877–1890.
45. Septien-Velez L, Pitrosky B, Padmanabhan SK, Germain JM, Tourian KA. A randomized, double-blind, placebo-controlled trial of desvenlafaxine succinate in the treatment of major depressive disorder. *Int Clin Psychopharmacol* 2007;22:338–347.
46. Ozmenler NK, Karlidere T, Bozkurt A, Yetkin S, Doruk A, Sutcigil L, et al. Mirtazapine augmentation in depressed patients with sexual dysfunction due to selective serotonin reuptake inhibitors. *Hum Psychopharmacol* 2008;23:321–326.
47. Ravindran LN, Eisfeld BS, Kennedy SH. Combining mirtazapine and duloxetine in treatment–resistant depression improves outcomes and sexual function. *J ClinPsychopharmacol* 2008;28:107–108.
48. Kopeykina I, Kim H-J, Khatun T, et al. Hypersexuality and couple relationships in bipolar disorder: A review. *J Affect Disord* 2016;195:1–14.
49. Vanwesenbeeck I, Have MT, de Graaf R. Associations between common mental disorders and sexual dissatisfaction in the general population. *Br J Psychiatry* 2014;205:151–157.
50. Haddad PM, Wieck A. Antipsychotic-induced hyperprolactinaemia: Mechanisms, clinical features and management. *Drugs* 2004;64:2291–2314.
51. Raja M, Azzoni A. Sexual behavior and sexual problems among patients with severe chronic psychoses. *Eur Psychiatry* 2003;18:70–76.
52. Spalt, L. Sexual behavior and affective disorders. *Disease of the Nervous System* 1975;36(12):644–647.
53. Downey J, Friedman RC, Haase E, et al. Comparison of sexual experience and behavior between bipolar outpatients and outpatients without mood disorders. *Psychiatry J* 2016;2016:5839181.
54. Chen LP, Murad MH, Paras ML, et al. Sexual abuse and lifetime diagnosis of psychiatric disorders: Systematic review and meta-analysis. *Mayo Clin Proc* 2010;85:618–629.

55. Romero S, Birmaher B, Axelson D, et al. Prevalence and correlates of physical and sexual abuse in children and adolescents with bipolar disorder. *J Affect Disord* 2009;112:144–150.
56. Mazza M, Harnic D, Catalano V, et al. Sexual behavior in women with bipolar disorder. *J Affect Disord* 2011;131:364–367.
57. Fountoulakis KN, Kasper S, Andreassen O, et al. Efficacy of pharmacotherapy in bipolar disorder: A report by the WPA section on pharmacopsychiatry. *Eur Arch Psychiatry Clin Neurosci* 2012;262:1–48.
58. Elnazer HY, Sampson A, Baldwin D. Lithium and sexual dysfunction: An under-researched area. *Hum Psychopharmacol Clin Exp* 2015;30:66–69.
59. Zuncheddu C, Carpiniello B. Sexual dysfunctions and bipolar disorder: A study of patients submitted to a long-term lithium treatment. *Clin Ter* 2006;157:419–424.
60. Dols A, Sienaert P, van Gerven H, et al. The prevalence and management of side effects of lithium and anticonvulsants as mood stabilizers in bipolar disorder from a clinical perspective. *Int Clin Psychopharmacol* 2013; 28:287–296.
61. Kesebir S, Toprak B, Baykaran B, et al. The level of awareness on sexually transmitted diseases of patients with bipolar mood disorder and patients with heroine dependence. *N€oro Psikiyatr Ars ivi* 2014;51:242–247.
62. Pacchiarotti I, Murru A, Kotzalidis GD et al. Hyperprolactinemia and medications for bipolar disorder: Systematic review of a neglected issue in clinical practice. *Eur Neuropsychopharmacol* 2015;25:1045–1059.
63. Verrotti A, Mencaroni E, Cofini M, et al. Valproic acid metabolism and its consequences on sexual functions. *Curr Drug Metab* 2016;17:573–581.
64. Murru A, Popovic D, Pacchiarotti I, et al. Management of adverse effects of mood stabilizers. *Curr Psychiatry Rep* 2015;17:66.
65. Pavone C, Giacalone N, Vella M, et al. Relation between sexual dysfunctions and epilepsy, type of epilepsy, type of antiepileptic drugs: a prospective study. *Urologia* 2017;84:88–92.
66. Figueira I, Possidente E, Marques C, Hayes K. Sexual dysfunction: A neglected complication of panic disorder and social phobia. *Arch Sex Behav* 2001;30:369–377.
67. Bodinger L, Hermesh H, Aizenberg D, Valevski A, Marom S, Shiloh R, Gothelf D, Zemishlany Z, Weizman A. Sexual function and behavior in social phobia. *J Clin Psychiatry* 2002;63:874–879.
68. Kotler M, Cohen H, Aizenberg D, Matar M, Loewenthal U, Kaplan Z, Miodownik H, Zemishlany Z. Sexual dysfunction in male posttraumatic stress disorder patients. *Psychother Psychosom* 2000;69:309–315.
69. Raboch J, Faltus F. Sexuality of women with anorexia nervosa. *Acta Psychiatr Scand* 1991;84:9–11.
70. Pelsser R. Separation anxiety and intrusion anxiety in borderline personality. *Information Psychiatrique* 1989;65:1001–1009.
71. Zeiss AM, Davis HD, Wood M, Tinklenberg JR. The incidence and correlates of erectile problem in patient with Alzheimers disease. *Arch Sex Behav* Aug 1990;19(4):325–331.
72. Sathyanarayana Rao TS, Ismail S, Darshan MS, Tandon A. Sexual disorders among elderly: An epidemiological study in south Indian rural population. *Indian J Psychiatry* 2015;57:236–241.
73. Sathyanarayana Rao TS, Ismail S, Darshan MS, Tandon A. Sexual disorders among elderly: An epidemiological study in south Indian rural population. *Indian J Psychiatry* 2015;57:236–241.
74. Hartmans C, Comijs H, Jonker C. Cognitive functioning and its influence on sexual behavior in normal aging and dementia. *Int J Geriatr Psychiatry* 2014;29:441–446.

11
Optimising Patient Care in Psychiatry With Autonomy and Choice

Richard M. Duffy, Deshwinder S. Sidhu and Brendan D. Kelly

Introduction	110
Limiting Coercive Practices: General Principles	111
Capacity	*111*
Capacity Assessments	*112*
Informed Consent	*112*
Limiting Coercive Practices for Individuals With Severe Illness	113
Advance Directives	*113*
Ulysses Clause	*113*
Nominated Representatives	*114*
Decision-Making	*114*
The Case for Involuntary Treatment	115
Limiting Coercion for Individuals Receiving Involuntary Treatment	116
Special Consideration	118
Women's Reproductive and Sexual Health	*118*
Minors	*119*
Conclusion	119
Acknowledgements	120

INTRODUCTION

Historically, much of the treatment for mental health conditions occurred without an individual's consent (Killaspy, 2006). Many of the old asylums only admitted individuals on an involuntary basis, and only later were provisions made for individuals who chose to be there. Consequently, much early mental health legislation addressed substitute decision-making and supported involuntary admission and treatment. Even today, many jurisdictions' mental health law only considers involuntary patients in detail (e.g., Ireland's Mental Health Act, 2001). This may be partly explained as a remnant from a time when the majority of psychiatric practice occurred on an inpatient basis.

Not until the deinstitutionalisation at the end of the asylum era were comprehensive outpatient services developed for individuals with mental health problems. While the majority of coercive practices now occur in inpatient settings, significant coercion can be present in community-based treatment too (Sheehan, 2009; World Health Organization, 2019a). This has been legally formalised in over 75 jurisdictions through community treatment orders (Rugkåsa, 2016).

The role of involuntary treatment is falling under increased scrutiny since the beginning of the twenty-first century. This is predominantly driven by the United Nations (UN) Convention on the Rights of Persons with Disabilities (CRPD) (2006). The first of the 'General principles' affirmed in Article 3 of the CRPD is 'respect for inherent dignity, individual autonomy including the freedom to make one's own choices, and independence of persons'. This has clear relevance in psychiatry.

The most important article in terms of protecting autonomy is Article 12, which refers to equal recognition before the law. It appears to be possible to comply with Article 12 and still make provisions for involuntary treatment (Caldas de Almeida, 2019; Callaghan and Ryan, 2014). However, the UN Committee on the Rights of Persons with Disabilities, which interprets the CPRD, states that Article 12 prohibits *all* involuntary treatment *and* substitute decision-making (2014). It is unclear how this *non sequitur* was arrived at by the Committee (Craigie et al., 2019). Many countries ratified the CRPD with formal reservations against this article, thus stripping it of some of its power (Dawson, 2015).

In addition to these two articles, Article 14 of the CRPD addresses liberty and the security of the person; Article 15 provides protection from torture or cruel, inhuman or degrading treatment or punishment; Article 16 addresses freedom from exploitation, violence and abuse, and Article 17 protects the integrity of the person. The World Health Organisation (WHO) has embraced this emphasis on autonomy and patient choice. Its QualityRights initiative aims to realise an individual-centred, rights-based approach to mental healthcare (WHO, 2012).

Against this background, this chapter examines how individuals' autonomy and preferences can be maximised both in general and during episodes of illness. It puts forward the case for involuntary treatment and discusses how individuals can continue to exercise agency during episodes of such treatment. Women in the perinatal period and minors are given particular consideration due to their vulnerability to coercive practices. Finally, key general underlying principles are highlighted, and consideration is given to local legislation.

LIMITING COERCIVE PRACTICES: GENERAL PRINCIPLES

Capacity

As described, autonomy and choice are key to empowering individuals with mental health difficulties. The concept of capacity is central to helping an individual exercise their autonomy. Many psychiatrists are familiar with assessing capacity, but to optimise the treatment of individuals attending mental health services, psychiatry needs to focus instead on building capacity. Before this discussion is developed, it is important to define both mental and legal capacity, as the term 'capacity' can refer to either concept (UN Committee on the Rights of Persons with Disabilities, 2014). 'Mental capacity' is a measure of someone's ability to make decisions and is dependent on many factors. 'Legal capacity' is 'the ability to hold rights and duties (legal standing) and to exercise those rights and duties (legal agency)' (p. 3).

Historically, these two concepts of capacity were treated synonymously, and capacity was often seen as both global and static. Indeed, this is still the case in many jurisdictions. An individual was either judged to have decision-making capacity or to lack it. This approach hugely limited, or removed, the individual's legal capacity, and once this determination was made, it was very hard to reverse (Zaubler et al., 1996). Thankfully, mental capacity is increasingly seen as decision specific and something that changes over time. Also, the concept of mental capacity itself is coming under increased scrutiny (WHO, 2019b), and its direct implications for legal capacity are being reduced. Much of what is discussed in this chapter can be conceptualised as steps to promote the legal capacity of individuals with impaired decision-making capacity.

Capacity is widely discussed and emphasised in the CRPD (UN, 2006), and it is given further attention in the UN Committee on the Rights of Persons with Disabilities (2014). These provisions are affirmed by the WHO, which promotes individuals' 'right to exercise their legal capacity on other issues affecting them, including their treatment and care' (p. 8) (WHO, 2013). Many of the practicalities of building capacity are also discussed by the QualityRights Initiative (WHO, 2012, 2019b).

As a result of these provisions, it is important that mental health services promote decision-making ability even when individuals are receiving involuntary treatment. Active encouragement to make decisions and state preferences may be necessary, as individuals may be reluctant to express their views, especially if they feel they might be controversial (Woltmann and Whitley, 2010). Mental health professionals also have a role in advocating for individuals to make choices outside of those relating to treatment options. This may be uncomfortable, as professionals may feel that some of this lies outside of their range of expertise. Additional support may therefore be needed to help people make decisions in relation to, *inter alia*, employment, housing, property ownership, financial matters, parenting and family life. Collaboration with social workers, mental health advocacy groups or legal professionals may be of benefit in this context.

In a manner similar to assessing capacity, building capacity can focus on four key areas: understanding, reasoning, appreciation and expression of choice (Grisso et al., 1997). To promote understanding, information can be presented in a manner that is easily understandable and consideration given to the person's level of educational attainment, learning styles, literacy and culture (Marcus, 2014). The other domains of capacity can be supported by providing individuals with additional time, optimising their treatment and facilitating informal support from friends, family and advocates. It is important to be aware that the relationship between the decision-maker and health professional can be more influential than the information provided; this situation has both advantages and disadvantages (Woltmann and Whitley, 2010). More formal supports are discussed in the following.

Capacity Assessments

Before any assessment of capacity occurs, it is vital that individuals be given every opportunity to accurately represent themselves. As mentioned, the WHO's QualityRights Initiative holds that mental capacity testing is an invalid concept, as it cannot be measured scientifically, often leads to a denial of legal capacity and is often considered a permanent state (WHO, 2019b). Even with the benefit of the CRPD, the assessment of capacity is a highly complex endeavour, and a large element of subjectivity is inescapable (Keene, 2017). Researchers have attempted to overcome the lack of scientific validity through the use of standardised tools such as the MacArthur Competence Assessment Tool (Grisso et al., 1997).

Capacity assessments are also disproportionately applied to people with mental health problems (Series and Nilsson, 2018). An individual without a mental illness is often free to make a choice perceived by others as poor without having their mental capacity called into question. Even in individuals with illnesses that are seen as chronic and enduring, a high level of mental capacity is still retained (Hostiuc et al., 2018). Consequently, it is vital that capacity assessments not be influenced by the diagnosis but by objective findings.

Informed Consent

Informed consent is the main mechanism through which autonomy is protected in the context of healthcare (Murray, in press). Once a mental health professional has supported an individual in optimising their decision-making capacity, it is important that informed consent be sought for any proposed treatment. The clinician is required to convey information that a judicious patient would require, including risks, benefits and alternative options (Cordasco, 2013; Darby and Weinstock, 2018). Seeking informed consent facilitates the therapeutic alliance, enhances trust and increases both patient and doctor satisfaction (Wolf-Braun and Wilke, 2015).

Even when an individual is unable to give fully informed consent, it is important that their perspective be considered. An individual's decision-making capacity may change over time, so it may be important to revisit the decision when indicated. As people improve clinically, they may be able to provide fuller consent, understand more of their treatment options or change their mind. It is important that a lack of decision-making capacity not deprive an individual of treatment options.

LIMITING COERCIVE PRACTICES FOR INDIVIDUALS WITH SEVERE ILLNESS

The measures described in this section can be used with all individuals attending mental health services. They are, however, of greater relevance to people with severe mental illness, who are more likely to experience coercive practices. These measures should also be considered for individuals who have been subject to involuntary treatment in the past and for those at increased risk of involuntary treatment in the future (Barnett et al., 2019). In these circumstances, creating an advance directive (AD), appointing nominated representatives and considering a framework for supporting decision-making may be of great value. Even in jurisdictions where there is no legal provision for such tools, these steps can still inform treatment and reduce coercion.

Advance Directives

An AD is a statement made by an individual with decision-making capacity that states how they would like to be treated and/or who they would like to support them should they lose their decision-making ability (Zelle et al., 2015). The QualityRights Initiative is supportive of advance planning documents (WHO, 2019c), and many jurisdictions are making formal legal provisions to this end; India is a good example (Duffy and Kelly, 2019). The use of coercive measures is reduced in individuals with ADs and, in addition to promoting autonomy during an episode of illness, there is evidence that creating an AD within a therapeutic alliance enhances autonomy (Nicaise et al., 2013).

Individuals find the experience of creating an AD to be meaningful and often express positive choices that can inform difficult decisions in the future (Lenagh-Glue et al., 2020; Shields et al., 2013). Despite clinicians' concerns (Duffy et al., 2019), the majority of people make ADs that are in line with the advice of their treating team (Gowda et al., 2018; Shields et al., 2013). While ADs are well accepted by patients, however, rates of utilisation are low (Gowda et al., 2018). Making an advance directive does not need to be time consuming (Philip et al., 2019a), and uptake can be greatly enhanced by assistance from clinicians (Zelle et al., 2015).

Careful consideration needs to be given to when an individual makes an AD because poor insight or residual symptoms can influence the directive (Gowda et al., 2018). It is important that ADs be as comprehensive as possible and include treatments that the person does not want to receive as well as other domains outside of mental healthcare (e.g., children, property) (WHO, 2019c). Both legislation and individual ADs should consider the contexts in which they want the directives to come into force and the process of deactivating an AD.

Ulysses Clause

For ADs to give meaningful protection, they arguably require a mechanism to prevent individuals from voiding them during an episode of illness. This may take the form of a capacity assessment or a 'Ulysses clause' (Dresser, 1984). In a Ulysses clause, an individual declares 'that what they have stated in their advance plan should take precedence over their stated wishes and preferences during specific future events' (p. 50) (WHO, 2019c). This tool is yet to be established as a commonly used legal mechanism, and the clear limitations of such clauses need to be clarified. It is beneficial to discuss context in which individuals would like to reconsider their ADs and what protections would they like to see in place should they wish to revoke them during an episode of illness. ADs, including Ulysses clauses, should be regularly reviewed, in particular following an episode of illness.

Nominated Representatives

An NR is a trusted person who best interprets a mental health service-user's will and preference where all other actions have failed to directly obtain the will and preference of the person (WHO, 2019c). This may be due to situations where the service-user is in a state of coma or has profound communication impairment. The WHO (2019b) highlights that, even in such challenging circumstances, 'we must always strive to find ways to ensure that people have the final say in all decisions concerning their lives' (p. 2). The articulation of preference might not always be verbal and might involve close family or relatives who were aware of an individual's preferences, an NR and/or an AD.

It is important to note that NRs are not substitute decision-makers. Rather, they play a supportive role in clarifying and advocating for the service-user's will and preference (WHO, 2019c). An NR can be elected in an AD or included in separate document, such as a care plan or clinical notes. NRs can be revoked and replaced by another preference at any time, although protections like those discussed in relation to a Ulysses clause might need to be considered. An additional NR should be selected if the primary NR is unreachable. An NR is generally a close friend or relative who respects the will and preference of the service-user; they should be easily available and accessible (Jeste et al., 2018). It should be possible for individuals to choose who does and does not support them in their decision-making. If someone wishes not to have a family member support their decision, this should be respected, especially where this view is consistently held outside the context of illness (Duffy and Kelly, 2017a). To avoid any conflict of interest, the WHO recommends excluding mental health and social service staff (WHO, 2019c). In circumstances where no supportive person is available, an independent person such as an advocate can be appointed temporarily. All measures are then taken to obtain information about the service-user's beliefs, will and preferences (WHO, 2019c).

A good model that has adopted many of these principles is seen in Ireland's new mental capacity legislation (which has yet to be implemented). Ireland's Assisted Decision-Making (Capacity) Act, 2015, recognises a three-level model of decision-making support, depending on the needs of the decider. This support ranges from assistance and provision of information to a court-appointed representative attempting to ascertain the decider's will and preference (Kelly, 2017). The Indian Mental Healthcare Act 2017 provides another example of legislative provisions for NRs (Philip et al., 2019b).

NRs have the potential to significantly enhance service-user care, satisfaction and autonomy during periods of severe illness. They may help reduce the risk of conflict within families, ensure prompt interventions and avoid the exploitation of vulnerable service-users. Careful protections are, however, required to ensure that an NR does not abuse their role.

Decision-Making

ADs and NRs are two of the key constructs in promoting the transition from substitute to supported decision-making. Moving from acting in someone's 'best interests' to acting in line with their 'rights, will and preference' is integral to this transition. Article 12 of the

CRPD mandates states to ensure that service-users have access to a range of supports to make their own decisions. This includes friends, family, advocates and many others. The QualityRights Initiative suggests a number of additional mechanisms, including a circle of support (Australia and United Kingdom), personal ombudsperson (Sweden), personal assistance and open dialogue (Finland) (WHO, 2019c).

A circle of support revolves around the service-user who invites people to be part of the circle and navigates the direction of the circle. The group supports and helps the service-user towards their goal. Formal research on this topic is highly limited, but these circles are extensively used in the United Kingdom (Circles Network, 2018).

Personal ombudsperson is a model used by non-governmental organisations in Sweden and involves a long-term relationship of trust in which a skilled person supports and assists the service-user with a range of matters relating to family, housing, employment and accessibility to services (Jesperson, 2013).

Open dialogue is a needs-based, service-user–initiated approach to mental healthcare that emphasises dialogue and shared understanding between service-users and their support networks (Twamley et al., 2020). It involves an open discussion between all participants, with an emphasis on the service-user's voice. This process enables sharing of information and better understanding to grow within the group. It has been used to attempt to reduce medication use and hospital admission for people with mental illness.

All of these constructs revolve around the fundamental idea of supporting the service-user to exercise their autonomy and replacing the substitute decision-making model. Mental health services can further facilitate supported-decision making by ensuring accessibility to relevant NGOs, advocates and peer support groups. Supported decision-making is a voluntary process and requires appropriate safeguarding measures that may include limiting the time-period of the acting supporter; involving non-profiting, non-conflicting supporters; and electing independent supporters only.

THE CASE FOR INVOLUNTARY TREATMENT

A full exploration of the case for involuntary treatment is outside the boundaries of this chapter. However, some of the key arguments are put forward here. Not all UN and WHO organisations agree with the current position of the Committee on the Rights of Persons with Disabilities (Szmukler, 2019). The interpretation of the committee might well exceed the intent of the CRPD (Craigie et al., 2019; Independent Review of the Mental Health Act 1983, 2018). Freeman and colleagues (2015) argue that its interpretation might actually undermine the rights of people with mental illness. Untreated illness would erode rights to health, liberty, justice and even possibly life.

It is unclear if the total prohibition of involuntary treatment is what the majority of people receiving treatment want. Surveys of service-users have shown support for the possibility of coercive measures when other options have been exhausted (Szmukler, 2019). Pathare and colleagues (2015) found that a significant majority of service-users recognise the need for a degree of coercion during periods of impaired decision-making. This supports the argument that there has been a lack of consultation between the Committee on the Rights of Persons with Disabilities and the full range of service-users (Freeman et al., 2015). The committee also excluded experienced clinicians. The UN and WHO agenda appears to be more ideologically driven than evidence based (Craigie et al., 2019). It is also unclear what would replace involuntary treatment and what the implications of such a change would be for people with severe mental illness.

The false belief that mental illness is untreatable and the overestimation of the association between mental illness and violence contribute to discrimination against, and stigmatisation of, people with experience of mental illness. Allowing individuals with very severe mental illness to remain untreated may perpetuate these stigmatising stereotypes (Appelbaum, 2019). Posing a risk to others remains one of the common grounds for involuntary treatment internationally, and the removal of this legal provision could lead to an increase in violence associated with mental illness.

In addition to contributing to fear and stigmatisation, this would also lead to the criminalisation of individuals with mental illness – something of which the WHO's QualityRights programme appears to be worryingly accepting (Duffy and Kelly, in press). Even in the absence of increased violence, a significant increase in the prevalence of untreated psychosis in the community would feed the myth that mental illness is untreatable and increase levels of fear and marginalisation. Scholten and Gather (2017) convincingly argue that this actually diminishes the autonomy of the person deprived of treatment.

If formal involuntary treatment were to be abolished, there is a high likelihood that coercion would be shifted from independent professionals to family members, who might engage in coercive practices when medical professionals cannot (Duffy and Kelly, 2017b). Untreated illness puts a further burden on families and cares and could curtail their rights to health or life either directly (through violence) or indirectly in other ways (Freeman, 2015).

LIMITING COERCION FOR INDIVIDUALS RECEIVING INVOLUNTARY TREATMENT

The absolutist stance concerning autonomy adopted by the QualityRights initiative and the Committee on the Rights of Persons with Disabilities does not reflect the legal reality in many jurisdictions, where involuntary treatment remains a core component of mental healthcare. Until clear alternative pathways for the management of individuals with severe mental illness are found, involuntary treatment will remain a feature in many jurisdictions. Consequently, it is important to consider protections during involuntary care. The WHO's 'Resource Book on Mental Health, Human Rights and Legislation' was published before the CRPD and considers protections in this context (WHO, 2005).

It is vital that the assessment on which involuntary admission is based be comprehensive and carried out by appropriately trained senior clinicians, acting within the local legislative provisions (WHO, 2005). Where this has not occurred during the admission process, it is essential that the admitting team rectify this situation immediately. Ideally, the assessment should be done by two independent practitioners. There must be clear evidence of a mental disorder, but admission should be based on the current clinical presentation rather than the diagnosis. Particularly careful consideration should be given to the involuntary admission of individuals with substance misuse or a personality disorder, even in jurisdictions that permit these as grounds for involuntary admission (Opsal et al., 2019; Stapleton and Wright, 2019).

Once the individual no longer meets the criteria for involuntary detention, their admission status should be changed, and they should be informed. Involuntary treatment should last only for as short a period as possible (WHO, 2005).

It is essential that people who are subject to involuntary admission have a right to appeal any admission or treatment that they feel is unwarranted or unjust. This appeal process should be both timely and independent. The involuntary patient themselves might not be in a position to initiate the appeal, so it is important that there be mandatory automatic independent review procedures (Deshpande et al., 2008; WHO, 2005). Where this is not necessitated by legislation, it can be conducted informally. This process should include an initial evaluation followed by periodic reviews. Free legal representation is needed for the review and appeal process to be effective.

The least restrictive practice should always be adopted and, as part of this, community-based and voluntary treatment options should be exhausted prior to considering involuntary admission and treatment. An individual who is subject to involuntary treatment still has a right to comprehensive information about the proposed treatment plan, and their assent should still be sought (WHO, 2005). Some of the harmful effects of coercive treatments can be mitigated by the establishment of supportive relationships with the individual, creating a sense of safety, protecting their rights and fostering a sense of agency (Wyder et al., 2016).

Seclusion or restraint, if used, should occur under close scrutiny, the indications should be recorded and details of each episode should be carefully documented. The use of seclusion and restraint can be reduced through staff counselling and training; enhanced communication and risk assessment; service-user participation; and careful analysis of all episodes of violence, seclusion and restraint (Dahm et al., 2017; Black et al., 2020). Additional layers of review should be present for electro-convulsive therapy or psychosurgery, and these processes should, again, be comprehensive and independent.

Community treatment orders (CTOs) have long been controversial, not least because the evidence in favour of them is sparse (Kisely et al., 2017), and there is significant evidence against effectiveness (Pai and Vella, 2016). Notwithstanding these facts, CTOs still have a degree of face validity owing to the fact that the community appears to be a less restrictive environment than a hospital. As a result, and despite their questionable evidence base, CTOs are used in over 70 jurisdictions worldwide (Mikellides et al., 2019).

Pridham and colleagues (2016) usefully highlight the fact that coercive elements of CTOs can be minimised, even when CTOs are used. In order to do this, they suggest enhancing patient access to information, fostering better relationships between service-providers and service-users and making the CTO process fair and transparent. Even when a CTO is in place, extensive consideration should still be given to the individual's preferences, and, where possible, these should be accommodated. For example, a person who is on an antipsychotic and unhappy about weight gain could be switched to an alternative medication, as clinically indicated (Alonso-Pedrero, 2019).

Where CTOs exist, it is important that their procedural protections mirror those received by individuals who are admitted on an involuntary basis so that deinstitutionalisation is not undermined by CTOs (WHO, 2005). CTOs should be an alternative to involuntary inpatient care rather than an alternative to voluntary community care. The use of CTOs in the context of the criminal justice system is outside the scope of this chapter but presents a range of complex issues of its own.

In jurisdictions that permit coercive treatments, clinicians should consider using them if and only if they are needed, especially in incidences associated with risk or adverse outcomes. However, extensive steps should be taken where possible to minimise restrictive practices and to facilitate the agency of the individual. This process can take a variety of forms (as discussed above) and is often most effective during periods of remission.

It is also important to consider the position of non-protesting patients who lack mental capacity who are considered voluntary patients in many jurisdictions (such as Ireland). These individuals might remain in hospital without protest, but this might not be the result of a fully informed decision. While 'voluntary' status in this situation might appear less restrictive, these people might be deprived of the statutory review and protective processes available to involuntary patients.

As a result, it is essential that 'voluntary' non-protesting patients who lack mental capacity receive the same level of protection as involuntary patients (WHO, 2005). This can occur through the periodic review of non-protesting patients or by acknowledging that they are not voluntary patients. India's Mental Healthcare Act, 2017 requires that an individual seeking an independent (voluntary) admission has the 'capacity to make mental healthcare and treatment decisions' or requires minimal support in doing so (Section 85).

This kind of protection enhances the rights of non-protesting patients, although it could also be seen as more restrictive, because such patients might now be classified as supported (involuntary) patients. In a similar manner, voluntary patients who would be detained in the event that they express a desire to leave might be considered to have more legal protection (e.g., a right to review, appeal or legal representation) if they are formally detained. It is important that voluntary patients know their rights and that they are free to leave but that they can be detained if they meet certain, clearly defined criteria (WHO, 2005).

SPECIAL CONSIDERATION

Women's Reproductive and Sexual Health

'Women with disabilities may face even more denial of their right to legal capacity as a result of multiple discrimination', according to the WHO (2019b, p. 7). While Article 6 of the CRPD places an onus on states to address this issue, many barriers still limit female reproductive and family rights. Women with mental illness often experience additional restrictions that impact, *inter alia*, access to family planning services, obstetric interventions (Halliday, 2019; Murray, in press) and custody of children (Weller, 2019). Historically, the limitation of these rights was overtly stated in laws such as British Columbia's Sexual Sterilization Act, 1933, and India's Special Marriage Act, 1954. Fourteen countries had legislation permitting involuntary sterilisation, many on the grounds of mental illness (Amy and Rowlands, 2018). This form of discrimination has not totally ended: as recently as the 1990s, China introduced legislation permitting the sterilisation of individuals with mental illness (Pearson, 1995).

The complexity of ethics in relation to pregnancy cannot be underestimated and is often done a great disservice by reductionistic ideological perspectives (Kingma, 2018). For the pregnant woman, there is a complex, nuanced balancing of rights and duties which different jurisdictions, cultures and philosophies commonly seek to influence, often by utilising blunt instruments (Rosamund, 2002). While many jurisdictions (e.g., United Kingdom) have established that pregnancy should not inhibit any legal protections for the woman, this position is still far from universally accepted (Murray, in press).

It is essential that women's reproductive health, sexual health and potential role as a parent be considered during interactions with mental health services, not just in a *post hoc* manner when an issue arises (McGuire et al, in press). Women's preferences about contraception, pregnancy, breastfeeding, sexual health, sexual expression and parenting may need to be part of a mental health assessment and, where necessary, should inform their treatment. By considering these during initial assessment, choice and autonomy can be greatly enhanced. Services also need to identify if they limit access to termination of pregnancy and, while this is highly heterogeneous internationally, it is important that mental illness not be used as grounds to reduce access to services.

Article 23 of the CRPD protects the rights to marry, found a family and access family planning; it also prohibits forced sterilisation. An onus is placed on states to 'render appropriate assistance to persons with disabilities in the performance of their child-rearing responsibilities'. The CRPD states that children should only be separated from their parents 'when competent authorities subject to judicial review determine, in accordance with applicable law and procedures, that such separation is necessary for the best interests of the child'.

Another key principle with respect to the right to a family is that parenting ability should not be called into question on the basis of a diagnosis alone. Until recently the majority of the literature on this theme focused on the risk posed by mothers with mental illness, but this approach has now shifted towards describing the capabilities of mothers with mental illness (Weller, 2019). Paradoxically, it can be fear of appraisal and judgement that prevents mothers from seeking treatment for mental illness; this can lead to a major relapse resulting in concerns being raised about child safety. It is important that mental health services emphasise their desire to support mothers in parenting and advocate on their behalf. All of these considerations are even more complex when providing healthcare to individuals with intellectual disability. Kong (2019) discusses the many injustices, competing guiding principles and highly nuanced balances that arise in this context.

Minors

Minors also deserve specific consideration. The general shift from substitute to supported decision-making is more ambiguous and complex in minors, with respect to whom greater degrees of substitute decision-making still occur. When dealing with adults, the guiding principle is the 'rights, will and preference' of the individual, but when dealing with minors, the CRPD states that the 'best interests' of the child shall be paramount (Articles 7 and 23).

Article 7 of the CRPD gives children with disabilities

> the right to express their views freely on all matters affecting them, their views being given due weight in accordance with their age and maturity, on an equal basis with other children, and to be provided with disability and age-appropriate assistance to realize that right.

Children and adolescents have demonstrated high levels of decision-making capacity from the age of 12 years, suggesting that additional weight should be given to their preferences at younger ages than is currently common practice (Hein et al., 2015).

The final general principle in Article 3 of the CRPD is 'respect for the evolving capacities of children with disabilities and respect for the right of children with disabilities to preserve their identities.' This highlights the need to include minors in the decision-making process. Assent to treatment should be sought and, where this is not given, a clear rationale provided for clinical decisions. Katz et al. (2016) provide a comprehensive discussion of this topic in a medical context. The presence of mental health difficulties adds an additional layer of complexity. Preferences have to be balanced with the views of parents, guardians and professionals and considered in the context of the child's capacity and local legislation.

CONCLUSION

The WHO QualityRights initiative and CRPD provide valuable guidance on protecting the rights of persons with mental illness. They promote the realisation of increased autonomy and choice for individuals with mental illness and offer protection from coercion and exploitation. Healthcare providers have a key role to play in building and promoting the decision-making capacity of individuals attending services, thus optimising care. Mental capacity is a dynamic, decision-specific concept, so, even in jurisdictions that do not conceptualise it in this way, efforts should continually be made to enhance capacity through both formal and informal supports.

Individuals who have experienced coercive practices or who are likely to have episodes of severe illness should be encouraged to take practical steps to plan for future episodes of illness in order to maximise their future autonomy. These practical steps might include making advance directives, nominating individuals who can support their decision-making and undertaking educational activities that will promote self-advocacy and insight and reduce risk of relapse. Substitute decision-making should be replaced with supported decision-making wherever possible, and an individual's rights, will and preference should be the guiding principles. Individuals should not be prohibited from making decisions simply because others perceive them as unwise.

There is currently no coherent, implementable framework for the complete abolition of all involuntary treatment. Situations may arise that necessitate coercive measures, and where this occurs, it is vital that procedures be in place to protect the rights of individuals receiving treatment. These include a right to appeal decisions, an automatic review process and free legal representation.

Legislation is an inherent part of psychiatry. Consequently, it is vital that we advocate for positive change in legislation that promotes individual autonomy and ensures access to treatment for individuals with mental illness. It is unacceptable and unjust that individuals can have no entitlement to treatment for mild symptoms of mental illness but can be treated against their will when symptoms reach a certain threshold. If involuntary treatment is permitted within a jurisdiction, it is vital that there also be a right to voluntary mental healthcare.

ACKNOWLEDGEMENTS

The authors are very grateful to everyone who assisted them with their research work and to the editors of this volume for inviting this chapter. We are particularly grateful to Soumitra Pathare for his time and wisdom and to the Centre for Mental Health Law & Policy. We would also like to thank the Ethics, Law and Pregnancy in Ireland Network based out of University College Cork.

References

Alonso-Pedrero L, Bes-Rastrollo M, Marti A. Effects of antidepressant and antipsychotic use on weight gain: A systematic review. *Obesity Reviews* 2019;20:1680–1690.
Amy JJ, Rowlands S. Legalised non-consensual sterilisation—eugenics put into practice before 1945, and the aftermath. Part 1: USA, Japan, Canada and Mexico. *European Journal of Contraception Reproductive Health Care* 2018;23:121–129.
Appelbaum PS. Saving the UN convention on the rights of persons with disabilities–from itself. *World Psychiatry* 2019;18:1–2.
Barnett P, Mackay E, Matthews H, Gate R, Greenwood H, Ariyo K, Bhui K, Halvorsrud K, Pilling S, Smith S. Ethnic variations in compulsory detention under the Mental Health Act: A systematic review and meta-analysis of international data. *Lancet Psychiatry* 2019;6:305–317.
Black V, Bobier C, Thomas B, Prest F, Ansley C, Loomes B, Eggleston G, Mountford H. Reducing seclusion and restraint in a child and adolescent inpatient area: Implementation of a collaborative problem-solving approach. *Australasian Psychiatry* 2020:1039856220917081.
Caldas de Almeida JM. The CRPD Article 12, the limits of reductionist approaches to complex issues and the necessary search for compromise. *World Psychiatry* 2019;18:46–47.
Callaghan SM, Ryan C. Is there a future for involuntary treatment in rights-based mental health law? *Psychiatry, Psychology and Law* 2014;21:747–766.
Circles Network. *2017–2018 Impact report.* Rugby: Circles Network, 2018.
Cordasco KM. Obtaining informed consent from patients: Brief update review. *Making Health Care Safer II: An Updated Critical Analysis of the Evidence for Patient Safety Practices* 2013:461–470.
Craigie J, Bach M, Gurbai S, Kanter A, Kim SYH, Lewis O, Morgan G. Legal capacity, mental capacity and supported decision-making: Report from a panel event. *International Journal of Law and Psychiatry* 2019;62:160–168.
Dahm KT, Steiro AK, Leiknes KA, Husum TL, Kirkehei I, Dalsbø TK, Brurberg KG. *Interventions for reducing seclusion and restraint in mental health care for adults: A systematic review.* Oslo: Knowledge Centre for the Health Services at The Norwegian Institute of Public Health, 2017.

Darby WC, Weinstock R. The limits of confidentiality: Informed consent and psychotherapy. *Focus* 2018;16:395–401.

Dawson J. A realistic approach to assessing mental health laws' compliance with the UNCRPD. *International Journal of Law and Psychiatry* 2015;40:70–79.

Deshpande N, Morton T, Haque S, Oyebode F. Appeals to the mental health review tribunal in an ageing population. *Medicine, Science and the Law* 2008;48:246–250.

Dresser R. Bound to treatment: The Ulysses contract. *The Hastings Center Report* 1984;14:13–16.

Duffy RM, Gulati G, Paralikar V, Kasar N, Goyal N, De Sousa A, Kelly BD. A focus group study of Indian psychiatrists' views on electroconvulsive therapy under India's Mental Healthcare Act 2017: "The ground reality is different". *Indian Journal of Psychological Medicine* 2019;41:507–515.

Duffy RM, Kelly BD. Privacy, confidentiality and carers: India's harmonization of national guidelines and international mental health law. *Ethics, Medicine and Public Health* 2017a;3:98–106.

Duffy RM, Kelly BD. Concordance of the Indian Mental Healthcare Act 2017 with the World Health Organization's checklist on mental health legislation. *International Journal of Mental Health Systems* 2017b;11:48.

Duffy RM, Kelly BD. India's mental healthcare act, 2017: Content, context, controversy. *International Journal of Law and Psychiatry* 2019;62:169–178.

Duffy RM, Kelly BD. The world health organization and mental health law. In: *India's Mental Healthcare Act, 2017: Building laws, protecting rights*. Ramanujam: Springer Nature, in press.

Freeman MC, Kolappa K, De Almeida JM, Kleinman A, Makhashvili N, Phakathi S, Saraceno B, Thornicroft G. Reversing hard won victories in the name of human rights: A critique of the general comment on article 12 of the UN Convention on the Rights of Persons with Disabilities. *Lancet Psychiatry* 2015;2:844–850.

Gowda GS, Noorthoorn EO, Lepping P, Kumar CN, Nanjegowda RB, Math SB. Factors influencing advance directives among psychiatric inpatients in India. *International Journal of Law and Psychiatry* 2018;56:17–26.

Grisso T, Appelbaum PS, Hill-Fotouhi C. The MacCAT-T: A clinical tool to assess patients' capacities to make treatment decisions. *Psychiatric Services* 1997;48:1415–1419.

Halliday S. Court-ordered obstetric intervention: insight and capacity, a tale of loss. In: C. Pickles, J. Herring (Eds.), *Childbirth, vulnerability and law: Exploring issues of violence and control*. New York: Routledge, 2019.

Hein IM, De Vries MC, Troost PW, Meynen G, Van Goudoever JB, Lindauer RJ. Informed consent instead of assent is appropriate in children from the age of twelve: Policy implications of new findings on children's competence to consent to clinical research. *BMC Medical Ethics* 2015;16:76.

Hostiuc S, Rusu MC, Negoi I, Drima E. Testing decision-making competency of schizophrenia participants in clinical trials: A meta-analysis and meta-regression. *BMC Psychiatry* 2018;18:2.

Independent Review of the Mental Health Act 1983. *Modernising the Mental Health Act: Increasing choice, reducing compulsion*. London: Department of Health and Social Services, 2018.

Jesperson M. Personal ombudsman and supported decision making. *Vertex* 2013;24:460–464.

Jeste DV, Eglit GML, Palmer BW, Martinis JG, Blanck P, Saks ER. Supported decision making in serious mental illness. *Psychiatry* 2018;81:28–40.

Katz AL, Webb SA, Committee on bioethics: Informed consent in decision-making in pediatric practice. *Pediatrics* 2016;138:1–18.

Keene AR. Is mental capacity in the eye of the beholder? *Advances in Mental Health and Intellectual Disabilities* 2017;11:30–39.

Kelly BD. The assisted decision-making (capacity) act 2015: What it is and why it matters. *Irish Journal of Medical Science* 2017;186:351–356.

Killaspy H. From the asylum to community care: Learning from experience. *British Medical Bulletin* 2006;79–80:245–258.

Kingma E. Lady parts: The metaphysics of pregnancy. *Royal Institute of Philosophy Supplement* 2018;82:165–187.

Kisely SR, Campbell LA, O'Reilly R. Compulsory community and involuntary outpatient treatment for people with severe mental disorders. *Cochrane Database of Systematic Reviews* 2017;3:CD004408.

Kong C. Constructing female sexual and reproductive agency in mental capacity law. *International Journal of Law and Psychiatry* 2019;66:101488.

Lenagh-Glue J, Thom K, O'Brien A, Potiki J, Casey H, Dawson J, Glue P. The content of mental health advance preference statements (MAPs): An assessment of completed advance directives in one New Zealand health board. *International Journal of Law and Psychiatry* 2020;68:101537.

Marcus C. Strategies for improving the quality of verbal patient and family education: A review of the literature and creation of the EDUCATE model. *Health Psychology and Behavioural Medicine* 2014;2:482–495.

McGuire E, Curtis C, Duffy RM. Fertile ground: Reproductive health consideration in mental health ward policy. *Irish Journal of Psychological Medicine*, in press.

Mikellides G, Stefani A, Tantele M. Community treatment orders: International perspective. *BJPsych International* 2019;16:83–86.

Murray C. Troubling consent: Pain and pressure in labour and childbirth. In: C. Pickles, J. Herring (Eds.), *Women's birthing bodies and the law: Unauthorised intimate examinations, power and vulnerability*. London: Hart Publishing, in press.

Nicaise P, Lorant V, Dubois V. Psychiatric advance directives as a complex and multistage intervention: A realist systematic review. *Health and Social Care in the Community* 2013;21:1–14.

Opsal A, Kristensen Ø, Clausen T. Readiness to change among involuntarily and voluntarily admitted patients with substance use disorders. *Substance Abuse Treatment, Prevention and Policy* 2019;14:47.

Pai N, Vella SL. Are community treatment orders counterproductive? *Asian Journal of Psychiatry* 2016;23:125–127.

Pathare S, Shields L, Nardodkar R, Narasimhan L, Bunders J. What do service users want? A content analysis of what users may write in psychiatric advance directives in India. *Asian Journal of Psychiatry* 2015;14:52–56.

Pearson V. Population policy and eugenics in China. *British Journal of Psychiatry* 1995;167:1–4.

Philip S, Chandran D, Stezin A, Viswanathaiah GC, Gowda GS, Moirangthem S, Kumar CN, Math SB. EAT-PAD: Educating about psychiatric advance directives in India. *International Journal of Social Psychiatry* 2019a;65:207–216.

Philip S, Rangarajan SK, Moirangthem S, Kumar CN, Gowda MR, Gowda GS, Math SB. Advance directives and nominated representatives: A critique. *Indian Journal of Psychiatry* 2019b;61:S680–S685.

Pridham KM, Berntson A, Simpson AI, Law SF, Stergiopoulos V, Nakhost A. Perception of coercion among patients with a psychiatric community treatment order: A literature review. *Psychiatric Services* 2016;67:16–28.

Rosamund S. The relation of the pregnant woman to the fetus: The interface between her moral rights and duties. In: *Rights, duties and the body: Law and ethics of the maternal – fetal conflict* (pp. 61–106). London: Hart Publishing, 2002.

Rugkåsa J. Effectiveness of community treatment orders: The international evidence. *Canadian Journal of Psychiatry* 2016;61:15–24.

Scholten M, Gather J. Adverse consequences of article 12 of the UN convention on the rights of persons with disabilities for persons with mental disabilities and an alternative way forward. *Journal of Medical Ethics* 2017;4:226–233.

Series L, Nilsson A. Article 12 CRPD: Equal recognition before the law. In I. Bantekas, M. I. Stein, and D. Anastasiou (Eds.), *The UN convention on the rights of persons with disability, a commentary* (pp. 339–382). Oxford: Oxford University Press, 2018.

Sheehan KA. Compulsory treatment in psychiatry. *Current Opinion in Psychiatry* 2009;22:582–586.

Shields LS, Pathare S, van Zelst SD, Dijkkamp S, Narasimhan L, Bunders JG. Unpacking the psychiatric advance directive in low-resource settings: An exploratory qualitative study in Tamil Nadu, India. *International Journal of Mental Health Systems* 2013;7:29.

Stapleton A, Wright N. The experiences of people with borderline personality disorder admitted to acute psychiatric inpatient wards: A meta-synthesis. *Journal of Mental Health* 2019;28: 443–457.

Szmukler G. "Capacity", "best interests", "will and preferences" and the UN convention on the rights of persons with disabilities. *World Psychiatry* 2019;18:34–41.

Twamley I, Dempsey M, Keane N. An open dialogue-informed approach to mental health service delivery: Experiences of service users and support networks. *Journal of Mental Health* 2020;13:1–6.

United Nations. *Convention on the Rights of Persons with Disabilities*. New York: United Nations, 2006.

United Nations Committee on the Rights of Persons with Disabilities. *General comment No. 1: Article 12: Equal recognition before the law*. New York: United Nations, 2014.

Weller P. Mothers and mental illness: Breaking the silence about child loss. *International Journal of Law Psychiatry* 2019;67:101500.

Wolf-Braun B, Wilke HJ. Patientenautonomie und Aufklärung – Ethische und rechtliche Aspekte der Aufklärung. *AINS – Anästhesiologie Intensivmedizin Notfallmedizin Schmerztherapie* 2015;50:202–210.

Woltmann EM, Whitley R. Shared decision making in public mental health care: Perspectives from consumers living with severe mental illness. *Psychiatric Rehabilitation Journal* 2010;34:29–36.

World Health Organization. *WHO resource book on mental health, human rights, and legislation.* Geneva: World Health Organization, 2005.

World Health Organization. *WHO quality rights tool kit to assess and improve quality and human rights in mental health and social care facilities.* Geneva: World Health Organization, 2012.

World Health Organization. *Mental health action plan 2013–2020.* Geneva: World Health Organization, 2013.

World Health Organization. *Freedom from coercion, violence, and abuse: WHO quality rights core training: Mental health and social services: Course guide.* Geneva: World Health Organization, 2019a.

World Health Organization. *Legal capacity and the right to decide: WHO quality rights core training: Mental health and social services: Course guide.* Geneva: World Health Organization, 2019b.

World Health Organization. *Supported decision-making and advance planning: WHO quality rights specialized training: Course guide.* Geneva: World Health Organization, 2019c.

Wyder M, Bland R, Crompton D. The importance of safety, agency and control during involuntary mental health admissions. *Journal of Mental Health* 2016;25:338–342.

Zaubler TS, Viederman M, Fins JJ. Ethical, legal, and psychiatric issues in capacity, competency, and informed consent: An annotated bibliography. *General Hospital Psychiatry* 1996;18:155–172.

Zelle H, Kemp K, Bonnie RJ. Advance directives in mental health care: Evidence, challenges and promise. *World Psychiatry* 2015;14:278–280.

12
Neurocognitive Rehabilitation Program for People With Mild Cognitive Impairment – "Memory Clinic"

*Victor Savilov, Olga Karpenko,
Marat Kurmyshev, George Kostyuk*

Introduction	124
Memory Clinics Within Moscow Mental Health Service	125
General Characteristics of Neurocognitive Rehabilitation Program	126
Neurocognitive Rehabilitation Program	*127*
Neurocognitive Rehabilitation Program Effectiveness	*131*
Electronic Neurocognitive Rehabilitation Program	132
Conclusions	132
Acknowledgements	132

ABBREVIATIONS

CDT – clock drawing test
CT – cognitive training
e-NCRP – electronic neurocognitive rehabilitation program
HADS – Hospital Anxiety and Depression Scale
MCI – mild cognitive impairment
MHIS – Modified Hachinski Ischemic Score
MMSE – mini-mental state examination
MoCA – Montreal Cognitive Assessment
NCRP – neurocognitive rehabilitation program
SF-36 – 36-Item Short Form Health Survey
WHO – World Health Organization

Funding: Russian Foundation of Basic Research, grant 20–04–60546.

INTRODUCTION

The WHO suggests fighting dementia should be a priority of healthcare systems worldwide (WHO, 2012). The prevalence of dementia in 2019 was 50 million cases, with an annual incidence of 10 million cases. In Russia, cognitive deterioration is prevalent in 25% of elderly people (>65 years old); among them, 6–8% have dementia and 16–19% mild and moderate cognitive impairment (Gavrilova, 2014).

Aging of the population is the strongest known risk factor for dementia and cognitive decline. Chronic diseases (cerebrovascular and heart diseases, diabetes, obesity, depression) together with the lifestyle risk factors like social isolation, low cognitive and physical activity, smoking and alcohol consumption are considered modifiable risk factors of cognitive impairment. Although the evidence of preventing dementia by interventions focused on modification of the risk factors remains controversial, attempts at early interventions in the case of cognitive decline have been undertaken (WHO, 2019).

Mild cognitive impairment (MCI) is a condition when preventive interventions might be effective and dementia development might be stopped or postponed. Memory clinics are designed for early detection and treatment of old age cognitive decline. Rehabilitation services for elderly people with cognitive deterioration are available in memory clinics in some countries of the world (Jolley et al., 2006; Gavrilova et al., 2021 in press).

In this chapter, we share our experience of implementation of a neurocognitive rehabilitation program (NCRP and e-NCRP) in memory clinics in Moscow designed for people with MCI.

MEMORY CLINICS WITHIN MOSCOW MENTAL HEALTH SERVICE

Memory clinics in Moscow are based in the rehabilitation departments of the public community mental-health service and organized for the treatment of age-related MCI (Burygina et al., 2019). The staff of one clinic consists of three psychiatrists (one of them is the head of the clinic), six clinical psychologists, one exercise physiologist, three nurses and five paramedics. One clinic has a capacity to treat 50 people within one rehabilitation course. The pilot project of the memory clinic started in 2016 in Moscow (Kostyuk et al., 2017); by 2020 Moscow had eight memory clinics in different parts of the city. All clinics work using the unified treatment algorithm that was developed in the first memory clinic of Moscow. The director of this clinic monitors the work of other clinics in order to maintain the unified methodology of care delivery.

Patients can apply to the treatment program themselves or get a referral from a local general practitioner or the district psychiatrist. Treatment is free of charge for the patients, but they need to meet inclusion criteria for the rehabilitation program: diagnosis of MCI and absence of severe health problems or concurrent mental disorders.

Contraindications for participation are the following:

1. Mild or moderate dementia
2. Acute phase of somatic diseases
3. Pelvic organ dysfunction
4. Anxiety or depression (HADS-A, HADS-D > 10)
5. Severe mental disorders
6. Epilepsy

The eligibility assessment of the patient has several steps. At the first step, all patients who applied for the program undergo a telephone interview with a psychiatrist. The goal of this step is to reveal major contraindications for the program and to inform patients about the rules of participation, content and goals of rehabilitation program. Patients who do not have contraindications and are ready to participate in the program are invited for clinical assessment by the psychiatrist.

At the consultation with the psychiatrist, the medical history is collected and primary scale assessment with MMSE (Folstein et al., 1975), CDT (Eddy and Sriram, 1977) and MHIS (Rosen et al., 1980) is performed. If the patient meets the clinical and scale diagnostic criteria of MCI (24–27 MMSE scores, 8–9 CDT scores), he/she is included in the treatment group.

GENERAL CHARACTERISTICS OF NEUROCOGNITIVE REHABILITATION PROGRAM

All therapeutic interventions in the memory clinic are designed to work with the cognitive, physical and social activation of the patients.

The treatment cycle lasts for 6 weeks, 50–55 people simultaneously participate in the treatment cycle and new participants are enrolled only when the new treatment cycle begins.

During the first week, all participants undergo assessment of cognitive functions using MoCa (Nasreddine et al., 2005), the "remembering of 10 words" test (Luria, 1962). Exclusion of current depression or anxiety is performed using clinical methods and HADS (Zigmond and Snaith, 1983), and assessment of health-related quality of life is performed with the SF-36 scale (Ware Jr and Sherbourne, 1992). An exercise physiologist assess physical activity of the patients; additionally, the Bartel scale is applied (Mahoney and Bartel, 1965). Upon the results of the diagnostics, people who don't meet inclusion criteria of the program are discharged at this point and referred for treatment of the revealed disorders, if needed.

Members of the treatment team distribute participants into six closed groups (8–9 participants in each) according to the diagnostics results. Personality, gender, level of cognitive performance and physical activity are taken into consideration.

The neurocognitive rehabilitation program lasts for 5 weeks, 5 days a week (Monday–Friday) and includes different types of scheduled activities (see Table 12.1):

1. Cognitive training
2. Group psychotherapy
3. Medical gymnastics
4. Medical management

On the sixth week before the discharge from the program, all participants undergo follow-up cognitive assessment using the MoCA, MMSE, CDT scales and SF-36. The desired treatment outcome of the NCRP is improvement of the patients' cognitive functions and cognitive performance, remediation of declined or lost cognitive skills, increase of social

Table 12.1 Daily schedule in a memory clinic.

Time	Activity
08.30–09.00	Breakfast
09.00–09.30	Medical gymnastics
10.00–11.00	Cognitive training
11.00–12.00	Break (cognitive games)
12.00–13.00	Cognitive training
13.00–14.00	Group psychotherapy
14.00–14.30	Lunch

activity and social functioning and quality of life improvement. The operationalized criteria of cognitive improvement is an increase of the total score of all cognitive scales on 3 points or more.

At discharge from the program, all participants receive a workbook with exercises that they should practice at home. The exercises in the workbook are scheduled for 3 months of work: twice a week, 1 hour a day.

Neurocognitive Rehabilitation Program

Cognitive Training

Neurocognitive training includes exercises focused on the higher mental functions (attention, thinking, memory, gnosis, praxis, etc.).

COGNITIVE TRAINING STIMULATES

- visual gnosis in normal and sensitized conditions;
- auditory gnosis;
- tactile gnosis and somatognosis;
- spatial and quasi-spatial analysis and synthesis (perception of spatial stimuli, actualization of spatial representations, counting operations skills, drawing skills, copying, constructive activity, improvement of logical and grammatical structures of the language);
- kinetic, kinesthetic and spatial organization of praxis;
- phonemic, kinesthetic, kinetic and nominative functions of speech;
- arbitrary memory (direct and delayed recall, semantic memory, memory for the past);
- voluntary attention;
- skills of goal setting and self-control;
- understanding of cause and effect relationships;
- skills of structuring current and future activities.

All neurocognitive exercises are divided into four cognitive training courses (CT-1, CT-2, CT-3 and CT-4) that address different cognitive functions. Each cognitive training course includes 10 sessions. Each patient undergoes all training courses according to the group schedule and receives two different neurocognitive sessions per day (Table 13.1). Further, we describe the focus of each training session within four training courses.

Cognitive Training-1 Sessions (CT-1)

The CT-1 course includes exercises that focus on programming, regulation and control of complex actions.

SESSIONS

1. Training the patient's action program; the skill of setting goals and objectives; their implementation, regulation and self-control.
2. Training of voluntary attention.
3. Training to establish cause-effect relationships.
4. Generalizing functions of a word, polysemy and hierarchy of concepts.
5. Increasing the plasticity of the sensorimotor support of mental processes.
6. Mnestic processes training.
7. Training of somatognostic, tactile and kinesthetic processes. Visual gnosis training.
8. Spatial perception training.

9. Training of auditory gnosis and phonemic hearing. Activation of the nominative function of speech.
10. Training the skill of setting goals and objectives, methods of their implementation, regulation and self-control in the process of performing a task (making a postcard using a scrapbooking technique for a birthday).

Cognitive Training-2 Sessions (CT-2)

The CT-2 course focuses on memory training.

SESSIONS

1. Recovery of the skill of associative and logical memorization and reproduction of the information.
2. Training the skills of mediated-logical memorization.
3. Training the skills of associative recall of events.
4. Training the skills of formulating an action program. Differentiation between causes and consequences. Increasing the plasticity of the sensorimotor support of mental processes.
5. Training the skill of purposeful recollection of a planned action. Action control training.
6. Training of somatognostic, tactile and kinesthetic processes. Visual gnosis training.
7. Training of spatial representations. Description of personal experiences while listening to the story.
8. Training the skills of identifying the cause and effect of an action. Kinetic process training.
9. Training of auditory gnosis and phonemic hearing. Training of the nominative function of speech.

Cognitive Training-3 Sessions (CT-3)

CT-3 focuses on attention training and perception.

SESSIONS

1. Training of programming the patients' action, skills of attention, regulation and self-control.
2. Perception training.
3. Training of mnestic processes, spatial perception.
4. Training of impressive and expressive speech.
5. Training of the nominative function of speech.
6. Training of visual gnosis.
7. Operational support of thought processes and algorithm of actions.
8. Spatial perception training.
9. Summing up session.

Cognitive Training-4 Sessions (CT-4)

CT-4 includes special art-therapy sessions with a focus on cognitive training.

SESSIONS

1. Portraying the mood as a combination of color, shapes and figures in space (formation of the skill of comprehending experienced emotions).
2. Portraying basic emotions as a combination of color, shapes and figures.

3. Drawing up personal palette of basic emotion colors.
4. Determination of the nature (mood) of the image.
5. Perception of the emotional meaning of the picture.
6. Drawing up a story describing the mood of the proposed picture.
7. Perception of the emotional meaning of the painting and expression of own emotions by drawing using the personal color palette.
8. Restoring the skill of performing a program of sequential actions.
9. Training of mnestic, sense-forming function and voluntary regulation in emotional experiences.
10. Training the skill of emotional experience depiction without reference to a sample.

Group Psychotherapy

The goal of psychotherapy as a part of the NCRP course is to reduce the intensity of destructive emotional states (fear, anxiety, anger, resentment) and to develop the skill to accept uncomfortable emotional experiences, including the fact of memory decline. Different psychotherapy approaches and technics are applied. The topics and structure of group psychotherapy sessions are adjusted to the common requests of elderly people with cognitive problems. All sessions are short and problem focused; psychotherapy is performed in a closed group format.

STRUCTURE OF THE PSYCHOTHERAPY SESSION

1. Introduction and feedback about previous session (5–10 minutes).
2. Main part (30 minutes).
3. Feedback about the session (10 minutes).
4. Relaxation (10 minutes).

The psychotherapy course includes five types of sessions (blocks). Each block uses a certain psychotherapy mode: body-oriented psychotherapy, cognitive-behavioral therapy, existential psychotherapy and psychodrama.

Patients get psychotherapy sessions on the daily basis. In all, the course includes 25 group sessions, 60 minutes each.

1. The first block consist of four sessions that focus primarily on the skills of muscle relaxation, breathing and attention switches. Participants acquire following skills:
   - Learn to selectively fix attention on muscle sensation, on the dynamics of contraction-relaxation of individual muscle groups of the limbs and body.
   - Learn to rhythmize smooth breathing (inhalation-exhalation) with a slow contraction-relaxation of individual muscle groups of the limbs and body.
   - Master "paradoxical" breathing with muscle contractions as a way to end the "mental dialogue".
   - Integration of visual and auditory images with positive emotions and emotional states (interest, surprise, overcoming, courage, etc.).
2. The second block includes four sessions with a focus on speech and articulation training, reading, learning to use reading as a means of emotional and cognitive self-support.
3. In the third block (six sessions), cognitive-behavioral therapy approaches are implemented with an emphasis on dealing with memory problems.

- Voluntary regulation of activity, programming, forecasting, operational support of mental activity.
- Awareness about the connection between behavior, emotions, thoughts and memory.
- Awareness about illogical, hasty or rigid conclusions and beliefs, dysfunctional stereotypes of perception and thinking.
- Finding the relationship between memory, motor activity and emotions; dependence of remembering process on physical and mental conditions of an individual.
- Finding the dependence of memory and external stimuli and the need to "transfer" memorization to internal stimuli.
- Master psychotherapeutic techniques that promote, develop and improve memory in old age.
- To shape an attitude towards memory as a natural and dynamic process that can be changed.

4. The fourth block uses elements of existential therapy (six sessions).
    During the group sessions, participants discuss such topics as self, personality, relations with others, support, fear, love, loneliness and limited physical capacities. Coping strategies are discussed in this regard using the examples from the literature and from participants' personal experience.
5. Cognitive psychodrama.
    Cognitive psychodrama for patients with MCI is a psychotherapeutic technique developed especially for patients of memory clinics by the members of the treatment team (Savilov et al., 2017). It is conducted during the sixth week of the NCRP course and includes five sessions, 60 minutes each. During the sessions, participants read and discuss popular short novels in the empathic environment of group members. Participants are welcomed to share their impressions about the story, and bodily and emotional liberation of all group members is encouraged by the therapist; emotions can be expressed both in words and in gestures.
    In the process of training, participants are encouraged:
- To solve a simulated problem together with the group using the principle of "here and now".
- To compare the impressions about the novel that they had reading it in youth and in the present time.
- To model and correct the protagonists' behavior of the novel.
- To discuss possible unconscious motives of protagonists.
- To perform multidimensional analysis of the story and find associations with one's life situations.
- To develop an adaptive attitude towards age-related changes and find "functional" behavior style in a simulated psychodrama situation with the help of the group members.

Medical Gymnastics

Gymnastics sessions are held daily; the duration of the session is 30 minutes. Participants are divided into two groups upon the results of physical activity evaluation using the Bartel scale: a group with a moderate load (85–102 scale score) and a group with a light load (70–85 scale score). The workload during the session depends on the patients' age, physical condition, trauma history and concurrent physical illnesses.

EXERCISES ARE AIMED AT

1. Improving the function of external respiration, prevention of congestion in the lungs.
2. Improving mobility in small and medium joints.
3. Strengthening the muscles of the arms and shoulder girdle.

4. Strengthening the muscles of the legs and pelvic floor. Prevention of prolapse and incontinence.
5. Strengthening the core muscles.
6. Strengthening the heart muscle.
7. Strengthening the abdominal muscles.

SESSION STRUCTURE

1. Preparation for the session. Pulse counting (5 min).
2. Introductory part. Breathing exercises aimed to activate the brain cortex (3 min).
3. The main part. A set of exercises aimed to maintain the optimal functional state of organs and body systems (15 min).
4. The final part. Breathing, static exercises (3 min).
5. Counting the pulse. Recommendations about the set of exercises for training at home (3–4 minutes).

Medical Management

All NCRP participants receive a consultation from a psychiatrist who specializes in old age psychiatry at admission and discharge. Medication treatment plays a secondary role in memory clinics and is prescribed additionally in the NCRP if needed.

Neurocognitive Rehabilitation Program Effectiveness

The effectiveness of the NCRP delivered in the memory clinics can be estimated both from the consumers' perspective and by the clinical effects.

From the memory clinic foundation, the request of consumers for the treatment were very high and resulted in waiting list formation. Moreover, the drop-out rate during the program is very low (does not exceed 5%). Patients never leave the program of their own free will, only due to external circumstances. According to the patients' and their relatives' narrative feedback, patients become more socially active and more involved in the communication with other family members and in the household.

The clinical effect can be measured by the dynamics in cognitive test performance and quality of life assessment (SF-36). These parameters were measured in the focus groups of program participants.

SF-36 parameters were compared before and after the NCRP in 87 patients. Statistically significant difference was estimated in two subscales of SF-36: general health and mental health. The general health perception improved by the end of the program from 51.56 ± 18.4, Me 55.0 (40.0; 67.0; CI 95%) to 54.9 ± 18.0, Me 55.0 (40.0; 67.0; CI 95%) scores, $p = 0.041$, Wilcoxon test. Although the standardized effect size was small, that can be explained by the low power of this particular research (Es = 0.18; $P = 0.25$). Meanwhile, effects observed in the self-estimation of mental health were more powerful (Es = 0.36. P = 0.68). Mental health perception improved by the end of the program from 60.3 ± 17.4, Me 60.0 (44.0; 72.0; CI 95%) to 66.4 ± 17.0, Me 68.0 (56.0; 76.0; CI 95%) scores, p = 0.0003, Wilcoxon test (Kurmyshev et al., 2018).

Difference in the cognitive performance was calculated in 115 patients using MMSE. According to this test, cognitive performance increased significantly by the end of the program from 24.0 ± 3; Me 25.0 (23.0; 26.0; CI 95%) to 26.0 ± 2; Me 26.0 (26.0; 28.0; CI 95%) scores, Wilcoxon test $p < 0.001$; effect size Es = 1.11 (Kostyuk et al., 2017).

Thus, the results of pilot studies are encouraging, as is service users' feedback. Prospective research on the larger samples of NCRP participants is ongoing with support from a Russian Foundation of Basic Research grant.

ELECTRONIC NEUROCOGNITIVE REHABILITATION PROGRAM

The COVID-19 pandemic and lockdown dramatically affected the population over 65 years old (Karpenko et al., 2020) and led to limitations in memory clinics' routine work. Therefore, the need for alternative methods of care delivery became a high-priority issue. The remote electronic NCRP (e-NCRP) was developed by the staff of memory clinics to enable patients to receive NCRP via Internet. e-NCRP includes only cognitive training in the form of video lessons led by psychologists of the memory clinic; all tasks double the exercises of the offline program. Participants receive an Internet link to the course. e-NCRP can be performed by patients at home without an instructor; the patient can follow electronic sessions himself/herself or with the help of relatives or a social worker. No special computer skills or equipment are required.

To pass e-NCRP, a patient needs to follow video lessons 3 days a week (total course duration 12 weeks) and do tasks in the workbook 2 days a week. The workbook can be downloaded from the memory clinic web site and printed out.

The impact of e-NCRP on the cognitive function and well-being of the patients is evaluated in the ongoing research program granted by the Russian Foundation of Basic Research.

CONCLUSIONS

Memory clinics organized in Moscow beautifully targeted the demand of the population for interventions aimed to deal with age-related cognitive decline. Being the part of the mental health service, memory clinics nonetheless do not experience any stigma-related problems. That can be explained both by their relevance and by the psychotherapeutic environment created in memory clinics.

The feasibility of the NCRP applied in memory clinics was proved within 5 years of successful work. Waiting lists, low drop-out rates and positive feedback from the patients and their relatives can be regarded as a feasibility confirmation from the service consumers.

The preliminary results of clinical effects assessment are also encouraging. Moreover, the NCRP can be flexibly adjusted to remote implementation using telemedicine technologies. However, the clinical effects of NCRP and e-NCRP are waiting to be estimated in ongoing clinical trials.

ACKNOWLEDGEMENTS

The authors express their gratitude to Dr. Daria Smirnova, MD, PhD, Associate Professor of the Department of Psychiatry, Deputy-Director on Clinical Issues, Neurosciences Research Institute & Head, International Research Lab in Neuropsychiatry, Samara State Medical University, Samara, Russian Federation, for the encouragement and support in writing this chapter.

References

Burygina L, Gavrilova S, Kostyuk G, Pak M, Kourmyshev M, Savilov V, et al. *Psychosocial therapy and neurocognitive rehabilitation of elderly patients with cognitive impairment*/Kostyuk G. Moscow: University Book House; 2019, 332 p (in Russ.).

Eddy JR, Sriram S. Clock-drawing and telling time as diagnostic aids. *Neurology*. 1977;27:595.

Folstein MF, Folstein SE, McHugh PR. "Mini-mental state": A practical method for grading the cognitive state of patients for the clinician. *J Psychiatr Res*. 1975 Nov;12(3):189–198. doi: 10.1016/0022-3956(75)90026-6. PMID: 1202204.

Gavrilova S, Kolykhalov I, Tukhvatullina D, Smirnova D. *Implementation of psychogeriatric services in Russia: Current state and challenges*, Book chapter, Ed. M. Kapur. India: Springer; 2021 (in press).

Gavrilova SI. Demencia. V kn.: SI Gavrilova. Rukovodstvo po geriatricheskoy psychiatrii. Pod red. SI Gavrilovoi.M.: Puls. 2014: 23–145 [Гаврилова С. И. Деменция. В кн.: Руководство по гериатрической психиатрии. Под ред. С.И. Гавриловой. М: Пульс, 2014: 23–145.] (in Russ.)

Jolley D, Benbow SM, Grizzell M. Memory clinics. *Postgraduate Medical Journal* 2006;82(965):199–206. https://doi.org/10.1136/pgmj.2005.040592

Karpenko OA, Syunyakov TS, Kulygina MA, Pavlichenko AV, Chetkina AS, Andrushchenko AV. Impact of COVID-19 pandemic on anxiety, depression and distress—Online survey results amid the pandemic in Russia. *Consortium Psychiatricum*. 2020;1(1):8–20. https://doi.org/10.17650/2712-7672-2020-1-1-8-20

Kostyuk GP, Kurmyshev MV, Savilov VB, Pak MV, Burygina LA. Restoration of cognitive functions in elderly persons in the conditions of specialized medical-rehabilitation division "Clinic of memory". *Socialnaya i clinicheskaya psichiatria*. 2017;27(4):25–31. (In Russ.).

Kurmyshev MV, Savilov VB, Kostyuk GP. Dynamics of life quality perception among patients with cognitive decline during an integrated rehabilitation process. 2018;3:47–52. doi: 10.31363/2313-7053-2018-3-47-52 (in Russ.)

Luria AR. *Higher cortical functions of humans and their impairment in local brain injuries*/Luria AR. Moscow: Moscow University Publishing House; 1962, 432 p. [Лурия А.Р. Высшие корковые функции человека и их нарушения при локальных поражениях мозга/А.Р. Лурия. Москва: Издательство Московского университета; 1962, 432 с.] (in Russ.).

Mahoney FI, Barthel DW. Functional evaluation: The Barthel Index. *Md State Med J*. 1965 Feb;14:61–65. PMID: 14258950.

Nasreddine ZS, Phillips NA, Bédirian V, Charbonneau S, Whitehead V, Collin I, Cummings JL, Chertkow H. The Montreal cognitive assessment, MoCA: A brief screening tool for mild cognitive impairment. *Journal of the American Geriatrics Society* 2005;53:695–699. https://doi.org/10.1111/j.1532-5415.2005.53221.x

Rosen WG, Terry RD, Fuld PA, Katzman R, Peck A. Pathological verification of ischemic score in differentiation of dementias. *Annals of Neurology*. 1980;7(5):486–488.

Savilov V., Dmitriev A. Application of the psychodrama technics in elderly patients with mild cognitive impairment. *Sovremennaya terapia v psychiatrii I nevrologii*. 2017;1:15–19. [Савилов В.Б., Дмитриев А.Л., Особенности применения метода когнитивной психодрамы для людей пожилого возраста с мягким когнитивным снижением // Научно-практический журнал: Современная терапия в психиатрии и неврологии. №1, 2017. С. 15–19.] (in Russ.)

Ware JE Jr, Sherbourne CD. The MOS 36-item short-form health survey (SF-36). I. Conceptual framework and item selection. *Med Care*. 1992 Jun;30(6):473–483. PMID: 1593914.

World Health Organization. (2012). *Dementia: A public health priority*. World Health Organization. https://apps.who.int/iris/handle/10665/75263

Zigmond AS, Snaith RP. The hospital anxiety and depression scale. *Acta Psychiatr Scand*. 1983;67:361–370. doi: 10.1111/j.1600-0447.1983.tb09716.x.

13
Huntington's Disease as a Multi-System Disorder
Current "Must Know" for Better Patient Management

Svetlana Kopishinskaia, Mariia Korotysh, Sergey Svetozarskii, Mikhail Sherman, Ivan Velichko, Paul Cumming and Daria Smirnova

Introduction	135
Endocrine Disorders in HD	136
Hypothalamic Dysfunction in HD	136
Impaired Glucose Tolerance in HD	136
Lesion of the Sex Glands in HD	137
Metabolic Disorders in HD: Weight Loss	137
Damage to the Autonomic Nervous System in HD	137
Sleep Disturbances in HD	138
Cardiovascular System Impairments in HD	138
Gastrointestinal Disorders in HD	139
Damage of the Skeletal System in HD	139
Haematological Disorders in HD	140
Skeletal Muscle Atrophy in HD	140
Ophthalmic Manifestations of HD	141
Visual Function	141
Oculomotor Disorders	141
Retinal Changes	142
Lesion of the Cortical Part of the Visual Pathway	142
Visual Hallucinations	142
Conclusions	143

ABBREVIATIONS

ANS – Autonomous Nervous System
BMI – body mass index
CAG-repeats – repeats of the cytosine-adenine-guanine triplets
CART – Cocaine and Amphetamine Regulated Transcript
CT – computer tomography
DACH2 – Dachshund Family Transcription Factor 2
HD – Huntington's Disease

HDAC4 – Histone deacetylase 4
HDDS – Huntington's Disease Dysphagia Scale
LH – luteinizing hormone
MRI – magnetic resonance imaging
mRNA – messenger ribonucleic acid
PD – Parkinson's Disease
PNS – peripheral nervous system
VIP – vasoactive intestinal polypeptide

INTRODUCTION

Huntington's disease (HD) is an inexorably progressing neurodegenerative disease caused by the accumulation of an excessive number of cytosine-adenine-guanine (CAG) repeats in the huntingtin gene (McColgan & Tabrizi, 2018; Mills et al., 2020). The motor, cognitive, and mental impairments of HD have typical onset from 35 to 44 years of age, with progression leading to disability and death, usually with 20 years of the first motor symptoms (McColgan & Tabrizi, 2018). HD occurs worldwide, with an estimated prevalence of 4.64–13.7 per 100,000 (Demetriou et al., 2018). The disease has an autosomal dominant inheritance mechanism, with late onset (after 65 years) for those having 36–39 CAG repeats but complete penetrance and typical onset in middle age in those with more than 39 repeats and rare cases of adolescent onset (Westphal variant) when there are more than 60 repeats (Cubo et al., 2016). In familial HD, there tends to be a generational increase in the number of repeats, known as anticipation.

Huntingtin is a multifunctional protein with a molecular weight of about 350 kDa, which has abundant expression in neurons and glial cells of the brain but also having high expression in the testes, skeletal muscle, and many other tissues. The normal or "wild" type of huntingtin protein is involved in nuclear and axoplasmic transport, regulation of transcription, and apoptosis and performs a number of functions in pre- and postsynaptic terminals; huntingtin is also associated with the regulation of microglia activity. A number of proteins (i.e., huntingtin-bound protein-1) mediate the interaction of huntingtin with cellular transport systems, in particular with kinesin, dynactin, and dynein of the microtubule network, thus determining its role in antero- and retrograde axonal transport. Expansion of the CAG repeats leads to a mutant protein carrying a polyglutamine tract that is vulnerable to proteolysis, which gives rise to protein conglomerates in the cytoplasm and nucleus of the cell. The mutant protein forms aggregate with other proteins involving different cellular systems, and the resultant intracellular deposits are toxic to the cell (Calabresi et al., 2016; Chouksey & Pandey, 2020). Conversely, the polyglutamine tract is especially toxic to cancer cells, which may well account for the extremely low incidence of cancer among HD patients (Murmann et al., 2018). Neuronal loss results in progressive atrophy of brain structures occurs, first evident in the striatum and subsequently affecting the cerebral cortex (Chouksey & Pandey, 2020). The selective loss of GABA-ergic medium spiny neurons of the striatum is responsible for the main motor disturbances of HD. A recent study showed that short polyadenylated mRNA, which arises from abnormal splicing of huntingtin exon 1, occurs in many peripheral tissues such as the heart, skeletal muscles, kidneys, and liver, with expression levels comparable to those in the brain. Thus, the broader clinical picture of HD is not simply due to neurodegeneration but involves the formation of toxic aggregates in many tissues, ultimately causing multiorgan dysfunction and consequent somatic symptoms (Bayati & Berman, 2017; Critchley et al., 2018). Indeed, there are many peripheral or somatic abnormalities in HD, which seem to arise independently of the primary striatal pathology. We wish in this chapter to focus on the relatively subtle and diverse non-motor manifestations of the disease.

ENDOCRINE DISORDERS IN HD

Hypothalamic Dysfunction in HD

Pathology of the hypothalamus in HD can give rise to secondary changes in peripheral tissues due to altered secretion of pituitary hormones. Peripheral manifestations such as a weight loss can complicate the clinical picture of HD, Alzheimer's disease, and other neurodegenerative diseases, which implies a role of brain dysfunction in driving certain peripheral symptoms. In the hypothalamus of HD model mice, the expression of vasopressin, oxytocin, cocaine and amphetamine-regulated transcriptional peptide (CART), gonadotropin-releasing hormone, vasoactive intestinal polypeptide (VIP), and VIP receptors are all reduced (Cheong et al., 2019), which would predict for pervasive effects on neuroendocrine function. Structural imaging studies of patients with HD at the preclinical stage have shown involvement of the hypothalamus even before the onset of movement disorders (Bartlett et al., 2018).

Hypothalamic damage in HD can manifest in dysfunction of energy metabolism in the body (Polo et al., 2015). Damage to the hypothalamus includes loss of dopamine D_2 receptors as well as microglia activation, which may precede the onset of motor symptoms (Vercruysse et al., 2018). Prolactin can protect against stress-induced neuron loss in the rodent hippocampus (Torner et al., 2009), and elevated prolactin levels in circulation have an association with diabetic pathology, metabolic syndrome, and inflammatory conditions (Balbach et al., 2013; Chirico et al., 2013). Reduced serum prolactin levels suggest that HD patients may experience dysfunction of the hypothalamic-pituitary neuroendocrine axis, which potentially affects food intake and energy balance, leading to further weight loss and metabolic changes (Wang et al., 2014). In line with this, neuropathological analyses of post-mortem human HD hypothalamic tissue have demonstrated loss of such neuropeptides as oxytocin and vasopressin (Cheong et al., 2020). HD model mice have shown alterations these peptides manifesting in an abnormal behavioural that was partially rectified by intranasal administration of oxytocin (Cheong et al., 2020). Indeed, HD patients showed reduced fMRI activation in various brain regions upon viewing emotionally disturbing faces, but this blunted response normalized upon administration of oxytocin (Labuschagne et al., 2017).

In general, there is a need for further research to identify the degree, selectivity, and importance of hypothalamic and neuroendocrine changes in the HD clinical picture. Most of the pathological aggregates and the greatest loss of neurons occur in the lateral hypothalamus of HD patients, which is the site of orexinergic neurons that regulate food intake and other physiological functions. Male HD patients have decreased plasma testosterone concentrations, but the extent of the individual decrease did not correlate with plasma concentrations of luteinizing hormone (LH), which is produced and released by the anterior pituitary gland under regulation by gonadotropin-releasing hormone. Indeed, male HD patients with the lowest testosterone concentrations had normal LH concentrations, suggesting that changes in testosterone production arise from a primary testicular pathology rather than from the neuroendocrine axis per se. A study of hypothalamic-pituitary functioning in HD patients also failed to link some of the observed peripheral symptoms with neuroendocrine pathology (Kalliolia et al., 2015). Taken together, these results suggest that peripheral symptoms in HD do not necessarily appear due to pathology of the hypothalamic-pituitary system but are sometimes associated with primary defects in peripheral organs (Nambron et al., 2016).

Impaired Glucose Tolerance in HD

High BMI is associated with a slower progression of HD disease (van der Burg et al., 2017). The incidence of Alzheimer's disease, Parkinson's disease, and HD fell by 50% in elderly diabetic patients treated with the insulin-sensitizer metformin (Shi et al., 2019). On the other hand, metabolic indicators of glucose tolerance were not conspicuously abnormal in non-diabetic

HD patients (Nambron et al., 2016). Thus, the metformin results may indicate exacerbation of HD progression by untreated diabetes rather than indicating a protective effect per se.

The causal relationship between greater body weight, glucose tolerance, and slower progression of neurological symptoms in HD is not yet clear. According to the results of one study, treatment with the hypoglycemic drug glibenclamide did not affect the clinical course or life expectancy in R6/2 HD model mice (Hunt et al., 2005). Conversely, metformin prolonged lifespan and decreased motor symptoms in male R6/2 mice. The antidiabetic agent exendin-4 (a glucagon-like peptide-1 agonist) also had beneficial effects in R6/2 mice, leading to better motor function and longer survival. The mechanism of this action of exendin-4 is unclear but could be attributable to its anti-inflammatory effects and resultant increased neuronal plasticity in the face of a neurodegenerative process (Montojo et al., 2017).

Lesion of the Sex Glands in HD

The testes have among the highest level of huntingtin expression in the body and testes. Although fertility is not impaired in patients with HD (Blancato et al., 2017), as noted, male patients have reduced testosterone levels, although symptoms such as gynecomastia are not typically reported in HD. Nonetheless, male HD patients show pathology of the testicles, with a reduced number of germ cells and abnormal morphology of the seminiferous tubules. A decrease in plasma testosterone concentration correlates with clinical worsening of the disease. Similarly, the mouse R6/2 and YAC128 HD models also show testicular atrophy, albeit to a greater extent than seen in patients. This pathology is probably a consequence of the direct toxic effect of mutant huntingtin on the testes (Novati et al., 2018). Results of rat studies suggests that male HD patients may benefit from hormone replacement therapy, as has been reported for Parkinson's disease patients (Okun et al., 2006).

Metabolic Disorders in HD: Weight Loss

Involuntary weight loss is one of the most common complaints in HD patients but is not necessarily associated with neuropathology per se (Gardiner et al., 2017). This weight loss is of a progressive character, being insignificant in preclinical carriers but progressing to profound cachexia in late-stage patients and of a severity correlating with the number of CAG repeats (Süssmuth et al., 2015). A number of studies has shown that the weight loss was not secondary to hyperactivity, swallowing difficulties, or anorexia but rather results from increased basal metabolic rate as calculated by the Harris-Benedict method (Harris et al., 1918). As noted, HD patients with a higher BMI at onset tend to have slower disease progression (Süssmuth et al., 2015). Patients at an early stage of the disease have an increased total energy expenditure, with higher basal energy expenditure during rest. In addition, asymptomatic HD carriers tend to consume more calories (Adanyeguh et al., 2018), possibly to compensate for an increase in metabolism. HD patients showed higher energy consumption as measured by indirect calorimetry after insulin challenge as compared to healthy controls. It is well known that insulin stimulates the sympathetic nervous system, which is the main regulator of resting metabolism. In fact, the sympathetic nervous system is overactive in HD patients, such that effect of insulin in stimulating energy metabolism in HD patients may be a consequence of sympathetic hyperactivity.

DAMAGE TO THE AUTONOMIC NERVOUS SYSTEM IN HD

The integrity of the myocardial sympathetic innervations was unaffected in an [^{123}I]-MIBG SPECT study of HD patients (Assante et al., 2020). Nonetheless, dysfunction of the autonomic nervous system (ANS) can be a sign of HD, clinically manifesting as gastrointestinal, genitourinary, and cardiovascular disorders. For example, dysautonomia of HD can give rise to neurogenic arrhythmias and sudden cardiac death (Abildtrup & Shattock, 2013). Indeed, there are subtle signs of ANS dysfunction even in the prodromal period of HD, although the underlying pathologies remain unclear.

Sleep Disturbances in HD

Sleep disturbances are one of those first symptoms of HD, often with onset a decade before the clinical diagnosis. Sleep disturbances in HD include insomnia, poor sleep efficiency, prolonged sleep retention, frequent awakenings at night, and slow wave sleep deficit. Chronic dyssomnia in these patients can contribute to the deterioration of cognitive functions and other neuropsychiatric symptoms, as well as an increase in the rate of neurodegeneration (Baker et al., 2016). Sleep disturbance becomes worse in the later stages of the disease, and the extent of delay in the sleep phase in patients with symptomatic HD correlates with a decrease in cognitive functions (Leblanc et al., 2015). A number of studies have shown that sleep disorders in HD are associated with hypothalamic atrophy and increased psychiatric symptoms. However, in one study, there were no significant differences in the volume of the hypothalamus or caudate nucleus in HD patients with complaints of sleep disturbances compared to patients without sleep disturbances (Poudel et al., 2015). Actigraphy studies have shown abnormal night-day ratios in HD patients (Maskevicha et al., 2017). In addition, patients with HD have a delayed sleep phase and an increased latency of the REM sleep phase. This is consistent with a delay in the circadian rhythm phase, as evidenced by the delay in the timing of peak melatonin concentrations in blood (Piano et al., 2015). Excessive daytime sleepiness is not a common feature in HD patients, as evidenced by the unchanged mean scores on the Epworth Sleepiness Scale compared to healthy controls, although some daytime sleepiness is present in 27% of patients (Baker et al., 2016). Several studies have shown abnormal movements during sleep, including periodic leg movements, in about 7% of patients (Piano et al., 2015). However, nocturnal choreic movements due to HD may sometimes be misidentified as periodic leg movements. In addition, nocturnal arousal in HD patients appears to be associated with voluntary movement during arousal. Moreover, the incidence of sleep apnoea was only 6.6% in HD patients (Piano et al., 2015).

The suprachiasmatic nucleus is a cluster of 20,000 neurons near the optic chiasm. It is responsible for regulating circadian rhythms, under the control of signals arising directly from the retina, and via downstream regulation of the pineal gland (Bennaroch, 2008). As noted, HD patients can have reduced production of several key neuropeptides of the suprachiasmatic nucleus such as VIP and vasopressin, perhaps due to a primary failure of circadian rhythms. Furthermore, PD patients have low blood plasma levels of melatonin, despite the absence of changes in the density of melatonin receptors in the suprachiasmatic nucleus (Cheong et al., 2020). Treatment with agomelatine, a dual melatonin receptor agonist, protected against pathology and behavioural changes in the 3-nitropropionic acid (3-NPA) rat model of HD (Gupta & Sharma, 2014), but it is not yet known if melatonin or its agonist remedies the sleep disturbances of human HD patients.

Cardiovascular System Impairments in HD

HD has been associated with an increased risk of cardiovascular disease. Early autonomic dysfunction in HD may be associated with the toxic effects of mutant huntingtin on cortical autonomic centres, which leads to sympathetic and parasympathetic dysregulation, as well as a combination of metabolic and neuroendocrine factors arising from damage to the myocardial vasculature. In HD, dyautonomia can manifest in abnormal parasympathetic activity or increased activity of the sympathetic nervous system. Sympathetic hyperactivity may be a secondary response to early neurodegeneration and decreased inhibition of higher autonomic centres (Veerabhadrappa & Schutte, 2017; Terroba-Chambi et al., 2020). Recent studies indicate sympathetic hyperfunction in asymptomatic carriers of the HD gene and early HD patients with a clinical picture of mild impairment of cognitive and motor functions (Cheong et al., 2019).

Heart failure occurs in about 30% of HD patients (compared to only 2% in the age-matched control group) and is thus the leading cause of death in these patients. Experimental data indicates that heart failure in HD may be a direct consequence of the expression of mutated huntingtin in cardiomyocytes (Schroeder et al., 2016). Prevention of heart failure in HD can improve quality of life and prevent early death. Ultrasonography is necessary to monitor this serious peripheral manifestation of HD. Hypertension is a risk factor for rapid progression of HD (Schultz et al., 2020), perhaps due to a general exacerbation of neurodegenerative processes. Given their great risk for cardiovascular disease, we suppose that counselling for smoking cessation is important for patients with HD.

Gastrointestinal Disorders in HD

HD patients suffer from xerostomia, which can affect taste, chewing, and swallowing, all of which can contribute to the typical weight loss. Pancreatic function is often impaired in patients with HD, resulting in impairments in insulin secretion as well as insulin sensitivity (Montojo et al., 2017). In patients, dysregulation of insulin transcription in islet cells may underlie the development of impaired glucose tolerance. Mutant huntingtin can also affect liver function in rodents, manifesting in reduced methionine catabolism, and gluconeogenesis (Procaccini et al., 2016). Indeed, the liver has a crucial role in whole-body energy balance and serves two especially notable roles in maintaining brain health. First, the liver removes toxins such as ammonia, thereby preventing damage to brain tissue. Second, liver maintains plasma glucose concentrations during fasting via gluconeogenesis and glycogenolysis, and this modulation is essential for the glucose-dependent brain. Both of these brain-relevant metabolic roles of liver seem to be impaired in patients with HD (Caroll et al., 2015). Indeed, treatment of liver and pancreatic pathologies decreases the severity of brain pathology and neurological symptoms in HD mice (Montojo et al., 2017). Studies in transgenic HD model mice indicate perturbations in the gut microbiome (Kong et al., 2020). Similarly, gut microbiome changes occur in HD patients, which correlate with aspects of the cognitive changes (Wasser et al., 2020).

Dysphagia occurs in HD patients at all stages of their disease, and aspiration, and pneumonia due to dysphagia is, after heart disease, the most common cause of death in HD. This motivated the development of the Huntington's Disease Dysphagia Scale (HDDS) for monitoring dysphagia in HD (Pizzorni et al., 2020). The HDDS is applicable at any stage of HD and is typically administrable by a caregiver to provide risk assessment of dysphagia.

DAMAGE OF THE SKELETAL SYSTEM IN HD

Osteoporosis is part of the HD phenotype, and its severity correlates with the number of CAG repeats (Costa de Miranda et al., 2019). The reason for decreased bone mineral density is unknown but could be secondary to antipsychotic treatment or a result of immobility rather than a direct consequence of the disorder itself. Alternatively, it may be that osteoporosis in HD results from a direct action of the mutant huntingtin gene on osteoblasts or osteoclasts in bone tissue (Costa de Miranda et al., 2019). There is evidence that HD patients are at elevated risk for vitamin D deficiency (Homann et al., 2020), and the increased fracture risk from osteoporosis and the propensity for falls call for vigilance about bone health in HD patients.

HAEMATOLOGICAL DISORDERS IN HD

Haematological findings in HD indicate subtle membrane damage in red blood cells that leads to metabolic dysfunction and mitochondrial dysfunction in leukocytes, resulting in increased apoptosis and features of autophagy, as well as transcription disorders. Furthermore, the release of immunomodulatory cytokines associated with monocytes and macrophages is impaired in HD, and there are conflicting reports of abnormal protein aggregation and impaired mitochondrial/metabolic metabolism in platelets (Di Pardo et al., 2017). A disturbance in platelets may contribute to aspects of the HD phenotype such as vascular permeability, inflammation, thrombosis, and impaired angiogenesis (Denis et al., 2018). Plasma samples from HD patients show signs of immune activation such as increased concentrations of interleukins 8 and 6, long preceding the onset of motor symptoms (Bouwens et al., 2016, Niranjan, 2018). Changes in the concentrations of immune system proteins such as clusterin and interleukin 6 also indicate disease progression. Blood cell dysfunction is another potential HD biomarker (Niranjan, 2018). An A_{2A} receptor dysfunction has been previously demonstrated in striatal cells engineered to express mutant huntingtin. A similar dysfunction (i.e., the binding and functional parameters of A_{2A} adenosine receptors) is present in peripheral blood cells (platelets, lymphocytes, and neutrophils) of subjects carrying the mutant gene (Varani et al., 2007). Furthermore, $A_{2A}R$ density in blood platelets correlates with the age of onset and CAG repeat expansion in HD patients (Maglione et al., 2005). These data highlight the need for further investigation of abnormal $A_{2A}R$ signalling in white blood cells of HD patients as a potential biomarker for disease prognosis and drug efficacy.

SKELETAL MUSCLE ATROPHY IN HD

Skeletal muscle wasting is one of the most important signs of HD, despite the often-excessive muscular activity of patients due to their hyperkinesis. At the molecular level, mitochondrial dysfunction, PPAR alpha signalling, and HSF1 activation are major players in skeletal muscle HD-related pathology (Quintanilla et al., 2009; Lin et al., 2005). Skeletal muscle atrophy in HD may result from any of the following mechanisms:

1. Impaired transcription of contractile proteins (Bondulich et al., 2017).
2. Mitochondrial dysfunction in myocytes (Farshbaf & Ghaedi, 2017).
3. Abnormal epigenetic activity HDAC4 (Histone deacetylase 4-dachshund family transcription factor 2-myogenin) in muscle remodelling. Interestingly, HD-related skeletal muscle weakness correlates directly with expression of the HDAC4-DACH2-myogenin axis (Mielcarek, 2015).
4. Decreased ionic currents through chloride and potassium channels of myocytes (Miranda et al., 2017). The resulting increased muscle excitability causes involuntary and prolonged contractions that can contribute to the chorea, rigidity, and dystonia that characterize HD.

Muscle mass of HD patients and HD carriers can be quantified by methods such as dual energy X-ray absorptiometry, MRI, and CT (Costa de Miranda et al., 2019). A rodent HD model did not recapitulate the finding of significant muscle wasting in patients at an early stage of HD (Bozzi et al., 2020). However, under certain circumstances, skeletal muscle mass can decline without changes in BMI.

OPHTHALMIC MANIFESTATIONS OF HD

Visual Function

Damage to the central and peripheral parts of the visual pathways leads to impaired acuity in various hereditary and sporadic neurodegenerative diseases (Heidary, 2017). There is evidence of visual-spatial impairments, a decrease in contrast sensitivity (one of the basic visual functions that determines the minimum contrast required to distinguish objects), although changes in visual fields have not been established. There is some evidence for nonspecific colour vision disorders due to retinal pathology in HD (Kersten et al., 2015), as likewise described in Parkinson's disease.

Oculomotor Disorders

Oculomotor symptoms are among the earliest manifestations of neurodegenerative diseases such as PD and HD (Winder & Roos, 2018). In HD, gaze fixation and the vestibulo-ocular reflex are impaired; at the clinical stage, there is a deficit in slow tracking eye movements. Saccadic eye movements are also disturbed, making it more difficult for the HD patient to start and complete saccades, as required, for example, in reading. Saccadic movements become progressively slower in the horizontal and vertical directions, with increasing time delays to onset, along with increasing hypometria or insufficient trajectory of the saccades. Visual-motor disintegration is evident in HD long before clinical motor manifestation, resulting in decreased speed and accuracy of vision-controlled movements and impaired correction of motor errors. A summary of the available information on oculomotor disorders in HD is presented in Table 13.1.

Table 13.1 Types of eye movements and their disturbances in Huntington's disease.

Type of eye movements	Functions	Disturbances in HD
Fixations	Retaining the image of a stationary object in the fovea area by reducing the drift and suppressing saccades	Interruption by unsuppressed saccades
Tracking movements	Slow conjugate eye movements that accompany the movement of an object in the field of view, keeping its image on the fovea	Decrease in speed, interruption by unsuppressed saccades
Saccades	Rapid conjugate eye movements that move the image of the object of interest to the fovea	Violation of initiation, slowing down, amplitude limitation
Vergences	Disconjugate eye movements directed towards each other (convergence) or away from each other (divergence) ensure simultaneous positioning of the object image in the fovea of both eyes	Weakness/absence of convergence

(Contintued)

Table 13.1 (Continuted)

Type of eye movements	Functions	Disturbances in HD
Vestibulo-ocular reflex	Conjugate eye movements that hold the image in the fovea during head movement consist of a slow and fast phase	Speed decrease of a slow phase
Optokinetic reflex	Conjugate eye movements: fix the gaze on objects moving in one direction, consist of a slow and fast phase	Speed decrease in a slow or fast phase, disappearance of optokinetic nystagmus

Retinal Changes

According to general electroretinography, damage to photoreceptor cells develops simultaneously with the appearance of neurological symptoms, with greater and earlier damage of cone cells as compared to rods, perhaps consistent with the colour vision deficits noted previously. Dopaminergic amacrine cells of the retina remain relatively intact in HD (Ouk et al., 2016). Specific retinal damage includes protein degradation, photoreceptor degeneration, and retinal remodelling. Due to the inconsistency and the small number of studies, it is not yet possible to propose a synopsis of the detailed cellular changes across retinal layers in HD; large-scale studies with optical coherence tomography of the retinal structure in HD are not yet available (Di Maio et al., 2020).

Intracranial hemodynamics suffers an early stages of HD development due to deposits of mutant huntingtin in the endothelium of microvessels of the brain and spinal cord (Lim et al., 2017; Sciacca & Cicchetti, 2017) and resultant damage to the blood-brain barrier (Di Pardo et al., 2017). In HD patients, there is an increase in the density of the vascular wall and a decrease in the diameter of the vessels in the retina, based on *post-mortem* examination.

Lesion of the Cortical Part of the Visual Pathway

HD patients show thinning of high order visual cortices in the occipital lobe, which is already present at the preclinical stage. Structural MRI indicate a loss of grey matter and underlying white matter in the occipital lobe. Functional MRI reveals changes in the activity in the occipital lobe both at rest and during visual stimulation in HD patients (Coppen et al., 2018).

Visual Hallucinations

Psychotic symptoms arise in at least 11% of patients with HD. The study of visual hallucinations in HD has not received special attention, but they may occur in 4.5% of patients (Rocha et al., 2018; Rossi et al., 2020). The negative impact of hallucinations on the quality of life of patients and caregivers calls for special attention in the clinical management of HD and is a neglected topic in the research literature, compared, for example, with hallucinations in Parkinson's disease (Borek & Friedman, 2014).

CONCLUSIONS

The most common systemic non-motor symptoms of HD are weight loss, skeletal muscle atrophy, ophthalmic disorders, damage to the cardiovascular and gastrointestinal systems, osteoporosis, and sleep disturbances. This wide range of systemic non-motor manifestations can appear in HD many years before the onset of movement disorders or diagnosis (Ghosh & Tabrizi, 2018). There is no doubt that these manifestations of the disease are clinically very important, since they reduce the quality of life and, in some cases, correlate with the progression of the disease, leading to early mortality, especially in the case of cardiovascular disease. With the aim of obtaining a deeper understanding of the pathogenesis of non-motor manifestations of HD, and to guide a search for new methods of treatment, there is a need for further research to study the relationship between the concentration of pro-inflammatory cytokines in the blood and muscle changes. Developing new diagnostic criteria and treatment approaches for HD cardiomyopathy and mitochondrial dysfunction of skeletal muscles would have tangible benefits from patient care.

References

Abildtrup M., Shattock M. Cardiac dysautonomia in Huntington's disease. *J Huntingtons Dis.* 2013;2(3):251–261. doi: 10.3233/JHD-130054. PMID: 25062674.

Adanyeguh I.M., Monin M.L., Rinaldi D., Freeman L., Durr A., Lehéricy S., Henry P.G., Mochel F. Expanded neurochemical profile in the early stage of Huntington disease using proton magnetic resonance spectroscopy. *NMR Biomed.* 2018 Mar;31(3). doi: 10.1002/nbm.3880.

Assante R., Salvatore E., Nappi C., Peluso S., De Simini G., Di Maio L., Palmieri G.R., Ferrara I.P., Roca A., De Michele G., Cuocolo A., Pappatà S., De Rosa A. Autonomic disorders and myocardial 123I-metaiodobenzylguanidine scintigraphy in Huntington's disease. *J Nucl Cardiol.* 2020 Aug 16. doi: 10.1007/s12350-020-02299-7. Epub ahead of print. PMID: 32803674.

Baker C.R., Domínguez D.J.F., Stout J.C., Gabery S., Churchyard A., Chua P., Egan G.F., Petersén Å., Georgiou-Karistianis N., Poudel G.R.J. Subjective sleep problems in Huntington's disease: A pilot investigation of the relationship to brain structure, neurocognitive, and neuropsychiatric function. *Neurol. Sci.* 2016 May 15;364:148–153. doi: 10.1016/j.jns.2016.03.021.

Balbach L., Wallaschofski H., Völzke H., Nauck M., Dörr M., Haring R. Serum prolactin concentrations as risk factor of metabolic syndrome or type 2 diabetes? *BMC Endocr Disord.* 2013 Mar 21;13:12. doi: 10.1186/1472-6823-13-12. PMID: 23517652; PMCID: PMC3614874.

Bartlett D.M., Domínguez D.J.F., Reyes A., Zaenker P., Feindel K.W., Newton R.U., Hannan A.J., Slater J.A., Eastwood P.R., Lazar A.S., Ziman M., Cruickshank T. Investigating the relationships between hypothalamic volume and measures of circadian rhythm and habitual sleep in premanifest Huntington's disease. *Neurobiol Sleep Circadian Rhythms.* 2018 Jul 3;6:1–8. doi: 10.1016/j.nbscr.2018.07.001.

Bayati A., Berman T. Localized vs. systematic neurodegeneration: A paradigm shift in understanding neurodegenerative diseases. *Front Syst Neurosci.* 2017;11:62. doi: 10.3389/fnsys.2017.00062

Blancato J.K., Wolfe E.M., Sacks P.C. Preimplantation genetics and other reproductive options in Huntington disease. *Handb Clin Neurol.* 2017;144:107–111. doi: 10.1016/B978-0-12-801893-4.00009-2. PMID: 28947109; PMCID: PMC5837037.

Bondulich M.K., Jolinon N., Osborne G.F., Smith E.J., Rattray I., Neueder A., Sathasivam K., Ahmed M., Ali N., Benjamin A.C., Chang X., Dick J.R.T., Ellis M., Franklin S.A., Goodwin D., Inuabasi L., Lazell H., Lehar A., Richard-Londt A., Rosinski J., Smith D.L., Wood T., Tabrizi S.J., Brandner S., Greensmith L., Howland D., Munoz-Sanjuan I., Lee S.J., Bates G.P. Myostatin inhibition prevents skeletal muscle pathophysiology in Huntington's disease mice. *Sci. Rep.* 2017;7(1):14275. doi: 10.1038/s41598-017-14290-3.

Borek L.L., Friedman J.H. Treating psychosis in movement disorder patients: A review. *Expert Opin Pharmacother.* 2014 Aug;15(11):1553–1564. doi: 10.1517/14656566.2014.918955. Epub 2014 May 20. PMID: 24846479.

Bouwens J.A., van Duijn E., Cobbaert C.M., Roos R.A., van der Mast R.C., Giltay E.J.J. Plasma cytokine levels in relation to neuropsychiatric symptoms and cognitive dysfunction in Huntington's disease. *Huntingtons Dis.* 2016 Dec 15;5(4):369–377. doi: 10.3233/JHD-160213

Bozzi M., Sciandra F. Molecular mechanisms underlying muscle wasting in Huntington's disease. *Int J Mol Sci.* 2020;21(21):8314. Published 2020 Nov 5. doi: 10.3390/ijms21218314.

Calabresi P., Pisani A., Rothwell J., Ghiglieri V. Hyperkinetic disorders and loss of synaptic downscaling. *Nat Neurosci.* 2016;19(7):868–875. doi: 10.1038/nn.4306.

Cheong R.Y., Gabery S., Petersén Å. The role of hypothalamic pathology for non-motor features of Huntington's disease. *J Huntingtons Dis.* 2019;8(4):375–391. doi: 10.3233/JHD-190372.

Cheong R.Y., Tonetto S., von Hörsten S., Petersén Å. Imbalance of the oxytocin-vasopressin system contributes to the neuropsychiatric phenotype in the BACHD mouse model of Huntington disease. *Psychoneuroendocrinology.* 2020 Sep;119:104773. doi: 10.1016/j.psyneuen.2020.104773.

Chirico V., Cannavò S., Lacquaniti A., Salpietro V., Mandolfino M., Romeo P.D., Cotta O., Munafò C., Giorgianni G., Salpietro C., Arrigo T. Prolactin in obese children: A bridge between inflammation and metabolic-endocrine dysfunction. *Clin Endocrinol (Oxf).* 2013 Oct;79(4):537–544. doi: 10.1111/cen.12183. Epub 2013 Apr 1. PMID: 23445298.

Chouksey A., Pandey S. Phenotypic variability in Huntington's disease. *Ann Indian Acad Neurol.* 2020;23(2):153–154. doi: 10.4103/aian.AIAN_543_19.

Coppen E.M., van der Grond J., Hart E.P., Lakke E.A.J.F., Roos R.A.C. The visual cortex and visual cognition in Huntington's disease: An overview of current literature. *Behav. Brain Res.* 2018 Oct 1;351:63–74. doi: 10.1016/j.bbr.2018.05.019.

Costa de Miranda R., Di Lorenzo N., Andreoli A., Romano L., De Santis G.L., Gualtieri P., De Lorenzo A. Body composition and bone mineral density in Huntington' disease. *Nutrition.* 2019 Mar;59:145–149. doi: 10.1016/j.nut.2018.08.005.

Critchley B.J., Isalan M., Mielcarek M. Neuro-cardio mechanisms in Huntington's disease and other neurodegenerative disorders. *Front. Physiol.* 2018 May 23;9:559. doi: 10.3389/fphys.2018.00559.

Cubo E., Ramos-Arroyo M.A, Martinez-Horta S., Martínez-Descalls A., Calvo S. Clinical manifestations of intermediate allele carriers in Huntington disease. *American Academy of Neurology Neurology.* 2016;87:1–8. doi: 10.1212/WNL.0000000000002944.

Demetriou C.A., Heraclides A., Salafori C., Tanteles G.A., Christodoulou K., Christou Y., Zamba-Papanicolaou E. Epidemiology of Huntington disease in Cyprus: A 20-year retrospective study. *Clin Genet.* 2018 Mar;93(3):656–664. doi: 10.1111/cge.13168.

Denis H.L., Lamontagne-Proulx J., St-Amour I., Mason S.L., Rowley J.W., Cloutier N., Tremblay M.È., Vincent A.T., Gould P.V., Chouinard S., Weyrich A.S., Rondina M.T., Barker R.A., Boilard E., Cicchetti F.J. Platelet abnormalities in Huntington's disease. *Neurol. Neurosurg. Psychiatry.* 2018 Dec 19. doi: 10.1136/jnnp-2018-318854.

Di Maio L.G., Montorio D., Peluso S., Dolce P., Salvatore E., De Michele G., Cennamo G. Optical coherence tomography angiography findings in Huntington's disease. *Neurol Sci.* 2020 Jul 22. doi: 10.1007/s10072-020-04611-2.

Di Pardo A., Amico E., Scalabrì F., Pepe G., Castaldo S., Elifani F., Capocci L., De Sanctis C., Comerci L., Pompeo F., D'Esposito M., Filosa S., Crispi S., Maglione V. Impairment of blood-brain barrier is an early event in R6/2 mouse model of Huntington disease. *Sci Rep.* 2017 Jan 24;7:41316. doi: 10.1038/srep41316.

Epping E.A., Kim J.I., Craufurd D., Brashers-Krug T.M., Anderson K.E., McCusker E., Luther J., Long J.D., Paulsen J.S. Longitudinal psychiatric symptoms in prodromal Huntington's disease: A decade of data. *Am. J. Psychiatry.* 2016;173:184–192. doi: 10.1176/appi.ajp.2015.14121551.

Farshbaf M.J., Ghaedi K. Huntington's disease and mitochondria. *Neurotox Res.* 2017;32(3):518–529. doi: 10.1007/s12640-017-9766-1.

Gardiner S.L., Ludolph A.C., Landwehrmeyer G.B. Body weight is a robust predictor of clinical progression in Huntington disease. *Ann Neurol.* 2017 Sep;2(3):479–483. doi: 10.1002/ana.25007.

Ghosh R., Tabrizi S.J. Clinical features of Huntington's disease. *Adv Exp Med Biol.* 2018;1049:1–28. doi: 10.1007/978-3-319-71779-1_1.

Gupta S., Sharma B. Pharmacological benefits of agomelatine and vanillin in experimental model of Huntington's disease. *Pharmacol Biochem Behav.* 2014 Jul;122:122–135. doi: 10.1016/j.pbb.2014.03.022. Epub 2014 Apr 3. PMID: 24704436.

Harris J.A., Benedict F.G. A biometric study of human basal metabolism. *Proc Natl Acad Sci U S A.* 1918 Dec;4(12):370–373. doi: 10.1073/pnas.4.12.370. PMID: 16576330; PMCID: PMC1091498.

Heidary G. Neuro: Ophthalmic manifestations of pediatric neurodegenerative disease. *Journal of Neuro-Ophthalmology.* 2017;37:S4–S13. doi: 10.1097/WNO.0000000000000549.

Homann C.N., Ivanic G., Homann B., Purkart T.U. Vitamin D and hyperkinetic movement disorders: A systematic review. *Tremor Other Hyperkinet Mov (NY).* 2020 Aug 25;10:32. doi: 10.5334/tohm.74. PMID: 32908795; PMCID: PMC7453965.

Hunt M.J., Morton A.J. Atypical diabetes associated with inclusion formation in the R6/2 mouse model of Huntington's disease is not improved by treatment with hypoglycaemic agents. *Exp Brain Res.* 2005 Oct;166(2):220–229. doi: 10.1007/s00221-005-2357-z. Epub 2005 Jul 21. PMID: 16034568.

Kalliolia E., Silajdžić E., Nambron R., Costelloe S.J., Martin N.G., Hill N.R., Frost C., Watt H.C., Hindmarsh P., Björkqvist M., Warner T.T. A 24-hour study of the hypothalamo-pituitary axes in Huntington's disease. *PLoS One.* 2015 Oct 2;10(10). doi: 10.1371/journal.pone.0138848

Kersten H., Danesh-Meyer H., Kilfoyle D., Roxburgh R. Optical coherence tomography findings in Huntington's disease: A potential biomarker of disease progression. *J. Neurol.* 2015;262(11):2457–2465. doi: 10.1007/s00415-015-7869-2

Kong G., Ellul S., Narayana V.K., Kanojia K., Ha H.T.T., Li S., Renoir T., Cao K.L., Hannan A.J. An integrated metagenomics and metabolomics approach implicates the microbiota-gut-brain axis in the pathogenesis of Huntington's disease. *Neurobiol Dis.* 2021 Jan;148:105199. doi: 10.1016/j.nbd.2020.105199. Epub 2020 Nov 26. PMID: 33249136.

Labuschagne I., Poudel G., Kordsachia C., Wu Q., Thomson H., Georgiou-Karistianis N., Stout J.C. Oxytocin selectively modulates brain processing of disgust in Huntington's disease gene carriers. *Prog Neuropsychopharmacol Biol Psychiatry.* 2018 Feb 2;81:11–16. doi: 10.1016/j.pnpbp.2017.09.023. Epub 2017 Sep 23. PMID: 28947180.

Leblanc M.F., Desjardins S., Desgagne A. Sleep problems in anxious and depressive older adults. *Psychol. Res. Behav. Manag.* 2015;8:161–169. doi: 10.2147/PRBM.S80642.

Lim R.G., Quan C., Reyes-Ortiz A.M., Lutz S.E., Kedaigle A.J., Gipson T.A., Wu J., Vatine G.D., Stocksdale J., Casale M.S., Svendsen C.N., Fraenkel E., Housman D.E., Agalliu D., Thompson L.M. Huntington's disease iPSC-derived brain microvascular endothelial cells reveal wnt-mediated angiogenic and blood-brain barrier deficits. *Cell Rep.* 2017 May 16;19(7):1365–1377. doi: 10.1016/j.celrep.2017.04.021.

Lin J., Handschin C., Spiegelman B.M. Metabolic control through the PGC-1 family of transcription coactivators. *Cell Metab.* 2005;1:361–370. doi: 10.1016/j.cmet.2005.05.004.

Maglione V., Cannella M., Martino T., De Blasi A., Frati L., Squitieri F. The platelet maximum number of A2A-receptor binding sites (Bmax) linearly correlates with age at onset and CAG repeat expansion in Huntington's disease patients with predominant chorea. *Neurosci. Lett.* 2006 Jan 23;393(1):27–30. doi: 10.1016/j.neulet.2005.09.037. Epub 2005 Oct 10. PMID: 16221531.

Maskevicha S., Jumabhoya R., Daoa P.D.M., Stouta J.C., Drummond S.P.A. Pilot validation of ambulatory activity monitors for sleep measurement in Huntington's disease gene carriers. *Journal of Huntington's Disease.* 2017;6:249–253. doi: 10.3233/JHD-170251.

McColgan P., Tabrizi S. Huntington's disease: A clinical review. *Eur. J. Neurol.* 2018:25(1):24–34. doi: 10.1111/ene.13413.

Mielcarek M. Huntington's disease is a multi-system disorder. *Rare Dis.* 2015;3(1):e1058464. doi: 10.1080/21675511.2015.1058464.

Mills J.A., Long J.D., Mohan A., Ware J.J., Sampaio C. Cognitive and motor norms for Huntington's disease. *Arch Clin Neuropsychol.* 2020 Aug 28;35(6):671–682. doi: 10.1093/arclin/acaa026

Miranda D.R., Wong M., Romer S.H., McKee C.J. Progressive Cl-channel defects reveal disrupted skeletal muscle maturation in R6/2 Huntington's mice. *Gen. Physiol.* 2017;149(1):55–74. https://dx.doi.org/10.1085/jgp.201611603.

Montojo M.T., Aganzo M., González N.J. Huntington's disease and diabetes: Chronological sequence of its association. *Huntington's Dis.* 2017;6(3):179–188. doi: 10.3233/JHD-170253.

Murmann A.E., Gao Q.Q., Putzbach W.E., Patel M., Bartom E.T., Law C.Y., Bridgeman B., Chen S., McMahon K.M., Thaxton C.S, Peter M.E. Small interfering RNAs based on huntingtin trinucleotide repeats are highly toxic to cancer cells. *EMBO Rep.* 2018 Mar;19(3):e45336. doi: 10.15252/embr.201745336. Epub 2018 Feb 12. PMID: 29440125; PMCID: PMC5836092.

Nambron R., Silajdzi˘c E., Kalliolia E., Ottolenghi C., Hindmarsh P., Hill N.R, Costelloe S.J., Martin N.G., Positano V., Watt H.C., Frost C., Björkqvist M., Warner T.T. A metabolic study of Huntington's disease. *PLoS. One.* 2016;11. doi: 10.1371/journal.pone.0146480.

Niranjan R. Recent advances in the mechanisms of neuroinflammation and their roles in neurodegeneration. *Neurochem. Int.* 2018 Nov;120:13–20. doi: 10.1016/j.neuint.2018.07.003

Novati A., Yu-Taeger L., Gonzalez Menendez I., Quintanilla Martinez L., Nguyen H.P. Sexual behavior and testis morphology in the BACHD rat model. *PLoS One.* 2018 Jun 8;13(6). doi: 10.1371/journal.pone.0198338.

Okun M.S., Fernandez H.H., Rodriguez R.L., Romrell J., Suelter M., Munson S., Louis E.D., Mulligan T., Foster P.S., Shenal B.V., Armaghani S.J., Jacobson C., Wu S., Crucian G. Testosterone therapy in men with Parkinson disease: Results of the TEST-PD study. *Arch Neurol.* 2006 May;63(5):729–735. doi: 10.1001/archneur.63.5.729. PMID: 16682542.

Ouk K., Hughes S., Pothecary C., Peirson S., Morton A. Attenuated pupillary light responses and downregulation of opsin expression parallel decline in circadian disruption in two different mouse models of Huntington's disease. *Human Molecular Genetics*. 2016;25(24):5418–5432. doi: 10.1093/hmg/ddw359.

Piano C., Losurdo A., Della Marca G. Polysomnographic findings and clinical correlates in Huntington disease: A cross-sectional cohort study. *Sleep*. 2015;38(9):1489–1495. doi: 10.5665/sleep.4996.

Pizzorni N., Pirola F., Ciammola A., Schindler A. Management of dysphagia in Huntington's disease: A descriptive review. *Neurol Sci*. 2020 Jun;41(6):1405–1417. doi: 10.1007/s10072-020-04265-0.

Polo C.G., Delgado E. C., Cachorro A.M., Posadas J. R., Pérez N. M., Formoso D.A. Energy balance in Huntington's disease. *Ann. Nutr. Metab*. 2015;67:267–273. doi: 10.1159/000441328.

Poudel G.R., Stout J.C., Dominguez D.J. Churchyard A., Chua P., Egan G.F., Georgiou-Karistianis N. Longitudinal change in white matter microstructure in Huntington's disease: The IMAGE-HD study. *Neurobiol. Dis*. 2015;74:406–412. doi: 10.1016/j.nbd.2014.12.009.

Procaccini C., Santopaolo M., Faicchia D., Colamatteo A., Formisano L., de Candia P., Galgani M., De Rosa V., Matarese G. Role of metabolism in neurodegenerative disorders. *Metabolism*. 2016 Sep;65(9):1376–1390. doi: 10.1016/j.metabol.2016.05.018.

Quintanilla R.A., Johnson G.V. Role of mitochondrial dysfunction in the pathogenesis of Huntington's disease. *Brain Res Bull*. 2009;80(4–5):242–247. doi: 10.1016/j.brainresbull.2009.07.010.

Rocha N., Mwangi B., Gutierrez Candado C., Sampaio C., Furr Stimming E., Teixeira A. The clinical picture of psychosis in manifest Huntington's disease: A comprehensive analysis of the Enroll-HD database. *Front. Neurol*. 2018;9:930. doi: 10.3389/fneur.2018.00930.

Rossi M., Farcy N., Starkstein S.E., Merello M. Nosology and phenomenology of psychosis in movement disorders. *Mov Disord Clin Pract*. 2020 Jan 7;7(2):140–153. doi: 10.1002/mdc3.12882.

Schroeder A.M., Wang H.B., Park S., Jordan M.C., Gao F., Coppola G., Fishbein M.C., Roos K.P., Ghiani C.A., Colwell C.S. Cardiac dysfunction in the BACHD mouse model of Huntington's disease. *PLoS One*. 2016 Jan 25;11(1). doi: 10.1371/journal.pone.0147269.

Schultz J.L., Harshman L.A., Langbehn D.R., Nopoulos P.C. Hypertension is associated with an earlier age of onset of Huntington's disease. *Mov Disord*. 2020 Sep;35(9):1558–1564. doi: 10.1002/mds.28062. Epub 2020 Apr 27. PMID: 32339315.

Sciacca G., Cicchetti F. Mutant huntingtin protein expression and blood: Spinal cord barrier dysfunction in Huntington disease. *Ann Neurol*. 2017;82(6):981–994. doi: 10.1002/ana.25107.

Shi Q., Liu S., Fonseca V.A., Thethi T.K., Shi L. Effect of metformin on neurodegenerative disease among elderly adult US veterans with type 2 diabetes mellitus. *BMJ Open*. 2019 Jul 30;9(7):e024954. doi: 10.1136/bmjopen-2018-024954. PMID: 31366635; PMCID: PMC6677947.

Süssmuth S.D., Müller V.M., Geitner C., Landwehrmeyer G.B., Iff S., Gemperli A., Orth M. Fat-free mass and its predictors in Huntington's disease. *J. Neurol*. 2015;262:1533–1540. doi: 10.1007/s00415-015-7753-0.

Terroba-Chambi C., Bruno V., Vigo D.E., Merello M. Heart rate variability and falls in Huntington's disease. *Clin Auton Res*. 2020 Feb 6. doi: 10.1007/s10286-020-00669-2.

Torner L., Karg S., Blume A., Kandasamy M., Kuhn H.G., Winkler J., Aigner L., Neumann I.D. Prolactin prevents chronic stress-induced decrease of adult hippocampal neurogenesis and promotes neuronal fate. *J. Neurosci*. 2009 Feb 11;29(6):1826–1833. doi: 10.1523/JNEUROSCI.3178-08.2009. PMID: 19211889; PMCID: PMC6666278.

van der Burg J.M.M., Gardiner S.L., Ludolph A.C., Landwehrmeyer G.B., Roos R.A.C., Aziz N.A. Body weight is a robust predictor of clinical progression in Huntington disease. *Ann Neurol*. 2017 Sep;82(3):479–483. doi: 10.1002/ana.25007. Epub 2017 Aug 22. PMID: 28779551.

Varani K., Bachoud-Lévi A.C., Mariotti C., Tarditi A., Abbracchio M.P., Gasperi V., Borea P.A., Dolbeau G., Gellera C., Solari A., Rosser A., Naji J., Handley O., Maccarrone M., Peschanski M., DiDonato S., Cattaneo E. Biological abnormalities of peripheral A(2A) receptors in a large representation of polyglutamine disorders and Huntington's disease stages. *Neurobiol Dis*. 2007 Jul;27(1):36–43. doi: 10.1016/j.nbd.2007.03.011. Epub 2007 Apr 5. PMID: 17512749.

Veerabhadrappa P., Schutte A.E. Homocysteine and nighttime blood pressure dipping: Is there a connection? *Hypertens Am. J*. 2017 Nov 6;30(12):1151–1152. doi: 10.1093/ajh/hpx141.

Vercruysse P., Vieau D., Blum D., Petersén Å., Dupuis L. Hypothalamic alterations in neurodegenerative diseases and their relation to abnormal energy metabolism. *Front Mol Neurosci*. 2018;11:2. Published 2018 Jan 19. doi: 10.3389/fnmol.2018.00002.

Wang R., Ross C.A., Cai H., et al. Metabolic and hormonal signatures in pre-manifest and manifest Huntington's disease patients. *Front Physiol*. 2014;5:231. Published 2014 Jun 23. doi: 10.3389/fphys.2014.00231.

Wasser C.I., Mercieca E.C., Kong G., Hannan A.J., McKeown S.J., Glikmann-Johnston Y., Stout J.C. Gut dysbiosis in Huntington's disease: Associations among gut microbiota, cognitive performance and clinical outcomes. *Brain Commun*. 2020 Jul 24;2(2):fcaa110. doi: 10.1093/braincomms/fcaa110. PMID: 33005892; PMCID: PMC7519724.

Winder J.Y., Roos R.A.C. Premanifest Huntington's disease: Examination of oculomotor abnormalities in clinical practice. *PLoS One*. 2018 Mar 1;13(3):e0193866. doi: 10.1371/journal.pone.0193866.

Section 3
High-Risk Groups

14
Optimizing Patient Care in Psychiatry – Bipolar Mood Disorder

Riteeka Deshpande and Anuja Bendre

Introduction	151
Effective Methods of Management	151
Motivational Pharmacotherapy	152
Automation	153
Telepsychiatry	153
Effective Patient Engagement in Therapeutic Alliance	153

INTRODUCTION

Mood disorders are characterized by disturbances of one's mood, thoughts and behavior, resulting in severe distress and loss of control.

Bipolar disorder is one type of mood disorder characterized as being episodic and recurrent in nature and often manifested by two diametrically opposed moods: mania and depression.

Both manic and depressive episodes result in significant impairment in social and occupational functioning, an inability to work and subsequent loss of employment and social alienation. Patients often present with poor insight and judgement, resulting difficulty in treatment and optimizing care. This chapter discusses various strategies like monitoring adherence, tele-psychiatry, automation and motivational pharmacotherapy to optimize care of bipolar mood disorder.

EFFECTIVE METHODS OF MANAGEMENT

Effective methods of managing symptoms and minimizing the suffering associated with this disorder include:

1. Medications
2. Psychosocial interventions
3. Managing associated medical and psychiatric comorbidities
4. Medication optimization – a broad approach aimed at ensuring the safest and most effective use of medications
5. After drug prescription – optimization includes support for adherence and medication reconciliation
6. Potential for financial savings is a strong motivator for medication optimization

DOI: 10.4324/9780429030260-17

The efficacy-effectiveness gap in clinical practice suggests that lack of adherence is a major problem in the treatment of bipolar disorder and contributes substantially to functional disability and sometimes mortality. Suicide rates among people with bipolar disorder are 12 times higher than those in the general population

Hassan and colleagues noted that "the quality of the professional-patient relationship in the treatment of mental illness predicts patient outcomes."

A collaborative relationship in the treatment of individuals with psychiatric disorders has been found to predict treatment outcomes across a range of therapeutic settings. This may be particularly important for successfully engaging patients who have previously demonstrated reluctance to engage in mental health services.

In treatment, therapeutic alliance was associated with a higher variance in outcome (21%) compared to any specific psychotherapy or pharmacotherapy. The medication optimization approach is intrinsically patient-centric, and medication review can provide an opportunity to explore patient beliefs and preferences and to reach shared treatment decisions.

The therapeutic relationship is a nonspecific, positive factor in treatment response; it provides a "holding environment" in which issues related to taking medication can be addressed. A National Depression and Manic-Depression Association survey reported that patients who were more satisfied with their provider were able to come to terms with their illness more readily, felt more able to cope with their illness, were less angry and ashamed about the illness and were more likely to adhere to their medication regimen.

In a study of patient experience by Bilderbeck et al., individuals with symptoms of unstable mood described the importance of receiving an explanation for their symptoms. They also noted the value of having a collaborative relationship with their clinicians, of being listened to and acknowledged and of being informed about and involved in clinical decisions regarding their care. It is important to discover the patient's goals and values regarding his or her care in the development of a strong therapeutic relationship.

MOTIVATIONAL PHARMACOTHERAPY

Balán, Moyers, and Lewis-Fernández described a therapeutic approach – motivational pharmacotherapy – where the physician and patient are equal co-decision makers; This improves medication adherence and incorporates elements of motivational interviewing into a standard pharmacotherapy session.

Motivational pharmacology uses four central processes: engaging the patient, focusing on the patient's desired behavior change, evoking and reinforcing the patient's own stated reasons for wanting to change and planning steps to achieve this goal.

The basics of motivational pharmacotherapy are:

1. Welcome the patient
2. Affirm the commitment to treatment
3. Suggest a brief overview of the forthcoming session

The psychiatrist asks directly about what steps the patient has taken to stay adherent to the treatment and what obstacles may be interfering with optimal adherence. The patient is encouraged to suggest strategies he or she may use to improve adherence. The session wraps up with a review of the treatment regimen and a collaborative decision about any changes to the medication treatment.

Motivational pharmacotherapy needs to be culturally congruent with the patient's worldview, hopes and fears.

AUTOMATION

Automation can be defined as the use of technology to perform four classes of functions: information acquisition, information analysis, decision and action selection and action implementation.

Effective automation for bipolar mood disorder to optimize psychiatrist treatment of individual patients can include:

1. Electronic medical records (EMRs)
2. Effects of complex system integration on e-prescribing
3. Use of clinical decision support to assist clinical decision making

Secure remote access to EMRs allows psychiatry to work remotely on tasks such as patient visits and clinical team meetings and provides improved back-up coverage. If a patient moves or changes hospitals for personal reasons, it will be easy to track details of previous treatment given through the EMR channel. Also, if patient loses or misplaces records, which could be common with mental illness patients, the treating psychiatrist can get access to the old history and management from an EMR.

TELEPSYCHIATRY

Telepsychiatry is a process that uses a telecommunications device to provide psychiatric services to people who are separated from a psychiatrist by a distance and those who feel more comfortable at home.

Telepsychiatry (e.g., assessment via video conferencing) could help reach patients living in rural and underserved areas. It offers several benefits, including convenience and better accessibility. It can provide an easy way for bipolar mood disorder patients to access psychiatric services if they are unable to travel. It may also result in a reduction in the need to take time off work.

EFFECTIVE PATIENT ENGAGEMENT IN THERAPEUTIC ALLIANCE

Effective ways for enhancing engagement with individuals in treatment for bipolar disorder:

1. Welcome the patient warmly each visit.
2. Emphasize from the first interactions the importance of honesty and trust (on both sides) in the therapeutic relationship; specify the treatment approach clearly; define areas of choice, limits of confidentiality and safety management plans.
3. The patient's aspirations, beliefs and concerns should be heard carefully and acknowledged regularly.
4. Help the patient clarify desired life goals and the behavior changes required to reach those goals.
5. Support "change talk," in which the patient discusses his or her reasons for wanting to change and perception of his or her ability to change.
6. Reinforce that your role as physician or clinician is to support the healthy change that the patient desires.
7. Clearly state that decisions are made jointly and encourage the patient to discuss methods of feeling more empowered.
8. Be realistic. Help the patient take on small and achievable goals. Success is the best motivator. Predict "bumps in the road," and normalize them to decrease the risk of a sense of failure if a patient does not meet his or her goals.

9. Write down the specific steps the patient has decided to take between sessions. This can motivate and allows discussion of what went well and what did not.
10. Inquire about treatment adherence and what helped or hindered this.
11. Specify a safety plan, ask regularly about safety (e.g., presence of weapons, pills, etc. in the home) and review the coverage and plan for the patient if he or she is not feeling safe.
12. Acknowledge your appreciation of the patient's honesty and efforts toward illness management.
13. Work in a collaborative team whenever possible, with regular and specified methods of team communication. Integrate the patient into these discussions whenever possible.

References

1) Optimizing adherence: Bipolar disorder and the therapeutic motivational alliance, Dorothy E. Stubbe, MD, *Focus*. 2019 Summer;17(3), Page No. 262–264, focus.psychiatryonline.org
2) Urgent need for improved mental health care and a more collaborative model of care, James Lake, MD; Mason Spain Turner, MD, *The Permanente Journal/Perm J*. 2017;21:17–024, E-pub: 08/11/2017
3) Openness of patients' reporting with use of electronic records: Psychiatric clinicians' views, Ronald M. Salomon; Jennifer Urbano Blackford; S. Trent Rosenbloom; Sandra Seidel; Ellen Wright Clayton; David M. Dilts; Stuart G. Finder, *J Am Med Inform Assoc*. 2010 Jan-Feb;17(1):54–60. doi:110.1197/jamia.M3341
4) Implementation and impact of psychiatric electronic medical records in a public medical center, Anna Q. Xiao, MD, MHA, assistant professor; Frank X. Acosta, PhD, associate professor emeritus, *Perspect Health Inf Manag*. 2016;13(Fall):1e. Published online 2016 Oct 1.
5) Usefulness of telepsychiatry: A critical evaluation of videoconferencing-based approaches, Subho Chakrabarti, *World J Psychiatry*. 2015 Sep 22;5(3):286–304. Published online 2015 Sep 22. doi:10.5498/wjp.v5.i3.286
6) What about telepsychiatry? A systematic review, Francisca García-Lizana, MD, PhD; Ingrid Muñoz-Mayorga, MS, *Prim Care Companion J Clin Psychiatry*. 2010;12(2):PCC.09m00831. doi:10.4088/PCC.09m00831whi
7) Automation to optimize physician treatment of individual patients: examples in psychiatry, Prof Michael Bauer MD, Scott Monteith MD, Prof John Geddes MD, Prof Michael J Gitlin MD, Prof Paul Grof MD, Prof Peter C Whybrow MD et al., *The Lancet Psychiatry VOLUME 6, ISSUE 4, P338–349, APRIL 01, 2019*

15

Optimising Patient Care – Pharmacogenetics in the Management of Addictions

Evgeny Krupitsky, Elvina Akhmetova, Dina Tukhvatullina, Daria Smirnova, Paul Cumming and Azat Asadullin

Introduction	155
The Use of Genetic Methods to Personalise Pharmacotherapy (Increasing Its Efficacy and Minimising Side Effects)	156
Pharmacogenetics of Drugs for the Treatment of Opioid Dependence Syndrome	*156*
Pharmacogenetics of Drugs for the Treatment of Alcohol Dependence Syndrome	*157*
Pharmacogenetics of Drugs for the Treatment of Nicotine Dependence Syndrome	*162*
Pharmacogenetics of the Use of Disulfiram in the Treatment of Cocaine Addiction	*162*
Genetic Engineering in Chemical Addiction Treatment	163
Anti-Catalase RNAs	*163*
RNAs Blocking Aldehyde Dehydrogenase Synthesis	*163*
Dopamine Receptor RNA	*164*
Conclusions	164

CORRESPONDING AUTHOR

Evgeny Krupitsky, Vice-Director for Research at V.M. Bekhterev National Medical Research Center for Psychiatry and Neurology, Bekhtereva Street, 3, Saint Petersburg, 192019, Russian Federation; e-mail: kruenator@gmail.com

INTRODUCTION

There are relatively few officially registered medications with proven efficacy in the treatment of psychoactive drug dependence (Krupitsky, 2003; Latt et al., 2009). This chapter is dedicated to a review of the impact of pharmacogenetics on the efficacy of pharmacological treatments for substance abuse, with a focus on opioids, alcohol, and nicotine/smoking. Notably, the opioid receptor antagonist naltrexone (in oral, injectable, and implantable sustained-release forms), the partial agonist-antagonist buprenorphine, and the full opioid receptor agonist methadone are officially registered for substitution therapy for opiate dependence syndrome in most countries in the world. Law in the Russian Federation (WHO, 2008) forbids the latter two compounds due to their abuse potential, while the need for effective treatments for drug dependence is especially acute in Russia. Naltrexone is also an approved medication for the treatment of alcohol dependence, as are compounds from several other pharmacological classes, such as disulfiram, acamprosate, and nalmefene. Furthermore, several novel drugs have shown efficacy for alcohol use disorder (AUD), including certain anticonvulsants (topiramate, pregabalin, gabapentin), serotonin reuptake inhibitor antidepressants (in particular, sertraline), baclofen, and ondansetron. The stringent requirements for proof of efficacy are such that these latter compounds have not yet found approval for the indication of AUD. Various forms of nicotine replacement therapy (patch, chewing gum, nasal spray, etc.), the antidepressant bupropion, and partial agonist-antagonists of nicotine cholinoreceptors (varenicline and cytisine) are registered for the treatment of nicotine dependence (Moerke et al., 2020). While there is substantial literature for the pharmacotherapy of opioid, ethanol, or nicotine dependence, the evidence for the efficacy of pharmacological treatments for psychostimulant dependence is relatively sparse. We do note that the classical treatment for ethanol abuse, disulfiram, has shown promising results in the treatment of cocaine dependence, particularly when supported by cognitive psychotherapy (Carroll et al., 2016).

Pharmacogenetics is the study of how hereditary factor influence the response to drugs (Pirmohamed et al., 2001). In the context of addiction medicine, pharmacogenetics commonly involves two main areas: (1) the use of genetic methods for personalisation of pharmacotherapy aiming to increase its effectiveness and minimise side effects and (2) the experimental use of genetic engineering methods for the treatment of addiction. This chapter provides a brief overview of both of these applications of pharmacogenetics in addiction medicine.

THE USE OF GENETIC METHODS TO PERSONALISE PHARMACOTHERAPY (INCREASING ITS EFFICACY AND MINIMISING SIDE EFFECTS)

Pharmacogenetics of Drugs for the Treatment of Opioid Dependence Syndrome

Opioid Receptor Antagonists: Naltrexone

The number of studies in this area is very limited. Krupitsky et al. (2015) demonstrated a specific role of polymorphisms associated with the genes for mu-opioid receptors (OPRK1), the D_2 and D_4 subtypes of dopamine receptors), the plasma membrane dopamine transporter (DAT), and the catecholamine metabolism enzyme catechol-ortho-methyltransferase (COMT) in modulating the stability of the remission of opiate dependence syndrome obtained with naltrexone administered as a subcutaneous implant. In particular, a number of polymorphic variants were associated with increased risk of relapse, despite naltrexone treatment. These variants included DRD4120bpm long allele of the dopamine D4 receptor with two repeats of 120 base pairs, DRD2NcoI the dopamine D2 C allele, and the DATVNTR40bp genotype of DAT. These results imply that individual differences in dopaminergic signalling mediate aspects of the rewarding properties of opiates (Cumming et al., 2019), or the aversive aspects of opioid withdrawal induced by naltrexone.

Furthermore, carriers of the (CC+CT)-(TT) polymorphism variant of the OPRK1-DRD2NcoI gene combination showed a greater likelihood of completing a naltrexone treatment program. In an oral naltrexone treatment group, carriers of the same variants (OPRK1-drd2ncol) were more likely to complete the treatment program, although this relationship was reversed in the double placebo group and was absent in the group treated by naltrexone via subcutaneous implant (Krupitsky et al., 2015). This suggests that timing and cues arising from oral naltrexone contributes to the efficacy of opioid receptor antagonism in supporting abstinence.

Opioid Receptor Agonists: Methadone

Methadone is a long-acting mu-selective agonist and NMDA antagonist with little affinity for other receptor subtypes (Codd et al., 1995). Treatment with opioid dependence with agonists such as methadone, or with partial agonists, is known as replacement therapy, which can be viewed as a harm reduction approach or a means for weaning the dependent individual from their use of illicit narcotics. There is evidence that polymorphisms of genes encoding certain cytochrome enzymes (CYP2B6, CYP2D6, CYP3A4) (Kharasch et al., 2015), as well as the dopamine D2 receptor Taq1 A1/A2 polymorphism (rs1800497) in association with protein kinases and signal transduction pathways, affect the compliance and retention of opioid-addicted patients in methadone replacement programs (Sturgess et al., 2011). The ratio of the plasma methadone concentration to its metabolites provides an index of individual differences in the rate of methadone metabolism, which can provide a rational basis to selecting treatment doses (McCarthy et al., 2020).

Partial Opioid Receptor Agonist-Antagonists: Buprenorphine

Buprenorphine is a high affinity partial agonist for mu- and kappa-opioid receptors (Cumming et al., 2019). Theoretically, a partial agonist may have lower abuse potential or higher safety margin due to the ceiling effect in receptor activation. In humans, CYP3A enzymes metabolise approximately 90% of buprenorphine, predicting that genetic variations due to gender or ancestry could modulate exposure to buprenorphine exposure (Zanger and Schwab, 2013). The START (Starting Treatment with Agonist Replacement Therapy) group concentrated on studying gender differences in the efficacy of buprenorphine for opioid addiction. In particular, polymorphic variants in the delta-opioid receptor OPRD1 gene (rs581111 and rs529520) were associated with continued opioid use during buprenorphine treatment in women, but not in men (Clarke et al., 2014). However, irrespective of gender, African-American patients with the CC polymorphism of the rs678849 gene showed poorer outcomes on buprenorphine treatment for opioid dependence compared to patients with the CT or TT alleles of this gene (Crist et al., 2019).

Pharmacogenetics of Drugs for the Treatment of Alcohol Dependence Syndrome

Disulfiram

As a non-competitive inhibitor of the ethanol catabolism enzyme, aldehyde dehydrogenase, disulfiram treatment causes acetaldehyde intoxication upon subsequent ingestion of ethanol, supposedly resulting in aversive conditioning against further ethanol use (Haass-Koffler et al., 2017). However, disulfiram is also an inhibitor of the noradrenaline-synthesising enzyme dopamine-beta-hydroxylase (DBH). Conceivably, the inhibitory effect of disulfiram on DBH in noradrenergic neurons could shift the bias of catecholamine signalling towards dopamine in the frontal cortex, which might have consequences for executive function in alcohol-dependent individuals (Devoto et al., 2015). A functional polymorphism of the gene for DBH has been associated with an increased risk of side effects of disulfiram therapy and consequently lower compliance. In a study of alcohol dependent veterans with comorbid depression, the DBH genotype interacted with disulfiram on the number of drinks per drinking day, with greater abstinence in among those with the CC genotype (Arias et al., 2014).

Acamprosate (Calcium Homotaurinate)

Acamprosate (N-Acetyl homotaurine) is not metabolised in the liver, but is excreted unchanged in the urine (Mason and Heyser, 2010). In the brain, acamprosate acts as a prodrug, being metabolised the neuroactive substances GABA, glutamate, und taurine. The mechanism of action of acamprosate in alcohol addiction may thus involve modulation of inhibitory and or glutamatergic neurotransmission. Genetic markers associated with the ionotropic NMDA receptor have shown an association with duration of sobriety maintenance in alcohol dependent patients (Karpyak et al., 2014), whereas variants or markers of the natriuretic peptide transcription factor GATA4 were associated with relapse probability in patients undergoing acamprosate treatment for alcohol dependence (Kiefer et al., 2011). In particular, the duration of sobriety was associated with two polymorphisms (rs2058878 and rs2300272) of the GRIN2B gene encoding the NR2B subunit of the NMDA receptor. Among alcoholism patients treated with acamprosate, the minor A allele of the rs2058878 polymorphism was associated with a longer period of sobriety, while the minor G allele of the rs2300272 polymorphism was associated with more rapid relapse (Karpyak et al., 2014). Attilia et al. (2018) identified polymorphisms serving as markers of the response to acamprosate treatment: the C1412T polymorphism of the GABA-B receptor gene GABRB2, the rs13273672 polymorphism of the GATA4 gene (which encodes a transcriptional activator), and the per2brdm1 mutation of the PER2 gene (which encodes a protein involved in a circadian rhythm). The first two genes are related to the physiological response to alcohol and the PER2 gene to the response to acamprosate (Attilia et al., 2018).

Naltrexone

As mentioned, naltrexone is an opioid receptor antagonist. Treatment with naltrexone may reduce the euphoria caused by ethanol intoxication by inhibiting the effects of endogenous opioid neuropeptides (primarily endorphins) released by alcohol, which, in turn, may reduce the release of dopamine in the brain's reward system (Anton, 2001). Naltrexone pharmacogenetics in alcoholism is one of the most well-researched areas of pharmacogenetics in addiction medicine. David Oslin of the University of Pennsylvania was the first to demonstrate the pronounced effect of the mu-opiate receptor type 1 polymorphism A118G (OPRM1, Asp40 allele) on the outcomes of oral naltrexone treatment for alcoholism (Oslin et al., 2003). Findings in that study were later confirmed by other researchers (Anton et al., 2008). While retrospective analyses of the mu-opiate receptor gene polymorphisms were highly conclusive, the only prospective study to date failed to demonstrate an association between the A118G polymorphism of the OPRM1 gene and persistence of abstinence in alcoholism (Oslin et al., 2015), a result causing great frustration among investigators of alcoholism pharmacogenetics. In a recent systematic review and meta-analysis by Hartwell et al. (2020), the authors conclude that it remains unclear whether the rs1799971 polymorphism of the OPRM1 Asn40Asp gene is in fact a predictor of the response to naltrexone therapy for alcohol dependence. This persisting uncertainty may be due to the complex interaction of genes regulating opioidergic and dopaminergic neurotransmission in the context of alcoholism, as shown recently in the work of Anton et al. (2020). Notably, a study by Ooteman et al. (2009) showed an association between dopamine and GABAA receptor gene polymorphisms (DRD2, GABRA6 and GABRB2) and the efficacy of naltrexone and acamprosate in the treatment of alcohol dependence.

Nalmefene

Nalmefene is an antagonist of mu-and delta-opioid receptors and a partial agonist-antagonist of kappa receptors (Bart et al., 2005). This drug may present a new paradigm in the treatment of ethanol addiction, with prophylactic administration a few hours before expected alcohol consumption, with the aim of reducing consumption rather than strictly maintaining sobriety. Arisa et al. (2008) investigated the effect of polymorphisms of several opioid receptor subtypes on the outcome of nalmefene treatment for alcoholism. That multicentre, randomised, placebo-controlled study did not reveal any relationship between the A118G (rs561720) polymorphism of the mu-opioid receptor OPRM1 gene, as well as the rs2234918 (T921C) and rs678849 polymorphisms of the delta-opioid receptor (OPRD1) gene and the rs963549 polymorphism of the kappa-opioid receptor (OPRK1) gene. Since nalmefene therapy has potential for harm reduction, we contend that further study of the pharmacogenetics of nalmefene is justified (Arias et al., 2008).

Topiramate

Topiramate is an anticonvulsant that reduces glutamatergic neurotransmission by interacting with GluK1 and GluK2 subunits of kainate receptor genes (GRIK1 and GRIK2) and blocking calcium channels of the L-type neuronal membrane (which also reduces glutamate release from neurons), while increasing GABAergic neurotransmission. Topiramate is mainly eliminated untransformed in the urine, but previous treatment with CYP450 inducers such as phenytoin can increase topiramate clearance (PMID: **12973408**). Kranzler et al. (2014) provide convincing data on the effect of the rs2832407 polymorphism of the kainite receptor gene (GRIK1) on the effectiveness of alcohol dependence therapy with topiramate. SS homozygotes showed better results compared to AS heterozygotes and AA homozygotes in both of the main indices of therapy effectiveness used in this study, namely the average number of days of heavy drinking (according to WHO criteria) and the average number of sober days per week. To a certain extent, the patterns discovered by Kranzler et al. can be explained by findings of Ray et al. (2009) that a polymorphism in intron 9 of the GRIK1 (rs2832407) kainate receptor gene is associated with the severity of side effects during treatment of alcoholism with topiramate. Topiramate side effects, most commonly dizziness, transient paresthesia, somnolence, and weight loss, and cognitive symptoms such as concentration/attention difficulties, slow thinking, and mood changes (Smeralda et al., 2020), are often a limiting factor in adherence among patients with alcohol dependence (Ray et al., 2009). Thus, the lower severity of side effects in SS-homozygotes of the rs2832407 polymorphism could promote better adherence of patients to the therapy, and consequently impart higher effectiveness of topiramate in this subgroup of alcohol-dependent patients.

Pregabalin

Like topiramate, pregabalin is an anticonvulsant, and is likewise eliminated unchanged in the urine (PMID: **15315511**). The underlying mechanism of action of pregabalin is through blockade of L-type neuronal membrane calcium channels, which significantly reduces the release of glutamate from hyperexcited glutamatergic neurons. The efficacy of pregabalin against alcohol dependence syndrome was first demonstrated in a double-blind, randomised placebo-controlled trial conducted by Krupitsky et al. (2017, 2019). The results of pharmacogenetic studies revealed a significant number of associations of polymorphisms of various genes with the outcomes of alcohol dependence therapy with pregabalin (Kibitov et al., 2018). Thirty polymorphic loci of 19 genes of several neurotransmitter systems were studied, including the dopamine, norepinephrine, opioid, GABA, and glutamate systems as well as voltage dependent calcium channels and neurotrophins. Pharmacogenetic markers of remission persistence included the GG allele of the BDNF polymorphism V66M rs6265 (neurotrophin system), CC DRD2–141C rs1799732 (dopamine system), and CC GRiK-GluR5 rs2832407 (GABA-glutamate system). The CC DRD2–141C variant rs1799732 was a specific predictor of long-term retention in the abstention program, and the CC GRiK-GluR5 rs2832407 was a specific predictor of therapy completion success with pregabalin. The duration of remission (time to relapse) was associated with GG allele of the DRD2 genetic polymorphism Nco I rs6275 (dopamine system), which was a high-risk marker of rapid relapse, whereas LL DRD4 48 bp acted as a low-risk dopaminergic marker of rapid relapse. Pharmacogenetic markers associated with the number of days of heavy drinking included GG DRD2 Nco I rs6275, CC DRD2–141C rs1799732, GG DBH Bst rs1108580, and TT CACNA2D1 rs17155798, all involving the dopamine system. Polymorphisms associated with the number of days of sobriety included GG DRD2 Nco I rs6275, TT CACNA2D1 rs17155798, and CC DBH Fau −1021 C−>T rs1611115 (also dopamine system).

The number of grams of pure ethanol consumed per day was associated with the following genetic markers: TT CACNA2D1 rs17155798, CC DBH Fau −1021 C − >T rs1611115 (dopamine system), and CC GRIN2A rs2072450 (glutamate system). The CACNA2D1 rs17155798 TT genotype (calcium channel α2δ2 subunit) turned out to be a pharmacogenetic marker with unique properties: in the placebo group, the effects of the genotype were the inverse of those seen in the pregabalin treatment group (Kibitov et al., 2018).

Serotonin Reuptake Inhibitor Antidepressants

Among serotonin reuptake inhibitors, the pharmacogenetics of sertraline in the treatment of alcoholism is the best studied to date. The predominant pathway for sertraline metabolism is CYP2C19, and its functional alleles influence the plasma pharmacokinetics of sertraline (PMID: **31066578**). Polymorphisms caused by repeat insertions in the promotor-region of the plasma membrane serotonin transporter (5-HTTLPR) gene are associated with the outcomes of alcohol dependence treatment with sertraline. Specifically, homozygotes for the L (long) allele of this gene had significantly lower mean rates of heavy drinking days and more sobriety days per week than did carriers of the S (short) allele (LS heterozygotes and SS homozygotes) (Kranzler et al., 2011). This seems reminiscent of similar associations in the context of seasonal affective disorder (PMID: 20110086), which may have some bearing on the strong association between seasonality and alcoholism reported in a Finnish population (PMID: **28364591**).

Ondansetron

Ondansetron is a centrally acting anti-emetic, which acts via blockade of the ionotropic 5-HT3 subtype of serotonin receptors, which are involved (*inter alia*) in the regulation of dopamine release in the brain. While acute ethanol causes an increase in striatal dopamine release, ondansetron can block this effect through its antagonism of 5-HT3 receptors. Johnson et al. (2011) investigated the role of the polymorphism (SLC6A4) of the 5-HTTLPR in the treatment of alcoholism with ondansetron (Kranzler et al., 2011). Homozygotes for the L allele of the 5-HTTLPR gene had significantly more sobriety days per week and lower daily consumption rates than S allele carriers (heterozygotes LS and homozygotes SS) who were treated with ondansetron (Johnson et al., 2011). In a model considering five alleles of the 5-HT3 receptor genes, those individuals carrying one or more of the genotypes rs1150226-AG and rs1176713-GG in HTR3A and rs17614942-AC in HTR3B showed a significant interaction between ondansetron treatment and the number of drinks per drinking day (Johnson et al., 2013).

Baclofen

Baclofen is a GABAB receptor ligand of the inhibitory GABAergic system of the brain, which finds uses primarily in neurology as a centrally acting muscle relaxant. Findings for the effectiveness of baclofen in treating alcoholism are contradictory; some studies showed it effective in stabilising remission, while others had negative results (Addolorato et al., 2013). These discrepant results for baclofen treatment in alcoholism may arise from effects of the rs29220functional polymorphism of the GABA B-receptor (GABBR1), which can alter the therapeutic and side effects of baclofen. Accordingly, only a certain proportion of patients with alcohol dependence respond positively to therapy with this medication (Morley et al., 2018), although the link with GABA B-receptor polymorphisms is not formally established.

In concluding this section, we note that the pharmacogenetics of therapy for alcohol dependence is quite well developed and can have practical benefits in improving the effectiveness of treatments (Seneviratne et al., 2015), as shown by our summary of effect sizes reported in the literature (Table 15.1).

Table 15.1 Effect sizes in pharmacogenetic and nonpharmacogenetic alcohol use disorder treatment trials.

Name of drug and efficacy criteria	Effect sizes*	
	Non-pharmacogenetic studies	Pharmacogenetic studies (gene polymorphisms)
Naltrexone		
Relapse to heavy drinking	0.247 (Del Re et al., 2013)	
Percentage of abstinence days	0.143 (Del Re et al., 2013)	
• Good clinical outcomes	Not measured	>0.8 among carriers of the G allele of the rs1799971 polymorphism (Anton et al., 2008)
Ondansetron		
Number of standard drinks on days of alcohol consumption	Statistically not significant; ondansetron vs. placebo (Correa et al., 2013; Johnson et al., 2000, 2011)	0.87 among carriers of one or more of the following genotypes: rs1150226:AG, rs1176713:GG and rs17614942:AC; 0.59 when carriers of SLC6A4: LL and rs1042173: TT were added to the previous group (Johnson et al., 2013)
% days of heavy drinking	Statistically not significant; ondansetron vs. placebo (Correa et al., 2013; Johnson et al., 2000, 2011)	0.78 among carriers of one or more of the following genotypes: rs1150226:AG, rs1176713: GG and rs17614942: A; 0.42 when carriers of SLC6A4: LL and rs1042173: TT were added to the previous group (Johnson et al., 2013)
% days sober	Statistically not significant; ondansetron vs. placebo (Correa et al., 2013; Johnson et al., 2000, 2011)	0.68 among carriers of any one or more of the following genotypes: rs1150226:AG, rs1176713:GG and rs17614942:AC; 0.43 when carriers of SLC6A4: LL and rs1042173: TT were added to the previous group (Johnson et al., 2013)
Topiramate		
Number of standard drinks on days of alcohol consumption	0.45 (Johnson et al., 2003, 2009)	
% days of heavy drinking	0.62 (Johnson et al., 2003, 2007; Kranzler et al., 2014; Rubio et al., 2009)	Effective only among rs2832407:CC carriers, but not among rs2832407: AC/AA carriers (Kranzler et al., 2014)
% days sober	0.46 (Johnson et al., 2003, 2007; Kranzler et al., 2014; Rubio et al., 2009)	Effective only among rs2832407:CC carriers, but not among rs2832407: AC/AA carriers (Kranzler et al., 2014)

Note: * The effect size estimate is given in Cohen's d.

Pharmacogenetics of Drugs for the Treatment of Nicotine Dependence Syndrome

The pharmacogenetics of drugs used to treat nicotine dependence mainly concerns genes encoding proteins involved in drug catabolism, as well as polymorphisms and variants of nicotinic acetylcholine (nACh) receptors.

Nicotine Replacement Therapy (Nicotine Patches, Chewing Gums, Intranasal Sprays, etc.)

Genetic markers associated with nicotine replacement therapy include certain polymorphisms of cytochrome enzymes involved in nicotine metabolism (CYP2B6, CYP2A6), nAChR genes (CHRNB2 and CHRNB4) genes. Other markers include polymorphisms of genes connected with the brain dopaminergic system, namely dopamine D2 receptor (DRD2–141C Ins/Del (rs1799732), COMT (Val108/158met) and ANKK1 Taq1A (a polymorphism associated with Ser/Thr kinase signal transduction pathways (Salloum et al., 2018; Sturgess et al., 2011). In particular, patients with at least one Taq1A A1 allele and one 1368A allele of the DBH enzyme demonstrated better smoking cessation outcomes by the end of 12 weeks of nicotine replacement therapy (Johnstone et al., 2004). It is noteworthy that AA homozygotes of the mu-opioid receptor OPRM1 A118G (rs561720) polymorphism, the same genetic feature associated with longer sobriety in the treatment of alcohol dependence with naltrexone, also showed better outcomes from NRT relative to placebo, as opposed to the carriers of the G-allele (Tutka et al., 2019; Munafo et al., 2007).

Bupropion

Bupropion is an antidepressant with the primary mechanism of action through inhibition of the reuptake of dopamine and noradrenaline, augmented by a non-competitive antagonism at nAChRs, mainly of the a3β4 subtype. Bupropion has official registration in many countries as a treatment for nicotine addiction. The results of pharmacogenetic studies of the efficacy and tolerability of bupropion for nicotine dependence are very extensive, such that we shall only list the most notable findings in this literature. Thus, the efficacy and tolerability of bupropion therapy for tobacco/nicotine dependence was affected by polymorphisms of the CYP2B6 and CYP2A6 cytochrome genes, which are involved in xenobiotic catabolism. Other relevant factors were genes for the nAChR genes (CHRNB2 rs2072661), dopamine D2 receptors (DRD2,-141 Ins/Del, and intron 8 VNTR and C957T), DAT (SLC6A3/DAT1 3 UTR VNTR), COMT (COMT-GG genotype polymorphism rs165599), and the ANKK1 Taq1A polymorphism of the Ser/Thr kinase second messenger pathway (King et al., 2012; Seneviratne et al., 2015; Sturgess et al., 2011). We also note that gender moderated the association of genetic variation in bupropion pharmacokinetics or pharmacodynamics and treatment response to bupropion (Schnoll and Paterson, 2009).

Varenicline

Varenicline is the perhaps most effective treatment for nicotine addiction. It acts as a partial agonist-antagonist of the alpha7 nAChR subtype. Certain nAChR polymorphisms (CHRNB2, CHRNA5, and CHRNA4 subgenes) are predictors of tobacco abstinence at 9–12 weeks of varenicline therapy (King et al., 2012). The frequency of nausea, the most common side effect of varenicline therapy, has been associated predominantly with polymorphisms of genes located at the loci of chromosome 15q25 (rs555018 of the nAChR CHRNA5 gene and rs1190449 of the nAChR CHRNG gene) (King et al., 2012).

Pharmacogenetics of the Use of Disulfiram in the Treatment of Cocaine Addiction

Disulfiram is not yet an officially registered drug for the treatment for cocaine dependence, and, indeed, there are no accepted pharmacological treatments for cocaine or other psychostimulant addictions. Nonetheless, several evidence-based studies have demonstrated a certain efficacy of disulfiram for cocaine addiction, which might relate to the dual action as an inhibitor of aldehyde dehydrogenase and DBH noted previously. Blockade of noradrenaline synthesis, in combination with cocaine effects, might potentiate cortical or striatal dopamine neurotransmission, conceivably provoking dysphoria and akathisia instead of euphoria (Gaval-Cruz et al., 2009). Indeed rats studies with pharmacological or genetic ablation of brain noradrenaline showed potentiation of the behavioural and neurochemical effects of methamphetamine. Several studies have associated polymorphisms of the DBH gene (DBH C-1021T (rs1611115)) with its enzyme activity. Thus, TT homozygotes have lower DBH activity and show a better response to disulfiram-based cocaine dependence therapy, possibly due to their lesser requirement for disulfiram to inhibit DBH in these patients (Bhaduri et al., 2008; Deinum et al., 2004; Köhnke et al., 2002; Zabetian et al., 2001).

GENETIC ENGINEERING IN CHEMICAL ADDICTION TREATMENT

Research into the potential of genetic engineering technologies for treating substance dependence has so far focused mainly on the use of different types of RNA.

Anti-Catalase RNAs

A group of scientists from Chile transfected the ventral tegmental region of the rat brain (part of the brain reward system) with a lentiviral vector carrying short hairpin RNA (shRNA) to inhibit the processing of the protein-coding RNA for the enzyme catalase, to block synthesis of this enzyme and change ethanol metabolism (Israel et al., 2015; Karahanian et al., 2011). Within 50 days of a single injection of the anti-catalase shRNA, dopamine release in the nucleus accumbens in response to ethanol consumption and the quantity ethanol consumption itself were almost completely blocked. While it is unclear how such an approach might ever find translational application, the proof of principle opens new vistas for the treatment of alcoholism by confirming the fundamental role of dopaminergic reward pathways in the maintenance of ethanol dependence.

RNAs Blocking Aldehyde Dehydrogenase Synthesis

As mentioned, disulfiram inhibits the aldehyde dehydrogenase enzyme, thus making ethanol consumption subjectively unpleasant. Thus, disulfiram may mimic the genetically determined effects of aldehyde dehydrogenase that are invoked to explain the "Asian flush," frequently reported among individuals of Asian descent after consuming alcohol (Chan, 1986). The main problem with disulfiram therapy of alcoholism is the low adherence rate due to reluctance to take daily disulfiram tablets. There have been numerous (unsuccessful) attempts to develop a formulation of disulfiram with prolonged action, which might ameliorate the problem of low adherence to therapy. In Russia, the lack of effective treatments has led to the emergence of numerous "quack" methods of treating alcoholism based on the exploitation of myths widespread among people addicted to alcohol, who may take pseudodrugs such as "Capsule," "Torpedo," "Esperali Implant," and the like. Unfortunately, these products are little more than scientifically decorated shamanism, albeit reflecting the popular perception among patients and their relatives that there *should* be some treatment causing long-term desensitisation to ethanol (Krupitsky, 2010). Recent research in the field of molecular genetics and genetic engineering offers new prospect for eventually creating such a method. Thus, a single injection of a shRNA to rats, blocking the transcription of mRNA coding for aldehyde dehydrogenase and thus blocking the synthesis of this enzyme, resulted in a persistent decrease in ethanol consumption (Israel et al., 2015; Karahanian et al., 2015). A major pharmaceutical company has investigated this approach to the treatment of alcoholism (Harris et al., 2013).

Dopamine Receptor RNA

Nora Volkow, the current director of the National Institute of Drug Addiction of the United States (NIDA) has led a series of study using positron emission tomography (PET) to measure the availability of dopamine D2 receptors in the brain of individuals with addictions to diverse substances (ethanol, opioids, cocaine, amphetamine, and food) (Volkow et al., 2010). There is a consistent finding of reduced dopamine receptor availability in reward regions of the brain of dependent subjects, suggesting a common mechanism for drug dependence through blunting of dopaminergic transmission. Conversely, transfection of RNA encoding the D2 receptor into the brain of rats, significantly increasing its expression, associated with a significant decrease in alcohol consumption in alcohol-dependent rats (Thanos et al., 2001). These findings may be the first steps towards an eventual genetic treatment for substance dependence.

CONCLUSIONS

1. A pharmacogenetic marker system allows the construction of polygenic predictive systems to predict efficacy and tolerability within the framework of personalised pharmacotherapy of addictions.
2. Genetic engineering methods may be a promising new approach to pathogenetic therapy of addiction diseases.
3. Pharmacogenetics of drug addiction is a relatively young discipline, spanning barely two and a half decades. The research findings on the treatment of chemical dependencies nonetheless provide convincing evidence that the efficacy and tolerability of medications relate to polymorphisms of genes determining the processes of drug catabolism in the body. Other genetic markers pertain to specific neuroreceptors or transporters, especially those involved dopamine, acetylcholine and opioid signalling. This constitutes compelling evidence of the congruence of current scientific understanding of the neurobiological mechanisms underlying substance dependence development, the mechanisms of action of therapeutic drugs, and the molecular mechanisms of genome functioning.

References

Addolorato G., Mirijello A., Leggio L. Alcohol addiction: Toward a patient-oriented pharmacological treatment. *Expert Opin Pharmacother*. 2013 Nov;14(16):2157–60. doi:10.1517/14656566.2013.83 4047. Epub 2013 Aug 29. PMID: 23984836; PMCID: PMC4465082.

Anton R.F. Pharmacologic approaches to the management of alcoholism. *J Clin Psychiatry*. 2001;62(Suppl 20):11–17. PMID: 11584870.

Anton R.F., Oroszi G., O'Malley S., Couper D., Swift R., Pettinati H., Goldman D. An evaluation of μ-opioid receptor (OPRM1) as a predictor of naltrexone response in the treatment of alcohol dependence: Results from the Combined Pharmacotherapies and Behavioral Interventions for Alcohol Dependence (COMBINE) study. *Archives of General Psychiatry*. 2008;65(2):135–44. doi:10.1001/archpsyc.65.2.135

Anton R.F., Voronin K.E., Book S.W., Latham P.K., Randall P.K., Glen W.B., Schacht J.P. Opioid and dopamine genes interact to predict naltrexone response in a randomized alcohol use disorder clinical trial. *Alcoholism: Clinical and Experimental Research*. 2020;44(10):2084–96. doi:10.1111/acer.14431

Arias A.J., Armeli S., Gelernter J., Covault J., Kallio A., Karhuvaara S., Kranzler H.R. Effects of opioid receptor gene variation on targeted nalmefene treatment in heavy drinkers. *Alcoholism: Clinical and Experimental Research*. 2008;32(7):1159–66. doi:10.1111/j.1530–0277.2008.00735.x

Arias A.J., Gelernter J., Gueorguieva R., Ralevski E., Petrakis I.L. Pharmacogenetics of naltrexone and disulfiram in alcohol dependent, dually diagnosed veterans. *Am J Addict*. 2014 May-Jun;23(3):288–93. doi:10.1111/j.1521–0391.2014.12102.x. PMID: 24724887; PMCID: PMC4600600.

Attilia F., Perciballi, R., Rotondo C., Capriglione I., Iannuzzi S., Attilia M.L., Ceccanti M. Pharmacological treatment of alcohol use disorder: Scientific evidence. *Rivista di psichiatria*. 2018;53(3):123–7. doi:10.1708/2925.29414

Bart G., Schluger J.H., Borg L., Ho A., Bidlack J.M., Kreek M.J. Nalmefene induced elevation in serum prolactin in normal human volunteers: Partial kappa opioid agonist activity? *Neuropsychopharmacology*. 2005 Dec;30(12):2254–62. doi:10.1038/sj.npp.1300811. PMID: 15988468.

Bhaduri N., Mukhopadhyay K. Correlation of plasma dopamine β-hydroxylase activity with polymorphisms in DBH gene: A study on Eastern Indian population. *Cellular and Molecular Neurobiology*. 2008;28(3):343–50. doi:10.1007/s10571-007-9256-8

Carroll K.M., Nich C., Petry N.M., Eagan D.A., Shi J.M., Ball S.A. A randomized factorial trial of disulfiram and contingency management to enhance cognitive behavioral therapy for cocaine dependence. *Drug Alcohol Depend*. 2016 Mar 1;160:135–42. doi:10.1016/j.drugalcdep.2015.12.036. Epub 2016 Jan 13. PMID: 26817621; PMCID: PMC4767616.

Chan A.W. Racial differences in alcohol sensitivity. *Alcohol Alcohol*. 1986;21(1):93–104. PMID: 2937417.

Clarke T.K., Crist R.C., Ang A., Ambrose-Lanci L.M., Lohoff F.W., Saxon A.J., Berrettini W.H. Genetic variation in OPRD1 and the response to treatment for opioid dependence with buprenorphine in European-American females. *The Pharmacogenomics Journal*. 2014;14(3):303. doi:10.1038/tpj.2013.30

Codd E.E., Shank R.P., Schupsky J.J., Raffa R.B. Serotonin and norepinephrine uptake inhibiting activity of centrally acting analgesics: Structural determinants and role in antinociception. *J Pharmacol Exp Ther*. 1995 Sep;274(3):1263–70. PMID: 7562497.

Correa Filho J.M., Baltieri D.A. A pilot study of full-dose ondansetron to treat heavy-drinking men withdrawing from alcohol in Brazil. *Addictive Behaviors*. 2013;38(4):2044–51. doi:10.1016/j.addbeh.2012.12.018

Crist R.C., Phillips K.A., Furnari M.A., Moran L.M., Doyle G.A., McNicholas L.F., Berrettini W.H. Replication of the pharmacogenetic effect of rs678849 on buprenorphine efficacy in African-Americans with opioid use disorder. *The Pharmacogenomics Journal*. 2019;19(3):260. doi:10.1038/s41397-018-0065-x

Cumming P., Marton J., Lilius T.O., Olberg D.E., Rominger A. A survey of molecular imaging of opioid receptors. *Molecules*. 2019 Nov 19;24(22):4190. doi:10.3390/molecules24224190. PMID: 31752279; PMCID: PMC6891617.

Deinum J., Steenbergen-Spanjers G.C.H., Jansen M., Boomsma F., Lenders J.W.M., van Ittersum F.J., Wevers, R.A. DBH gene variants that cause low plasma dopamine β hydroxylase with or without a severe orthostatic syndrome. *Journal of Medical Genetics*. 2004;41(4):e38. doi:10.1136/jmg.2003.009282

Del Re A.C., Maisel N., Blodgett J., Finney J. The declining efficacy of naltrexone pharmacotherapy for alcohol use disorders over time: A multivariate meta-analysis. *Alcoholism: Clinical and Experimental Research*. 2013;37(6):1064–68. doi:10.1111/acer.12067

Devoto P., Flore G., Saba P., Frau R., Gessa G.L. *Brain Behav*. 2015 Sep 24;5(10):e00393. doi:10.1002/brb3.393. eCollection 2015 Oct. PMID: 26516613.

Gaval-Cruz M., Weinshenker D. Mechanisms of disulfiram-induced cocaine abstinence: Antabuse and cocaine relapse. *Molecular Interventions*. 2009;9(4):175. doi:10.1124/mi.9.4.6

Haass-Koffler C.L., Akhlaghi F., Swift R.M., Leggio L. Altering ethanol pharmacokinetics to treat alcohol use disorder: Can you teach an old dog new tricks? *Journal of Psychopharmacology*. 2017;31(7):812–18. doi:10.1177/0269881116684338

Harris J.F., Micheva-Viteva S., Li N., Hong-Geller E. Small RNA-mediated regulation of host: Pathogen interactions. *Virulence*. 2013;4(8):785–95. doi:10.4161/viru.26119

Hartwell E.E., Feinn R., Morris P.E., Gelernter J., Krystal J., Arias A.J., Kranzler H.R. Systematic review and meta-analysis of the moderating effect of rs1799971 in OPRM1, the mu-opioid receptor gene, on response to naltrexone treatment of alcohol use disorder. *Addiction*. 2020;115:1426–37. doi:10.1111/add.14975

Israel Y., Quintanilla, M.E., Karahanian, E., Rivera-Meza, M., Herrera-Marschitz, M. The "first hit" toward alcohol reinforcement: Role of ethanol metabolites. *Alcoholism: Clinical and Experimental Research*. 2015;39(5):776–86. doi:10.1111/acer.12709

Johnson B.A., Ait-Daoud N., Bowden C.L., et al. Oral topiramate for treatment of alcohol dependence: A randomized controlled trial. *Lancet.* 2003;361(9370):1677–85. doi:10.1016/s0140-6736(03)13370-3

Johnson B.A., Ait-Daoud N., Seneviratne C., Roache J.D., Javors M.A., Wang X.Q., Li M.D. Pharmacogenetic approach at the serotonin transporter gene as a method of reducing the severity of alcohol drinking. *American Journal of Psychiatry.* 2011;168(3):265–275. doi:10.1176/appi.ajp.2010.10050755

Johnson B.A., Roache J.D., Javors M.A., et al. Ondansetron for reduction of drinking among biologically predisposed alcoholic patients: A randomized controlled trial. *JAMA.* 2000;284(8):963–71. doi:10.1001/jama.284.8.963

Johnson B.A., Rosenthal N., Capece J.A., et al. Topiramate for treating alcohol dependence: A randomized controlled trial. *JAMA.* 2007;298(14):1641–51. doi:10.1001/jama.298.14.1641

Johnson B.A., Seneviratne C., Wang X.Q., et al. Determination of genotype combinations that can predict the outcome of the treatment of alcohol dependence using the 5-HT(3) antagonist ondansetron. *American Journal of Psychiatry.* 2013;170(9):1020–31. doi:10.1176/appi.ajp.2013.12091163

Johnstone E.C., Yudkin P.L., Hey K., Roberts S.J., Welch S.J., Murphy M.F., Griffiths S.E., Walton R.T. Genetic variation in dopaminergic pathways and short-term effectiveness of the nicotine patch. *Pharmacogenetics and Genomics.* 2004;14(2):83–90. doi:10.1097/00008571-200402000-00002

Karahanian E., Quintanilla M.E., Tampier L., Rivera-Meza M., Bustamante D., Gonzalez-Lira V., Morales P., Herrera-Marschitz M., Israel Y. Ethanol as a prodrug: Brain metabolism of ethanol mediates its reinforcing effects. *Alcoholism: Clinical and Experimental Research.* 2011;35(4):606–12. doi:10.1111/j.1530-0277.2011.01439.x

Karahanian E., Rivera-Meza M., Tampier L., Quintanilla M.E., Herrera-Marschitz M., Israel Y. Long-term inhibition of ethanol intake by the administration of an aldehyde dehydrogenase-2 (ALDH 2) coding lentiviral vector into the ventral tegmental area of rats. *Addiction Biology.* 2015;20(2):336–44. doi:10.1111/adb.12130

Karpyak V.M., Biernacka J.M., Geske J.R., Jenkins G.D., Cunningham J.M., Rüegg J., Loukianova L.L. Genetic markers associated with abstinence length in alcohol-dependent subjects treated with acamprosate. *Translational Psychiatry.* 2014;4(10):1–7. doi:10.1038/tp.2014.103

Kharasch E.D., Regina K.J., Blood J., Friedel C. Methadone pharmacogenetics: CYP2B6 polymorphisms determine plasma concentrations, clearance, and metabolism. *Anesthesiology.* 2015 Nov;123(5):1142–53. doi:10.1097/ALN.0000000000000867. PMID: 26389554; PMCID: PMC4667947.

Kibitov A.O., Brodyansky V.M., Rybakova K.V., Solovva M.G., Skurat E.P., Chuprova N.A., Nikolishin A.E., Krupitsky E.M. Pharmacogenetic markers of the effectiveness of alcohol dependence therapy with pregabalin, a modulator of GABA and glutamate systems. *Voprosy narkologii.* 2018;10–11:101–50. (In Russ.)

Kiefer F., Witt S.H., Frank J., Richter A., Treutlein J., Lemenager T., Wodarz N. Involvement of the atrial natriuretic peptide transcription factor GATA4 in alcohol dependence, relapse risk and treatment response to acamprosate. *The Pharmacogenomics Journal.* 2011;11(5):368. doi:10.1038/tpj201051

King D.P., Paciga S., Pickering E., Benowitz N.L., Bierut L.J., Conti D.V., Park P.W. Smoking cessation pharmacogenetics: Analysis of varenicline and bupropion in placebo-controlled clinical trials. *Neuropsychopharmacology.* 2012;37(3):641. doi:10.1038/npp.2011.232

Köhnke M.D., Zabetian C.P., Anderson G.M., Kolb W., Gaertner I., Buchkremer G., Cubells J.F. A genotype-controlled analysis of plasma dopamine β-hydroxylase in healthy and alcoholic subjects: Evidence for alcohol-related differences in noradrenergic function. *Biological Psychiatry.* 2002;52(12):1151–8. doi:10.1016/S0006-3223(02)01427-0

Kranzler H.R., Armeli S., Tennen H., Covault J., Feinn R., Arias A.J., Oncken C. A double-blind, randomized trial of sertraline for alcohol dependence: Moderation by age of onset and 5-HTTLPR genotype. *Journal of Clinical Psychopharmacology.* 2011;31(1):22. doi:10.1097/JCP.0b013e31820465fa

Kranzler H.R., Covault J., Feinn R., Armeli S., Tennen H., Arias A.J., Kampman K.M. Topiramate treatment for heavy drinkers: Moderation by a GRIK1 polymorphism. *American Journal of Psychiatry.* 2014;171(4):445–52. doi:10.1037/a0037309

Krupitsky E.M. Short-term intensive psychotherapeutic intervention in narcology from the standpoint of evidence-based medicine. *Nevrologicheskiy vestnik.* 2010;42(3):25–7. (In Russ.)

Krupitsky E.M. The use of pharmacological agents to stabilize remissions and prevent relapse in alcoholism: Foreign studies. *Voprosy narkologii.* 2003;1:51–61. (In Russ.)

Krupitsky E.M., Kibitov A.O., Blokhina E.A., Verbitskaya E.V., Brodyansky V.M., Alekseeva N.P., Bushara N.M., Yaroslavtseva T.S., Palatkin V.Ya., Masalov D.V., Burakov A.M., Romanova T.N., Sulimov G.Yu., Kosten T., Nielsen D., Zvartau E.E., Woody D. Stabilization of remissions in patients with opium addiction Naltrexone implant: Pharmacogenetic aspect. *Zhurnal nevrologii i psikhiatrii im. S.S. Korsakova*. 2015;115(4):14–23. (In Russ.)

Krupitsky E.M., Rybakova K.V., Skurat E.P., Mikhailov A.D., Neznanov N.G. Double-blind, randomized, placebo-controlled study of the effectiveness of the use of pregabalin for the treatment of alcohol dependence syndrome. *Voprosy narkologii.* 2017;8: 81–2. (In Russ.)

Krupitsky E.M., Rybakova K.V., Skurat E.P., Mikhailov A.D., Neznanov N.G. Pregabalin reduces smoking and drinking in alcohol dependent subjects. *European Neuropsychopharmacology.* 2019;29(1):S176–7. doi:10.1016/j.euroneuro.2018.11.300

Latt N., Conigrave K., Saunders J., Marshall E.J., Nutt D. *Addiction Medicine.* Oxford University Press, 2009, 459 p.

Mason B.J., Heyser C.J. Acamprosate: A prototypic neuromodulator in the treatment of alcohol dependence. *CNS Neurol Disord Drug Targets.* 2010 Mar;9(1):23–32. doi:10.2174/187152710790966641. PMID: 20201812; PMCID: PMC2853976.

McCarthy J.J., Graas J., Leamon M.H., Ward C., Vasti E.J., Fassbender C. The use of the Methadone/Metabolite Ratio (MMR) to identify an individual metabolic phenotype and assess risks of poor response and adverse effects: Towards scientific methadone dosing. *J Addict Med.* 2020 Sep/Oct;14(5):431–6. doi:10.1097/ADM.0000000000000620. PMID: 32032212.

Moerke M.J., McMahon L.R., Wilkerson J.L. More than smoke and patches: The quest for pharmacotherapies to treat tobacco use disorder. *Pharmacol Rev.* 2020 Apr;72(2):527–57. doi:10.1124/pr.119.018028. PMID: 32205338; PMCID: PMC7090325.

Morley K.C., Luquin N., Baillie A., Fraser I., Trent R.J., Dore G., Haber P.S. Moderation of baclofen response by a GABAB receptor polymorphism: Results from the BacALD randomized controlled trial. *Addiction.* 2018;113(12):2205–13. doi:10.1111/add.14373

Munafo M.R., Elliot K.M., Murphy M.F., Walton R.T., Johnstone E.C. Association of the mu-opioid receptor gene with smoking cessation. *The Pharmacogenomics Journal.* 2007;7(5):353–61. doi:10.1038/6500432

Ooteman W., Michael N., Koeter M., Verheul R., Schippers G., Houchi H., Van den Brink W. Predicting the effect of naltrexone and acamprosate in alcohol-dependent patients using phenotypic, endophenotypic and genetic indicators. *Behavior Genetics.* 2007;37(6):781–2. doi:10.1111/j.1369–1600.2009.00159.x

Oslin D.W., Berrettini W., Kranzler H.R., Pettinati H., Gelernter J., Volpicelli J.R., O'Brien C.P. A functional polymorphism of the μ-opioid receptor gene is associated with naltrexone response in alcohol-dependent patients. *Neuropsychopharmacology.* 2003;28(8):1546–52. doi:10.1038/1300219

Oslin D.W., Leong S.H., Lynch K.G., Berrettini W., O'Brien C.P., Gordon A.J., Rukstalis M. Naltrexone vs placebo for the treatment of alcohol dependence: A randomized clinical trial. *JAMA Psychiatry.* 2015;72(5):430–7. doi:10.1001/jamapsychiatry.2014.3053

Pirmohamed M. Pharmacogenetics and pharmacogenomics. *Br J Clin Pharmacol.* 2001;52(4):345–7. doi:10.1046/j.0306–5251.2001.01498.x

Ray L.A., Miranda R. Jr., MacKillop J., McGeary J., Tidey J.W., Rohsenow D.J., Gwaltney C., Swift R.W., Monti P.M. A preliminary pharmacogenetic investigation of adverse events from topiramate in heavy drinkers. *Exp Clin Psychopharmacol.* 2009 Apr;17(2):122–9. doi:10.1037/a0015700. PMID: 19331489; PMCID: PMC3682424.

Rubio G., Martinez-Gras I., Manzanares J. Modulation of impulsivity by topiramate: Implications for the treatment of alcohol dependence. *Journal of Clinical Psychopharmacology.* 2009;29(6):584–9. doi:10.1097/JCP.0b013e3181bfdb79

Salloum N.C., Buchalter E.L., Chanani S., Espejo G., Ismail M.S., Laine R.O., Vance E. From genes to treatments: A systematic review of the pharmacogenetics in smoking cessation. *Pharmacogenomics.* 2018;19(10):861–71. doi:10.2217/pgs-2018–0023

Schnoll R.A., Patterson F. Sex heterogeneity in pharmacogenetic smoking cessation clinical trials. *Drug Alcohol Depend.* 2009 Oct 1;104(Suppl 1):S94–9. doi:10.1016/j.drugalcdep.2008.11.012. Epub 2009 Jan 8. PMID: 19135319; PMCID: PMC2810256.

Seneviratne C., Johnson B.A. Advances in medications and tailoring treatment for alcohol use disorder. *Alcohol Research: Current Reviews.* 2015;37(1):15. doi:10.0000/www.ncbi.nlm.nih.gov/PMC44

Smeralda C.L., Gigli G.L., Janes F., et al. May lamotrigine be an alternative to topiramate in the prevention of migraine with aura? Results of a retrospective study. *BMJ Neurology Open* 2020;2:e000059. doi:10.1136/bmjno-2020–000059

Sturgess J.E., George T.P., Kennedy J.L., Heinz A., Müller D.J. Pharmacogenetics of alcohol, nicotine and drug addiction treatments. *Addiction Biology.* 2011;16(3):357–76. doi:10.1111/j.1369–1600.2010.00287.x

Thanos P.K., Volkow N.D., Freimuth P., Umegaki H., Ikari H., Roth G., Hitzemann R. Overexpression of dopamine D2 receptors reduces alcohol self-administration. *Journal of Neurochemistry.* 2001;78(5):1094–103. doi:10.1046/j.1471-4159.2001.00492.x

Tutka P., Vinnikov D., Courtney R.J., Benowitz N.L. Cytisine for nicotine addiction treatment: A review of pharmacology, therapeutics and an update of clinical trial evidence for smoking cessation. *Addiction.* 2019 Nov;114(11):1951–69. doi:10.1111/add.14721. Epub 2019 Jul 19. PMID: 31240783.

Volkow N.D., Wang G.J., Fowler J.S., Tomasi D., Telang F., Baler R. Addiction: Decreased reward sensitivity and increased expectation sensitivity conspire to overwhelm the brain's control circuit. *Bioessays.* 2010;32(9):748–55. doi:10.1002/bies.201000042

World Health Organization. The methadone fix. *Bull World Health Organ.* 2008;86(3):162. doi:10.2471/blt.08.052100

Zabetian C.P., Anderson G.M., Buxbaum S.G., Elston R.C., Ichinose H., Nagatsu T., Cubells J.F. A quantitative-trait analysis of human plasma – dopamine β-hydroxylase activity: Evidence for a major functional polymorphism at the DBH locus. *The American Journal of Human Genetics.* 2001;68(2):515–22. doi:10.1086/318198

Zanger U.M., Schwab M. Cytochrome P450 enzymes in drug metabolism: Regulation of gene expression, enzyme activities, and impact of genetic variation. *Pharmacol Ther.* 2013 Apr;138(1):103–41. doi:10.1016/j.pharmthera.2012.12.007. Epub 2013 Jan 16. PMID: 23333322.

16
Optimizing Patient Care in Psychiatry – Behavioral Addictions

Elvin Lukose

Similarities Between Substance Use Disorder and Behavioral Addiction	169
Pathological Gambling	170
Fallacies Observed in Gamblers	*170*
Other Behavioral Addictions	*171*
Internet Addiction	172
Compulsive Shopping and Buying	*172*
Compulsive Sexual Behavior/Sex Addiction	*174*
Assessment and Screening	175
Psychopharmacological Treatments	176
Interventional Modalities	176
Conclusions	178

Pathological behaviors like pathological gambling, online gaming, excessive internet use, compulsive shopping, non-paraphilic hypersexuality and kleptomania were classified under the chapter of 'Impulse Control Disorders' in DSM IV-TR. Recent findings of translational research and neuro-imaging have provided a gross similarity between the neurobiological models of pathological gambling and substance use disorder that eventually led to inclusion of gambling disorder under 'Non-Substance Use Disorder' in DSM V. Despite clinical similarities between all the mentioned behaviors and substance addiction, much research evidence is at best inconclusive; hence, they remain classified under the rubric of impulse control disorders even in DSM V.

SIMILARITIES BETWEEN SUBSTANCE USE DISORDER AND BEHAVIORAL ADDICTION

The common phenomenological denominators of both substance use disorder and pathological behaviors are positive anticipation of increasing rewards, decreased pleasure from previously achieved levels of reward, urge to continue engaging in the behavior despite negative consequences to self, negative emotional responses to thwarted rewards or their unavailability and the failure to resist an impulse to perform the act. The physiological withdrawal syndrome and the associated medical complications seen in substance use disorder are not observed in behavioral addictions. Symptoms of emotional dysregulation like dysphoria are noted in response to craving. Like drug tolerance, people engaged in pathological gambling, kleptomania, compulsive sexual behavior and compulsive buying do report a decrease in these positive mood effects on repeating the same level of behavior, accompanied by a need to increase the intensity and frequency of behavior to achieve the same desirable mood states. Similar to substance use disorders, behavioral addictions have led to marital conflicts and frequent conflicts with law as well as professional and financial losses.

Cognitive similarities include a tendency to discount rewards rapidly and perform disadvantageously on decision-making tasks on account of impulsivity.

Jentsch and Taylor founded the classic neuropsychological model of addictions that emphasizes on the balance between a subcortical *accelerator* system (comprising the nucleus accumbens and amygdala) and a prefrontal cortical *braking* system. As a person transitions from harmful drug abuse to addiction, the reflexive system becomes sensitized through learning processes, while the efficacy of prefrontal brake is gradually weakened by the toxic effects of the offending drug. Later extensions of this model usefully separate the substrates for initial intoxication and subsequent craving and highlight the involvement of the hippocampus in holding drug-related memories and conditional place preference. Recent neuroscientific findings have shown the insula as an important node in addiction. Insula act as a thermostat in a three-system model where the insula represents a gateway between the subcortical reward system and the prefrontal system responsible for decision making and inhibitory control.

PATHOLOGICAL GAMBLING

Gambling disorder is the only behavioral addiction that has currently achieved a place in the DSM5; hence, it will provide a neurobiological model for research on other similar behavioral addictions that include excessive online gaming, internet addiction and compulsive shopping.

Oldman claimed pathological disorder was produced by a defective relationship between a strategy of play and a way of managing one's finances. 'Losers' in gambling were assumed to lie on a continuum, with pathological gambling occupying the extreme end of it. Hayano claimed gamblers lost money due to 1) inexperience and imperceptive/bad play; 2) erroneous ideas about cards, dice and so forth; and 3) inept money management ('chasing').

Moran classified gamblers into five types based on the predominant personality trait: 1) 'sub-cultural' variety (gambling dependent on social setting), 2) 'neurotic' variety (gambling with money rather than for money), 3) 'impulsive' variety (loss of control and ambivalence about play), 4) 'psychopathic' variety (gambling as a part of a global disturbance) and 5) 'symptomatic' variety (gambling associated with mental illness).

Fallacies Observed in Gamblers

Gamblers also experience the 'Gambler's fallacy' or 'Monte Carlo fallacy' wherein previous wins convince them of possible future wins with minimum weight on statistical probabilities. It also leads the gambler into a false belief that number of wins and losses are finite and both add up to nullify each other, hence suggesting to the gambler that a series of losses implies that the prospective bets will be a series of 'wins', which further traps the player in the game and prevents him from quitting when he has lost a significant amount of money already. 'Hot hand fallacy' is observed when a gambler achieves a 'series of wins' which skews his subjective estimation of further wins. Similarly, 'beginner's luck' is seen, where a novice gambler may view a big initial win as suggestive of his talent or gift or expertise, pushing him to bet higher and continue gambling. All these fallacies revolve around a sense of 'illusory control', convincing the gambler that the probabilities are in his favor and that he has 'control' over them. Other specific phenomena within gambling games can be considered under the rubric of these two effects. The role of intermittent or partial reinforcement effects occurs when most *near misses* are perceived as having been close to a win, despite being objective losses. Near misses are perceived as more aversive than complete misses but increase the desire to continue the game.

Gambling has become a significant problem with the proliferation of lottery tickets, casinos and Internet gambling sites with the accommodation and gradual acceptance of gambling as a legitimate form of entertainment. Epidemiological studies show that men represent the majority of pathological gamblers and that being male appears to be a risk factor for developing a gambling disorder during adolescence. The telescoping phenomenon (the rapid rate of progression from initial to problematic behavior in women compared with men) has been observed in pathological gambling, similar to alcohol use disorder. High rates of pathological gambling and substance abuse have been reported during adolescence and young adulthood, supporting a relationship between behavioral and substance addictions. Adolescents who are moderate- to high-frequency drinkers are more likely to gamble frequently than those who are not, suggesting a behavioral interaction between alcohol and gambling. Substance use co-morbidity may affect gambling in two ways: by disinhibiting a range of inappropriate behaviors (including those identified as addictive) or acting as a substitute for drinking. Problem gamblers with frequent alcohol use have higher gambling severity and more psychosocial problems resulting from gambling than those without alcohol use disorder. Problem gamblers who use tobacco daily are more likely to have alcohol and drug use problems.

Other Behavioral Addictions

The Diagnostic and Statistical Manual Fifth Edition (DSM-V) task force proposed two important changes related to compulsive buying: distinguishing obsessive-compulsive disorder from the anxiety disorders and placing it in a separate category – the obsessive-compulsive disorder spectrum disorders and classifying several new autonomous disorders from those currently described as impulse control disorders not otherwise specified. The task force suggested including in this group of disorders compulsive-impulsive varieties of shopping, internet use disorder, sexual behaviour and skin-picking.

Of these, gaming disorder (online) as a type of internet use disorder has achieved the status of a formal diagnosis in ICD 11, although it is still in the pipeline for the next batch of non-substance use disorders as proposed by DSM V taskforce.

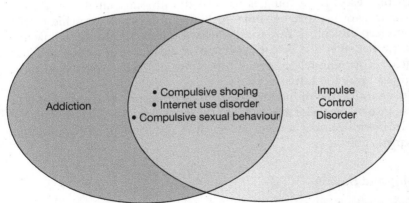

Figure 16.1 Phenomenological and neurobiological relationships of behavioral addictions with impulse control disorders and addiction disorders (substance use disorders).

INTERNET ADDICTION

There have been differences in opinion regarding diagnosis of excessive internet use as a form of addiction amidst the stigma of psychiatrists having the tendency to pathologize everyday behavior practiced in an overindulgent fashion. Due to multiple reports of substance abuse–like behavioral syndromes in people addicted to gaming, ICD 11 classified gaming disorder under disorders due to addictive behaviors. Young classified internet addiction into three subtypes: gaming, email/texting and online sexual preoccupations.

There have been numerous studies correlating internet addiction to underlying depression, anxiety and adjustment issues to environmental stressors. Conducted a survey in a sample of 275 high school students in Florence, Italy, through administering the Shorter PROMIS Questionnaire and the Internet Addiction Scale in the assessment of multiple addictions, and 5.4% of the students were found to qualify for internet addiction, similar to other countries. Disability strongly correlated to the subscale of alcohol, gambling, sex, tobacco, food starving and bingeing, shopping, exercise and internet addiction. A first large-scale epidemiological study of problematic internet use through a random-digit-dial telephone survey of 2,513 adults in the United States by Aboujaoude et al. showed 3.7% to 13% of respondents endorsing ≥1 markers consistent with problematic internet use. Internet use has a significant effect on vegetative functions like sleep; for example, a meta-analysis by Alimoradi et al. revealed a significantly increased odds ratio for sleep problems and significant sleep contraction among individuals experiencing internet addiction.

Internet gaming disorder (IGD) has been viewed as a separate disorder on its own as compared to other internet-related behavioral addictions. Video game play is also associated with substantial physiological arousal similar to gambling. The analysis of 3,000 massively multiplayer online role-playing game (MMORPG) players' gaming motivations revealed that MMORPGs provide a hyper-real virtual environment for players not only to achieve game goals but to provide opportunities to be social and immerse oneself in the game, allowing an 'escapist' route from the mundanities and problems of daily life. Achievement is implied in advancing in the game, progressing or 'leveling up' and acquiring status and power in the game, which, along with the game's mechanics, like the possibilities for optimizing game play, competition with the added prospect of dominating others and the admiration and opportunities for status signaling, is highly contingent on reinforcement within the construct of the game, thus fueling the intensity and frequency of involvement of the gamer in the game. The game environment is uncertain, with rewards delivered on a variable-ratio schedule of reinforcement, identical to gambling. In fact, the structural features of video games lend themselves to a very similar analysis to gambling games.

There is evidence that excessive gaming is associated with substantial impairment, associated with a wide array of negative outcomes including poor scholastic achievement, oppositional behavior, sleep difficulties and suicidal behavior. IGD has also been linked to depression, social difficulties, attention deficit hyperactivity disorder and substance abuse. The stroboscopic effect of gaming-related visual experience has been reported to cause game-induced seizures as a rare and extreme case.

Compared to other excessive uses of internet use, gaming problems are symptomatically closest to typical substance use behavior and hence at the highest risk for adverse effects. It is possible that problems with gaming account for much of the relation between internet addiction and problematic outcomes.

Compulsive Shopping and Buying

Although the lines between buying and pathological levels of buying are arbitrary, when it is repetitive and associated with adverse consequences, psychological or financial or both, this kind of buying is known as compulsive buying. Compulsive buyers experience repetitive, irresistible and overpowering urges to purchase goods, perhaps similar to the approach behavior in substance addiction. The bought goods are frequently unnecessary, out of proportion to the need, maybe even useless and tend to remain unused or minimally used. Availability of the online megastores and retail environment may promote compulsive buying because it permits avoidance of direct, confrontational face-to-face social contact and maintains secrecy of the transactions within the privacy of the shopper's account, which remains practically invisible from scrutiny by family or spouses.

Compulsive buyers strongly focus on the buying process itself; that is, they are more interested in the acquisition than in possession or use of the item purchased and are always vigilant about sales and seasonal deals and hence more susceptible to the 'scarcity error', that is, the bias that one will lose the opportunity to buy and experience the product because of limited stocks. McElroy et al. noted that 70% of patients presenting with compulsive buying described buying as 'a high', 'a buzz', 'a rush': the positive feeling (e.g., pleasure, excitement) experienced while buying. For compulsive buyers, money and the opportunities to buy could be considered a drug equivalent. For compulsive buyers, the focus is the buying process, not the item, so they usually lose interest in their purchase and keep it hidden (e.g., in a closet) or give or throw it away, which differentiates them from collectors.

Many psychiatric disorders may present with compulsive buying as a symptom. Excessive buying in mania or hypomania, which disappears during euthymic periods, is driven by grandiosity and loss of impulse control, without any focus on the buying process itself. Unnecessary and even bizarre purchases may be seen in psychotic disorders and are usually congruent to their delusional content, for example, purchasing window blinds to avoid outsiders or 'suspected' people of spying on the patient or special helmets to avoid 'thought withdrawal' by external sources that constitute the patient's delusional system.

For compulsive shopping, the major link to the neurobiology of drug addiction comes from Parkinson's disease, where this syndrome can appear alongside gambling disorder and hypersexuality in a constellation of reward-driven, impulsive behaviors that are seen as occasional side effects of dopamine agonist medications. Recent work has found that trait-reward sensitivity predicted compulsive buying tendencies differentially from either depression or obsessive-compulsive disorder.

Following internet use disorder, compulsive shopping shows some possibility of acquiring the status of behavioral addiction; however, evidence remains to be obtained in research.

Table 16.1 Research criteria used by McElroy et al. for compulsive shopping.

Inappropriate preoccupations with buying or shopping, or inappropriate buying or shopping impulses or behavior, as indicated by at least one of the following:

- *Frequent preoccupations with buying or impulses to buy that are experienced as irresistible, intrusive, and/or senseless*
- *Frequent buying of more than can be afforded, frequent buying of items that are not needed, or shopping for longer periods of time than intended*
- *The buying preoccupations, impulses, or behaviors cause marked distress, are time-consuming significantly interfere with social or occupational functioning, or result in financial problems (e.g., indebtedness or bankruptcy)*
- *The excessive buying or shopping behavior does not occur exclusively during periods of hypomania or mania*

Compulsive Sexual Behavior/Sex Addiction

It was in the mid-1970s when the concept of excessive non-paraphilic sexual behavior as a form of sexual dependence was introduced. Orford identified this out-of-control sexual behavior as some form of sexual addiction and pointed out the similarities between the behavior and alcohol addiction. He described the behavior as a maladaptive pattern of use and impaired control over a behavior associated with adverse consequences to self and intimate relationships. Patrick Cames, in his seminal book *Out of the Shadows*, observed sex addiction as a psychopathological condition. Although the DSM V makes no separate diagnosis for hypersexual behavior or sex addiction, ICD 11 classifies compulsive sexual behavior disorder under the chapter on 'Impulse Control Disorders'.

Drawing boundaries between problematic sexuality, excessive or hypersexuality and sex addiction has been controversial due to different models proposed for their existence as psychopathological conditions and their criticisms. A lack of a statistically sound neurobiological model may explain the dilemma between sex addiction being a form of compulsive-impulsive behavior and being a form of behavioral addiction. A dysfunctional attachment during childhood has been a consistent risk factor hallmark for sexual addiction. Negative or traumatic childhood attachment experiences may negatively impact individuals' affective, cognitive, and behavioral development, and interfere with the maturation of sexual behavior, thus favoring the development and maintenance of sexual addiction.

Table 16.2 Proposed criteria for sexual addiction.

A) Recurrent failure to resist impulses to engage in a specified sexual behavior;
B) Increasing sense of tension immediately prior to initiating the sexual behavior;
C) Pleasure or relief at the time of engaging in the sexual behavior;
D) At least five of the following criteria:
  (1) Frequent preoccupations with sexual behavior or with activity that is preparatory to the sexual behavior;
  (2) Frequent involvement in sexual behavior to a greater extent or over a longer period than intended;
  (3) Repeated efforts to reduce, control, or stop sexual behavior;
  (4) A great amount of time spent in activities necessary for engaging in sexual behavior, or for recovering from its effects;
  (5) Frequent involvement in sexual behavior when the subject is expected to fulfill occupational, academic, domestic, or social obligations;
  (6) Important social, occupational, or recreational activities given up or reduced because of the behavior;
  (7) Continuation of the behavior despite knowledge of having a persistent or recurrent social, financial, psychological, or physical problem that is caused or exacerbated by the sexual behavior;
  (8) Tolerance: need to increase the intensity or frequency of the sexual behavior to achieve the desired effect, or diminished effects obtained with sexual behavior of the same intensity;
  (9) Restlessness or irritability if unable to engage in sexual behavior
E) Some symptoms have persisted for at least one month or have occurred repeatedly over a longer period of time.

Studies estimate the prevalence of sexual addiction to be 3% to 6% in the general adult population. Higher rates have been suggested in specific populations, such as sexual offenders, HIV patients and people with hypersexual disorders and paraphilias. The evidence suggests a male preponderance in the affected population over female.

ICD 11 defines a core symptom of compulsive sexual behavior disorder as 'a persistent pattern of failure to control intense, repetitive sexual impulses or urges resulting in repetitive sexual behavior'. Such a pattern of sexual activity becomes a central focus of the person's life to the point of neglecting personal health and care and other interests. More than 70% of sexual addiction patients report withdrawal symptoms in the form of nervousness, insomnia, sweating, nausea, palpitations, shortness of breath and fatigue during urges and prior to engaging in the sexual act.

More than 90% of people who are categorized as having a compulsive, impulsive, addictive sexual disorder or a hypersexual disorder reported having thoughts and behaviors or sexual fantasies of 'obsessional' quality. Research has found that some hypersexual persons are cognitively dissociated from their sexual behavior when in high states of sexual arousal and hence, experience difficulty identifying their feelings.

Problems with compulsive sexual behavior can be analyzed via two dimensions, 1) behavioral symptoms and 2) cognitive/emotional symptoms. *Behavioral symptoms* include seeking new sexual partners, engaging in frequent sexual encounters and compulsive masturbation, frequent use of pornography, failed attempts to reduce or stop excessive sexual behaviors, lack of adequate physiological arousal during sexual activities, engaging in risky sexual activities, decreased self care and disregard for risk of sexually transmitted diseases. Cognitive and emotional symptoms include obsessive thoughts of sex; guilt about thoughts or engagement in excessive sexual behavior; the desire to escape from or suppress unpleasant emotions like loneliness, boredom or low self esteem; embarrassment and secrecy regarding sexual behaviors; rationalization about the continuation of sexual behaviors; and an absence of control in many aspects of life.

ASSESSMENT AND SCREENING

PATHOLOGICAL GAMBLING

- South Oaks Gambling Screen
- Gambling Symptom Assessment Scale
- Gambling-Yale-Brown Obsessive Compulsive Scale
- Pathological Gambling-Clinical Global Impression

INTERNET/GAMING ADDICTION

- Young's Internet Addiction Test (IAT)
- Compulsive Internet Use Scale (CIUS)
- Chen's Internet Addiction Scale

COMPULSIVE SHOPPING

- Compulsive Buying Scale
- Questionnaire about Buying Behavior (QABB)
- Canadian Compulsive Buying Measurement Scale
- Edwards Compulsive Buying Scale
- Minnesota Impulsive Disorder Interview
- Ridgway's Compulsive Buying Scale

COMPULSIVE SEXUAL BEHAVIOR/SEX ADDICTION

- Kalichman and Rompa's Sexual Compulsivity Scale (SCS)
- Sexual Addiction Screening Test (SAST)
- Sexual Outlet Inventory (SOI)
- Sexual Dependence Inventory (SDI-R)
- The Garos Sexual Behavior Index (GSBI)
- Yale-Brown Obsessive Compulsive Scale-Compulsive Sexual Behavior (YBOCS-CSB)

PSYCHOPHARMACOLOGICAL TREATMENTS

PHARMACOTHERAPY FOR PATHOLOGICAL GAMBLING

- Selective serotonin reuptake inhibitors (SSRIs) (more statistical evidence for fluvoxamine)
- Lithium (in cases with comorbid bipolar mood type II disorder and cyclothymic disorder)
- Naltrexone (more effective in gamblers with more severe urges)
- N-acetyl cysteine

While selective serotonin reuptake inhibitors such as fluvoxamine are effective in pathological gamblers, they may exacerbate gambling behavior and mood symptoms in a subgroup of patients with comorbid cyclothymia or bipolar spectrum condition, necessitating the addition of a mood stabilizer.

PHARMACOTHERAPY FOR INTERNET ADDICTION AND INTERNET GAMING DISORDER

- Methylphenidate/atomoxetine (in cases with comorbid ADHD)
- Bupropion (in cases with comorbid depression)
- Escitalopram (significant improvement but inferior to bupropion in internet addiction with comorbid depression)

PHARMACOTHERAPY FOR COMPULSIVE SHOPPING

- Selective serotonin reuptake inhibitors (open-label studies)
- Naltrexone (open-label studies)

PHARMACOTHERAPY FOR COMPULSIVE SEXUAL BEHAVIOR

- Selective serotonin reuptake inhibitors (open-label studies)
- Naltrexone (open-label studies)
- Topiramate

INTERVENTIONAL MODALITIES

FOR PATHOLOGICAL GAMBLING

1. Imaginal desensitization
2. Exposure and response prevention
3. Cognitive behavior therapy
   - Understanding the concept of randomness
   - Understanding the erroneous beliefs held by gamblers

- Awareness of inaccurate perceptions,
- Cognitive correction of erroneous perceptions
4. Support groups (Gamblers' Anonymous)

Grant et al. provided a diagnostic and treatment approach for gambling disorder as follows.

Table 16.3 Screen all patients for pathological gambling. For those who screen positive, perform the following diagnostic assessment.

1. RIf the person is reporting urges or cravings to gamble, consider a trial of an opioid antagonist.
2. RIf the person is having a co-occurring substance use disorder, consider a trial of an opioid antagonist.
3. RIf the person gambles because of depression or anxiety, or has co-occurring depressive or anxiety symptoms, consider an SRI trial.
4. RIf the person gambles when hypomanic or manic or has symptoms of subsyndromal (hypo)mania, consider a trial of lithium.
5. RAlways consider cognitive-behavioral therapy alone or in addition to medication.

FOR INTERNET ADDICTION
1. Digital detoxification
2. Group therapy
3. Cognitive behavioral therapy
   - Self monitoring of thoughts triggering addictive behavior
   - Eliciting cognitive distortions
   - Challenging core beliefs and thinking styles
   - Activation/facilitation of offline behaviors and hobbies
4. Applied behavioral analysis–based approaches
   - Altering antecedents (breaking or building pauses into the behavioral chain, re-ordering the links)
   - Habit reversal (awareness of craving, distraction and use of competing responses)
   - Changing response effort (amount of effort required to perform the addictive task)
5. Maintaining 'daily internet log' to monitor internet use
6. Home-based daily journaling
   - Tracking their smart phone use daily for amount of time spent, content, location used
   - Reflective self-evaluations
7. Reality therapy
   - Using the WDEP model, W = wants, D = direction and doing, E = evaluation, P = planning and commitment)

In South Korea, where internet gaming addiction is viewed as a significant concern for public health, up to 24% of children diagnosed with internet addiction have been hospitalized. In Japan, following a study by the Ministry of Education, the government initiated the development of 'fasting camps' where individuals suffering from internet and gaming addiction are cut off from technology completely. Specialized treatment centers and programs have been established in Europe. Established in 2008, the Sabine M. Grüsser-Sinopoli Outpatient Clinic for Behavioral Addictions, Mainz, has been the first outpatient clinic in Germany to offer group therapy for computer game and internet addiction in addition to therapy for pathological gambling. The Capio Nightingale Hospital in London, UK, also caters to the mental healthcare needs of those with behavioral addiction. Inpatient centers like the RESTART Internet Addiction Recovery Program in Seattle and the recently opened digital detoxification programs at the Bradford Regional Medical Centre in Pennsylvania reflect the growing need for professional help and legitimization of behavioral addictions.

Campaign for Commercial Free Childhood (CCFC) is a collective active attempt to inform and educate the masses about the potential harms of technology and the internet on the newer generations.

FOR COMPULSIVE SHOPPING

1. Cognitive behavioral therapy
2. Applied behavioral analysis
   - Altering antecedents (breaking or building pauses into the behavioral chain, re-ordering the links
   - Deactivating shopping accounts and credit cards
   - Using cash for purchases
3. Purchase log for self monitoring

FOR COMPULSIVE SEXUAL BEHAVIOR

1. Cognitive behavioral therapy
2. Family/couples therapy
3. Support groups (Sex and Love Addicts Anonymous a.k.a. SLAA)

CONCLUSIONS

Growing evidence indicates that behavioral addictions resemble substance addictions in many domains, simulating the chronic, relapsing course with higher incidence and prevalence in adolescents and young adults, phenomenology of craving, intoxication and withdrawal, tolerance, co-morbidity, overlapping genetic contribution, neurobiological mechanisms and response to treatment. However, existing data are most supportive for pathological gambling, with only limited data for compulsive buying, internet and video/computer game addiction. Due to an obvious dearth of knowledge, especially in the absence of validated diagnostic criteria and prospective, longitudinal studies, it would be premature to consider other behavioral addictions full-fledged independent non-substance use disorders, much less classify them all as similar to substance addictions rather than as impulse control disorders.

Substantial translational research in both human and animal studies is needed in the future to accommodate the status of behavioral addictions to the level of that for substance addictions, especially in the domains of genetics, neurobiology and treatment.

Bibliography

- Aboujaoude E, Koran LM, Gamel N, Large MD, Serpe RT. Potential markers for problematic internet use: A telephone survey of 2,513 adults. *CNS Spectrums*. 2006 Oct 1;11(10):750.
- Alimoradi Z, Lin CY, Broström A, Bülow PH, Bajalan Z, Griffiths MD, Ohayon MM, Pakpour AH. Internet addiction and sleep problems: A systematic review and meta-analysis. *Sleep Medicine Reviews*. 2019 Oct 1;47:51–61.

- Bostwick JM, Bucci JA. Internet sex addiction treated with naltrexone. In *Mayo Clinic Proceedings* (Vol. 83, No. 2, pp. 226–30). Elsevier; 2008 Feb 1.
- de Castro V, Fong T, Rosenthal RJ, Tavares H. A comparison of craving and emotional states between pathological gamblers and alcoholics. *Addict Behav*. 2007;32(8):1555–64. [PubMed: 17174480]
- Freimuth M, Waddell M, Stannard J, Kelley S, Kipper A, Richardson A, Szuromi I. Expanding the scope of dual diagnosis and co-addictions: Behavioral addictions. *Journal of Groups in Addiction & Recovery*. 2008 Nov 3;3(3–4):137–60.
- Grant JE, Brewer JA, Potenza MN. The neurobiology of substance and behavioral addictions. *CNS Spectr*. 2006;11(12):924–30. [PubMed: 17146406]
- Grant JE, Kim SW. Medication management of pathological gambling. *Minnesota Medicine*. 2006 Sep;89(9):44.
- Hayano DM. *Poker Faces: The Life and Work of Professional Card Players*. Univ of California Press; 1982.
- Kafka MP, Prentky R. Fluoxetine treatment of nonparaphilic sexual addictions and paraphilias in men. *The Journal of Clinical Psychiatry*. 1992 Oct.
- Khazaal Y, Zullino DF. Topiramate in the treatment of compulsive sexual behavior: Case report. *BMC Psychiatry*. 2006 Dec;6(1):1–4.
- Ko CH, Hsiao S, Liu GC, Yen JU, Yang MJ, Yen CF. The characteristics of decision making, potential to take risks, and personality of college students with Internet addiction. *Psychiatry Res*. 2010;175:121–5. [PubMed: 19962767]
- Krueger RB, Kaplan MS. The paraphilic and hypersexual disorders: An overview. *Journal of Psychiatric Practice*. 2001 Nov 1;7(6):391–403.
- McElroy SL, Keck PE, Pope HG, Smith JM, Strakowski SM. Compulsive buying: A report of 20 cases. *The Journal of Clinical Psychiatry*. 1994 Jun.
- Moran E. Varieties of pathological gambling. *The British Journal of Psychiatry*. 1970 Jun;116(535):593–7.
- Oldman D. Compulsive gamblers. *The Sociological Review*. 1978 Feb;26(2):349–72.
- Orford J. Hypersexuality: Implications for a theory of dependence. *British Journal of Addiction to Alcohol & Other Drugs*. 1978 Mar;73(3):299–310.
- Pallanti S, Bernardi S, Quercioli L. The Shorter PROMIS Questionnaire and the Internet Addiction Scale in the assessment of multiple addictions in a high-school population: Prevalence and related disability. *CNS Spectr*. 2006 Dec 1;11(12):966–74.
- Petry NM, Casarella T. Excessive discounting of delayed rewards in substance abusers with gambling problems. *Drug Alcohol Depend*. 56(1):25–32. [PubMed: 10462089]
- Stein DJ, Hollander E, Anthony DT, Schneier FR, Fallon BA, Liebowitz MR, Klein DF. Serotonergic medications for sexual obsessions, sexual addictions, and paraphilias. *The Journal of Clinical Psychiatry*. 1992 Aug.
- Zajac K, Ginley MK, Chang R, Petry NM. Treatments for Internet gaming disorder and Internet addiction: A systematic review. *Psychology of Addictive Behaviors*. 2017 Dec;31(8):979.

17
Optimizing Patient Care in Psychiatry – Eating Disorders

Avinash De Sousa and Shorouq Motwani

Introduction	180
Epidemiology	181
Causes	181
Genetics	*181*
Developmental Influences	*181*
Environmental Influences	*182*
Other Psychiatric Illnesses	*182*
Complications	182
Classification and Types	183
Anorexia Nervosa	*183*
Bulimia Nervosa	*184*
Binge Eating Disorder	*184*
Avoidant/Restrictive Food Intake Disorder	*184*
Pica	*185*
Other Specified and Unspecified Feeding and Eating Disorders	*185*
Treatment of Eating Disorder	185
Goal of Treatment	185
Pharmacological Treatment of Eating Disorder	185
Anorexia Nervosa	*185*
Bulimia Nervosa	*186*
Binge Eating Disorder	*186*
Night Eating Disorder	*186*
Non-Pharmacological Treatment Options	186
Nutritional Rehabilitation	*187*
Psychotherapy	*187*
Inpatient Programs	*187*
Self-Help Groups	*187*

INTRODUCTION

Eating disorders are characterized by persistent disturbances in feeding and eating behaviors that significantly interfere with the individual's life, severely impacting physical health as well as impairing psychosocial functioning and causing intense distress. As a result of the associated medical complications seen in feeding and eating disorders, these illnesses are serious and often dangerous, making their early identification and intervention extremely important, although it is common for them to go unrecognized and thus untreated.

The "Feeding and Eating Disorders" chapter of the Diagnostic and Statistical Manual of Mental Disorders, Fifth Edition (DSM-5), includes six diagnoses: anorexia nervosa, bulimia nervosa, binge eating disorder (BED), avoidant/restrictive food intake disorder (ARFID), pica, and rumination disorder.[1]

After a brief classification per clinical features for easy identification of eating disorders, causes, and prevalence, the major focus will be on management: both pharmacological as well as nonpharmacological.

EPIDEMIOLOGY

Binge eating disorder affects about 1.6% of women and 0.8% of men in a given year.[5] Anorexia affects about 0.4%, and bulimia affects about 1.3% of young women in a given year.[5] Anorexia and bulimia occur nearly ten times more often in females than males, while binge eating disorder is twice as common in women.[5] Typically, eating disorders begin in late childhood or early adulthood.[6]

CAUSES

Predisposed individuals of any age can be affected by pressure from their peers, the online world, and even their families, but it is especially difficult for a teenager. There are many genetic, environmental, social, and psychological issues that could trigger and perpetuate eating disorders.[4]

In recent times social media has often been blamed for the rise in the incidence of eating disorders due to the idealized body images of models and celebrities that motivate or even force people to attempt to achieve unattainable body standards.

Genetics

Numerous studies show a genetic predisposition toward eating disorders.[8,9] A genetic link has been found on chromosome 1 in multiple family members of an individual with anorexia nervosa.[7] A first-degree relative of someone who has had or currently has an eating disorder is 7 to 12 times more likely to have an eating disorder themselves.[10] Twin studies also show that at least a portion of the vulnerability to develop eating disorders can be inherited.[10] About 50% of eating disorder cases are attributable to genetics.[11] Other cases are due to socio-environmental stressors. There are neurobiological factors at play tied to emotional reactivity and impulsivity that could lead to binging and purging behaviors.[12]

Developmental Influences

The psychological and social stressors of puberty and adolescence may put teenagers at risk for anorexia nervosa as well as also for bulimia nervosa. Research suggests that hormonal changes during this time, especially shifts in estrogen levels, may be an even greater risk factor in bulimia nervosa than in anorexia nervosa.[1]

Environmental Influences

Child Maltreatment

Child abuse, which includes physical, psychological, and sexual abuse, as well as neglect, has been shown to approximately triple the risk of an eating disorder.[13]

Parental Influence

Parental influence is manifested by a variety of diverse factors such as familial genetic predisposition, dietary choices as dictated by cultural or ethnic preferences, the parents' own body shape and eating patterns, and the presence or absence of a nurturing stable environment at home. A direct link has been shown between obesity and parental pressure to eat more. Young women in overbearing families lack the ability to be independent, often resulting in rebellion. Controlling their food intake may make them feel better, as it provides them with a sense of control.[14]

Peer and Internet Pressure

Pro-ana refers to the promotion of behaviors related to the eating disorder anorexia nervosa. Several websites promote eating disorders and can provide a means for individuals to communicate in order to maintain eating disorder.[15] Dieting is reported to be influenced by peer behavior.[16,17,18] Elite athletes have a significantly higher rate in eating disorders. Female athletes in sports such as gymnastics, ballet, and diving are found to be at the highest risk among all athletes.

Social Isolation

Social isolation can be stressful, depressing, and anxiety provoking. In an attempt to ameliorate these distressing feelings, an individual may engage in comfort eating. This is especially important during the current COVID pandemic, as social interactions have been hampered.

Other Psychiatric Illnesses

Other psychological problems that could possibly trigger or worsen an eating disorder are depression and low self-esteem.[19] Many people with eating disorders also have body dysmorphic disorder (BDD), which alters the way a person sees oneself.[2,3] Studies have found that a high proportion of individuals diagnosed with BDD also have some type of eating disorder, with 15% of individuals having either anorexia nervosa or bulimia nervosa.[2] This link stems from the fact that both BDD and anorexia nervosa are characterized by a preoccupation with physical appearance and a distortion of one's body image.[3] Other co morbidities include substance use; alcoholism;[21] anxiety disorder;[23] obsessive compulsive disorder;[25] and personality disorders – obsessive compulsive,[20] borderline,[22] narcissistic,[24] and histrionic.

Certain personality traits including high levels of perfectionism, self-discipline, harm-avoidance, and self-criticism are common in individuals with eating disorders.[1]

COMPLICATIONS

Individuals with eating disorders may present with multiple health complications – underweight to obesity, malnutrition, severe muscle and fat loss, hypothermia, hair thinning, calluses on hands due to self induced vomiting – Russell's sign, skin yellowing due to carotenemia, arrhythmias, hypotension, gastric distension, dental caries, electrolyte imbalance, hypoglycemia, deranged liver and renal functions, and oligomenorrhea/amenorrhea.[1]

CLASSIFICATION AND TYPES

Although feeding and eating disorders suggestively revolve around disturbed feeding patterns, the etiology, manner of clinical presentation, course, treatment, and prognosis behind the disorders vary significantly, thus indicating the need for specific diagnostic criteria for each of classified eating disorders.[26] Based on the previously mentioned parameters, the Diagnostic and Statistical Manual of Mental Disorders 5 has classified feeding and eating disorders into six different diagnoses. These include but are not exclusive to the following:

1. Anorexia nervosa
2. Bulimia nervosa
3. Binge eating disorder
4. Avoidant/restrictive food intake disorder (ARFID)
5. Pica
6. Other specified and unspecified feeding and eating disorders[27]

A major change recorded in the classification of eating disorders has been the cohesion of all feeding and eating disorders into one common diagnosis in DSM 5, unlike that seen in the previous editions of the DSM. (28) We will be attempting to highlight some of the prominent features of each of these feeding and eating disorders as we classify them based on DSM 5 diagnostic criteria.

Anorexia Nervosa

The most significant aspect of anorexia nervosa that puts the disorder in the limelight is the remarkably low weight seen in patients when compared to other age-appropriate peers and for their developmental stage and height. An incessant and persistent desire for thinness accompanied by behaviors to reinforce weight loss helps restrict anorexic patients from gaining weight. However, this aspect of the illness is more commonly seen in growing teenagers and in the later stages of the disorder.[29] The disordered thought process behind this deviant behavior is the obsessive fear of becoming fat and major body image issues manifested as a sense of believing that they are fat in spite of having a low body weight. The pathological thought process also extends beyond excessive weight issues and even encroaches into issues like low self-esteem, with weight playing a vital part in an individual's self-evaluation.[30]

In order to lose significant amount of weight, patients with anorexia nervosa not only restrict their food intake but also occasionally resort to methods which affect weight. These medically dangerous methods include:

Purging (a form of self-induced vomiting by usually shoving one's fingers down one's throat)
Laxative use (in an attempt to pass stool frequently and in greater quantity than normally induced)
Diuretic use (in an attempt to pass urine frequently and in greater quantity than normally induced)
Rigorous and compulsive exercise

Unfortunately, patients suffering from anorexia nervosa fail to recognize the impending medical complications of their current weight status and their deviant behaviours.[31]

Bulimia Nervosa

Often confused with anorexia nervosa, though bulimia nervosa admittedly does share some features with anorexia nervosa, its distinguishing features are defined by recurrent episodes of binge or excessive eating followed by compensatory behaviors trying to maintain or reduce body weight.

These pathological and medically compromising behaviors include and are not exclusive to:

1. Purging or self induced vomiting
2. Laxative/diuretic/enema use
3. Intense exercise
4. Fasting
5. Medications misuse or abuse

The defining concept of bulimia nervosa is, however, binge eating which is characterized by the consumption of excessively large quantities of food at one go associated with a lack of self control, meaning the persons eats a large amount of food, feeling that she cannot stop eating.[32]

The differentiating feature of bulimia nervosa from anorexia nervosa is that patients suffering from bulimia often maintain their body weight at or above normal for their age and height, in contrast to anorexia patients who are abnormally thin for their development and height. The common ground shared by anorexia and bulimia patients is the fact that patients of both disorders display an obsessive preoccupation with their weight or shape. They let weight become the deciding factor in their self-evaluation, which leads to harsh self-judgement.[33]

Binge Eating Disorder

Like bulimia nervosa, the central concept of binge eating disorder is repeated episodes of uncontrollable eating or, in simpler terms, binge eating. However, the differentiating feature of BED from bulimia nervosa is the fact that these binge eating episodes are not followed by the various compensatory behaviors typically seen in bulimia nervosa.

Certain restrictive behaviors like diet restrictions are often observed in binge eating disorders, but such patients never engage in expulsive behaviors or compulsive exercise meant to specifically reduce the weight that is gained by overeating.

Individuals with binge eating disorders often maintain their body weight at or above normal for their height and age and often are also in the overweight or obese category.[34]

Avoidant/Restrictive Food Intake Disorder

According to past nomenclature, ARFID was referred to as feeding disorder of infancy or early childhood, but the term was changed to avoidant/restrictive food intake disorder in DSM 5. Characterized by eating disturbances manifesting in medical consequences like nutritional deficiencies and/or psychosocial impairment, there are multiple etiological concerns to the disorder like concern with texture/consistency/smell of certain food items, anxiety associated with eating due to a pathological history of choking, vomiting, or stressful mealtimes.[35]

The highlight of this disorder is the differentiating feature from anorexia and bulimia, where weight issues must not motivate the restrictive behavior of ARFID. Also, ARFID should not be diagnosed if the restrictive eating habits are seen as part of developmental delay unless requiring clinical attention. A point also to be noted is that culturally acceptable eating or feeding behaviors should not be a part of ARFID.[36]

Pica

Consumption of inedible items which fall outside the culturally acceptable norms of the society that the patient is part of defines pica. These inedible items can include virtually anything, for example, paper, pebbles, mud, and so on. Other relevant medical or psychiatric disorders must also be ruled out before providing a diagnosis of pica.[37]

Other Specified and Unspecified Feeding and Eating Disorders

Due to insufficient research in describing and categorizing certain feeding and eating disorders, a novel class of disorders has been provided by DSM 5 to describe those eating disorders which do not fit into any of the previously defined categories in description or duration of illness.

These include the following illnesses:

1. Purging disorder
2. Atypical anorexia nervosa, bulimia nervosa, and BED of low frequency and/or limited duration
3. Night eating syndrome[38]

TREATMENT OF EATING DISORDER

- It is very difficult to treat eating disorders[39]
- Treatment of eating disorders remain a challenging task for the treating psychiatrist
- It is because of the following:
    1. There is a lack of empirically supported intervention in certain populations like adults with anorexia nervosa.[40]
    2. The rate of treatment non-response or relapse remain relatively high in the population for which there is evidence-based treatment available.
- Additional research efforts are required to identify effective interventions for eating disorders.[41]

GOAL OF TREATMENT

1. One of the goals of treatment is to disrupt the disordered behavior, which includes problematic patterns of eating and feeding.
2. The second goal of treatment is to alter the problematic cognition, attitudes, and beliefs associated with the eating disorder.
3. Treatment of accompanying co-morbidities.[42]

PHARMACOLOGICAL TREATMENT OF EATING DISORDER

Anorexia Nervosa

Many drugs have been studied for the treatment of anorexia, but no clear empirical support has been established for any

Selective Serotonin Reuptake Inhibitors

Treatment with selective serotonin reuptake inhibitors (SSRIs) has received significant attention;[43] for example, fluoxetine helps in weight gain and has a positive response in patients with accompanying depression.

Cyproheptadine

It is a drug with antihistaminic and anti-serotonergic properties. It is specifically used in restrictive type of anorexia nervosa.[44]

Amitriptyline

This drug belongs to the tricyclic antidepressants group.
Patient who have been treated with amitriptyline show some improvement in anorexia.

Other

This include various drugs like clomipramine,[45] chlorpromazine,[46] and pimozide.[47]
Patients also show a positive response when treated with these drugs.

Bulimia Nervosa

Antidepressants

Antidepressants have been shown to be helpful in treating bulimia; this includes selective serotonin reuptake inhibitors like fluoxetine.[48] Fluoxetine enhances the level of 5-hydroxytryptamine. It reduces binge eating as well as purging with a dose of 60mg/day.[49]

Others

Imipramine, desipramine,[50] trazadone, and monoamine oxidase inhibitors (MAOIs)[51] also seem to improve the condition.

Binge Eating Disorder

Symptoms of binge eating disorder respond well to medication like desipramine, imipramine, topiramate, and sibutramine[52,53,54]
Fluvoxamine, sertraline, and citalopram are SSRIs that have demonstrated improvement in mood as well as binge eating disorder.[55]
Fluoxetine is also reported to cause weight loss; initially, however, weight loss is transient. Amphetamine-like drugs may also helpful.[56]

Night Eating Disorder

SSRIs have been shown to improve symptoms of night eating disorder like night awakening, nocturnal eating, and post-evening calorie intake.[57]

NON-PHARMACOLOGICAL TREATMENT OPTIONS

A team approach is required for treatment of eating disorders; the team includes a psychiatrist, a therapist, and a dietician. Thus, the treatment options not only focus on pharmacological but also emphasize non-pharmacological options.[58] Nonpharmacologic treatments are the most likely to cause a response in patients suffering from eating disorders. This includes nutritional counseling, cognitive behavioral therapy (CBT), interpersonal psychotherapy, behavioral management, and family therapy.[59]

Nutritional Rehabilitation

The most widespread approach to weight restoration is oral refeeding. Adequate guidance is required, and a tailor-made dietary plan is to be given, keeping in mind the nutritional requirements of the patient. This includes use of liquid formulations, or, in extreme cases, nasogastric refeeding or parenteral nutrition is employed.[59]

Psychotherapy

Psychotherapies are a part of standard treatment of eating disorders. Various trials have showed the effectivity of psychotherapy in eating disorders.[60]

Various therapies can be used in the treatment of eating disorders:

Cognitive Behavioral Therapy

CBT provides positive support for weight gain. It assists patients in overcoming distorted thinking and helps change the patient's behavioral disturbances.[61] It also helps in reducing relapse rates.[62]

Family Therapy

Also known as the Maudsley method, family therapy is a specialized therapy used for treating adolescents. In it, the parents of the patient are supported by a family therapist. Parents are actively involved in making decisions about the eating and related behaviors of the patient, and as the patient improves gradually, control is shifted back to the patient. This also addresses issues with overall family dynamics and functioning.[61]

Motivational Interviewing

Motivational interviewing addresses the patient's hesitancy about change and their reasons for gaining weight and can motivate individuals to gain weight.[61]

Apart from the these, dialectical behavioral therapy, interpersonal psychotherapy, art therapy, and cognitive emotional behavior therapy can also be employed.[63]

Inpatient Programs

Most inpatient programs use a variety of psychosocial interventions, including family and individual psychotherapy, behaviorally formulated interventions, empathic nursing approaches, and several group therapies along with nutritional counseling.

Self-Help Groups

Self-help and guided self-help have been shown to be highly effective in eating disorders; this includes support groups such as Eating Disorders Anonymous and Overeaters Anonymous.[64,65,66]

References

1. Christine C, Call AB, Evelyn A, MD, Timothy Walsh B, M.D. *Kaplan and Sadock's Synopsis of Psychiatry: Behavioral Sciences/Clinical Psychiatry.* LWW, New York.
2. Ruffolo JS, Phillips KA, Menard W, Fay C, Weisberg RB. Comorbidity of body dysmorphic disorder and eating disorders: Severity of psychopathology and body image disturbance. *The International Journal of Eating Disorders.* 2006 Jan;39(1):11–19. doi:10.1002/eat.20219. PMID 16254870.
3. Grant JE, Kim SW, Eckert ED. Body dysmorphic disorder in patients with anorexia nervosa: Prevalence, clinical features, and delusionality of body image. *The International Journal of Eating Disorders.* 2002 Nov;32(3):291–300. doi:10.1002/eat.10091. PMID 12210643.
4. Bulik CM, Hebebrand J, Keski-Rahkonen A, Klump KL, Reichborn-Kjennerud T, Mazzeo SE, Wade TD. Genetic epidemiology, endophenotypes, and eating disorder classification. *The International Journal of Eating Disorders.* 2007 Nov;40(Suppl):S52–60. doi:10.1002/eat.20398. PMID 17573683. S2CID 36187776.
5. American Psychiatric Association. *Diagnostic and Statistical Manual of Mental Disorders* (5th ed.). Arlington, VA: American Psychiatric Association; 2013. pp. 329–54. ISBN 978-0-89042-555-8.
6. *What Are Eating Disorders?.* NIMH. Archived from the original May 23, 2015. Accessed May 24, 2015
7. DeAngelis T. A genetic link to anorexia. *Monitor on Psychology.* 2002;33(3):34.
8. Klump KL, Kaye WH, Strober M. The evolving genetic foundations of eating disorders. *The Psychiatric Clinics of North America.* 2001 Jun;24(2):215–25. doi:10.1016/S0193–953X(05)70218–5. PMID 11416922.
9. Mazzeo SE, Bulik CM. Environmental and genetic risk factors for eating disorders: What the clinician needs to know. *Child and Adolescent Psychiatric Clinics of North America.* 2009 Jan;18(1):67–82. doi:10.1016/j.chc.2008.07.003. PMC 2719561. PMID 19014858.
10. Patel P, Wheatcroft R, Park RJ, Stein A. The children of mothers with eating disorders. *Clinical Child and Family Psychology Review.* 2002 Mar;5(1):1–19. doi:10.1023/A:1014524207660. PMID 11993543. S2CID 46639789.
11. Trace SE, Baker JH, Peñas-Lledó E, Bulik CM. The genetics of eating disorders. *Annual Review of Clinical Psychology.* 2013;9:589–620. doi:10.1146/annurev-clinpsy-050212–185546. PMID 23537489. S2CID 33773190.
12. Iarovici D (2014). *Mental Health Issues & the University Student.* Baltimore: Johns Hopkins University Press. pp. 104. ISBN 9781421412382.
13. Caslini M, Bartoli F, Crocamo C, Dakanalis A, Clerici M, Carrà G. Disentangling the association between child abuse and eating disorders: A systematic review and meta-analysis. *Psychosomatic Medicine.* 2016 Jan;78(1):79–90. doi:10.1097/psy.0000000000000233. PMID 26461853. S2CID 30370150.
14. Nolen-Hoeksema S. *Abnormal Psychology* (6th ed.). London, UK: McGraw-Hill Education; 2014. pp. 359–360
15. Gailey J. Starving is the most fun a girl can have: The Pro-Ana subculture as edgework. *Critical Criminology.* 2009;17(2):93–108. doi:10.1007/s10612–009–9074-z. S2CID 144787200.
16. Page RM, Suwanteerangkul J. Dieting among Thai adolescents: Having friends who diet and pressure to diet. *Eating and Weight Disorders.* 2007 Sep;12(3):114–24. doi:10.1007/bf03327638. PMID 17984635. S2CID 28567423.
17. The Mcknight Investigators. Risk factors for the onset of eating disorders in adolescent girls: Results of the McKnight longitudinal risk factor study. *The American Journal of Psychiatry.* 2003 Feb;160(2):248–54. doi:10.1176/ajp.160.2.248. PMID 12562570.
18. Paxton SJ, Schutz HK, Wertheim EH, Muir SL. Friendship clique and peer influences on body image concerns, dietary restraint, extreme weight-loss behaviors, and binge eating in adolescent girls. *Journal of Abnormal Psychology.* 1999 May;108(2):255–66. doi:10.1037/0021–843X.108.2.255. PMID 10369035.
19. *Anorexia & Depression: When Eating Disorders Co-Exist with Depression.* Psycom.net – Mental Health Treatment Resource since 1986. Accessed May 5, 2020
20. Serpell L, Livingstone A, Neiderman M, Lask B. Anorexia nervosa: Obsessive-compulsive disorder, obsessive-compulsive personality disorder, or neither? *Clinical Psychology Review.* 2002 Jun;22(5): 647–69. doi:10.1016/S0272–7358(01)00112-X. PMID 12113200.
21. Bulik CM, Klump KL, Thornton L, Kaplan AS, Devlin B, Fichter MM, et al. Alcohol use disorder comorbidity in eating disorders: A multicenter study. *The Journal of Clinical Psychiatry.* 2004 Jul;65(7): 1000–6. doi:10.4088/JCP.v65n0718. PMID 15291691.

22. Larsson JO, Hellzén M. Patterns of personality disorders in women with chronic eating disorders. *Eating and Weight Disorders.* 2004 Sep;9(3):200–5. doi:10.1007/bf03325067. PMID 15656014. S2CID 29679535.
23. Swinbourne JM, Touyz SW. The co-morbidity of eating disorders and anxiety disorders: A review. *European Eating Disorders Review.* 2007 Jul;15(4):253–74. doi:10.1002/erv.784. PMID 17676696.
24. Ronningstam E. Pathological narcissism and narcissistic personality disorder in Axis I disorders. *Harvard Review of Psychiatry.* 1996;3(6):326–40. doi:10.3109/10673229609017201. PMID 9384963. S2CID 21472356.
25. Anderluh MB, Tchanturia K, Rabe-Hesketh S, Treasure J. Childhood obsessive-compulsive personality traits in adult women with eating disorders: Defining a broader eating disorder phenotype. *The American Journal of Psychiatry.* 2003 Feb;160(2):242–7. doi:10.1176/appi.ajp.160.2.242. PMID 12562569
26. Erzegovesi S, Bellodi L. Eating disorders. *CNS Spectrums.* 2016;21.
27. Hoek HW. Classification, epidemiology and treatment of DSM-5 feeding and eating disorders. *Current Opinion in Psychiatry.* 2013;26.
28. Call C, Walsh BT, Attia E. From DSM-IV to DSM-5: Changes to eating disorder diagnoses. *Current Opinion in Psychiatry.* 2013;26.
29. Davenport E, Rushford N, Soon S, McDermott C. Dysfunctional metacognition and drive for thinness in typical and atypical anorexia nervosa. *J Eat Disord.* 2015;3(1).
30. Woerwag-Mehta S, Treasure J. Causes of anorexia nervosa psychological factors. *Psychiatry.* 2008;7(4).
31. Steinglass JE, Berner LA, Attia E. Cognitive neuroscience of eating disorders. *Psychiatric Clinics of North America.* 2019;42.
32. Fairburn CG, Cooper PJ. The clinical features of bulimia nervosa. *Br J Psychiatry.* 1984;144(3).
33. Alvarenga MS, Koritar P, Pisciolaro F, Mancini M, Cordás TA, Scagliusi FB. Eating attitudes of anorexia nervosa, bulimia nervosa, binge eating disorder and obesity without eating disorder female patients: Differences and similarities. *Physiol Behav.* 2014;131.
34. Kessler RM, Hutson PH, Herman BK, Potenza MN. The neurobiological basis of binge-eating disorder. *Neuroscience and Biobehavioral Reviews.* 2016;63.
35. Katzman DK, Norris ML, Zucker N. Avoidant restrictive food intake disorder. *Psychiatric Clinics of North America.* 2019;42.
36. Sieke EH, Strandjord SE, Richmond M, Rome ES, Khadilkar AC. Avoidant/restrictive food intake disorder and anorexia nervosa subtypes: How do they compare? *J Adolesc Heal.* 2016;58(2).
37. Rajput N, Kumar K, Moudgil K. Pica an eating disorder: An overview. *Pharmacophore.* 2020;11(4).
38. Mancuso SG, Newton JR, Bosanac P, Rossell SL, Nesci JB, Castle DJ. Classification of eating disorders: Comparison of relative prevalence rates using DSM-IV and DSM-5 criteria. *Br J Psychiatry.* 2015;206(2).
39. Fassino S, Abbate-Daga G. Resistance to treatment in eating disorders: A critical challenge. *BMC Psychiatry.* 2013;13(1):1–4.
40. Peterson K, Fuller R. Anorexia nervosa in adolescents: An overview. *Nursing 2020.* 2019 Oct 1;49(10):24–30.
41. Kan C, Treasure J. Recent research and personalized treatment of anorexia nervosa. *Psychiat. Clin. N. Am.* 2019 Mar 1;42:11–19.
42. Marucci S, Ragione LD, De Iaco G, Mococci T, Vicini M, Guastamacchia E, Triggiani V. Anorexia nervosa and comorbid psychopathology. *Endocrine, Metabolic & Immune Disorders-Drug Targets* (Formerly *Current Drug Targets-Immune, Endocrine & Metabolic Disorders*). 2018 Jul 1;18(4):316–24.
43. Kruger S, Kennedy SH. Psychopharmacotherapy of anorexia nervosa, bulimia nervosa and binge-eating disorder. *Journal of Psychiatry and Neuroscience.* 2000 Nov;25(5):497.
44. Crow SJ. Pharmacologic treatment of eating disorders. *The Psychiatric Clinics of North America.* 2019 Apr 3;42(2):253–62.
45. Marvanova M, Gramith K. Role of antidepressants in the treatment of adults with anorexia nervosa. *Mental Health Clinician.* 2018 May;8(3):127–37.
46. Murray SB, Quintana DS, Loeb KL, Griffiths S, Le Grange D. Treatment outcomes for anorexia nervosa: A systematic review and meta-analysis of randomized-controlled trials: Corrigendum. *Psychological Medicine.* 2019 Mar;49(4):701–4.
47. Khalil RB. Targeting all psychopathological dimensions in the treatment of anorexia nervosa. *L'encephale.* 2021 Feb 1;47(1):79–81.

48. McElroy SL, Guerdjikova AI, Mori N, Romo-Nava F. Progress in developing pharmacologic agents to treat bulimia nervosa. *CNS Drugs*. 2019 Jan;33(1):31–46.
49. Krzystanek M, Pałasz A. The role of blocking serotonin 2C receptor by fluoxetine in the treatment of bulimia. *Pharmacotherapy in Psychiatry and Neurology/Farmakoterapia w Psychiatrii i Neurologii*. 2020;36(2):135–141.
50. Pope HG, Hudson JI, Jonas JM, Yurgelun-Todd D. Bulimia treated with imipramine: A placebo-controlled, double-blind study. *Am J Psychiatry*. 1983 May 1;140(5):554–8.
51. Walsh BT, Stewart JW, Wright L, Harrison W, Roose SP, Glassman AH. Treatment of bulimia with monoamine oxidase inhibitors. *The American Journal of Psychiatry*. 1982;139(12):1629–30.
52. Amodeo G, Cuomo A, Bolognesi S, Goracci A, Trusso MA, Piccinni A, Neal SM, Baldini I, Federico E, Taddeucci C, Fagiolini A. Pharmacotherapeutic strategies for treating binge eating disorder: Evidence from clinical trials and implications for clinical practice. *Expert Opinion on Pharmacotherapy*. 2019 Apr 13;20(6):679–90.
53. Cuesto G, Everaerts C, León LG, Acebes A. Molecular bases of anorexia nervosa, bulimia nervosa and binge eating disorder: Shedding light on the darkness. *Journal of Neurogenetics*. 2017 Oct 2;31(4):266–87.
54. Guerdjikova AI, Walsh B, Shan K, Halseth AE, Dunayevich E, McElroy SL. Concurrent improvement in both binge eating and depressive symptoms with naltrexone/bupropion therapy in overweight or obese subjects with major depressive disorder in an open-label, uncontrolled study. *Advances in Therapy*. 2017 Oct;34(10):2307–15.
55. Karth MD. *Effects of Serotonin Deficiency and Fluoxetine on Binge Eating Behavior and Gene Expression in the Hypothalamus*. USA: Villanova University; 2019.
56. Bello NT, Yeomans BL. Safety of pharmacotherapy options for bulimia nervosa and binge eating disorder. *Expert Opinion on Drug Safety*. 2018 Jan 2;17(1):17–23.
57. Kel L, Laura A. Approaches for night eating disorders. In: *Clinical Handbook of Complex and Atypical Eating Disorders*. London, UK: Springer; 2017 Aug 29. p. 205.
58. American Psychiatric Association. *American Psychiatric Association practice guidelines for the treatment of psychiatric disorders (PDF)* (3rd ed.). Arlington, VA: American Psychiatric Association; 2006. ISBN 978–0890423851.
59. Talbert RL, DiPiro JT, Matzke GR, Posey LM, Wells BG, Yee GC. Chapter 64 Multiple sclerosis. In: *Pharmacotherapy: A Pathophysiologic Approach* (8th ed.). New York: McGraw-Hill; 2011. www.accesspharmacy.com/content.aspx?aID=7984977. Accessed June 1, 2013
60. American Psychiatric Association. Treatment of patients with eating disorders, third edition. *Am J Psychiatry*. 2006;163(7 Suppl):4–54.
61. Forman SF. Eating disorders: Overview of treatment. UpToDate. www.uptodate.com/contents/eating-disorders-overview-of-treatment. Updated March 25, 2013. Accessed June 1, 2013.
62. Pike KM, Walsh BT, Vitousek K, et al. Cognitive behavior therapy in the posthospitalization treatment of anorexia nervosa. *Am J Psychiatry*. 2003;160(11):2046–9.
63. Safer DL, Telch CF, Agras WS. Dialectical behavior therapy for bulimia nervosa. *The American Journal of Psychiatry*. 2001 Apr;158(4):632–4. doi: 10.1176/appi.ajp.158.4.632. PMID 11282700. S2CID 16651053.
64. Perkins SJ, Murphy R, Schmidt U, Williams C. Self-help and guided self-help for eating disorders. *The Cochrane Database of Systematic Reviews*. 2006 Jul;3(3):D004191. doi:10.1002/14651858. CD004191.pub2. PMID 16856036. S2CID 45718608
65. Thiels C, Schmidt U, Treasure J, Garthe R. Four-year follow-up of guided self-change for bulimia nervosa. *Eating and Weight Disorders*. 2003 Sep;8(3):212–17. doi:10.1007/bf03325016. PMID 14649785. S2CID 25197396.
66. Peterson CB, Mitchell JE, Crow SJ, Crosby RD, Wonderlich SA. "The efficacy of self-help group treatment and therapist-led group treatment for binge eating disorder". *The American Journal of Psychiatry*. 2009 Dec;166(12):1347–54. doi:10.1176/appi.ajp.2009.09030345. PMC 3041988. PMID 19884223.

18
Optimising Patient Care in Psychiatry – Homeless Mentally Ill Patients

Adarsh Tripathi, Aathira J. Prakash

Introduction	191
Homelessness in Indian Context	192
Prevalence of Homelessness in India	192
Factors Contributing to Homelessness	193
Factors Related to Administration and Policy	*193*
Factors Related to Delivery of Service	*193*
Factors Related to Illness	*194*
Factors Related to Society	*194*
Challenges	194
Rehabilitation Services in India	195
Policies and Programmes	195
Future Directions for Optimising Care	196

INTRODUCTION

A home is not just a place of dwelling but an anchor in a person's life where one feels secure, happy and loved. Per article 25 of Universal Human Declarations Act,

> Everyone has the right to a standard of living adequate for the health and well-being of himself and of his family, including food, clothing, housing and medical care and necessary social services, and the right to security in the event of unemployment, sickness, disability, widowhood, old age or other lack of livelihood in circumstances beyond his control.

However, homelessness is still a major public crisis, with more than 100 million homeless people globally (1),(2). It has been found that this unique group of the population is more vulnerable to various health problems, including psychiatric illness (3). Hence, the homeless mentally ill form a more susceptible population with a high morbidity. It has been seen that poor socio-economic status is a risk factor for development of mental illness. The bidirectional aspect of this relationship of socio-economic status and mental illness is supported by two hypotheses. The social causation theory explains how economic hardship results in subsequent development and persistence of mental health problems, whereas the social drift hypothesis posits that mental health problems drive these individuals into poverty (4).

The homeless mentally ill (HMI) often present with a complex combination of physical, psychological and social problems. This population (HMI) can be subdivided into various groups: individuals with severe mental illness who have been rendered homeless because of the illness; those who have mental illness but have never approached treatment services, with the underlying illness contributing to drift; and those whose mental health problems are a consequence of becoming homeless. Especially in a developing country like India, this context becomes even more significant due to poor economic conditions, inadequacy in implementation of mental health policies, scarcity of resources and a pervasive presence of social stigma among the people. This prevailing situation further aggravates the vicious cycle of homelessness, moreover being homeless adds to the expanse of neglect, abuse and violation of human rights faced by people with mental illness.

HOMELESSNESS IN INDIAN CONTEXT

According to the census of India, homeless people are those "who do not live in census houses [a structure with a roof] which is either self-owned or rented" but instead reside in homeless households such as on roadsides, under flyovers or staircases, in places of worship or railway platforms; spend nights at transit homes, short stay homes or beggar homes; or reside in temporary structures without walls and roofs, such as under plastic sheets, in parks and in other common spaces (5). But the discussion of homelessness from a perspective of mental health and illness needs a broader dimension. Working definitions are adopted by non-governmental organisations in order to focus on and prioritise the most deprived population. The National Campaign for Housing Rights in India defines home as "a place where one lives with dignity, has security and can access basic essential housing resources like water, fuel, land, building materials etc." The Aashray Adhikar Abhiyan defines a homeless person as "an individual with no place which can be referred as a home in that city where home implies a shelter and also nurturance of one's cultural, social, health and economic needs" (6).

PREVALENCE OF HOMELESSNESS IN INDIA

It has been difficult to estimate the actual prevalence of homelessness in India; attempts made so far have had their share of methodological flaws owing to the nature of their estimation and difficulty in accessing the actual conditions owing to physical and linguistic barriers. The census of India in 2011 estimated the prevalence of the homeless population as 4,49,761 households/families by point in time estimation. The homeless number comes to 17,72,889 people, with a distribution of 8,34,541 in rural and 9,38,348 in urban settings. There has been a 28% drop from rural setting but a 20% rise in the urban setting since the 2001 census. Other epidemiological data available shows that there are 78 million homeless people (the Action Aid 2003) and 11 million homeless children in India (Child Relief and You-CRY-2006). UN-HABITAT (2005) says that 63% of all slum dwellers from South Asia are in India, which amounts to a figure of 170 million people (17% of the total slum dwellers in the world) (7). When it comes to homeless mentally ill, epidemiological data is even more scarce. The recently concluded National Mental Health Survey of India (2015–16) attempted to find the burden and status of HMI in India by conducting focus group discussions (FGDs) and key informant interviews (KIIs) in India. The participants of FGDs and KIIs were local stakeholders, media persons, family members of persons with mental illness, police personnel and doctors. It was found that the exact estimate of HMI was difficult to formulate. In urban areas, HMI are seen more commonly than in rural areas. Few epidemiological studies have been conducted in India concerning this vulnerable population. One of these studies included a retrospective chart review of inpatients admitted to department of psychiatry of a north Indian medical university from February 2005 to July 2011; out of the 140 patients admitted, about 90% were found to have mental illness, with the most common disorder being schizophrenia and other psychotic illnesses, and reintegration into society was made possible for about 68% of these individuals (8). Another north Indian study from Haryana on inmate girls of a female shelter home included 36 female participants who were runaways or throwaways. It was seen that more than 60% had received at least one psychiatric diagnosis: 22.2% had a diagnosis of depression, 13.88% had a diagnosis of post-traumatic stress disorder (PTSD), 11.11% had conversion disorder, 5.55% had panic disorder, 2.8% had generalised anxiety disorder and 11.11% had mental retardation (9). As part of "Know the Unknown" project, the National Institute of Mental Health and Neurosciences (NIMHANS), Bangalore, conducted a retrospective chart review of homeless mentally ill patients from 1st January 2002 to 31st December 2015 who were admitted to the Department of Psychiatry. The majority of the patients were diagnosed with schizophrenia and other psychotic illness, and it was possible to relocate about half of these patients to their families (10). A similar retrospective study conducted in western India also found that out of 78 institutionalised patients, the majority suffered from psychotic illness, and it was possible to establish ties with the family in only half of these patients (11). Hence, it may be concluded that the majority of the homeless mentally ill suffer from psychotic illness. This has also shed light on the difficulties that crop up during reintegration of these individuals into society.

FACTORS CONTRIBUTING TO HOMELESSNESS

Various factors are responsible for coexisting mental illness and homelessness. In the Indian context, the possible reasons may be placed in the following categories (12):

- Factors related to administration and policy
- Factors related to delivery of service
- Factors related to the illness
- Factors related to society

Factors Related to Administration and Policy

Lack of proper homes, rehabilitation centres and measures to reintegrate homeless individuals into society after de-institutionalisation from psychiatric hospitals leads to poor outcomes in these individuals.

Factors Related to Delivery of Service

A lack of rehabilitation services after acute management and poor follow-up and continuation of treatment increase the risk of persistence of mental illness in homeless individuals and their status of homelessness (13). The scarcity of adequate resources for mental health, including a lack of workforce, financial sources and mental healthcare delivery system which are not hospital-centred, are significant in this causation and especially significant in low- and middle-income countries (14). About 76–85% of the mentally ill received no treatment in less developed countries when compared to developed countries, where about 35–50% of these patients received no treatment (15). The Mental Health Atlas of 2017 found there are <2 mental health workers per 100,000 population in India and other low-income countries. The Mental Health Atlas 2014 depicted the ratio of mental health professionals as 0.07 clinical psychologists and psychiatric social workers and 0.12 psychiatric nurses per 100,000 population (16). The inadequacy of mental health resources in low- and middle-income countries like India is further complicated by the lack of political will (13).

Factors Related to Illness

The deteriorating nature of psychiatric illnesses if left untreated, trouble in maintaining self-care and managing daily life, disruptions in interpersonal relationships, cognitive deficits associated with mental illness, coexisting physical illness and use of addictive substances are all illness-related factors which are responsible for propagation of the poor economic conditions and health status of the homeless mentally ill (17,18).

Factors Related to Society

The stigma related to mental illness, which is very prevalent in society, plays a significant role in making those with mental illness social outcasts. This leads to their social isolation and, along with a lack of social support, is a cause of homelessness (19). In the Indian scenario, women are especially vulnerable, as it is not acceptable per social norms for a female to roam the streets, so homeless mentally ill women are not easily accepted back at their homes and thus may end up isolated from the family and maintain their homeless status (20). Poverty and low literacy lead to poor access to mental healthcare and lower awareness regarding mental health problems, which further contributes to deteriorating situation of people with mental illness (21). Rapid urbanisation and its subsequent effect on the societal structure has led to harmful effects on the mental health of people owing to various stressors like poor socio-economic conditions, overcrowding, pollution and rising crimes. This has made them more vulnerable to the development of mental health disorders and hence to the risk of homelessness. There is also a serious lack of affordable, accessible and appropriate dwellings, which contributes to poor residential stability. Moreover, people with mental illness have a higher chance of being unemployed or holding menial jobs with low wages, which may push them towards homelessness. The lack of employment is also prevalent among people abusing substances (22).

CHALLENGES

There are various issues that crop up in the management of the homeless mentally ill and their reintegration back into the community. The homeless and especially the homeless mentally ill seem to be living in a post-apocalyptic era with no ties to society. This is an even greater battle to be won, particularly in Indian settings, as community-level care is very difficult to achieve. Most people are not generally aware of the available facilities for restoration and rehabilitation of these individuals. Often such facilities are only located in major cities. People with mental illness who are found wandering on the streets are often ignored by people, and no action is taken to bring them to notice. Only when such individuals become violent or meet with accidents is any further action taken. The aftermath of such actions leads to admission to mental healthcare facilities; however, a lack of proper history, language barriers, unavailability of any information regarding the status of the individuals and lack of any offline or online data resources for identifying these individuals all lead to poor diagnosis and management issues. Management is based on the cross-sectional assessment of these individuals. These patients are only admitted when brought in by proper authorities and when accompanied by appointed caregivers; there is no provision in place to receive homeless mentally ill who may be brought to the hospital by civilians. In the case where some of these people are admitted to mental health institutions, in the absence of an appointed caregiver, there are no provisions to ensure the care of these individuals, often leading to their absconding from the hospital. There is a lack of financial support for the treatment of these patients, and the available resources involve cumbersome procedures. There is a concept of "critical time intervention" in preventing homelessness in mentally ill persons by ensuring continuity of care post-discharge until harmonious community living is restored. This critical intervention needs to be planned at the point of deinstitutionalisation (23). However, after beginning the treatment and symptomatic recovery, there are no available protocols in place for the long-term rehabilitation of these patients, and the outcome of homeless mentally ill is often unpredictable, with some ending up back on the streets. There is no systematised way to keep tabs on the homeless mentally ill and ensure their continuous care from mental health institutions. Owing to the limited resources and services available in India, most of the homeless mentally ill end up with their issues unaddressed and unaccounted for. The lack of integration of the homeless into the population registry, and the fact that they are completely nameless and do not appear in any offline or online records, makes it difficult to track and obtain knowledge of the whereabouts of these individuals, and they remain hidden. There is an acute shortage of community outreach programs, specifically those of mental health services, in the Indian scenario.

REHABILITATION SERVICES IN INDIA

The current scenario of rehabilitation services in India comprises limited options, most of which are voluntary agencies. The pioneers in psychosocial rehabilitation services are the Medico-Pastoral Association and the Richmond Fellowship Society–India (RFS-I) branch. These societies have opened halfway homes based on the model of "therapeutic community" and have established centres at Bengaluru, New Delhi, Siddlaghata (rural Bengaluru) and Lucknow. Other organisations which have functioned over the past three decades include the Ashray Adhikar Abhiyan in Delhi, the Banyan in Chennai, Navachetana in Guwahati, Paripurnata in West Bengal, Shraddha Foundation in Maharashtra, Ashadeep in Guwahati, Iswar sankalpa in Kolkata and many others. These organisations have each worked in unique ways to rehabilitate mentally ill homeless people and have worked towards the goal of their reintegration into society (24).

POLICIES AND PROGRAMMES

With the introduction of the National Mental Health Programme in 1982, India became the first nation among the low- and middle-income countries to take a step towards mental health care. The programme focused primarily on community-level care. The National Mental Health Policy 2014 addressed the issue of homelessness and its vicious effect on psychiatric illness and vice-versa. It brought attention to the issues of the need to reduce poverty and economic disparity, improve standards of living and develop universal access to mental healthcare and rehabilitation services. The National and District Mental Health Program has also focused a lot on community rehabilitation; however, it does not adequately address the burning problem of mental illness and homelessness (4). The Ayushman Bharat Campaign, launched in 2018, aimed at providing cashless access healthcare for up to 5 lakh rupees per family to the poor and vulnerable, population including the homeless (described as households without shelter in the socio-economic census of 2011). Legal provisions to homeless person with mental illness were provided in the Mental Health Act (MHA) 1987 and also in the Mental Healthcare Act (MHCA) 2017. The Mental Health Care Act 2017 provided some modifications of legal provisions for homeless mentally ill. The MHCA 2017 has simplified the process of providing care for HMI, as it has taken away the mandatory judiciary involvement, which will prevent untoward delays in providing care (16). Some of the provisions pertaining to care of homeless mentally ill in the MHCA Act 2017 are as follows (25):

1. **Chapter V Section 18,** states the "right to access mental healthcare," which signifies that all persons have the right to access the entire range of mental healthcare and treatment from any mental health service which is run or funded by the appropriate government. This includes sufficient provisions of rehabilitation services like halfway homes; sheltered accommodation; and home-, hospital- or community-based rehabilitation. Sub-clause 7 also specifies that destitute or homeless persons with mental illness are entitled to mental health treatment and services free of any charge and at no financial cost at any mental health establishment run or funded by the appropriate government and at other mental health establishments designated by it.
2. **Chapter V Section 19** concerns the right to community living. It states that every person with mental illness, including homeless persons, shall have a right to live in society, be part of and nor segregated from society and not continue to remain in a mental health establishment merely due to absence of community facilities.
3. **Chapter XIII Sections 100 and 102** cover the duties of police officers with respect to homeless persons with mental illness found wandering in the community.
4. **Chapter Section 27:** The treating mental health professional should educate the HMI about the right to free legal aid. This would help in situations when the family members are reluctant to take the patients home even after they have improved.
5. **Chapter Section 89 and 90:** For admitting a HMI patient, there is no availability of advanced directive or nominated representative (NR). A person appointed by the Mental Health Review Board/director of Department of Social Welfare/person from an organisation under Societies Registration Act (the NGOs mostly working with HMI)/a representative from Rogi Kalyan Samiti from the hospital can act as the NR for the time being.

FUTURE DIRECTIONS FOR OPTIMISING CARE

The Mental Health Care Act 2017 has taken into account the existing state of mental healthcare for homeless individuals and has given directions for them to lead better lives. An ideal integration and implementation of these policies will go a long way in optimising care of the homeless mentally ill. However, the ground reality is that there is a lack of adequate infrastructure to bring this to fruition. This will require all stakeholders involved in the healthcare system to work together for quick and efficient implementation of directives, which may also require public-private partnerships (16). There is an urgent need for well-organised surveillance of streets and identification of individuals who appear mentally ill by police officers and their institutionalisation. Better tagging of the homeless and their integration into records will help in identifying these individuals and bringing them back home. Tracing the families of the homeless mentally ill, encouraging their involvement by providing any needed support and the use of legal means to bring them onto the scene when they refuse to accept recovered patients can also improve outcomes for homeless mentally ill patients. There is a need to explore innovative approaches to ensure continuity of care by family, like incentivised care (16). It is a crucial need to invest in community facilities and rehabilitation centres like halfway homes, daycare centres, home again facilities and clustered group homes. Grassroots programmes and community drives aimed at recognising high-risk vulnerable people (like psychotic patients living alone and those with comorbidity of a severe mental disorder with substance use, lack of social support or intellectual disabilities with a severe mental disorder) can help in prevention of homelessness for these individuals.

References

1. Universal declaration of human rights [Internet]. 2015 [cited 2020 Nov 18]. Available from: www.un.org/en/universal-declaration-human-rights/
2. Together-EndHomelessness-Event-CN-13Feb-1.pdf [Internet]. [cited 2020 Nov 18]. Available from: www.un.org/development/desa/dspd/wp-content/uploads/sites/22/2020/02/Together-End Homelessness-Event-CN-13Feb-1.pdf
3. Scott J. Homelessness and mental illness. *Br J Psychiatry*. 1993;162(3):314–24.
4. Gopikumar V. Understanding the mental ill health – poverty – homelessness nexus in India: Strategies that promote distress alleviation and social inclusion. 2014 [cited 2020 Nov 27]. Available from: https://research.vu.nl/en/publications/understanding-the-mental-ill-health-poverty-homelessness-nexus-in
5. General R. Census Commissioner, India. Census India. 2011; 2000.
6. Tipple G, Speak S. Definitions of homelessness in developing countries. *Habitat Int*. 2005;29(2):337–52.
7. Kumar P. Homelessness and mental health: Challenging issue in an Indian context. *Am Int J Res Humanit Arts Soc Sci*. 2014;7(2):160–3.
8. Tripathi A, Nischal A, Dalal PK, Agarwal V, Agarwal M, Trivedi JK, et al. Sociodemographic and clinical profile of homeless mentally ill inpatients in a north Indian medical university. *Asian J Psychiatry*. 2013 Oct 1;6(5):404–9.
9. Gupta R, Nehra DK, Kumar V, Sharma P, Kumar P. Psychiatric illnesses in homeless (runaway or throwaway) girl inmates: A preliminary study. *Dysphrenia*. 2013;4(1):31–5.
10. Gowda GS, Gopika G, Kumar CN, Manjunatha N, Yadav R, Srinivas D, et al. Clinical outcome and rehabilitation of homeless mentally ill patients admitted in mental health institute of South India: "Know the Unknown" project. *Asian J Psychiatry*. 2017 Dec;30:49–53.
11. Singh G, Shah N, Mehta R. The clinical presentation and outcome of the institutionalized wandering mentally ill in India. *J Clin Diagn Res JCDR*. 2016 Oct;10(10):VC13–16.
12. Kukreti P, Khanna P, Khanna A. Chronic mental illnesses and homelessness. In: *Chronic Mental Illness and the Changing Scope of Intervention Strategies, Diagnosis, and Treatment*. IGI Global; 2017. pp. 1–20.
13. Saraceno B, Saxena S. Mental health resources in the world: results from Project Atlas of the WHO. *World Psychiatry*. 2002 Feb;1(1):40–4.
14. Thirunavukarasu M. Closing the treatment gap. *Indian J Psychiatry*. 2011;53(3):199–201.
15. WHO World Mental Health Survey Consortium. Prevalence, severity, and unmet need for treatment of mental disorders in the World Health Organization World Mental Health Surveys. *JAMA*. 2004 Jun 1;291(21):2581–90.
16. Swaminath G, Enara A, Rao R, Kumar KVK, Kumar CN. Mental Healthcare Act, 2017 and homeless persons with mental illness in India. *Indian J Psychiatry*. 2019 Apr;61(Suppl 4):S768–72.
17. Bines W. *The Health of Single Homeless People*. Centre for Housing Policy, University of York; 1994.
18. Cisneros HG. Searching for home: Mentally ill homeless people in America. *Cityscape*. 1996;155–72.
19. Trivedi JK, Jilani AQ. Pathway of psychiatric care. *Indian J Psychiatry*. 2011;53(2):97–8.
20. Lives without roots: Institutionalized homeless women with chronic mental illness. ProQuest [Internet]. [cited 2021 Jan 2]. Available from: https://search.proquest.com/openview/c35f399af3555c770db07a722d2cd0c4/1?pq-origsite=gscholar&cbl=226501
21. Lund C, Breen A, Flisher AJ, Kakuma R, Corrigall J, Joska JA, et al. Poverty and common mental disorders in low and middle income countries: A systematic review. *Soc Sci Med*. 2010 Aug 1;71(3):517–28.
22. Argeriou M, McCarty D. *Treating Alcoholism and Drug Abuse among Homeless Men and Women: Nine Community Demonstration Grants*. Psychology Press; 1990. 182 p.
23. Susser E, Valencia E, Conover S, Felix A, Tsai WY, Wyatt RJ. Preventing recurrent homelessness among mentally ill men: A "critical time" intervention after discharge from a shelter. *Am J Public Health*. 1997 Feb 1;87(2):256–62.
24. Thara R, Patel V. Role of non-governmental organizations in mental health in India. *Indian J Psychiatry*. 2010;52(Suppl 1):S389.
25. Final Draft Rules MHC Act, 2017 (1).pdf [Internet]. [cited 2021 Jan 11]. Available from: https://main.mohfw.gov.in/sites/default/files/Final%20Draft%20Rules%20MHC%20Act%2C%202017%20%281%29.pdf

19

Challenges in Community Psychiatry – Farmer Suicides and Their Survivors

Prakash B. Behere, Shruti Agarwal, Debolina Chowdhury, Aniruddh P. Behere and Richa Yadav

Introduction	198
Magnitude of the Problem	199
Indian Scenario for Rural Psychiatry	199
Challenges Faced in Community Psychiatry and Their Possible Solutions	200
Conclusion	201

INTRODUCTION

The word 'community' is used to refer to a particular geographical and administrative area with a well-integrated neighbourhood or simply society at large. In the context of community psychiatry, it refers to any locality outside of hospitals.[1] Szmukler and Thornicroft described community psychiatry as follows

> Community psychiatry comprises the principles and practices needed to provide mental health services for a local population by (i) establishing population-based needs for treatment and care; (ii) providing a service system linking a wide range of resources of adequate capacity, operating in accessible locations and (iii) delivering evidence based treatments to people with mental disorders.[2]

Caplan and Caplan gave us principles of community psychiatry, which came to be used as a guide in defining as well as understanding the nuances of the subject. The principles defined by them are as follows:

1. Responsibility to a population, usually a catchment area defined geographically
2. Treatment close to the patient's home
3. Multi-disciplinary team approach
4. Continuity of care
5. Consumer participation
6. Comprehensive services[3]

Community psychiatry has come a long way from when patients would be 'shackled' to developed countries now focusing on deinstitutionalisation of the mentally ill patients. Low- to middle-income countries, like India, need to focus on strengthening existing mental healthcare facilities and developing new mental health services as well as making these services easily accessible.[1] This chapter will provide an overview of the challenges faced and the attempts at finding possible solutions to these challenges.

MAGNITUDE OF THE PROBLEM

Mental illness contributed about 13% to the global disease burden in 2004, and more than 260 million people are affected by depression globally.[4] Depression contributes about one-third of the disease burden by mental illness, and by the year 2030, it is anticipated to be the leading cause of it.[5] Mental illnesses account for about one-fourth and one-third of the total years lived with disability in low-income and middle-income countries, respectively.[6] The economic loss is huge and is predicted to be about 16 trillion US dollars by 2030.[7]

Mental health disorders have been ignored and sidelined for many years, and the majority of nations, including India, spend less than 2% of their health budget on mental health illness treatment and prevention.[8] This has created a chasm between the required and available mental health services.

India has nearly 12% (150 million) of its population in need of active mental health service intervention.[9] A WHO report shows that the burden of mental health problems is around 2,443 disability adjusted life years per 100,000 population in India, and the age-adjusted suicide rate per 100,000 population is 21.1. The mental health workforce in India (per 100,000 population) includes psychiatrists (0.3), nurses (0.12), psychologists (0.07) and social workers (0.07).[10] The psychiatrist to patient ratio in India is abysmal, with only one trained psychiatrist catering to nearly 2.5 lakh population.[9] For every 1000 patients in need of hospitalisation, only 6 to 8 beds are dedicated to mental healthcare.[11] This disparity is further increased in small towns and villages, since most of these services are concentrated in major cities, resulting in a lack of specialised care by adequately trained professionals.[12] The primary point of contact for patients seeking help is therefore local healers or inadequately qualified professionals. It is very disheartening that the situation has not improved in the past 30 years despite policy intervention and programme implementation by the government.[9]

INDIAN SCENARIO FOR RURAL PSYCHIATRY

The majority of the Indian population, that is, nearly three-quarters of the total population, resides in villages. Per the Census of India, a village is "a rural settlement is one which has less than 5000 population, its population density is <400 persons/sq. km (in contrast to an urban area), and at least 75% of male working population is engaged in agriculture activities."[13] From this, we can ascertain that a majority of India's population is engaged in farming.

Farmer's suicide is a global problem plaguing many countries.[14-25] Although farming promotes a peaceful and healthy lifestyle, the mortality rate is extremely high.[23] Farming practices greatly vary across regions in type of farm, number of crops grown in a year, type of crop grown, manual or machine-based labour and organic farming or use of pesticides, and even then, there are many commonalities determining the mental health of the farmers.[14] The unpredictable and capricious nature of weather, global markets and regulations imposed by the government leave family-owned businesses with uncertainty and at the mercy of these changing trends. Productivity is also affected by global warming. This uncertainty and unpredictability create an extremely stressful situation for farmers and their families.[24]

Survivors of farmer's suicide were given ex gratia monetary help by the state. Eleven studies pertaining to farmer's suicide and nearly 200 media reports and government initiatives portrayed it as an economical problem and reduced it merely to a debt-driven crisis. This resulted in policies being drafted that only provided financial support to farmers.[25] This is equivalent to looking at the issue with blinders on and ignoring the multitude of factors that drive a person to commit this desperate act. Behere and Bhise explored these factors in their paper and found that farming is not just a profession for these farmers but a way of life and at times their only source of livelihood. Farmer's suicide differs in that they are mostly married, middle-aged men survived by a family which includes schoolgoing kids and no other earning member.[25] They use convenient and easily accessible methods to commit suicide. Pesticides are easily available in India for agricultural purposes, and their consumption the commonest method for farmers to commit suicide.[18,25] Bereaved families are in need of not just financial support but social support as well. Functioning is maintained despite such high stress, warning signs are often missed and families might blame themselves. Policies and support groups should be implemented which should include teaching farmers and surviving families economic management, diversifying sources of income and creating self-help groups within the farming community itself.

CHALLENGES FACED IN COMMUNITY PSYCHIATRY AND THEIR POSSIBLE SOLUTIONS

Myriad barriers are faced by mental healthcare providers as well as patients. Perceived stigma, lack of knowledge, superstitions, denial, inability to identify and recognise a mental disorder by family members, lack of availability of specialists, inaccessible or far-off centres of care and financial constraints are a few of the many challenges faced.

Developing countries need to realistically assess the needs of the community and develop healthcare skills which are pragmatic to meet these needs. Community participation like training volunteers from the community to identify common mental health disorders and clearly defining simple guidelines for referrals will go a long way in building a bridge between apt care and those in need of help.[26] Kilbourne et al. identify barriers that impede access to continuous standard mental healthcare like shortage of manpower, fewer institutes and government policies.[27] The burden of patient care due to these hindrances often fall on the families. Caregiver burden may increase due to a lack of proper instruction or training, and the caregiver themselves may be at risk of developing mental health problems.[28] Training non-specialists will reduce the burden on existing healthcare professionals and bridge the gap between patient and healthcare. The exponential value of task-shifting should be recognised.[26] Regular monitoring of these non-specialists is essential, and task shifting should not become task dumping by those in power.[29] A way of maintaining standard of care can be to give a checklist that the non-specialist has to fill out with every patient. The checklist can include questions to be asked to the patient and family member along with instructions and warnings about red flags. A standard method will reduce the possibility of misinformation or half-information being passed on.

The global pandemic of COVID-19 has caused a significant increase in stress, anxiety and depression. Earlier, distance was a barrier, but due to the pandemic, accessing healthcare has become even more difficult. Telemedicine has been of invaluable help during this crisis. Telepsychiatry can include primary assessment, patient education and counselling, medicine management and therapy, with a majority of clinically stable patients being managed by teleconsultation only.[30]

Possible solutions include non-governmental organisations helping to create awareness amongst the community as well as in training volunteers and monitoring them. SAWAB is an NGO which started a project in the Ganderbal district of Kashmir and Nashik district of Maharashtra for this. Per the national and district mental health programme, the aim is to train local mental health professionals to identify, manage and refer patients with mental health problems. Finally, mental health is integrated into the general health system. Studies show that it is a very low-cost and effective method.[31]

Mobile applications have been developed for ease of access to telepsychiatry. Peter Yellowlees and Steven Chan, in their paper "Mobile Mental Health Care – An Opportunity for India" suggested that mobile applications are the practical solution to the rural community in India. Telepsychiatry also has the advantage of allowing healthcare access anywhere and anytime without the restrictions of the traditional brick-and-mortar facilities. Telepsychiatry is more economical in terms of travel expenses and maintenance of huge facilities to cater to the need of such a massive population.[32] Mobile applications also have the advantage of a large number of patients being connected at the same time, so redundancy and effort and time required can be reduced. Psychoeducation of family members and general instructions regarding medicine side effects can be shared via online group meetings or pre-recorded videos, followed by a live session for dealing with any queries. An NGO called Atmiyata launched mobile phone apps for supporting community workers, self-help groups and farmers' clubs for common mental health disorders. The Schizophrenia Research Foundation (SCARF) launched a mobile tele-psychiatry project known as Scarf Telepsychiatry (STEP) in Pudukottai in 2010. This project provided free mental health services using mobile clinics to provide free mental healthcare in Pudukottai, a backward district in Tamil Nadu. It covers more than 156 villages with a population of more than 25 lakh and has helped 1500 people to date.[33]

In the era of digital India, smart phone apps can be innovatively used for diagnosis or at least screening for mental illness and identifying persons who should seek professional help. GMHAT PC is one such tool that enables paramedical workers to screen patients using handheld devices. This is a computer-based assessment which can identify a variety of mental health problems and generate possible clinical diagnosis. It also has a symptom rating and risk assessment system along with generation of a referral letter. The tool was feasible to use, as it took less than 15 minutes to apply. The GMHAT-PC has a sensitivity of 98.18% and specificity of 72.22%.[34] Staff can be trained to use this application, and appropriate screening of patients even in remote areas can be done. This will help in bridging the wide gap between mental health professionals and patients.

The government has already implemented certain policies on whose foundation we can further build and strengthen community psychiatry. The existing programmes and policies are the National Mental Health Programme, 1982; the Mental Health Act, 1987; and the District Mental Health Programme (DMHP), 1996.[35] The Mental Health Care Bill (MHCB) was passed on 27th March 2017 by the Indian Parliament to replace the Mental Health Act of 1987.[36] The universal health coverage's aim is that "all people have access to needed promotive, preventive, curative, and rehabilitative health services, of sufficient quality to be effective, while also ensuring that people do not suffer financial hardship while paying for these services."[37] The National Health Policy 2017 of India includes universal health coverage as one of its major points, and this should be used to as a way of making mental health more accessible and affordable.[38] It is important that these well-drafted policies be implemented with haste and that action on them is taken now rather than later. The right to mental health is an important milestone and can very well shape the future of Indian health.[9]

CONCLUSION

It is important to provide acceptable and accessible mental healthcare to the community to reduce social and economic loss. Overcoming barriers in community psychiatry is possible only by active participation of the community and integrating mental health with primary healthcare. Telepsychiatry is cost effective and time saving and should be looked into to make it more refined and safer.

References

1. Thara R, Rameshkumar S, Mohan CG. Publications on community psychiatry. *Indian J Psychiatry.* 2010 Jan;52(Suppl1):S274–7.
2. Thornicroft G, Szmukler G. *Textbook of Community Psychiatry.* Oxford, UK: Oxford Medical Publications; 2001.
3. Caplan G, Caplan R. Development of community psychiatry concepts. In: *Comprehensive Textbook of Psychiatry.* Baltimore, MD: Williams and Wilkins; 1967.
4. James SL, Abate D, Abate KH, Abay SM, Abbafati C, Abbasi N, et al. Global, regional, and national incidence, prevalence, and years lived with disability for 354 diseases and injuries for 195 countries and territories, 1990–2017: A systematic analysis for the Global Burden of Disease Study 2017. *The Lancet.* 2018 Nov 10;392(10159):1789–858.
5. Mahajan P, Rajendran P, Sunderamurthy B, Keshavan S, Bazroy J. Analyzing Indian mental health systems: Reflecting, learning, and working towards a better future. *J Curr Res Sci Med.* 2019 Jan 1;5:4.
6. World Health Assembly 65. Global burden of mental disorders and the need for a comprehensive, coordinated response from health and social sectors at the country level: Report by the Secretariat. 2012 [cited 2021 Mar 10]; Available from: https://apps.who.int/iris/handle/10665/78898
7. Bloom D, Cafiero E, Jané-Llopis E, Abrahams-Gessel S, Bloom L, Fathima S, et al. *The Global Economic Burden of Non-Communicable Diseases: A Report by the World Economic Forumn and the Harvard School of Public Health.* Geneva: World Economic Forum; 2011 Sep.
8. World Health Organization. *Mental Health Atlas 2017.* Geneva, Switzerland: World Health Organization; 2018. 68 p.
9. Lahariya C. Strengthen mental health services for universal health coverage in India. *J Postgrad Med.* 2018;64(1):7–9.
10. World Health Organisation. Mental health [Internet]. World Health Organisation India. 2021 [cited 2021 Mar 10]; Available from: www.who.int/westernpacific/health-topics/mental-health
11. Ravindran NR. 2 crore Indians need help for mental disorders. India Today [Internet]. 2011 Jul 1 [cited 2021 Mar 10]; Available from: www.indiatoday.in/magazine/health/story/20110711-2-crore-indians-need-help-for-mental-disorders-746701-2011-07-01
12. Lahariya C, Singhal S, Gupta S, Mishra A. Pathway of care among psychiatric patients attending a mental health institution in central India. *Indian J Psychiatry.* 2010 Oct 1;52(4):333.
13. Murthy R. Rural and community psychiatry. *Indian J Soc Psychiatry.* 2018;34:281–4.
14. Behere P, Bansal A. Farmer's suicide in Vidarbha everybody's concern: Guest editorial. *J Mahatma Gandhi Inst Med Sci.* 2009;14(2):3–5.
15. Behere P, Bhise M. Farmers' suicides in central rural India: Where are we heading?: Guest editorial. *Indian J Soc Psychiatry.* 2010;26:1–2.
16. Behere PB, Bhise M. Farmers suicide in rural India. In: *Comprehensive Text Book of Community Psychiatry in India.* Chandigarh: PGI Chandigarh; 2010.
17. Behere PB, Behere AP. Current themes farmers' suicide in Vidarbha region of Maharashtra state: A myth or reality? *Indian J Psychiatry.* 2008;50:124–7.
18. Behere PB, Reddy S. Clinical evaluation of suicide and related issues. In: *Psychiatry in India Training & Training Centers.* New Delhi, India: Indian Psychiatric Society; 2010. p. 457.
19. Behere PB. Families take years to cope with loss. *Times of India.* 2010 May 11;5.
20. Behere PB. Families of farmers who killed self also distressed. *Times of India.* 2010 May 11;1.
21. Bhise M, Behere PB. Prevention of farmer's suicide in central India: Barriers, boundaries and beyond. Winner of Dr. M. Murugappan Poster Award presented at: 66th ANCIPS 2013. Bangalore; 2014.
22. Behere PB, Bhise M, Behere AP. Suicide studies in India In: *Developments in Psychiatry in India: Clinical, Research and Policy Perspectives.* Springer; 2015.
23. McCurdy SA, Carroll DJ. Agricultural injury. *Am J Ind Med.* 2000;38(4):463–80.
24. Gibbens S. Why these farmers are protesting with skulls. National Geographic. 2017 Aug.
25. Behere PB, Bhise M. Psychological distress in survivors of farmers' suicides: A cross sectional comparative study from central part of rural India. In: 63rd ANCIPS. Delhi; 2012.
26. Srinivasa Murthy R, Kumar K. Challenges of building community mental health care. *World Psychiatry.* 2008 Jun;7(2):101–2.
27. Kilbourne AM, Beck K, Spaeth-Rublee B, Ramanuj P, O'Brien RW, Tomoyasu N, et al. Measuring and improving the quality of mental health care: A global perspective. *World Psychiatry.* 2018 Feb;17(1):30–8.

28. Von Kardorff E, Soltaninejad A, Kamali M, Eslami Shahrbabaki M. Family caregiver burden in mental illnesses: The case of affective disorders and schizophrenia: A qualitative exploratory study. *Nord J Psychiatry*. 2016;70(4):248–54.
29. Kottai SR, Ranganathan S. Task-shifting in community mental health in Kerala: Tensions and ruptures. *Med Anthropol*. 2020 Aug 17;39(6):538–52.
30. Bao Y, Sun Y, Meng S, Shi J, Lu L. 2019-nCoV epidemic: Address mental health care to empower society. *The Lancet*. 2020 Feb 22;395(10224):e37–8.
31. Malathesh BC, Gowda GS, Kumar CN, Narayana M, Math SB. Response to: Rethinking online mental health services in China during the COVID-19 epidemic. *Asian J Psychiatry*. 2020 Jun;51:102105.
32. Yellowlees P, Chan S. Mobile mental health care: An opportunity for India. *Indian J Med Res*. 2015 Oct 1;142:359–61.
33. Tharoor H, Thara R. Evolution of community telepsychiatry in India showcasing the SCARF model. *Indian J Psychol Med*. 2020 Oct 7;42(5 Suppl):69S–74S.
34. Behere P, Sinha S. Correlation of global mental health assessment tool (GMHAT-PC) in assessment of psychiatric patients as compared to the psychiatrist's diagnosis in a primary care of central India: Preliminary findings. *J Datta Meghe Inst Med Sci Univ*. 2014 Jan 1;9:1–4.
35. Press Information Bureau. *Country's First Ever Mental Health Policy Unveiled Society Needs to Change Perception on Mental Illness: Dr Harsh Vardhan*. New Delhi, India: Government of India Ministry of Health and Family Welfare. 2014 Oct 10.
36. Government of India. *New Pathway New Hope: National Mental Health Policy of India*. New Delhi, India: Ministry of Health and Family Welfare, Government of India; 2014.
37. World Health Organization, Etienne C, Asamoa-Baah A, Evans DB, editors. *The World Health Report: Health Systems Financing: The Path to Universal Coverage*. Geneva: World Health Organization; 2010. 96 p.
38. Government of India. *National Health Policy 2017*. New Delhi, India: Ministry of Health and Family Welfare, Government of India; 2017.

20
Optimizing Patient Care in Psychiatry – Geriatric Psychiatry

Elvin Lukose and Heena Merchant Pandit

Interview	204
History Taking	205
Presenting Complaints	*205*
Medical Complaints	*205*
Past Psychiatric History	*206*
Social History	*206*
Personality Assessment	*206*
Substance Use History	*206*
Physical Examination	207
Investigations	207
Psychotropic Drug Monitoring	209
Various Scales for Use in Geriatric Care	209
Scales for Adverse Drug Effects	*209*
Scales for Quality of Life	*210*
Scales for Depression	*210*
Various Models of Care in Mental Health for Geriatric Population	210
Improving Mood-Promoting Access to Collaborative Treatment	*210*
PEARLS	*210*
PRISM-E Study Model	210
Helping Older People Experience Success	211
Psycho-Geriatric Assessment and Treatment in City Housing	211
Wellness Recovery Action Planning	211
Providing Resources Early to Vulnerable Elders Needing Treatment	*212*
Special Models for Older Nursing Home Residents	212
Preadmission Screening and Resident Review	*213*
Minimum Data Set	*213*
Conclusions	214

INTERVIEW

Due to the higher prevalence of sensory impairments and cognitive deficits in the geriatric age group, the therapist has to ensure if the patient understands the questions and the implications of a psychiatric referral to enhance cooperation from the patient. The availability of an informant may help in clarifying and corroborating details on history, but in the event of a patient reporting alone, the following care can be taken while interviewing a geriatric patient.

- Using simple words and terminology with respect to the patient's educational background
- Speaking at a comfortable pace
- Use of non-verbal gestures to maximize comprehension while asking questions or eliciting answers
- Using leading questions if the patient experiences difficulty in recalling some details from memory

Most patients understand more clearly the psychosocial rather than the biological model of psychiatric illness. Depending on the cultural context, patients may minimize or under-report psychiatric illnesses, considering them part of normal ageing. Older adults might associate having depressive illness with feelings of shame, which results in under-reporting of psychopathology in the geriatric age group. Hence, directly eliciting psychiatric complaints can trigger defensiveness on the patient's part and thus undermine the objectives of the therapist. Building rapport and encouraging a narrative style from the patient can help pinpoint major life events and role transitions in the patient's life. This allows the therapist to use those epochs of personal significance and ask about the patient's emotional experience, which can provide clues to the possibility of a latent, sub-syndromal or undiagnosed psychiatric illness. Leading questions like "How was your sleep and appetite during that time?" or "Did you ever attempt or have thoughts of suicide following that incident?" can separate clinically relevant information from rest of the details for an adequate diagnosis.

HISTORY TAKING

Presenting Complaints

A geriatric case usually presents with complex intertwined social issues. Psychological factors like ongoing interpersonal disputes in the family, financial struggles or recent loss of a family member can exacerbate the patient's medical or psychiatric illness. Respecting the emotional involvement in social matters, leading questions regarding patient's mental status can help reveal any psychiatric illness that may have gone undiagnosed. Most patients will present to the general hospital for acute medical or surgical complications, and the dependency on healthcare along with the ambivalence of family caregivers may bring the patient's psychiatric problems to the surface. For example, a geriatric patient admitted for an acute surgical emergency may start experiencing crying spells and start voicing death wishes even after the surgery and warrant a psychiatric consultation. Another example would be a geriatric patient whose caregivers may not be around often or even abandon the person in a hospital, which may precipitate depressive or agitated behavior in the patient.

Medical Complaints

Ongoing stressors may trigger certain behaviors in the geriatric patient which may ultimately culminate in high healthcare-seeking behavior or dependency. Some common incidences of psychological factors affecting an underlying medical illness in the geriatric patient are as follows.

- Non-compliance with treatment, leading to relapse in chronic medical illnesses
- Non-cooperative behavior in indoor hospital settings, like refusal to eat food or take medications

- Overdosing on medical treatments as a possible or suspected suicidal attempt
- Refusal of life-saving procedures like hemodialysis or surgical interventions
- Substance use and related complications (for example, alcohol withdrawal) following a major life event or role transition in the patient's life

Such inimical behaviors may be the first indication of an underlying psychological conflict or a psychiatric illness and warrant medical attention along with a multi-disciplinary management and consequent psychosocial rehabilitation.

Past Psychiatric History

Due to difficulties in recalling details about past psychiatric treatments and maintaining documentation, the therapist may have to be well versed with certain peculiarities like the shape or colors of some drugs distributed in the region or colloquial names assigned to certain treatments like ECT or investigations like MRI scans to deduce the probable diagnosis or the nature of treatment that the geriatric patient was on. Enquiring about the patient's previous compliance with prescribed treatments, as well as the reasons for non-compliance, can reveal important information about patient's insight or possible deterioration of an underlying cognitive impairment. Poor compliance can stem from the following causes

- A sense of hopelessness and pessimism regarding treatments
- Lack insight into their illness
- Experiencing side effects or unpleasant effects from the drugs
- Inability to afford treatments or lack of adequate health insurance
- Greater travelling time or expenses and related inconveniences

Social History

Fluctuations in financial state or size of social support are common triggers of psychiatric symptoms in geriatric patients. The recent demise of a spouse or emigration of children from home can discourage a patient from seeking help for his/her healthcare needs. The state of living alone, unable to care for himself and under a significant risk to health may affect the short-term treatment plan for the patient from prescribing a treatment at home, on an outpatient basis or transferring to an in-patient healthcare facility.

Personality Assessment

The history of a patient's personality from the informant along with longitudinal observation can help in providing a useable sketch of the patient's personality. Knowledge of pre-morbid personality traits can be helpful in identifying personality change caused by mental illness and also gives an estimate of the patient's reserve of coping mechanisms that may influence the picture of psychiatric symptoms.

Substance Use History

Patient's substance use may be hidden due to the conspicuous manifestations of medical or surgical illness or decreased attention from family caregivers to the daily habits and whereabouts of the patient. Sudden onset of medical complications, lack of adequate response to ongoing treatment, delayed healing of wounds and frequent falls or major accidents should alert the treating physicians to the moderating influence or exacerbation of an underlying substance use or dependence. Substance use–related screening tools, for example, questionnaires for alcohol use like Michigan Alcohol Screening Test (MAST) and Alcohol Use Disorders Identification Test (AUDIT) help in assessment of harmful alcohol use in geriatric patients. Additional tools like the Readiness to Change questionnaire can help in assessment of motivation, and feedback reports like ASSIST could help in developing insight about the impact of substance use on health.

PHYSICAL EXAMINATION

A detailed physical examination of the geriatric patient is essential, as a high prevalence of physical illnesses in the patient may interfere with treatment choices and thus affect treatment outcomes. Undiagnosed medical illnesses result in high mortality rates in the geriatric age group. Labelling multiple vague somatic complaints as 'somatization' may steer attention away from a possible medical diagnosis and lead to up-titration of psychiatric medications, leading to debilitating side effects, further complicating the underlying medical illness.

INVESTIGATIONS

The geriatric population has a high prevalence of comorbid physical illnesses which necessitates complete blood workup and other ancillary investigations. However, as much as the treating physician might want to clinch a diagnosis, putting the geriatric patient through discomfort and pain needs to be balanced against the relevance and expected benefits of the corresponding treatment. Hence, investigations should be guided by relevant findings from history and mental state examination and on physical examination.

The following diagnostic possibilities coexist with psychiatric disorders in the geriatric patient.

- Depression (anemia, thyroid disease, malignancy, drug-induced)
- Mania (stroke, frontal dementia syndromes, drug side effects)
- Anxiety (thyroid disease, cardiovascular disorder)
- Delirium (infectious etiology, metabolic abnormalities, drug-induced)
- Dementia (thyroid disease, vitamin deficiencies, vascular disease)
- Psychosis (space occupying lesions in the brain, substance withdrawal/toxicity)
- Perceptual disturbances (visual defects, substance withdrawal, drug-induced).

A comorbid medical disorder or illness could amplify the existing cognitive deterioration, worsen treatment-induced side effects, create diagnostic difficulties and increase the risk of mortality.

ROUTINE BLOOD INVESTIGATIONS

- Hemogram and full blood count
- Erythrocyte sedimentation rate (ESR)
- C-reactive protein (CRP)
- Liver functions tests (bilirubin and enzymes)
- Renal function tests (blood urea nitrogen, creatinine)
- Thyroid function tests (free T_3, free T_4, TSH, thyroid antibodies)
- Lipid profile
- Blood glucose (fasting and post-prandial, HbA1c)

- Serum electrolytes (sodium, potassium, calcium, magnesium, phosphate)
- Urine microscopy
- Electro-cardiogram
- Chest X-ray
- CT/MRI brain scan

In addition to the previously mentioned investigations, the following specific tests may be required to pinpoint certain etiologies. Abnormalities of thyroid function and vitamin deficiencies are reversible and modifiable causes of cognitive decline, making blood investigations even more imperative in optimal care.

- Vitamin assays:
  - Serum B_{12}
  - Red blood cell folate levels
  - Vitamin D_3
- Thyroid function tests:
  - Free T_3, free T_4, TSH, thyroid antibodies
- Viral and fungal tests:
  - HIV-ELISA
  - Western blot test
  - CSF cryptococcal antigen
- Bacterial test:
  - Rapid plasma reagin test
  - VDRL
  - Blood cultures
  - CSF glucose, protein and counts
- Metal assays:
  - Serum copper
  - Ceruloplasmin
  - Serum heavy metals
  - Heavy metal urine screening
- Neuro-imaging (additional):
  - FDG-PET
  - SPECT
  - MRS
- Others:
  - EEG
  - Cortical evoked potentials
  - Polysomnography

Positron emission tomography (PET) and single photon emission computed tomography (SPECT) utilize radioactive isotopes to assess brain metabolism (PET) and perfusion (SPECT) and provide information about the functional status of brain tissue. These investigations are discussed in detail elsewhere. Compared to PET, SPECT is more specific in differentiating different types of dementia (Talbot) and so is recommended to aid in the differential in cases of doubt, especially in latter stages of dementia. Functional imaging like DAT (dopamine transporter) scanning can be helpful in distinguishing drug-induced Parkinsonism from idiopathic Parkinson's disease and aid in the diagnosis of Lewy body dementia. In the latter, low striatal DAT occurs, whereas DAT activity is normal in Alzheimer's disease.

PSYCHOTROPIC DRUG MONITORING

The geriatric age group is highly susceptible to the onset of side effects and toxicity even at clinical doses, which necessitates strict therapeutic drug monitoring and associated blood parameters. Therapeutic drug levels of mood stabilizers like lithium, carbamazepine and sodium valproate and anti-psychotics like clozapine can be obtained by their plasma levels. The following investigations are required before and during treatment with psychotropics.

VARIOUS SCALES FOR USE IN GERIATRIC CARE

Due to confounding factors in assessment of geriatric patients, scales provide an objective set of data on the patient's ongoing condition as well as its impact on his/her quality of life.

Scales for Adverse Drug Effects

- Abnormal Involuntary Movement Scale (drug-induced movement disorder)
- Simpson-Angus Scale (for drug-induced Parksinonism)
- Anti Cholinergic Cognitive Burden Scale (if on anti-cholinergic medications)

Table 20.1 Drug-monitoring parameters when prescribing psychotropics in the elderly.

Lithium	Complete blood counts
	Renal function (BUN, creatinine)
	Serum electrolytes
	ECG (Brugada syndrome, arrhythmias)
	Thyroid function
Carbamazepine	Full blood count
	Serum sodium and electrolytes
	Liver function (AST, ALT)
Sodium valproate	Full blood count
	Liver function (AST, ALT)
	Serum ammonia (if toxicity suspected)
Clozapine	Full blood count
	Fasting blood and post-prandial blood sugar
	Compete lipid profile
	ECG (myocarditis, arrhythmias)
	Chest X-ray (pneumonia)
Atypical anti-psychotics	Full blood count
	Fasting blood sugar, post-prandial blood sugar
	Compete lipid profile
	ECG (QTc prolongation)
Anti-depressants	ECG (QT prolongation, *Torsades de pointes*)
	Fasting and post-prandial blood sugar
	Complete lipid profile

Scales for Quality of Life

- WHO-QOL-OLD (WHO Quality of Life scale for the geriatric age group)
- GQOL (Geriatric Quality of Life)
- QUALID (Quality of Life in Late Stage Dementia)

Scales for Depression

- Geriatric Depression Scale
- Dementia Mood Assessment Scale

VARIOUS MODELS OF CARE IN MENTAL HEALTH FOR GERIATRIC POPULATION

Improving Mood-Promoting Access to Collaborative Treatment

Improving Mood-Promoting Access to Collaborative Treatment (IMPACT) was one of the largest Randomized Controlled Trials (RCTs), conducted at 18 primary care clinics in urban and semi-rural settings in five states of the United States. IMPACT included healthcare delivery systems like several health maintenance organizations (HMOs), traditional fee-for-service clinics, an independent provider association (IPA), an inner-city public health clinic and two Veterans Affairs (VA) clinics.

In the IMPACT model, potential patients are identified via routine depression screening or referred to treatment by their primary care provider (PCP). The pivotal member in the algorithm is the depression care manager (DCM), who discharges his/her duties under the supervision of a psychiatrist. The DCM assesses the patient during the first visit and provides treatment options of either pharmacotherapy with anti-depressant medications or a psychotherapeutic intervention like 'problem solving treatment' in primary care. The patient's preference is followed, and all patients are encouraged to engage in some form of behavioral activation, such as physical activity or scheduling tasks that provide self esteem. The total duration of the intervention is 1 year. Every 2 weeks during the intensive phase, the DCM follows up in person or by telephone and monitors progress.

Following the intervention, IMPACT patients reported greater improvement in depression, greater remission rates, improved quality of life and satisfaction with care.

PEARLS

The Program to Encourage Active and Rewarding Lives for Seniors (PEARLS) program is a home-based intervention specifically designed for homebound older adults with chronic medical conditions. Compared to the IMPACT model, the PEARLS model is prescriptive of counseling or psychotherapeutic interventions over medications.

Similar to the IMPACT study, the PEARLS program consisted of a depression care manager providing depression management sessions in the patient's home. The sessions usually ranged from 6–8 over a 5-month period with follow-ups of up to six brief monthly telephone contacts. The sessions include problem-solving treatment, which trains the patient to recognize depressive symptoms, to define problems associated with or contributory to their depression and to devise steps to solve those problems. Behavioral activation strategies such as social and physical activity planning and pleasant event scheduling are also advised.

PRISM-E STUDY MODEL

The PRISM-E study was a multisite, randomized trial which compared service use, outcomes and costs in integrated and enhanced referral models of mental healthcare for older persons with depression, anxiety or at-risk alcohol consumption. In the integrated care model, a mental health provider provided patients with corresponding mental health services, substance abuse services or both in the primary care clinic, whereas the enhanced specialty referral model provided mental health services, substance abuse services or both in a specialty setting that was physically separate and designated as a mental health or substance abuse clinic. Both referral models were associated with significant reductions in symptom severity for the aggregate group of patients with major depression, dysthymia, minor depression or depression not otherwise specified. Compared with integrated care, enhanced specialty referral showed a trend toward greater reduction in depression severity.

HELPING OLDER PEOPLE EXPERIENCE SUCCESS

The Helping Older People Experience Success (HOPES) model is an integrated health management program specifically developed to improve psychosocial functioning and to reduce the medical needs of older persons with serious mental illness.

The integrated model combines skills training (independent living skills, social skills) with management of medical care needs and promotion of preventive healthcare for older individuals. The total duration of intervention is 2 years. A curriculum that focuses on intensive skills training and health management is implemented in the first year. Monthly visits by psychiatric nurses are done for management of individual's overall healthcare needs. Rehabilitation specialists provide weekly group skills training in mental health clinics, rehabilitation centers and senior centers. The second year is the maintenance phase. Participants attend skills classes, go on community practice trips and meet with a nurse monthly. Compared with usual care, HOPES was more likely to engage individuals to remain in the program and to improve their social skills and functioning in the psychosocial and community while at the same time providing a sense of self efficacy.

PSYCHO-GERIATRIC ASSESSMENT AND TREATMENT IN CITY HOUSING

The foundation of the Psycho-Geriatric Assessment and Treatment in City Housing (PATCH) program is based on the concept underlying two proactive, community-based models for adults with serious mental illness, that is, the Assertive Community Treatment (ACT) model and the Gatekeeper model.

The Gatekeeper model utilizes lay community members, such as utility employees, bank tellers, postal carriers and others who are trained to identify older adults they come in contact with who may require appropriate mental health services. The Assertive Community model is designed for persons with serious mental illness who have a recent history of psychiatric hospitalizations, criminal justice involvement, homelessness or substance abuse.

In the PATCH model, the psychiatric nurse is the pivotal member. Nurses meet with building managers and other personnel to describe the program and initiate a structured educational program for building staff. Upon receiving a referral, the nurse contacts the concerned old resident to schedule a home visit and conducts a protocol-driven assessment. The nurse is later joined by the team psychiatrist on subsequent home visit to interview and evaluate the resident.

WELLNESS RECOVERY ACTION PLANNING

Self-management support – also referred to as self-care, self-help, and illness management is the core of the Wellness Recovery Action Planning (WRAP) program. In WRAP, the peer and professionals do not assume responsibility for the individual's care, which removes the implied hierarchy in the relationship between the healthcare professional and the person with the mental illness. Activities included in self-management support for mental health conditions include medication support, participation in self-directed components of psychotherapy, physical activity, recovery maintenance, relapse prevention or vocational skills training.

In the WRAP program, trained peer facilitators create an individualized plan for recovery based on which they teach individuals with serious mental illness the skills and behaviors to self-manage their condition independent of any more formal healthcare services they may receive. They are trained not to use psychiatric or medical jargon to describe individuals' needs.

The intervention sessions led by trained WRAP facilitators include lectures, group discussions, instructional materials and individual and group exercises. Self-guided wellness and recovery resources are also included.

Providing Resources Early to Vulnerable Elders Needing Treatment

Providing Resources Early to Vulnerable Elders Needing Treatment (PREVENT) was an Agency for Healthcare Research and Quality–funded RCT that assessed the psychiatric impact of a collaborative care management model on 153 older adults with Alzheimer's disease (and their caregivers).

The 153 eligible older adults with Alzheimer's disease and their self-identified caregivers were randomized by physicians to receive either collaborative care management or augmented usual care at primary care practices. Patients in the treatment group received 1 year of care management by an interdisciplinary team integrated within primary care led by an advanced practice nurse working with the patient's family caregiver.

Collaborative care for the treatment of Alzheimer's disease resulted in significant improvement in the quality of care and in behavioral and psychological symptoms of dementia among primary care patients as well as their caregivers. These improvements were achieved with minimal use of antipsychotics or sedative-hypnotics without significant dose escalations.

The geriatric nurse practitioners acted as care managers. The nurse practitioner focused on the patient's behavioral symptoms and coordinated with the primary care physician in the management of the patients' other chronic medical conditions. The patient's caregiver was treated as the primary conduit by which the patient received hands-on care. The standard protocols included methods to identify, monitor and treat behavioral and psychological symptoms of dementia (primarily without any prescription drugs) like repetitive behavior, mobility, sleep disturbances, depression, agitation or aggression, delusions or hallucinations. The necessary healthcare needs of the caregivers were also provided.

Collaborative care for the treatment of Alzheimer's disease resulted in significant improvement in the quality of care and in behavioral and psychological symptoms of dementia among primary care patients as well as their caregivers. These improvements were achieved with minimal use of antipsychotics or sedative-hypnotics without significant dose escalations.

The PREVENT protocol has been reengineered recently to improve its applicability and feasibility in the typical primary care practice and to facilitate its implementation in a real-world clinical practice. To accomplish these goals, the team developed a treatment manual with more attention to de novo implementation of the program in primary care, designed a new care model that delivers most of the intervention in the home while remaining a primary care – based service and developed a specialty dementia clinic designed to support co-management with primary care.

SPECIAL MODELS FOR OLDER NURSING HOME RESIDENTS

With more decentralization of mental healthcare, nursing homes have begun to use nurse-centered models in which a psychiatric nurse visits the nursing home to evaluate residents' mental health needs while coordinated by a psychiatrist who acts as an "extender" of the mental health services. Depending in the individual's need, the psychiatrist and nurse may come to the facility together and residents are triaged to either the nurse or psychiatrist.

Despite lack of significant effectiveness on RCTs, observational research suggests that 50 to 75% of residents who receive mental health services improve in some aspect.

Interdisciplinary team models allow for innovative approaches for providing ongoing care and addressing the needs of nursing homes in their means to train and educate staff.

The Nursing Home Reform Act (1987) introduced two federal programs in the United States with direct implications for the mental health status and care of nursing home residents:

- Preadmission Screening and Resident Review Program
- Minimum Data Set

Both programs have the potential to identify and to facilitate the appropriate care of older nursing home residents.

Preadmission Screening and Resident Review

Preadmission Screening and Resident Review (PASRR) requires all individuals to be screened for mental health conditions prior to admission to a nursing home. On identification of a mental illness, a mental health specialist must further assess the patient to determine if there is need for admission in the nursing home. The second level of screening involves a specialist who provides follow-up treatment recommendations for the patient's mental healthcare during the admission stay. The evaluation and recommendations of the specialist are reviewed by a consulting psychiatrist.

Minimum Data Set

The Minimum Data Set (MDS) is a mandatory nursing home patient data collection and screening instrument used to assess patients' physical and mental health status. Every nursing home resident receives an MDS assessment upon admission and every 90 days thereafter and whenever there is a major change in the resident's status. Compared to PASRR, the MDS provides a routine, regularly scheduled mechanism for identification of nursing home residents with mental health needs and their requirement. The MDS instrument has been updated and improved since its introduction. MDS 3.0 is the current format in use and contains better-validated assessments of cognition, quality of life and depression. The model also allows greater participation of the resident in the mental healthcare management.

Data on Integrated and Multi-Disciplinary Approaches

Care in Assisted Living Facilities

In an attempt to draw a relationship between social engagement in an assisted living facility (ALF) with patient depressive features, 82 patients were interviewed face to face in eight ALFs in a southern state of the United States. Results indicate life satisfaction and depressive symptoms were significantly associated with perceived friendliness of residents and staff, and pleasure in daily activities like enjoyment of mealtimes was related to low depressive symptoms. Thus, ALFs could foster psychological well-being by encouraging residents to develop meaningful relationships within the facility and by designing enjoyable mealtimes.

Yale Geriatric Care Program

The Yale Geriatric Care Program was designed as a nursing-centered model for developing optimum geriatric care. A study was conducted at a university hospital on 240 patients aged 70 years and older on four non–intensive care units. It utilized an integrated model of primary nurses, specially trained unit-based geriatric resource nurses, gerontological nurse specialists and geriatric physicians. It included surveillance and identification of frail older patients, unit-based geriatric educational programs for all nurses, special education and support for the geriatric resource nurses. The findings are yet to be published.

GRACE Model

The Geriatric Resources for Assessment and Care of Elders (GRACE) model uses an integrated model of a geriatrics team within the primary care environment, in-home assessment and care management. The GRACE interdisciplinary team consists of a nurse practitioner and social worker team, in affiliations with pharmacy, mental health, home health and community-based services. The first step involves the enrollment of the geriatric case, following which the GRACE support team conducts an in-home consultation for an initial comprehensive geriatric assessment. The support team then meets with the larger GRACE interdisciplinary team to develop an individualized care plan, including use of GRACE protocols for evaluating and managing common geriatric conditions. The GRACE support team then meets with the patient's primary care physicians to collaborate and make modifications in the plan, following which the plan is put into action. Using an electronic medical record and longitudinal tracking system, the GRACE support team provides ongoing care management and coordination of care across different sites of care for multiple geriatric syndromes. The GRACE model has been successfully implemented within diverse healthcare systems with positive results such as reduction in acute care service utilization and high patient and physician satisfaction.

CONCLUSIONS

Such interdisciplinary models allow for holistic management of the otherwise underserved healthcare needs of the geriatric population. Adoption of a particular model will be contingent on the resources of the relevant and corresponding healthcare system, feasibility and the prevalent healthcare-related policies of the state.

Bibliography

- Abou-Saleh MT, Katona CLE, Kumar A, eds. *Principles and practice of geriatric psychiatry*. LWW, New York, 2011.
- Bartels SJ, Moak GS, Dums AR. Models of mental health services in nursing homes: A review of the literature. *Psychiatric Services*. 2002;53(11):1390–1396.
- Bhugra D. Depression across cultures. *Prim Care Psychiatry*. 1996;2:155–65.
- Butler DE, Frank KI, Counsell SR. The GRACE model. In *Geriatrics models of care* (pp. 125–38). Springer, Cham. 2015.
- Callahan CM, Boustani MA, Unverzagt FW, Austrom MG, Damush TM, Perkins AJ, Fultz BA, Hui SL, Counsell SR, Hendrie HC. Effectiveness of collaborative care for older adults with Alzheimer disease in primary care: A randomized controlled trial. *JAMA*. 2006 May 10;295(18):2148–57.
- Committee on the Mental Health Workforce for Geriatric Populations, Board on Health Care Services, Institute of Medicine, Eden J, Maslow K, Le M, et al., eds. *The mental health and substance use workforce for older adults: In whose hands?* National Academies Press (US), Washington (DC). 2012 Jul 10;4. Workforce Implications of Models of Care for Older Adults with Mental Health and Substance Use Conditions.

- Counsell SR, Callahan CM, Buttar AB, Clark DO, Frank KI. Geriatric Resources for Assessment and Care of Elders (GRACE): A new model of primary care for low-income seniors. *Journal of the American Geriatrics Society*. 2006 Jul;54(7):1136–41.
- Inouye SK, Acampora D, Miller RL, Fulmer T, Hurst LD, Cooney Jr LM. The Yale Geriatric Care Program: A model of care to prevent functional decline in hospitalized elderly patients. *Journal of the American Geriatrics Society*. 1993 Dec;41(12):1345–52.
- Krahn DD, Bartels SJ, Coakley E, Oslin DW, Chen H, McIntyre J, Chung H, Maxwell J, Ware J, Levkoff SE. PRISM-E: Comparison of integrated care and enhanced specialty referral models in depression outcomes. *Psychiatric Services*. 2006 Jul;57(7):946–53.
- Levkoff SE, Cleary PD, Wetle T, Besdine RW. Illness behavior in the aged: Implications for clinicians. *Journal of the American Geriatrics Society*. 1988 Jul;36(7):622–9.
- Mueser KT, Pratt SI, Bartels SJ, Swain K, Forester B, Cather C, Feldman J. Randomized trial of social rehabilitation and integrated health care for older people with severe mental illness. *Journal of Consulting & Clinical Psychology*. 2010;78(4):561–73.
- Pink J, O'Brien J, Robinson L, Longson D. Dementia: Assessment, management and support: Summary of updated NICE guidance. *BMJ*. 2018 Jun 20;361.
- Pratt SI, Bartels SJ, Mueser KT, Forester B. Helping older people experience success: An integrated model of psychosocial rehabilitation and health care management for older adults with serious mental illness. *American Journal of Psychiatric Rehabilitation*. 2008;11(1):41–60.
- Sadock BJ. *Kaplan & Sadock's synopsis of psychiatry: Behavioral sciences/clinical psychiatry*. LWW, New York, 2007.
- Schonfeld L, King-Kallimanis BL, Duchene DM, Etheridge RL, Herrera JR, Barry KL, Lynn N. Screening and brief intervention for substance misuse among older adults: The Florida BRITE project. *American Journal of Public Health*. 2010 Jan;100(1):108–14.
- Talbot PR, Lloyd JJ, Snowden JS, Neary D, Testa HJ. A clinical role for 99mTc-HMPAO SPECT in the investigation of dementia? *Journal of Neurology, Neurosurgery & Psychiatry*. 1998 Mar 1;64(3):306–13.

21
Optimizing Patient Care in Psychiatry – Borderline Personality Disorder

Sayuri Perera

Introduction	216
Epidemiology	217
Pathogenesis	217
Child and Adolescent Temperament and Personality Factors	218
Factors Associated With Borderline Personality Pathology in Childhood	219
Clinical Features and Comorbidities	221
Borderline Personality Disorder and Bipolar Disorder	222
Borderline Personality Disorder and Early Trauma History	222
Borderline Personality Disorder and ADHD	222
Treatment	223
Lifetime Course	224
Adolescence	*224*
Adulthood	*225*
Treatment Implications	225

INTRODUCTION

The term borderline personality disorder (BPD) originated in 1938 in the United States. It was a term used by psychiatrists to describe patients they believed had a vulnerability to progress into a borderline schizophrenic state during certain situations[1].

Borderline personality disorder has since then been conceptualized as a severe psychiatric disorder, characterized by having a negative impact on affective stability and interpersonal relationships as well as self image. Those suffering from this disorder also show severe impulsivity, self harm, and suicidal behavior, which leads to distress and impairment in day-to-day life[2]. In addition to these symptoms, paranoid and dissociative states are also transient features of this disorder[3].

BPD is one of the most widely studied personality disorders owing to it being associated with increased clinical attention and having significant psychosocial impairments[4,5].

This chapter aims to cover the prevalence, symptomatology, and therapeutic options related to borderline personality disorder.

EPIDEMIOLOGY

The lifetime prevalence of BPD is approximately 5.9%, and the point prevalence of BPD is 1.6%[6,7]. Although the prevalence of BPD is not higher than other personality disorders in the general population, BPD has a high prevalence in treatment settings; It was present in 6.4% of primary care visits, 9.3% of psychiatric outpatients, and 20% of psychiatric inpatients according to the studies in clinical settings[8,9]. However, the ratio of females to males with the disorder is also greater in the clinical population. This result can be interpreted as women with BPD being more likely to seek treatment than men. About 80% of patients who receive treatment for BPD were reported to be women[10].

PATHOGENESIS

Although research has been conducted on the prognosis, course, consequences, and correlates of BPD, little is known about the emergence and early manifestations of this disorder. Theoretical models of the pathogenesis of BPD suggest that this disorder is best accounted for within the context of a diathesis-stress model, resulting from the interaction of environmental stressors and trait vulnerabilities[11].

With regard to the former, researchers have highlighted the role of adverse childhood experiences in the development of BPD, in particular childhood maltreatment, including sexual, physical, and emotional abuse[12] and emotional and physical neglect[13].

These experiences alone are not sufficient to account for the development of BPD, however, and are thought to lead to BPD only in the context of an underlying vulnerability.

However, given evidence that personality develops from an early age[14] and that adults with BPD report having experienced many borderline personality symptoms in childhood[15], early manifestations of borderline personality pathology can most likely be observed in childhood and warrant empirical attention. Indeed, research on the early manifestations of borderline pathology would have significant and important implications for the development of secondary prevention programs.

The cause of BPD is not known, and it is suggested that BPD is the product of an interaction between genetic, neurobiological, and psychosocial influences that affect brain development[16].

Although studies are rare and different values have been reported, there is evidence for the genetic transmission and heritability of BPD. According to two studies, the concordance rate for BPD was found to be higher in monozygotic twins compared with dizygotic twins (36 and 35% versus 19 and 7%)[17,18]. In summary, constitutional predisposition to emotional dysregulation with a non-supporting environment leads to the development of BPD[19].

According to neurobiological research data, it has been suggested that neuropeptide functions may predispose to interpersonal problems of BPD patients[20]. The hypothalamic pituitary adrenal (HPA) axis dysfunction has a central role in the development of BPD. Increased levels of stress hormones, such as basal cortisol, and reduced feedback sensitivity were reported in BPD patients[21]. However, maladaptive behaviors of self – others and relationships with others are believed to be modulated by the oxytocinergic system[22]. Increased HPA activity and decreased peripheral oxytocin levels are correlated with a history of early life maltreatment and insecure attachment in patients with BPD[23]. Moreover, few studies also reported increased testosterone levels in female and male patients with BPD[21].

Neuroimaging studies that have compared BPD patients with healthy controls have reported bilateral reductions in the hippocampus, amygdala, and medial temporal lobe[24,25]. The neurobiology of BPD can be conceptualized as abnormalities in the top-down control, provided by the orbitofrontal cortex and the anterior cingulate cortex, and the bottom-up control drives generated in the limbic system such as amygdala, hippocampus, and insular cortex. Top-down control provides cognitive control areas and bottom-up control provides salience detection[26]. In this circuitry, serotonin regulates the prefrontal regions by acting on 5-HT2 receptors in a different role[27]. Impulsive traits, a major component of BPD, are associated with deficits in central serotonergic functioning. More specifically, increased 5-HT2A receptors and decreased 5-HT2C receptors are related with impulsivity[26]. Impulsivity is a core feature of BPD, and it is related to reward and control circuits and deficient behavioral inhibition in prefrontal areas[28]. However, left amygdala hyperactivity was found in unmedicated patients with acute BPD. This feature is consistent with negative environmental stimuli[29]. Intense and variable emotions of BPD patients are related with amygdala hyperactivity. The role of the amygdala also reflects maladaptive top-down processes in evaluating negative environmental stimuli[30]. However, an enlarged hypothalamus and dysregulated HPA axis and a reduced volume of the amygdala and hippocampus are found in patients with a history of early trauma and posttraumatic stress disorder (PTSD)[31–33]. In addition, the finding of reductions in gray matter volume of amygdala in older BPD patients has been interpreted as reflecting a reversible progressive pathology[34]. Emotional regulation difficulties of BPD patients are related with insufficient capacity of cognitive processes of prefrontal cortex (PFC) activity[35]. Koenigsberg et al. reported hypoactivity in orbitofrontal cortex, ventrolateral cortex, and dorsal anterior cingulate cortex (ACC) in BPD patients compared with healthy individuals[36]. This result is related with maladaptive affective regulation in BPD patients. However, lower prefronto-limbic connectivity within the affect regulation circuitry was reported to be normalized after successful psychotherapy[37].

Life experiences are also known to be associated with the development of BPD[38]. Childhood trauma is the most significant risk factor for development of BPD[39]. Since childhood trauma is not always present in BPD, and individuals who had trauma do not always necessarily develop BPD, this relationship between childhood trauma and BPD is not clear. It can be interpreted that childhood trauma is not a mandatory precondition for the development of BPD. Childhood trauma in BPD patients can take many forms in prospective studies including sexual abuse, physical abuse and neglect, verbal abuse, and early parental separation or loss[40]. According to a prospective study with 500 individuals, more physically abused and/or neglected children met the criteria of BPD as adults. Interestingly, sexual abuse history is not found as a risk factor for BPD. However, having a parent with alcohol or substance use problems, having a diagnosis of drug abuse, major depressive disorder, and post-traumatic stress disorder have all been associated with the development of BPD but are also non-specific factors[41]. Another prospective, longitudinal study involving more than 600 children reported that childhood abuse/neglect was significantly associated with BPD in adulthood[42]. Meta-analyses have revealed that only a small effect size for the relationship between development of BPD and childhood maltreatment[43,44]. As with most psychiatric disorders, no single factor can explain the development of the disorder, multiple factors can help in explaining the development of BPD. Although, there were studies that reported that childhood trauma did not play a significant role in the development of BPD, it still remains an important risk factor for BPD and more studies are needed to elucidate this relationship.

CHILD AND ADOLESCENT TEMPERAMENT AND PERSONALITY FACTORS

The investigation of intrapsychic factors, including temperamental characteristics and personality traits in childhood and adolescence, is fundamental to recognize predictors of BPD at an early phase. Researchers identified several personality traits in children or adolescents, including affective instability, negative affectivity, negative emotionality, inappropriate anger, poor emotional control, impulsivity, and aggression, that could prepare to borderline pathology[45]. Few studies evaluated the relation of childhood personality traits to BPD in adulthood[46,47]. Across other temperamental traits, aggressive behaviors in childhood and early adolescence was associated to onset of BPD. Crick and collaborators[48] investigated different subtypes of aggression in a prospective study that recruited 400 children and found that relational aggression, but not physical aggression, emerged as a significant predictor for BPD features. This result was confirmed by Underwood[49] in a prospective study with the same objective.

Negative emotionality, in terms of negative affectivity and poor emotional control, is another important precocious factor associated to BPD onset. Lenzenweger and collaborators[50] conducted a community 3-year study with 250 adolescents/young adults, aimed to evaluate whether negative emotionality might impact early onset of BPD. Findings showed that negative emotionality predicted BPD at 19 years. Tragesser and collaborators[51] in a high-risk population of 353 subjects of 18 years reported a significant association of negative affectivity and impulsivity in childhood with BPD at 20 years. In addition, Hallquist and colleagues[52] found that low self-control may predict BPD at 14 years, and a worsening self-control increased BPD symptoms during the time.

Low self-control, impulsivity, and affective instability are three tightly connected dimensions that in very young age can be considered predictors for developing borderline pathology. Several investigations have assessed the influence of these constructs in childhood on later BPD symptoms. Tragesser and colleagues reported that affective instability and impulsivity predicted BPD onset at 20 years. Gratz et al.[52] highlighted, in a sample of 263 children, the importance of interrelationship among these two relevant personality traits (affective instability and impulsivity) with low self and emotion regulation, and with childhood borderline personality symptoms. Lower self-control and higher level of impulsivity were also identified as predictors of a diagnosis of BPD at 12 years in a 7-year twins study conducted in 1,116 children (around 5 years old)[53].

Five studies explored the interaction between child/adolescent personality traits and environmental or neurobiological factors in development of precocious BPD. Four investigations examined the effect of the relationships between temperamental characteristics and childhood maltreatment on the onset of BPD. Jovev et al[54] studied the interaction between emotional control, parental maltreatment and BPD in 245 children aged between 11 and 13 years. They observed that specific early temperamental features, particularly low emotional control, interact with familial maltreatment in promoting BPD symptoms across early to middle adolescence. Martin-Blanco and colleagues[55] found in 130 subjects with early BPD that neuroticism-anxiety, aggression-hostility dimensions, and emotional abuse were independent risk factors associated with BPD.

One study evaluated in 153 healthy adolescents the interaction of a temperamental risk factor and a neurobiological risk factor in predicting the emergence of BPD during early adolescence[56]. Authors examined several temperamental factors and volumetric measures of hippocampal asymmetry. Results showed that subjects were more likely to have BPD symptoms in presence of low effortful control and rightward hippocampal asymmetry.

FACTORS ASSOCIATED WITH BORDERLINE PERSONALITY PATHOLOGY IN CHILDHOOD

Although almost no research to date has examined the personality traits associated with childhood borderline personality symptoms, researchers have suggested that the trait vulnerabilities of affective dysfunction and disinhibition likely underlie the development of borderline personality pathology in children[22]. Further, studies of the likely behavioral manifestations of these traits provide suggestive evidence for the role of both affective dysfunction and disinhibition in childhood borderline personality pathology.

With regard to the relationship between affective dysfunction and childhood borderline personality pathology, studies have found that one aspect of affective dysfunction (i.e., emotional sensitivity) uniquely predicted borderline personality features in a community sample of children over time[23]. As for the potential manifestations of affective dysfunction, studies of primarily male psychiatric patients aged 6–12 have found higher levels of anxiety and depression among patients with a diagnosis of BPD[22,23]. Although this use of BPD diagnoses differs from the dimensional approach to the conceptualization and operationalization of childhood borderline personality symptoms used here, these findings provide suggestive support for a relationship between affective dysfunction[24–26] specifically, psychopathological manifestations of affective dysfunction) and childhood borderline personality pathology.

As for the relationship between disinhibition and childhood borderline personality pathology, research has shown that the presence of a BPD diagnosis among a sample of primarily male psychiatric patients aged 6–12 was associated with heightened levels of disinhibition (in the form of impulsivity)[29]. However, as with the aforementioned research on affective dysfunction, most research on the relationship between disinhibition and childhood borderline personality pathology has focused on behavioral manifestations of disinhibition, particularly aggressive and delinquent behavior. These studies have found that a diagnosis of BPD among samples of primarily male psychiatric patients aged 6–12 is associated with heightened levels of aggressive and delinquent behavior[31,33].

As was the case with the adult BPD literature, however, researchers have not examined explicitly the interaction of affective dysfunction and disinhibition in the risk for childhood borderline personality symptoms. Further, in regard to the potential mediating role of self- and emotion-regulation deficits in the relationship between these personality traits (and their interaction) and childhood borderline personality symptoms, no studies to date have examined the relationship between self- and emotion-regulation deficits and childhood borderline personality symptoms. However, researchers in the area of developmental psychology have long suggested that these capacities are integral to normative development[34,35] and research on the correlates of self- and emotion-regulation among children provides suggestive evidence for the importance of these phenomena to borderline personality symptoms in childhood (as deficits in each have been found to be associated with a range of negative borderline personality-relevant outcomes).

As such, preliminary evidence suggests a potential relationship between deficits in self- and emotion-regulation and borderline personality-relevant pathology among children and adolescents, although the extent to which these deficits are associated with childhood borderline personality symptoms per se remains unclear. Further, the extent to which deficits in these capacities mediate the relationship between affective dysfunction and disinhibition and childhood borderline personality symptoms is unknown. Nonetheless, lending support to the conceptualization of self- and emotion-regulation deficits as mediators of the relationship between the traits of interest and childhood borderline personality symptoms, research suggests that both affective dysfunction and disinhibition interfere with the development of self- and emotion-regulation capacities throughout childhood[38]. As such, these findings (in combination with the aforementioned findings that both the traits and proposed mediators predict borderline personality pathology and/or borderline personality-relevant outcomes) suggest that self- and emotion regulation deficits may mediate the relationship between these traits and borderline personality symptoms in childhood.

In summary, temperamental traits in childhood, including relational aggression, impulsivity, low emotional control, and negative affectivity, are robust predictors of early onset of BPD. Some evidences support the role of the interaction between temperamental features (low emotional control and negative affectivity) and familial environment (parental maltreatment, harsh discipline, and familial adversities) in developing BPD.

CLINICAL FEATURES AND COMORBIDITIES

BPD is a psychiatric disorder, which was initially thought to emerge during adolescence and continue into adulthood[57]. According to DSM-5 Section II, the diagnostic criteria of BPD are divided into four dimensions: (a) interpersonal instability dimension, which has the features of fear of abandonment and intense unstable relationships; (b) cognitive and/or self-disturbance, which consists of paranoid ideations, dissociative symptoms, and identity disturbances; (c) affective and emotional dysregulation; and (d) behavioral dysregulation dimension, which has impulsivity and suicidal behavior[58].

Affective instability has been shown to be the most specific, sensitive criteria for BPD[59]. Patients with BPD are emotionally labile, react strongly, and express dysphoric emotions such as depression, anxiety, and irritable mood[60]. However, a study that examined the associations of age with affective instability of BPD patients showed an inverse relationship between age and affective instability in patients with BPD[61]. Patients with BPD have unstable and conflicted relationships. They tend to view others as all good and bad, which is labeled as 'splitting'. They can easily become dependent on others, but they can also have dramatic shifts in their feelings toward others. Cognitive dysfunction in BPD patients has also been shown in a meta-analysis, where BPD patients scored poorer on tests of attention, cognitive flexibility, planning, learning, and memory[62].

Impulsive behavior is a core feature of BPD and might take many forms. Substance abuse, impulsive spending, binge eating, reckless driving, and self-damaging behavior are very common and put the patient at risk of harm[63]. Previous studies suggested that impulsivity, emotional dysregulation, and self-harm behaviors during childhood are predictive features of BPD[64].

Suicidal attempts and ideations are common manifestations of BPD and are one of the diagnostic criteria[58]. In retrospective studies, the rate of suicide is found to be 8–12% in BPD individuals[65]. Suicidal tendency is most common at age 20, and completed suicide attempts are more common after the age of 30 years in patients with BPD[66]. Patients may also engage in suicidal behaviors, such as cutting themselves. These behaviors, ideation or acts might be conceptualized as non-suicidal self-injury[67]. Since non-suicidal acts and suicide attempts are so common in BPD patients, it is quite difficult to assess the current risk of a patient's suicidal intent. Patients who have attempted suicide more than once have an increased risk for completed suicide. According to prospective studies, the predictors of suicide in patients with BPD were reported as co-occurring symptoms of dissociation, affective reactivity, self-harm, depression comorbidity, family history of suicide, and history of childhood abuse[68,69]. According to a recent study, which examined gender differences and similarities in aggression, psychiatric comorbidity, and suicidal behavior in patients with BPD, men with BPD were found more aggressive, impulsive and more impaired than women with BPD. Men with BPD were found at higher risk of dying due to a suicide attempt compared to women with BPD[70].

Comorbid psychiatric disorders are common in patients with BPD[71]. According to an epidemiologic survey, 85% of BPD patients have at least one comorbid psychiatric disorder[50]. Mood disorders, especially depressive disorder, bipolar disorder, anxiety disorder, posttraumatic stress disorder, substance use disorder, or other personality disorder and neurodevelopmental disorder such as attention-deficit/hyperactivity disorder (ADHD), might be present in patients with BPD[72]. According to several large patient samples, the rate of lifetime depression comorbidity ranges from 71% to 83%, and anxiety disorder comorbidity is as high as 88% in patients with BPD[73,74]. More recently in a genome-association study by Witt et al., genetic overlap has been found between BPD and bipolar disorder, major depressive disorder, and schizophrenia[75]. Their findings supported the role of genetic factors having a role in the development of BPD.

BORDERLINE PERSONALITY DISORDER AND BIPOLAR DISORDER

Borderline personality disorder (BPD) and bipolar disorder can co-occur in 10–20% of cases, and since symptomatology of these disorders is very similar, many patients with BPD have been mistakenly diagnosed with bipolar disorder[76]. It has also been suggested that BPD should be conceptualized as a part of the bipolar spectrum[77,78]. Smith et al. reported that a significant percentage of patients with BPD were in the bipolar spectrum[79], while Paris et al. reported that no empirical evidence supported BPD's link to the bipolar spectrum[80]. By reviewing neuroimaging studies, Sripada and Silk reported that there were both overlap and differences in certain brain regions between BPD and bipolar disorder individuals[81]. Vieta et al. reported that BPD was diagnosed twice as frequently in patients with bipolar II disorder and bipolar I disorder[82]. Zimmerman et al. reported that patients with major depressive disorder (MDD) and BPD had excess psychosocial morbidity compared to MDD patients without BPD, and that BPD was the third most frequent diagnosis in patients with bipolar disorder after obsessive-compulsive disorder and histrionic personality disorder, respectively[83]. In sum, these results can be interpreted as each disorder is diagnosed in the absence of the other and these findings challenge the notion that BPD can be conceptualized as the part of the bipolar spectrum[84].

BORDERLINE PERSONALITY DISORDER AND EARLY TRAUMA HISTORY

Trauma history is a central feature of both PTSD and BPD. The neurobiological impairments associated with the development of BPD can be conceptualized as the predisposing factor for BPD. Both environmental and neurobiological factors contribute to the development of BPD. Genetic predisposition becomes activated during environmental experiences of trauma history. It has been reported that trauma and neglect might exacerbate both biological and behavioral tendencies[85]. However, sufficient maternal care may buffer these vulnerabilities. These results might explain why some emotionally dysregulated individuals do not develop BPD despite their genetic tendencies. There is also evidence for a strong association between traumatic events and dissociative symptoms in BPD[86]. According to retrospective studies, borderline patients have high rates of childhood abuse and dissociation[87]. Depersonalization/derealization are core symptoms of BPD and dissociation can be a prominent feature in some individuals with BPD. Research in the dissociative subtype of PTSD and depersonalization suggested that dissociation might be a form of emotional over-modulation, promoting trauma-related stressful emotions[88]. Dissociation severity was predicted by the childhood traumas such as inconsistent care taking, sexual abuse, adult rape, and emotional neglect[89].

BORDERLINE PERSONALITY DISORDER AND ADHD

The comorbidity of ADHD has been reported in 20% of BPD patients in several studies[90]. Since impulsivity is considered to be a central feature of BPD and ADHD, impulsivity has been examined as part of adult ADHD symptomatology in BPD patients. According to Philipsen et al., ADHD should be considered a potential risk factor in patients with BPD with impulsivity[91]. In a recent study that has examined the association between impulsivity and

ADHD in BPD patients, we reported higher comorbidity of ADHD in BPD group, and motor impulsiveness has been shown as a potential predictor of ADHD symptoms in BPD group[92].

In sum, since BPD has been associated with chronic course of other psychiatric disorders, clinicians should carefully evaluate comorbid psychiatric conditions in patients with BPD in order to plan appropriate treatments.

TREATMENT

Since patients with BPD suffer considerable morbidity and mortality, BPD causes a therapeutic challenge for clinicians. First-line treatment for BPD is psychotherapy[93]. However, symptom-targeted medications have also been found effective[94].

The psychotherapies that have been adapted to treat patients with BPD are dialectical behavior therapy (DBT), mentalization-based therapy, transference-focused therapy, cognitive-behavioral therapy (CBT), and schema-focused therapy[95]. These therapies provide active and focused interventions that emphasize current functioning and relationships. These therapy modalities also (a) provide a structured manual that supports the therapist and provides recommendations for common clinical problems; (b) are structured so that they encourage increased activity, proactivity, and self-agency for the patients; (c) focus on emotional processing, particularly on creating robust connections between acts and feelings; and (d) show increased cognitive coherence in relation to subjective experience in the early phase of treatment by including a model of pathology that is carefully explained to the patient and encouraging an active stance by the therapist, which invariably includes an explicit intent to validate and demonstrate empathy and generate strong attachment relationships to create a foundation of alliance. Psychoeducation is also an important part of BPD treatment. It includes informing patients and families about the disorder, signs and the symptoms of the disorder, and also possible causes and treatment options[96]. According to a 2017 systematic review and meta-analyses of 33 clinical trials with 2256 participants that examined the efficacy of psychotherapies for BPD, DBT and psychodynamic approaches were found more effective compared to other psychotherapy modalities[97]. DBT is a well-studied form of CBT that puts emphasis on impulsive behavior and affective instability, and aims to regulate emotional lability using group or individual sessions.

DBT focuses on improving coping skills, self-destructive behavior and acting out. Mentalization-based and transference-focused therapies are primarily psychodynamic therapies. Mentalization therapy also includes cognitive techniques. For example, the patient is supported to observe her mind and create alternative perspectives of her thoughts to others. Transference-focused therapy includes confrontation, exploration and transference interpretations for the relationships of the BPD patients with other individuals. Schema-focused therapy is a form of CBT that includes skills training. Family education can be used adjunct to other therapies for BPD treatment 95.

According to the literature, the pharmacological treatment for BPD is limited. It is suggested that the patient with BPD who continues to experience severe, impairing symptoms (for example, affective dysregulation, impulsive-behavioral dyscontrol, perceptual symptoms) despite receiving psychotherapy should receive symptom-focused, adjunctive medication treatment60. According to clinical surveys and meta-analyses, low-dose antipsychotic drugs are more effective for cognitive and perceptual symptoms such as dissociation, paranoid ideation, and hallucinations compared with antidepressants or mood stabilizers. Mood stabilizers are found to be more effective for impulsivity, aggression, and behavior control in BPD[98]. Mood stabilizers in the meta-analyses were lamotrigine, topiramate, valproate, and lithium. Lithium is also found to be effective in preventing suicide in BPD patients, as reported by a retrospective study. However, according to preliminary evidence, omega-3 fatty acids are suggested as adjunct to primary medication treatment, with mood stabilizers to prevent recurrent self-harm[99]. Meta-analyses have also found that mood stabilizers and low-dose antipsychotics are more effective for affective dysregulations in BPD compared to antidepressants[98].

Since BPD has a high rate of psychiatric comorbidity, clinicians should be aware of co-occurring mood and anxiety disorders and substance use disorder for treating patients with BPD. For mood and anxiety disorders, clinicians should be careful to prescribe higher doses of antidepressant drugs for treating subthreshold symptoms. Thus, clinicians should focus on BPD treatment and effective treatment should be organized for comorbid psychiatric situations for patients with BPD. However, when it comes to substance use disorder, bipolar disorder comorbidity and treatment of the substance use disorder should take precedence over BPD for safety[100]. There is no evidence supporting the use of polypharmacy in personality disorder. In sum, treatment of BPD is multimodal. Psychotherapy is the first line treatment, and adjunctive, symptom-focused pharmacotherapy is essential. Comorbid psychiatric disorders should be assessed. A positive therapeutic alliance with patient and family, as well as psychoeducation about the nature of the disorder, are useful to maintain the treatment.

LIFETIME COURSE

Zanarini et al.[101] have demonstrated that patients with BPD begin their first treatment, typically individual psychotherapy, at the age of 18, although symptoms are likely to start earlier. As previously mentioned, DSM-5 permits the diagnosis of BPD in patients younger than 18 if symptoms persist for at least 1 year. Symptoms of BPD usually start prior to adulthood and the diagnosis can be made reliably.

Adolescence

While BPD in childhood is a relatively understudied topic, there is growing evidence that BPD can be reliably and validly diagnosed in adolescence. The course of adolescent-onset BPD is similar to what is seen in adult populations[102].

There are an increasing number of studies that examine the outcomes of patients diagnosed with BPD in adolescence. In general, the course of BPD during adolescence is not very stable. In particular, a prospective study[102] of a clinical population between the ages of 15 and 18 found that only 40% of patients with BPD met criteria at 2-year follow-up. However, this sample only included a smaller number of adolescents with BPD, as this study looked at the course of all PDs. A community study of self-reported symptoms in adolescent twins also found a decrease in rates of BPD diagnosis from 14 to 24 years of age, with significant reductions in symptoms at each 2- to 3-year interval throughout the 10-year follow-up[103]. A 2-year follow-up of adolescent inpatients also found a change of diagnosis, with an over 50% reduction in the number of patients with BPD at follow-up[104]. However, a large longitudinal community study of adolescents with 2- and 8-year follow-up[105–107] found that BPD symptoms tended to persist, even when formal diagnostic criteria were no longer met. When a sample of adolescents previously diagnosed with BPD were followed up about 4 years later, 65% remitted from the diagnosis, consistent with other studies[108]. Another research group attempted to identify risk factors for the development of BPD in a community sample of adolescents, and found that maternal – child discord, maternal BPD, paternal SUD, as well as depression, SUD, and suicidality in the adolescent, predict later development of BPD symptoms[109]. These risks may moderate the improvement of patients during this phase of development.

Adulthood

The course of BPD in adults has been a focus of research during the past two decades, with several longitudinal studies providing insights into its course. Measures focused on symptomatology, comorbidity, and functioning but also included several assessments of dimensional personality traits[110].

Both studies found that most patients with BPD improve with time. The CLPS provides evidence that, even when followed up 2 years after the initial assessment, about one-quarter of patients experience a remission of the diagnosis (defined here as meeting fewer than 2 symptoms for a period of 2 months or longer) during the prior 2 years. During a 10-year period of follow-up, 91% achieve at least a 2-month remission, with 85% achieving remission for 12 months or longer[111]. The MSAD has found similar results extended out to 16 years using a slightly different definition of remission (no longer meeting diagnostic criteria for a period of 2 years or longer) and found that by 16 years, 99% of patients have at least a 2-year period of remission and 78% have a remission lasting 8 years[112]. Both of these studies also demonstrated that BPD is slower to remit than other PDs and MDD. Finally, one study followed patients after 27 years and found that 92% of them no longer met criteria for BPD[113]

However, rates of recurrence were not quite consistent between studies. In the CLPS, recurrence rates for patients with BPD were 11% at 10-year follow-up in those who had achieved at least a 12-month remission. This was significantly lower than for the other PDs and also significantly lower than the recurrence rate for patients with MDD[111]. The MSAD found that recurrence rates decreased the longer the remission lasted; 36% of patients experienced a recurrence if their remission lasted only 2 years, but this declined to 10% if their remission lasted 8 years. In general, the BPD group was faster to remit than the comparison group of patients with other PDs.[112]. Taken together, these results suggest that patients with BPD are able to achieve remission of symptoms, and that the longer the remission lasts, the lower the risk of relapse.

When the course of individual symptoms of BPD are examined, studies have generally demonstrated an overall decrease in all symptoms, but with symptoms relating to impulsivity and behavioral manifestations of BPD remitting at a quicker rate than internal, primarily affective experiences[111,114]. In general, behavioral symptoms of PDs are less stable than the personality traits associated with BPD over time[115]. Despite early reductions in symptoms of self-harm and suicidality, the risk of completed suicide remains. After 27 years of follow-up, about 10% of patients completed suicide, typically when patients were in their 30s and after multiple failed treatments[113]. The MSAD found a suicide rate of about 5% and an identical rate of death by all other causes[112]. In this sample, several factors were associated longitudinally with suicide attempts, including comorbid MDD, SUD, post-traumatic stress disorder, family history of suicide, and some specific symptoms of BPD[116]. However, based on previous research in retrospective studies, the rate of suicide in BPD can be expected to fall between 8% and 10%[117,118].

TREATMENT IMPLICATIONS

Understanding the course of BPD can have a significant impact on the clinical management of patients with the disorder. One of the first issues is accurately diagnosing the disorder. As previously discussed, BPD can often be identified in adolescents and young adults, and it is at this age that clinicians should start to look for symptoms of the disorder. The course of the disorder appears unstable during adolescence, yet the long-term course for most patients is essentially identical to what is seen in adults. As evidence-based treatments are available – although evidence in youth is not as robust as it is in adults[119] – patients should be directed to these psychotherapies as early as possible. There is no rationale to wait to provide diagnosis and treatment, and many of the arguments for waiting (based on the assumption that symptoms are transient) are not based on evidence[120]. Finally, providing an accurate diagnosis and providing information on the generally positive outcomes for BPD can instill hope in patients who, all too often, feel completely hopeless[121]. Evidence suggests that even a single session of psychoeducation about the diagnosis can be beneficial[122].

One of the all-too-frequent reasons to avoid the diagnosis of BPD in all age groups is the fear of stigmatization. BPD is known to be highly stigmatized in mental health settings[123], particularly in youth mental health, and part of the reason for the stigma is that BPD is seen as a lifelong disorder that is untreatable. Actually, patients with BPD can be cautiously optimistic about their prognosis, and many treatments exist that can profoundly improve their lives. Much of the stigma occurs when clinicians encounter these patients in crisis settings, such as the emergency department, crisis clinics, and general psychiatric inpatient wards. As these are not the settings in which treatment occurs, clinicians develop a biased perspective on these patients. Few clinicians will have the opportunity to see these patients improve over time in specialized treatment clinics; nonetheless, these patients improve and are treatable. Awareness of the course of BPD is one effective way of reducing stigma against the diagnosis.

Although the course of BPD is generally positive, some patients do experience relapses over time. Most of the specialized treatments for BPD are time limited and generally of 1 to 3 years' duration. This makes them expensive, and some experts suggest that a better model of care for patients with BPD would be intermittent psychotherapy[124]. Intermittent treatment may allow patients to address different problems at different points in their lives. For example, DBT focuses primarily on self-harm and suicidality[125], which tend to be problems early on in the lives of patients with BPD. As these symptoms remit with time, patients who are older may want to deal with problems relating to emptiness and fear of abandonment, which are not directly addressed by DBT and are symptoms that are slower to remit[114]. An intermittent psychotherapy model would allow patients to focus on specific problems at specific times in their lives, using the therapeutic approach that has the best evidence for that problem.

A related issue is the poor long-term functional status of patients with BPD. Zanarini et al.[112] demonstrated that recovery is significantly less likely in patients with BPD than in an Axis II comparison group. Slightly more than one-half the patients with BPD achieved recovery, which was defined as remission from symptoms as well as good, full-time vocational or educational functioning and at least one stable and supportive relationship with a friend or partner. Patients with BPD were also quite likely to rapidly lose their recovery. Several factors were identified as predictors to recovery, including not being hospitalized (prior to the index hospitalization), higher IQ, prior good vocational functioning, absence of a cluster C comorbidity, and the trait measures of high extraversion and high agreeableness[126]. Recovery was also associated with both marriage and being a parent, although often at an older age than nonrecovered patients[127]. Another longitudinal study demonstrated that the Global Assessment of Functioning scores were lower in the BPD group and significantly fewer of these patients achieved levels that represent good functioning[111] and were also more likely to receive social assistance.

As functional recovery is so difficult for patients with BPD to attain and maintain, this becomes an important long-term goal for intervention. Currently, the only long-term study to directly assess vocational or educational functioning indicates that mentalization-based treatment, provided in an 18-month partial hospitalization setting, is associated with a greater chance of being employed or in school up to 8 years later[128]. Other studies have also demonstrated improved social and global functioning, but these were not primary outcomes and were not significantly different between the different treatments; also, duration of follow-up was too short[129]. Thus there is evidence that, while treatment is likely to lead to improvements in functional recovery, there is a notable absence of studies that focus on this as a primary outcome. Consideration should be given to providing patients with BPD as much support in attaining functional recovery as possible. This may include psychosocial programs aimed at returning to work, and evaluation and involvement from occupational therapists, vocational counsellors, or other specialists who can help patients develop the skills necessary for any sort of work.

References

1. González Vives S, Diaz-Marsa M, Fuentenebro F, Lopez-Ibor Aliño JJ, Carrasco JL. Historical review of the borderline personality disorder concept. *Actas Espanolas de Psiquiatria* 2006 Sep–Oct;34(5):336–334.
2. Lieb K, Zanarini MC, Schmahl C, Linehan MM, Bohus M. Borderline personality disorder. *Lancet*. 2004;364:453–461.
3. Brüne M. Borderline personality disorder why 'fast and furious'?. *Evolution, Medicine, and Public Health* 2016;1(2016):52–66.
4. Fonagy P, Target M, Gergely G. Attachment and borderline personality disorder: A theory and some evidence. *Psychiatr Clin North Am* 2000;23:103.
5. Zweig-Frank H, Paris J. Parents' emotional neglect and overprotection according to the recollections of patients with borderline personality disorder. *Am J Psychiatry* 1991;148:648–651.
6. Lenzenweger MF, Lane MC, Loranger AW, Kessler RC. DSM-IV personality disorders in the National Comorbidity Survey Replication. *Biol. Psychiatry* 2007;62:553–564.
7. Grant BF, Chou SP, Goldstein RB, Huang B, Stinson FS, Saha TD, Smith SM, Dawson DA, Pulay AJ, Pickering RP, et al. Prevalence, correlates, disability, and comorbidity of DSM-IV borderline personality disorder: Results from the Wave 2 National Epidemiologic Survey on Alcohol and Related Conditions. *J. Clin. Psychiatry* 2008;69:533–545.
8. Gross R, Olfson M, Gameroff M, Shea S, Feder A, Fuentes M, Lantigua R, Weissman MM. Borderline personality disorder in primary care. *Arch. Intern. Med.* 2002;162:53–60. [CrossRef] [PubMed].
9. Zimmerman M, Rothschild L, Chelminski I. The prevalence of DSM-IV personality disorders in psychiatric outpatients. *Am. J. Psychiatry* 2005;162:1911–1918.
10. Kulacaoglu F, Kose S. Borderline personality disorder (BPD): In the midst of vulnerability, chaos, and Awe. *Brain Sciences* 2018;8(11): 201.
11. Gratz KL, et al. Extending extant models of the pathogenesis of borderline personality disorder to childhood borderline personality symptoms: The roles of affective dysfunction, disinhibition, and self-and emotion-regulation deficits. *Development and Psychopathology* 2009;21(4): 1263.
12. Bornovalova MA, et al. Stability, change, and heritability of borderline personality disorder traits from adolescence to adulthood: A longitudinal twin study. *Development and Psychopathology* 2009;21(4):1335.
13. Gunderson JG, Berkowitz C, Ruiz-Sancho A. Families of borderline patients: A psychoeducational approach. *Bulletin of the Menninger Clinic* 1997;61(4):446.
14. Hartup WW, Cornelis FM Van Lieshout. Personality development in social context. *Annual Review of Psychology* 1995;46(1):655–687.
15. Reich DB, Zanarini MC. Developmental aspects of borderline personality disorder. *Harvard Review of Psychiatry* 2001;9(6):294–301.
16. Caspi A, McClay J, Moffitt TE, Mill J, Martin J, Craig IW, Taylor A, Poulton R. Role of genotype in the cycle of violence in maltreated children. *Science* 2002;297:851–854.
17. Herpertz SC, Bertsch K. A new perspective on the pathophysiology of borderline personality disorder: A model of the role of oxytocin. *Am. J. Psychiatry* 2015;172:840–851.
18. Bertsch K, Schmidinger I, Neumann ID, Herpertz SC. Reduced plasma oxytocin levels in female patients with borderline personality disorder. *Horm. Behav*. 2013;63:424–429.
19. Ruocco AC, Carcone D. A neurobiological model of borderline personality disorder: Systematic and integrative review. *Harv. Rev. Psychiatry* 2016;24:311–329.
20. Stanley B, Siever LJ. The interpersonal dimension of borderline personality disorder: Toward a neuropeptide model. *Am. J. Psychiatry* 2010;167:24–39.

21. Rausch J, Gabel A, Nagy K, Kleindienst N, Herpertz SC, Bertsch K. Increased testosterone levels and cortisol awakening responses in patients with borderline personality disorder: Gender and trait aggressiveness matter. *Psychoneuroendocrinology* 2015;55:116–127.
22. Herpertz SC, Bertsch K. A new perspective on the pathophysiology of borderline personality disorder: A model of the role of oxytocin. *Am. J. Psychiatry* 2015;172:840–851.
23. Bertsch K, Schmidinger I, Neumann ID, Herpertz SC. Reduced plasma oxytocin levels in female patients with borderline personality disorder. *Horm. Behav.* 2013;63:424–429.
24. Hansenne M, Pitchot W, Pinto E, Reggers J, Scantamburlo G, Fuchs S, Pirard S, Ansseau M. 5-HT1A dysfunction in borderline personality disorder. *Psychol. Med.* 2002;32:935–941.
25. Soloff P, Nutche J, Goradia D, Diwadkar V. Structural brain abnormalities in borderline personality disorder: A voxel-based morphometry study. *Psychiatry Res.* 2008;164:223–236.
26. Siever LJ. Neurobiology of aggression and violence. *Am. J. Psychiatry* 2008;165:429–442.
27. Barratt ES, Stanford MS, Kent TA, Felthous A. Neuropsychological and cognitive psychophysiological substrates of impulsive aggression. *Biol. Psychiatry* 1997;41:1045–1061.
28. Silbersweig D, Clarkin JF, Goldstein M, Kernberg OF, Tuescher O, Levy KN, Brendel G, Pan H, Beutel M, Pavony MT, et al. Failure of frontolimbic inhibitory function in the context of negative emotion in borderline personality disorder. *Am. J. Psychiatry* 2007;164:1832–1841.
29. Schulze L, Schmahl C, Niedtfeld I. Neural correlates of disturbed emotion processing in borderline personality disorder: A multimodal meta-analysis. *Biol. Psychiatry* 2016;79:97–106.
30. Dyck M, Loughead J, Kellermann T, Boers F, Gur RC, Mathiak K. Cognitive versus automatic mechanisms of mood induction differentially activate left and right amygdala. *Neuroimage* 2011;54:2503–2513.
31. Kuhlmann A, Bertsch K, Schmidinger I, Thomann PA, Herpertz SC. Morphometric differences in central stress-regulating structures between women with and without borderline personality disorder. *J. Psychiatry Neurosci.* 2013;38:129–137.
32. Kreisel SH, Labudda K, Kurlandchikov O, Beblo T, Mertens M, Thomas C, Rullkotter N, Wingenfeld K, Mensebach C, Woermann FG, et al. Volume of hippocampal substructures in borderline personality disorder. *Psychiatry Res* 2015;231:218–226.
33. Niedtfeld I, Schulze L, Krause-Utz A, Demirakca T, Bohus M, Schmahl C. Voxel-based morphometry in women with borderline personality disorder with and without comorbid posttraumatic stress disorder. *PLoS ONE* 2013;8:e65824.
34. Kimmel CL, Alhassoon OM, Wollman SC, Stern MJ, Perez-Figueroa A, Hall MG, Rompogren J, Radua J. Age-related parieto-occipital and other gray matter changes in borderline personality disorder: A meta-analysis of cortical and subcortical structures. *Psychiatry Res. Neuroimaging* 2016;251:15–25.
35. Silvers JA, Hubbard AD, Biggs E, Shu J, Fertuck E, Chaudhury S, Grunebaum MF, Weber J, Kober H, Chesin M, et al. Affective lability and difficulties with regulation are differentially associated with amygdala and prefrontal response in women with Borderline Personality Disorder. *Psychiatry Res. Neuroimaging* 2016;254:74–82.
36. Koenigsberg HW, Fan J, Ochsner KN, Liu X, Guise KG, Pizzarello S, Dorantes C, Guerreri S, Tecuta L, Goodman M, et al. Neural correlates of the use of psychological distancing to regulate responses to negative social cues: A study of patients with borderline personality disorder. *Biol. Psychiatry* 2009;66:854–863.
37. Schmitt R, Winter D, Niedtfeld I, Herpertz SC, Schmahl C. Effects of psychotherapy on neuronal correlates of reappraisal in female patients with borderline personality disorder. *Biol. Psychiatry Cogn. Neurosci. Neuroimaging* 2016;1:548–557.
38. Zanarini MC, Williams AA, Lewis RE, Reich RB, Vera SC, Marino MF, Levin A, Yong L, Frankenburg FR. Reported pathological childhood experiences associated with the development of borderline personality disorder. *Am. J. Psychiatry* 1997;154:1101–110.
39. Hengartner MP, Ajdacic-Gross V, Rodgers S, Muller M, Rossler W. Childhood adversity in association with personality disorder dimensions: New findings in an old debate. *Eur. Psychiatry* 2013;28:476–482.
40. Johnson JG, Cohen P, Gould MS, Kasen S, Brown J, Brook JS. Childhood adversities, interpersonal difficulties, and risk for suicide attempts during late adolescence and early adulthood. *Arch. Gen. Psychiatry* 2002;59:741–749.
41. Widom CS, Czaja SJ, Bentley T, Johnson MS. A prospective investigation of physical health outcomes in abused and neglected children: New findings from a 30-year follow-up. *Am. J. Public Health* 2012;102:1135–1144.
42. Johnson JG, Cohen P, Brown J, Smailes EM, Bernstein DP. Childhood maltreatment increases risk for personality disorders during early adulthood. *Arch. Gen. Psychiatry* 1999;56:600–606.

43. Fossati A, Madeddu F, Maffei C. Borderline personality disorder and childhood sexual abuse: A meta-analytic study. *J. Pers. Disord.* 1999;13:268–280.
44. Paris J. Childhood trauma as an etiological factor in the personality disorders. *J. Pers. Disord.* 1997;11:34–49.
45. Belsky DW, Caspi A, Arseneault L, Bleidorn W, Fonagy P, Goodman M, et al. Etiological features of borderline personality related characteristics in a birth cohort of 12-year-old children. *Dev Psychopathol* 2012;24(1):251–265.
46. Carlson EA, Egeland B, Sroufe LA. A prospective investigation of the development of borderline personality symptoms. *Dev Psychopathol* 2009;21(4):1311–1334.
47. Belsky DW, Caspi A, Arseneault L, Bleidorn W, Fonagy P, Goodman M, et al. Etiological features of borderline personality related characteristics in a birth cohort of 12-year-old children. *Dev Psychopathol* 2012;24(1):251–265.
48. Crick NR, Murray-Close D, Woods K. Borderline personality features in childhood: A short-term longitudinal study. *Dev Psychopathol* 2005;17(4):1051–1070.
49. Underwood MK, Beron KJ, Rosen LH. Joint trajectories for social and physical aggression as predictors of adolescent maladjustment: Internalizing symptoms, rule-breaking behaviors, and borderline and narcissistic personality features. *Dev Psychopathol* 2011;23(2):659–678.
50. Lenzenweger MF, Cicchetti D. Toward a developmental psychopathology approach to borderline personality disorder. *Dev Psychopathol* 2005;7(4):893–898.
51. Tragesser SL, Solhan M, Brown WC, Tomko RL, Bagge C, Trull TJ. Longitudinal associations in borderline personality disorder features: Diagnostic Interview for Borderlines-Revised (DIB-R) scores over time. *J Pers Disord* 2010;24(3):377–391.
52. Gratz KL, Tull MT, Reynolds EK, Bagge CL, Latzman RD, Daughters SB, et al. Extending extant models of the pathogenesis of borderline personality disorder to childhood borderline personality symptoms: The roles of affective dysfunction, disinhibition, and self- and emotion-regulation deficits. *Dev Psychopathol* 2009;21(4):1263–1291.
53. Belsky DW, Caspi A, Arseneault L, Bleidorn W, Fonagy P, Goodman M, et al. Etiological features of borderline personality related characteristics in a birth cohort of 12-year-old children. *Dev Psychopathol* 2012;24(1):251–265.
54. Jovev M, McKenzie T, Whittle S, Simmons JG, Allen NB, Chanen AM. Temperament and maltreatment in the emergence of borderline and antisocial personality pathology during early adolescence. *J Can Acad Child Adolesc Psychiatry* 2013;22(3):220–229.
55. Martín-Blanco A, Soler J, Villalta L, Feliu-Soler A, Elices M, Pérez V, et al. Exploring the interaction between childhood maltreatment and temperamental traits on the severity of borderline personality disorder. *Compr Psychiatry* 2014;55(2):311.
56. Jovev M, Whittle S, Yücel M, Simmons JG, Allen NB, Chanen AM. E relationship between hippocampal asymmetry and temperament in adolescent borderline and antisocial personality pathology. *Dev Psychopathol* 2014;26:275–285.
57. Chanen AM. Borderline personality disorder in young people: Are we there yet? *J. Clin. Psychol.* 2015;71:778–791.
58. American Psychiatric Association. *Diagnostic and statistical manual of mental disorders*, 5th ed. Arlington, VA, USA: American Psychiatric Association, 2013.
59. Zimmerman M, Multach MD, Dalrymple K, Chelminski, I. Clinically useful screen for borderline personality disorder in psychiatric out-patients. *Br. J. Psychiatry* 2017;210:165–166.
60. Gunderson JG, Herpertz SC, Skodol AE, Torgersen S, Zanarini MC. Borderline personality disorder. *Nat. Rev. Dis. Primers* 2018;4:18029.
61. Santangelo PS, Koenig J, Kockler TD, Eid M, Holtmann J, Koudela-Hamila S, Parzer P, Resch F, Bohus M, Kaess M, et al. Affective instability across the lifespan in borderline personality disorder: A cross-sectional e-diary study. *Acta Psychiatr. Scand.* 2018;138(5):409–419.
62. Ruocco AC. The neuropsychology of borderline personality disorder: A meta-analysis and review. *Psychiatry Res* 2005;137:191–202.
63. Links PS, Heslegrave R, van Reekum, R. Impulsivity: Core aspect of borderline personality disorder. *J. Pers. Disord.* 1999;13:1–9.
64. Zanarini MC, Frankenburg FR, Hennen J, Reich DB, Silk KR. Prediction of the 10-year course of borderline personality disorder. *Am. J. Psychiatry* 2006;163:827–832.
65. Pompili M, Girardi P, Ruberto A, Tatarelli R. Suicide in borderline personality disorder: A meta-analysis. *Nord. J. Psychiatry* 2005;59:319–324.
66. Paris J. Borderline personality disorder. *CMAJ* 2005;172:1579–1583.
67. Zanarini MC, Laudate CS, Frankenburg FR, Wedig MM, Fitzmaurice, G. Reasons for self-mutilation reported by borderline patients over 16 years of prospective follow-up. *J. Pers. Disord.* 2013;27:783–794.

68. Wedig MM, Silverman MH, Frankenburg FR, Reich DB, Fitzmaurice G, Zanarini MC. Predictors of suicide attempts in patients with borderline personality disorder over 16 years of prospective follow-up. *Psychol. Med.* 2012;42:2395–2404.
69. Soloff PH, Fabio A. Prospective predictors of suicide attempts in borderline personality disorder at one, two, and two-to-five year follow-up. *J. Pers. Disord.* 2008;22:123–134.
70. Sher L, Rutter SB, New AS, Siever LJ, Hazlett EA. Gender differences and similarities in aggression, suicidal behavior, and psychiatric comorbidity in borderline personality disorder. *Acta Psychiatr. Scand.* 2018;139(2):145–153.
71. Shea MT, Stout RL, Yen S, Pagano ME, Skodol AE, Morey LC, Gunderson JG, McGlashan TH, Grilo CM, Sanislow CA, et al. Associations in the course of personality disorders and Axis I disorders over time. *J. Abnorm. Psychol.* 2004;113:499–508.
72. Eaton NR, Krueger RF, Keyes KM, Skodol AE, Markon KE, Grant BF, Hasin DS. Borderline personality disorder co-morbidity: Relationship to the internalizing-externalizing structure of common mental disorders. *Psychol. Med.* 2011;41;1041–1050.
73. Zanarini MC, Skodol AE, Bender D, Dolan R, Sanislow C, Schaefer E, Morey LC, Grilo CM, Shea MT, McGlashan TH, et al. The collaborative longitudinal personality disorders study: Reliability of axis I and II diagnoses. *J. Pers. Disord.* 2000;14:291–299.
74. Zimmerman M, Mattia JI. Axis I diagnostic comorbidity and borderline personality disorder. *Compr. Psychiatry* 1999;40:245–252.
75. Witt SH, Streit F, Jungkunz M, Frank J, Awasthi S, Reinbold CS, Treutlein J, Degenhardt F, Forstner AJ, Heilmann-Heimbach S, et al. Genome-wide association study of borderline personality disorder reveals genetic overlap with bipolar disorder, major depression and schizophrenia. *Transl. Psychiatry* 2017;7:e1155.
76. Zimmerman M, Martinez JH, Morgan TA, Young D, Chelminski I, Dalrymple, K. Distinguishing bipolar II depression from major depressive disorder with comorbid borderline personality disorder: Demographic, clinical, and family history differences. *J. Clin. Psychiatry* 2013;74:880–886.
77. Akiskal HS, Bourgeois ML, Angst J, Post R, Moller H, Hirschfeld, R. Re-evaluating the prevalence of and diagnostic composition within the broad clinical spectrum of bipolar disorders. *J. Affect. Disord.* 2000, 59 (Suppl. 1):S5–S30.
78. Angst J, Cui L, Swendsen J, Rothen S, Cravchik A, Kessler RC, Merikangas KR. Major depressive disorder with subthreshold bipolarity in the National Comorbidity Survey Replication. *Am. J. Psychiatry* 2010;167:1194–1201.
79. Smith DJ, Muir WJ, Blackwood DH. Is borderline personality disorder part of the bipolar spectrum? *Harv. Rev. Psychiatry* 2004;12:133–139.
80. Paris J. Borderline or bipolar? Distinguishing borderline personality disorder from bipolar spectrum disorders. *Harv. Rev. Psychiatry* 2004;12:140–145.
81. Sripada CS, Silk KR. The role of functional neuroimaging in exploring the overlap between borderline personality disorder and bipolar disorder. *Curr. Psychiatry Rep.* 2007;9:40–45.
82. Vieta E, Colom F, Corbella B, Martinez-Aran A, Reinares M, Benabarre A, Gastó C. Clinical correlates of psychiatric comorbidity in bipolar I patients. *Bipolar Disord.* 2001;3:253–258.
83. Zimmerman M, Coryell, W. DSM-III personality disorder diagnoses in a nonpatient sample. Demographic correlates and comorbidity. *Arch. Gen. Psychiatry* 1989;46:682–689.
84. Zimmerman M, Morgan TA. The relationship between borderline personality disorder and bipolar disorder. *Dialogues Clin. Neurosci.* 2013;15:155–169.
85. Pally R. The neurobiology of borderline personality disorder: The synergy of "nature and nurture". *J. Psychiatr. Pract.* 2002;8:133–142.
86. Spiegel D, Cardena, E. Disintegrated experience: The dissociative disorders revisited. *J. Abnorm. Psychol.* 1991;100:366–378.
87. Sabo AN. Etiological significance of associations between childhood trauma and borderline personality disorder: Conceptual and clinical implications. *J. Pers. Disord.* 1997;11:50–70.
88. Lanius RA, Vermetten E, Loewenstein RJ, Brand B, Schmahl C, Bremner JD, Spiegel, D. Emotion modulation in PTSD: Clinical and neurobiological evidence for a dissociative subtype. *Am. J. Psychiatry* 2010;167:640–647.
89. Zanarini MC. Childhood experiences associated with the development of borderline personality disorder. *Psychiatr. Clin. N. Am.* 2000;23:89–101.
90. Asherson P, Young AH, Eich-Hochli D, Moran P, Porsdal V, Deberdt, W. Differential diagnosis, comorbidity, and treatment of attention-deficit/hyperactivity disorder in relation to bipolar disorder or borderline personality disorder in adults. *Curr. Med. Res. Opin.* 2014;30:1657–1672.

91. Philipsen A. Differential diagnosis and comorbidity of attention-deficit/hyperactivity disorder (ADHD) and borderline personality disorder (BPD) in adults. *Eur. Arch. Psychiatry Clin. Neurosci.* 2006;256(Suppl. 1):i42–i46.
92. Kulacaoglu FSM, Belli H, Ardic FC, Akin E, Kose, S. The relationship between impulsivity and attention-deficit/hyperactivity symptoms in female patients with borderline personality disorder. *Psychiatry Clin. Psychopharmacol.* 2017;27:255–261.
93. Paris J. The treatment of borderline personality disorder: Implications of research on diagnosis, etiology, and outcome. *Annu. Rev. Clin. Psychol.* 2009;5:277–290.
94. Ingenhoven T, Lafay P, Rinne T, Passchier J, Duivenvoorden H. Effectiveness of pharmacotherapy for severe personality disorders: Meta-analyses of randomized controlled trials. *J. Clin. Psychiatry* 2010;71:14–25.
95. Stoffers JM, Vollm BA, Rucker G, Timmer A, Huband N, Lieb K. Psychological therapies for people with borderline personality disorder. *Cochrane Database Syst. Rev.* 2012;(8).
96. Bateman AW. Treating borderline personality disorder in clinical practice. *Am. J. Psychiatry* 2012;169:560–563.
97. Cristea IA, Gentili C, Cotet CD, Palomba D, Barbui C, Cuijpers P. Efficacy of psychotherapies for borderline personality disorder: A systematic review and meta-analysis. *JAMA Psychiatry* 2017;74:319–328.
98. Ingenhoven T, Lafay P, Rinne T, Passchier J, Duivenvoorden H. Effectiveness of pharmacotherapy for severe personality disorders: Meta-analyses of randomized controlled trials. *J. Clin. Psychiatry* 2010;71:14–25.
99. Zanarini MC, Frankenburg FR. Omega-3 Fatty acid treatment of women with borderline personality disorder: A double-blind, placebo-controlled pilot study. *Am. J. Psychiatry* 2003;160:167–169.
100. Links PS, Ross J, Gunderson JG. Promoting good psychiatric management for patients with borderline personality disorder. *J. Clin. Psychol.* 2015;71:753–763.
101. Zanarini MC, Frankenburg FR, Khera GS, et al. Treatment histories of borderline inpatients. *Compr Psychiatry.* 2001;42:144–150.
102. Chanen AM, Jackson HJ, McGorry PD, et al. Two-year stability of personality disorder in older adolescent outpatients. *J Pers Disord* 2004;18(6):526–541.
103. Bornovalova MA, Hicks BM, Iacono WG, et al. Stability, change, and heritability of borderline personality disorder traits from adolescence to adulthood: A longitudinal twin study. *Dev Psychopathol* 2009;21(4):1335–1353.
104. Mattanah JJF, Becker DF, Levy KN, et al. Diagnostic stability in adolescents followed up 2 years after hospitalization. *Am J Psychiatry* 1995;152(6):889–894.
105. Bernstein DP, Cohen P, Velez CN, et al. Prevalence and stability of the DSM-III-R personality disorders in a community-based survey of adolescents. *Am J Psychiatry* 1993;150(8):1237–1243.
106. Crawford TN, Cohen P, Brook JS. Dramatic-erratic personality disorder symptoms: II. Developmental pathways from early adolescence to adulthood. *J Pers Disord* 2001;15(4):336–350.
107. Crawford TN, Cohen P, Brook JS. Dramatic-erratic personality disorder symptoms: I. Continuity from early adolescence into adulthood. *J Pers Disord* 2001;15(4):319–335.
108. Biskin RS, Paris J, Renaud J, et al. Outcomes in women diagnosed with borderline personality disorder in adolescence. *J Can Acad Child Adolesc Psychiatry* 2011;20(3):168–174.
109. Stepp SD, Olino TM, Klein DN, et al. Unique influences of adolescent antecedents on adult borderline personality disorder features. *Personal Disord* 2013;4(3):223–239.
110. Skodol AE, Gunderson JG, Shea MT, et al. The Collaborative Longitudinal Personality Disorders Study (CLPS): Overview and implications. *J Pers Disord* 2005;19(5):487–504.
111. Gunderson JG, Stout RL, McGlashan TH, et al. Ten-year course of borderline personality disorder: Psychopathology and function from the Collaborative Longitudinal Personality Disorders study. *Arch Gen Psychiatry* 2011;68(8):827–837.
112. Zanarini MC, Frankenburg FR, Reich DB, et al. Attainment and stability of sustained symptomatic remission and recovery among patients with borderline personality disorder and Axis II comparison subjects: A 16-year prospective follow-up study. *Am J Psychiatry* 2012;169(5):476–483.
113. Paris J, Zweig-Frank H. A 27-year follow-up of patients with borderline personality disorder. *Compr Psychiatry* 2001;42(6):482–487.
114. Zanarini MC, Frankenburg FR, Reich DB, et al. The subsyndromal phenomenology of borderline personality disorder: A 10-year follow-up study. *Am J Psychiatry* 2007;164(6):929–935.
115. Hopwood CJ, Morey LC, Donnellan MB, et al. Ten-year rank-order stability of personality traits and disorders in a clinical sample. *J Pers* 2013;81(3):335–344.

116. Wedig MM, Silverman MH, Frankenburg FR, et al. Predictors of suicide attempts in patients with borderline personality disorder over 16 years of prospective follow-up. *Psychol Med* 2012;42(11):2395–2404.
117. Oldham JM. Borderline personality disorder and suicidality. *Am J Psychiatry* 2006;163(1):20–26.
118. Paris J. Chronic suicidality among patients with borderline personality disorder. *Psychiatr Serv* 2002;53(6):738–742.
119. Biskin RS. Treatment of borderline personality disorder in youth. *J Can Acad Child Adolesc Psychiatry* 2013;22(3):230–234.
120. Kaess M, Brunner R, Chanen A. Borderline personality disorder in adolescence. *Pediatrics* 2014;134(4):782–793.
121. Biskin RS, Paris J. Diagnosing borderline personality disorder. *CMAJ* 2012;184(16):1789–1794.
122. Zanarini MC, Frankenburg FR. A preliminary, randomized trial of psychoeducation for women with borderline personality disorder. *J Pers Disord* 2008;22(3):284–290.
123. Miller AL, Muehlenkamp JJ, Jacobson CM. Fact or fiction: Diagnosing borderline personality disorder in adolescents. *Clin Psychol Rev.* 2008;28(6):969–981.
124. Paris J. Intermittent psychotherapy: An alternative to continuous long-term treatment for patients with personality disorders. *J Psychiatr Pract* 2007;13(3):153–158.
125. Linehan M. *Cognitive-behavioral treatment of borderline personality disorder.* New York (NY): Guilford Press; 1993. p. xvii, 558 p.
126. Zanarini MC, Frankenburg FR, Reich DB, et al. Prediction of time-to-attainment of recovery for borderline patients followed prospectively for 16 years. *Acta Psychiatr Scand* 2014;130(3):205–213.
127. Zanarini MC, Frankenburg FR, Reich DB, et al. The course of marriage/sustained cohabitation and parenthood among borderline patients followed prospectively for 16 years. *J Pers Disord* 2015;29(1):62–70.
128. Clarkin JF, Levy KN, Lenzenweger MF, et al. Evaluating three treatments for borderline personality disorder: A multiwave study. *Am J Psychiatry.* 2007;164(6):922–928.
129. McMain SF, Links PS, Gnam WH, et al. A randomized trial of dialectical behavior therapy versus general psychiatric management for borderline personality disorder. *Am J Psychiatry* 2009;166(12):1365–1374. Erratum in *Am J Psychiatry* 2010;167(10):1283.

22
Optimising Patient Care in Dementia

Shabbir Amanullah, Shiva K. Shivakumar, Catrin Thomas, Sarmishtha Bhattacharyya and Swar Shah

Introduction	233
International Scan of Guidelines on Management of Dementia	234
Biopsychosocial Model	236
Pharmacological Management of Dementia	236
Alzheimer's Dementia	236
Vascular Dementia	238
Lewy Body Dementia	238
Parkinson's Disease Dementia	239
Frontotemporal Dementia	239
Behavioural and Psychological Symptoms of Dementia	239
Agitation and Aggression	240
Management of Comorbidities in Dementia	240
Frailty	240
Delirium and Dementia	241
Optimising Support for Carers and Caregiver Burden	241
The Impact of COVID-19 on Dementia Care	243
Mortality	243
Antipsychotic Use	243
BPSD	243
Impact on Social Support and Carer Stress	244

INTRODUCTION

Dementia is a neurocognitive syndrome characterised by deterioration in memory, thinking, behaviour and the ability to perform everyday activities. Worldwide, around 50 million people have dementia, and there are nearly 10 million new cases every year.[1] It is one of the major causes of disability and dependency and has significant impact not only on people with dementia but their carers, families and society at large.

Alzheimer's dementia is the commonest form of dementia, affecting about 60–70% of diagnosed cases; however, there are several types of dementias such as vascular dementias, Lewy body dementias, dementia associated with Parkinson's disease, fronto temporal dementias and other secondary dementias of varied aetiology. Dementia is not typically associated with older adults and may affect all ages; however, age does remain a risk factor for developing dementias.

DOI: 10.4324/9780429030260-25

The basis of care for a person with dementia should be holistic and person centred, and it is important to involve carers and families in optimising care.

Neuropsychiatric symptoms in dementias include agitation, depression, delusions and hallucinations and are often the major cause of distress to person with dementia and their carer.

At the time of writing, the COVID pandemic continues and has significantly impacted how care is delivered to people with dementia and their carers. With government-imposed lockdowns, increasing virtual assessments and reduced face-to-face contacts, it has been a challenge in delivering and optimising patient centred care for person with dementia (PWD) and carers.

INTERNATIONAL SCAN OF GUIDELINES ON MANAGEMENT OF DEMENTIA

Given the complex nature of dementia, several pertinent clinical guidelines for the diagnoses and management of dementia and dementia-related disorders exist. A study by Ngo and Holroyd-Leduc identified a total of 12 distinct guidelines that were deemed moderate or high quality according to the AGREE-II tool.[2] Examples of guideline groups with strategies for management of dementia include NICE (UK), CCC (CAN), APA (US), AAN (US) and QUT (AUS). The guidelines follow similar recommendations on the diagnoses of dementia, but there is less consensus about management strategies. We will be presenting the ideal diagnoses and management strategy for dementia based upon consensus guidelines recommendations, primarily considering the NICE, CCC, QUT, APA and AAN guidelines.

Table 22.1 Various guidelines for the diagnosis and management of dementia.

Guideline	Diagnoses	Management
USA: American Academy of Neurology (AAN)[3]	• Extensive history from patient and care-taker • Cognitive screening (ex. MMSE, Memory Impairment Screen) • Cognitive assessments such as the clock-drawing test are considered weaker evidence • Lab testing (CBC, BUN, glucose, TFT, serum B12, LFT) • Depression screening • Structural neuroimaging (CT, MRI) • Genetic marker (Ex. APOE) testing is not recommended	• **Non-pharmacological:** • Exercise, music therapy • Environmental manipulation for problem behaviours • Care-giver educational programs (ex. computer support networks) • **Pharmacological:** • Donepezil, rivastigmine, galantamine (AChE inhibitors) or memantine for AD, Parkinson's dementia, VD • Vitamin E and selegiline also recommended for AD
USA: American Psychiatric Association (APA)[4]	• Extensive history from patient and care-taker • Functional screening (ex. Functional Activities Questionnaire)	• **Non-pharmacological:** • Exercise, recreational clubs • Psychotherapy (ex. address driving cessation) • Education of caregivers

Guideline	Diagnoses	Management
	• Cognitive screening (MMSE) • Depression assessment • Lab tests (CBC, BUN, glucose, TFT, serum B12, LFT) • Structural imaging (MRI, CT) • Measurement of caregiver strain • May consider CSF, syphilis serology and EEG	• Behavioural therapy • **Pharmacological:** • Donepezil, rivastigmine, galantamine (AChE inhibitors) for mild-to-moderate AD • Memantine or donepezil for moderate-to-severe AD • Aspirin and anti-hypertensives for risk-mitigation • Consider referral to local clinical trials for AD treatment • Vitamin E, ginkgo biloba, and selegiline are not recommended
CAN: **Canadian Consensus Conference (CCC)**[5]	• Extensive history from patient and care-taker • Cognitive screening (ex. Memory Impairment Screen + clock-drawing Test, MMSE) • Functional screening (ex. Disability Assessment for Dementia) • Referral to specialty memory clinic for sub-typing dementia (aided by lab tests, neuroimaging, gait tests)	• **Non-pharmacological:** • Exercise • Group cognitive stimulation therapy • Psychoeducational therapy for care-giver • Recommends adherence to Mediterranean diet • **Pharmacological:** • Donepezil, rivastigmine, galantamine (AChE inhibitors) or memantine for AD, Parkinson's dementia, VD • AChE inhibitors for mild-to-moderate dementia • Memantine for moderate-to-severe dementia • Treatment of hypertension (to minimise risk of VD)
UK: **National Institute for Health and Care Excellence (NICE)**[6]	• Extensive history from patient and care-taker (aided by Functional Activities Questionnaire) • Physical examination (ex. gait test) • Lab tests (ex. CBC, BUN, glucose, TFT, serum B12, LFT) • Structural tests (MRI/CT)	• **Non-pharmacological:** • Exercise • Group cognitive stimulation therapy (mild-to-moderate dementia) • Referral to support centres for patient and caregiver • **Pharmacological:**

(Continued)

Table 22.1 (Continuted)

Guideline	Diagnoses	Management
	• Cognitive testing (ex. Mini-cog, 6-item screener, Test Your Memory) • Refer to specialist services for sub-typing dementia diagnosis (aided by neuropsychological testing)	• AChE inhibitors: donepezil, rivastigmine and galantamine (mild to moderate AD, Lewy body dementia, and VD) • Memantine (severe AD) • Donepezil or rivastigmine for Lewy Body dementia • AChE inhibitors and memantine contraindicated in FTD, MS, and VD (unless VD has co-morbidity with AD, Lewy body or Parkinson's)
AUS: **Queensland University of Technology (QUT)**[7]	• Extensive history from patient and care-taker • Cognitive assessment (MMSE) • KIGA-Cognitive assessment tool is recommended for Australians >45 years in rural areas • Functional Assessment Questionnaire • Lab tests (ex. CBC, BUN, glucose, TFT, serum B12, LFT) • Distinguish between dementia and delirium (ex. usage of DRS-R98) • Referral to geriatrician or other specialist for sub-typing dementia	• **Non-pharmacological:** • Exercise • Music therapy • Behavioural management • Reminiscence therapy • Driving ability assessment recommended • **Pharmacological:** • Refers to NICE guidelines

BIOPSYCHOSOCIAL MODEL

The biopsychosocial approach to illness was first proposed by George Engel in 1977.[8] Numerous risk factors have been linked to the development of the different subtypes of dementias (Figure 22.1). The management of PWD can also be considered using the biopsychosocial approach (Figure 22.2).[9,10]

PHARMACOLOGICAL MANAGEMENT OF DEMENTIA

Alzheimer's Dementia

Two classes of drugs are currently approved for the treatment of Alzheimer's dementia. The first class is the acetylcholinesterase inhibitors (AChEI) – donepezil, rivastigmine and galantamine. The second class is the N-methyl-D-aspartate (NMDA) receptor antagonist memantine.

OPTIMISING PATIENT CARE IN DEMENTIA • 237

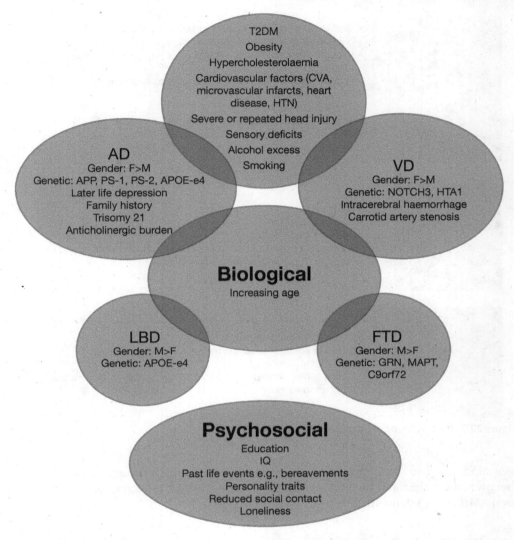

AD – Alzheimer's disease; VD – Vascular dementia; LBD – Lewy body dementia; FTD – frontotemporal dementia; T2DM – type 2 diabetes mellitus; CVA – cerebrovascular accident; HTn – htpertension; F – female; M – male; APP – amyloid precursor protein; PS-1 – presenilin-1; PS-2 – presenilin-2; APOE-e4 – apolipoprotein in E e4 allele; GRN – progranulin; MAPT – microtubule-associated protein tau; C9orf72 – chromosome 9 open reading frame 72.

Figure 22.1 Modifiable and non-modifiable risk factors for dementia.

Donepezil, rivastigmine and galantamine are all licenced for use in mild to moderate Alzheimer's dementia, and several randomised controlled trials have proven their efficacy. The National Institute for Health and Care Excellence (NICE) in the United Kingdom recommends the use of AChEIs in the management of mild to moderate Alzheimer's disease.[6] Comparative trials have not demonstrated significant differences in efficacy between the three AChEIs.[11] Up to 50% of people appear to both tolerate and benefit from switching to an alternative AChEI if they cannot tolerate one.[11]

Memantine has been recommended by NICE as monotherapy for the management of people with moderate Alzheimer's dementia who are either intolerant of or have a

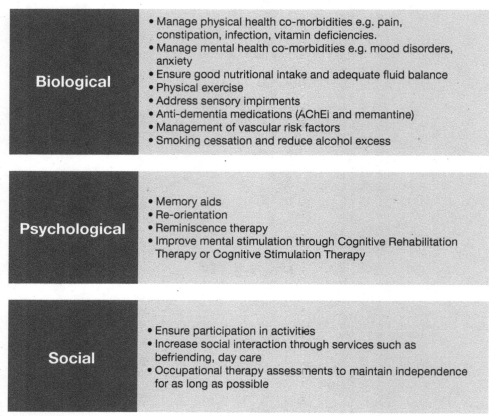

Figure 22.2 Biopsychosocial management of dementia.

contraindication to AChEI and of people with severe Alzheimer's dementia.[6] Combination therapy with AChEI and memantine has been recommended for those with moderate to severe Alzheimer's dementia.[6,11]

Vascular Dementia

AChEIs and memantine should only be used in people with vascular dementia if it's as part of a mixed-type dementia with Alzheimer's dementia, Lewy body dementia or Parkinson's disease dementia.[6] There are no licenced treatments for vascular dementia in the United Kingdom. Treatment strategies should focus on management of underlying cardiovascular and cerebrovascular risk factors based on national guidelines, including: diabetes, hypertension, hypercholesterolaemia, cardiac arrhythmias, heart disease, carotid artery stenosis, metabolic syndrome and obesity. For prevention of recurrent stroke, consideration should be given to the use of antihypertensive medications in haemorrhagic strokes and use of antiplatelets or anticoagulants, antihypertensive and lipid-lowering strategies in ischaemic strokes, based on national guidelines.[11]

Lewy Body Dementia

Pharmacological management of Lewy body dementia is challenging due to the combination of symptoms including cognitive, neuropsychiatric, autonomic dysfunction and parkinsonism. It's important to get the right balance between treating these different aspects, as treating one may exacerbate the symptoms of another.

NICE recommends the use of both rivastigmine and donepezil for people with Lewy body dementia.[6] Randomised controlled trials of rivastigmine have demonstrated benefits in cognition and also showed benefit for management of neuropsychiatric symptoms including hallucinations, apathy, anxiety and sleep disorders.[11] Caution is required, as AChEI can cause worsening of autonomic dysfunction, and people with Lewy body dementia are more likely to experience cardiac side effects, including bradycardia and QT prolongation, as well as gastrointestinal side effects.[12] People with Lewy body dementia frequently have sleep disorders, and AChEIs may worsen vivid dreams. This effect can be minimised by using a rivastigmine patch or, if using rivastigmine tablets, the second dose may be given in the afternoon.[12] Memantine can be considered for people with Lewy body dementia if AChEIs are either not tolerated or are contraindicated.[6]

The management of neuropsychiatric symptoms of Lewy body dementia are covered elsewhere in this book. It's important to note, however, that severe neuroleptic sensitivity occurs in 30–50% of patients with Lewy body dementia.[12] The best evidence for effectiveness and lower side effect profile is for quetiapine and clozapine.[12]

Parkinson's Disease Dementia

AChEIs are recommended for use in people with Parkinson's disease dementia.[13] The most evidence is for the effectiveness of rivastigmine.[12] The use of memantine is only recommended for those for who AChEIs are not tolerated or contraindicated.[13] Evidence of management of Parkinson's disease dementia tends to mirror that of Lewy body dementia.

Frontotemporal Dementia

AChEIs and memantine should not be used in the management of people with frontotemporal dementia.[6] There are currently no pharmacological therapies approved for use in frontotemporal dementia in the United Kingdom or United States. There is limited evidence that suggests that selective serotonin reuptake inhibitors, namely paroxetine, citalopram and sertraline, may be useful in the management of impulsivity, irritability, agitation, eating behaviour and disinhibition.[14,15] There is a small amount of evidence that trazodone is helpful in decreasing symptoms of problematic eating, agitation, irritability, dysphoria and depression when used in high doses of at least 300mg/day.[14,15] There are a limited number of trials that have looked into the use of stimulant medications to manage risk taking behaviours, disinhibition and apathy, but further trails are required.[14,15]

Behavioural and Psychological Symptoms of Dementia

Nearly all PWD will experience some form of behavioural and psychological symptoms of dementia (BPSD) at some stage of their illness. Common behavioural symptoms include restlessness, pacing, wandering, irritability, poor sleep, agitation and physical aggression. The psychological symptoms include anxiety, depression and psychotic symptoms such as hallucinations and delusions. Numerous factors have been linked as being contributing factors and causes of BPSD, and it's important to manage and treat these risk factors in the first instance. These include sensory impairments, social isolation, poor sleep, pain, constipation, reduced dietary and fluid intake, depression, boredom, acute physical health causes such as infections, side effects of medications and polypharmacy. The next sections cover management of agitation, aggression and other BPSD. Psychotic symptoms as part of dementia are covered in a separate chapter.

AGITATION AND AGGRESSION

Agitation is a common form of BPSD, occurring in approximately 20% of PWD at some stage of their illness.[10] Agitation can be displayed as numerous symptoms, including restlessness, pacing, repetitive speech and verbal or physical aggression. A behavioural management approach should be used as first-line management, including person-centred care, social engagement, sensory interventions, engagement in meaningful activities and music therapy.[10] Large randomised controlled trials have shown that citalopram is effective at managing less severe forms of agitation in mild to moderate stages of dementia.[10,16]

The use of antipsychotic agents in the management of agitation and aggression should be reserved for patients who are at significant risk to themselves or others. Although there is evidence confirming their effectiveness, they have been linked to a three-fold increased risk of stroke and mortality in the elderly population with dementia. Risperidone is the only antipsychotic licensed for short-term use in the treatment of BPSD in the United Kingdom, Europe and United States. At a dose of up to 1 mg, risperidone has the best evidence for reduction in agitation, especially when aggression was the main target symptom, during the first 12 weeks of use.[10,16] There is evidence to show that haloperidol is effective at managing aggression, but not agitation, and that aripiprazole can improve agitation. Olanzapine and quetiapine have not shown any benefit in the management of agitation or aggression.[10]

Randomised controlled trials show that anti-dementia medications, including AChEI and memantine, are not effective in reducing levels of agitation as a target symptom.[10]

Benzodiazepines have an increased risk of falls and cognitive decline in PWD. There is evidence showing effectiveness of lorazepam in the management of acute agitation, but it should only be used on a short-term basis.[17]

Several small studies have shown carbamazepine to be effective at managing agitation in dementia; however, slow titration is recommended, and its use is limited by its side effect profile, including dizziness, sedation, ataxia, confusion, and cardiac and hepatotoxicity.[16,17] Recent meta-analyses have not shown any benefit from valproic acid, and it may even increase agitation.[16,17] There is a lack of evidence for other antiepileptic medications such as levetiracetam and lamotrigine.

A recent randomised controlled trial of people with Alzheimer's dementia showed that the use of dextromethorphan and quinidine in combination improved levels of agitation and reduced caregiver burden,[16,17] with phase 3 trials currently under way. This shows promise of safer alternative medications for the management of agitation in PWD in the future.

Research into the use of cannabinoid receptor agonists such as THC, dronabinol and nabilone to reduce levels of agitation and aggression in PWD is ongoing. Both dronabinol and nabilone have been shown to reduce motor agitation and aggression, with the main side effect being sedation.[18] Although these small studies show promising results, larger studies are required prior to concluding on their efficacy and side effect profiles in PWD.

MANAGEMENT OF COMORBIDITIES IN DEMENTIA

Frailty

Frailty is a syndrome related to ageing and caused by a cumulative decline in multiple physiological systems as a person ages. However, frailty should not be seen as a normal part of ageing. It's estimated that between a quarter and a half of people over the age of 85 have frailty.[19]

Two models of characterising frailty have been widely accepted. The first is the phenotype model, which describes a number of patient characteristics to predict frailty and associated poor outcomes.[20] These characteristics include unintentional weight loss, reduced grip strength, self-reported exhaustion, slow gait speed and low energy expenditure. It's generally accepted that if a person has three or more of these characteristics they have frailty. The second model is the cumulative deficit model.[21] This model is based on the cumulative effect of individual deficits as listed in their frailty index (e.g., low mood, hearing loss, tremor), so the more deficits a person has, the more likely they are to have frailty. Rockwood has also developed a Clinical Frailty Scale to measure frailty based on a clinical judgement.

Observational studies have show an association between frailty and greater risk of developing mild cognitive impairment and an accelerated rate of cognitive decline.[22,23] There is an association between frailty and dementia both in terms of level of frailty and rate of change in frailty and that frailty is a significant predictor of dementia.[23,24,25,26,27]

There are different pathophysiological changes occurring in the brain of individuals with Alzheimer's disease with frailty compared to those without frailty. Hirose et al. found that individuals with Alzheimer's disease and frailty had significantly more small vessel disease pathology. They also found a decreased regional cerebral blood flow in the bilateral anterior cingulate gyrus of those with frailty and Alzheimer's disease and a decreased regional cerebral blood flow in the left dominant parietal lobe and precuneus in those without frailty on SPECT.[28] Frailty has also been shown to be associated with increased BPSD and caregiver burden in people with Alzheimer's disease.[29]

All people identified as having frailty should be offered a comprehensive geriatric assessment with a multidisciplinary team approach. The assessment should focus on management of physical health co-morbidities, optimising medications with reduction in anticholinergic burden and polypharmacy, review of nutritional and alcohol intake and physiotherapy assessment with tailored exercises.

DELIRIUM AND DEMENTIA

Delirium is under-recognised in older adults, particularly in PWD, and this is likely due to the great overlap of the signs and symptoms. A systematic review by Fick et al. noted the prevalence of delirium in PWD ranged from 22–89% of hospitalised and community populations.[30]

The relationship between delirium and dementia is two way. Delirium has been found to be an independent risk factor for dementia, and dementia has been associated with an increased risk of developing delirium.[30] Multiple studies have shown worse outcomes for people with delirium superimposed on dementia including accelerated decline in cognition and function, increased need for institutional based care and increased morbidity and mortality.

Delirium in PWD may manifest itself as a perceived worsening of BPSD. Management should focus on treating the underlying delirium rather than the BPSD especially given that medications used to treat BPSD such as antipsychotics or benzodiazepines lead to further masking of the symptoms of delirium and may potentially even worsen the underlying delirium. Benzodiazepines themselves have been linked to be a cause of delirium.[30]

The most important step in management of delirium superimposed on dementia is its recognition. Management of delirium in PWD is similar to that of people without dementia with a focus on non-pharmacological approaches including frequent visits from loved ones, re-orientation, ensuring adequate nutrition and hydration and treating any underlying sensory impairments.

OPTIMISING SUPPORT FOR CARERS AND CAREGIVER BURDEN

Dementia can be overwhelming for the families of affected people and for their carers. Physical, emotional and financial pressures can cause great stress to families and carers, and support is required from the health, social, financial and legal systems.[1]

Table 22.2 Characteristics of delirium and dementia.

Characteristics	Delirium	Dementia
Onset	Acute	Insidious
Duration	Hours to weeks	Months to years
Symptoms	Fluctuate throughout the day	Gradually progress
Orientation	Impaired	Intact in early stage; impaired in late stage
Attention	Impaired	Intact in early stage
Memory	Recent and immediate memory is impaired	Poor short-term memory
Speech	Incoherent (slow or rapid)	Word finding difficulty
Sleep-wake cycle	Day/night reversal	Fragmented sleep
Thoughts	Disorganised	Impoverished
Alertness	Hypervigilant or reduced	Usually normal
Perceptions	Hallucinations and illusions common	Usually intact in early stage

Caregivers of PWD are at significant risk of depression, anxiety and burden. Depression can occur in at least one in three caregivers of PWD, as reported in a recent meta-analysis, and this is comparatively higher than those found in the general population or in the caregivers of other physical or mental illnesses.[31]

Supporting informal caregivers of PWD is an effective strategy for improving the wellbeing of caregivers and for delaying nursing home placement. Day care services are effective in decreasing caregiver burden and behavioural problems in PWD, but they also accelerate time to nursing home admission.[32]

NICE guidance for dementia aims to improve care by making recommendations on training staff and helping carers to support people living with PWD.[6] It highlights education and training for carers to develop personalised strategies and skills to manage non-cognitive symptoms of dementia.

Carers should be made aware of relevant local services both statutory and third sector to be able to access for support. In United Kingdom, legally, carers also need to be informed of their rights and a formal assessment of their own needs including their physical and mental health (known as 'Carer's Assessment') to happen.

Support provided to carers is tailored to their needs and preferences, designed to help them support people living with dementia, available at a location they can get to easily, provided in a format suitable for them. Assistive technologies have a role in supporting both formal and informal carers of PWD and in maintaining the independence and quality of life of both PWD and their carers.[33]

More recently, the COVID pandemic has exacerbated the situation with increased social isolation and lack of face-to-face contact and support during government imposed lockdowns and possibly increased the invisibility of informal carers for PWD. During the pandemic, therefore, digital technology and communication developed exponentially to support during isolation, and to connect PWD and their carer.

The diagram below shows the support available for carers in UK

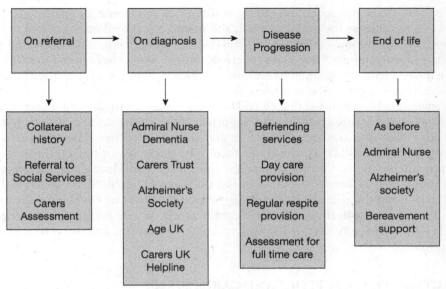

Figure 22.3 Support available for carers in the United Kingdom.

THE IMPACT OF COVID-19 ON DEMENTIA CARE

Mortality

Recent systematic reviews and meta-analyses have shown that dementia is associated with increased risk of severity and mortality in people with COVID-19.[34,35,36]

The reasons for this increased mortality are multifactorial and represent the shared risk factors for both dementia and severity and mortality of COVID-19, including increasing age and co-morbidities such as hypertension, diabetes and cardiovascular diseases.[35,36] The ApoE e4 allele increases the risk of severe COVID-19 infection, which is likely in part linked to the increased risk seen in people with Alzheimer's disease.[37] PWD also have higher baseline inflammatory markers, including tumour necrosis factor-alpha, interleukin-1 and interleukin-6, elevation of all of which have also been linked to the cytokine storm associated with COVID-19.[35] Last, PWD are less likely to be able to follow public health recommendations such as wearing face coverings, frequent handwashing and maintaining social distancing.

Antipsychotic Use

Antipsychotic prescribing for PWD has increased in the United Kingdom during the COVID-19 pandemic. It is possible to relate some of this increase to the management of co-occurring delirium and to end of life care however the majority is likely due to an increase in BPSD secondary to the lockdown.[38]

BPSD

Several studies have shown that COVID-19 quarantine is linked with an increase in BPSD. The symptoms with the highest reported increase include irritability, anxiety, apathy and agitation.[39,40,41,42] Quarantine has also been linked to a worsening in cognitive symptoms, with an increase in forgetfulness and confusion most commonly reported.[42]

As a result of the pandemic and the social distancing requirements, many non-pharmacological interventions had to be adapted, and many recreational activities had to be suspended. Studies have shown that reduced visits from loved ones is linked to increased anxiety and depressive symptoms.[43] Some non-pharmacological approaches can continue to be used during the pandemic and should be encouraged, such as physical exercise, music, doll therapy, relaxation therapy and regular teleconferencing with loved ones.

It's increasingly recognised that COVID-19 in a systemic disease, and increasing numbers of neuropsychiatric symptoms are reported. It's therefore unsurprising that individuals with BPSD who contract COVID-19 are likely to experience at least a temporary worsening of their BPSD. This leads to them potentially requiring additional pharmacological interventions. Caution should be used when considering the use of sedating medications such as benzodiazepines in the management of BPSD in individuals with COVID-19 given the risk of respiratory depression.[43] Extra caution should also be used when prescribing medications that have cardiovascular effects such as QT prolongation, as COVID-19 infection has been linked to numerous cardiac complications, including arrhythmias.[43]

IMPACT ON SOCIAL SUPPORT AND CARER STRESS

In the United Kingdom, in the first national lockdown in March 2020, all over-70s were advised to isolate – a significant proportion of these were PWD and their carers. Hospital discharges happened to care homes, initially raising transmission and deaths. Care homes were locked down to prevent the transmission of the virus, and this caused distress to people who could not see their close relatives.

The COVID-19 pandemic has had a significant negative impact on the availability of social support services for PWD and their carers, with closure of day centres and suspension of support groups. There was less of an effect on the number of paid home carers, but PWD and their unpaid carers were apprehensive about having paid carers enter their homes due to the risk of COVID-19 transmission.[44]

Day care and respite options for carers were closed in March 2020 – again to prevent transmissibility of the virus, but this had significant psychological effect on carers trying to manage PWD and neuropsychiatric symptoms with little support from other sectors. Studies have also shown a significant rise in carers stress and a decline in their wellbeing during the COVID-19 pandemic, in up to as much as two-thirds of caregivers in one study.[39] Other studies also showed that during quarantine, carers reported a significant increase in anxiety, depression, irritability and distress, even those with high resilience levels, and that these should be addressed by psychological interventions.[42,45]

Reference List

1. World Health Organisation (2020). Dementia. who.int/news-room/fact-sheets/detail/dementia. Last accessed 26th February 2021.
2. Ngo J, Holroyd-Leduc JM. (2014). Systematic review of recent dementia practice guidelines. *Age and Ageing*. 44(1):25–33.
3. Knopman DS, et al. (2001). Practice parameter: Diagnosis of dementia (an evidence-based review). *Neurology*. 56(9):1143.
4. Reus VMD, et al. (2016). The American psychiatric association practice guideline on the use of antipsychotics to treat agitation or psychosis in patients with dementia. *American Journal of Psychiatry*. 173(5):543–546.
5. Ismail Z, Black SE, Camicioli R, et al. (2020). Recommendations of the 5th Canadian Consensus Conference on the diagnosis and treatment of dementia. *Alzheimer's Dement*. 16:1182–1195. https://doi.org/10.1002/alz.12105

6. National Institute for Health and Care Excellence NICE (NICE). (2018). Dementia: Assessment, management and support for people living with dementia and their carers. www.nice.org.uk/guidance/ng97. Last accessed 26th February 2021.
7. Queensland University of Technology (QUT). (2008). Clinical practice guidelines and care pathways for people with dementia living in the community. http://eprints.qut.edu.au/17393/. Last accessed 22nd February 2021.
8. Engel G. (1977). The need for a new medical model: A challenge for biomedicine. *Science*. Apr 8;196(4286):129–136.
9. Spector A, Orrell M. (2010). Using a biopsychosocial model of dementia as a tool to guide clinical practice. *Int Psychogeriatr*. Sep;22(6):957–965.
10. Livingston G, Sommerlad A, Orgeta V, Costafreda S, Huntley J, et al. (2017). Dementia prevention, intervention, and care. *Lancet*. Dec 16;390(10113):2673–2734.
11. O'Brien J, Holmes C, Jones M, Jones R, Livingston G, et al. (2017). Clinical practice with anti-dementia drugs: A revised (third) consensus statement from the British Association for Psychopharmacology. *J Psychopharmacol*. Feb;31(2):147–168.
12. Boot B. (2015). Comprehensive treatment of dementia with Lewy bodies. *Alzheimers Res Ther*. May 29;7(1):45.
13. National Institute for Health and Care Excellence NICE (NICE). (2017). Parkinson's disease in adults. www.nice.org.uk/guidance/ng71. Last accessed 26th February 2021.
14. Pompanin S, Jelcic N, Cecchin D, Cagnin A. (2014). Impulse control disorders in frontotemporal dementia: Spectrum of symptoms and response to treatment. *Gen Hosp Psychiatry*. Nov–Dec;36(6):760.e5–7.
15. Nardell M, Tampi R. (2014). Pharmacological treatments for frontotemporal dementias: A systematic review of randomised controlled trials. *Am J Alzheimers Dis Other Demen*. Mar;29(2):123–132.
16. Cummings J, Ritter A, Rothenberg K. (2019). Advances in management of neuropsychiatric syndromes in neurodegenerative diseases. *Curr Psychiatry Rep*. Aug 8;21(8):79.
17. Phan S, Osae S, Morgan J, Inyang M, Fagan S. (2019). Neuropsychiatric symptoms in dementia: Considerations for pharmacotherapy in the USA. *Drugs R D*. Jun;19(2):93–115.
18. Marcinkowska M, Sniecikowska J, Fajkis N, Pasko P, Franczyk W, et al. (2020). Management of dementia-related psychosis, agitation and aggression: A review of the pharmacology and clinical effects of potential drug candidates. *CNS Drugs*. Mar;34(3):243–268.
19. Clegg A, Young J, Iliffe S, Rikkert M, Rockwood K. (2013). Frailty in elderly people. *Lancet*. 381(9868):752–762.
20. Fried L, Tangen C, Walston J, Newman A, Hirsch C, et al. (2001). Frailty in older adults: Evidence for a phenotype. *J Gerontol a Biol Sci Med Sci*. Mar;56(3):M146–M156.
21. Rockwood K, Song X, MacKnight C, Bergman H, Hogan D, et al. (2005). A global clinical measure of fitness and frailty in elderly people. *CMAJ*. Aug 30; 173(5):489–495.
22. Boyle P, Buchman A, Wilson R, Leurgans S, Bennett D. (2010). Physical frailty is associated with incident mild cognitive impairment in community-based older persons. *J Am Geriatr Soc*. Feb;58(2):248–255.
23. Buchman A, Boyle P, Wilson R, Tang Y, Bennett D. (2007). Frailty is associated with incident Alzheimer's disease and cognitive decline in the elderly. *Psychosom Med*. Jun;69(5):483–489.
24. Wallace L, Hunter S, Theou O, Flemin J, Rockwood K, et al. (2021). Frailty and neuropathology in relation to dementia status: The Cambridge city over-75s cohort study. *Int Psychogeriatr*. Feb 15;1–9.
25. Wallace L, Theou O, Darvesh S, Bennett D, Buchman A, et al. (2020). Neuropathological burden and the degree of frailty in relation to global cognition and dementia. *Neurology*. Dec 15;95(24) e3269–e3279.
26. Li M, Huang Y, Liu Z, Shen R, Chen H, et al. (2020). The association between frailty and incidence of dementia in Beijing: Findings from 10/66 dementia research group population-based cohort study. *BMC Geriatr*. Apr 15;20(1):138.
27. Kojima G, Taniguchi Y, Iliffe S, Walters K. (2016). Frailty as a predictor of Alzheimer disease, vascular dementia, and all dementia among community-dwelling older people: A systematic review and meta-analysis. *J Am Med Dir Assoc*. Oct 1;17(10):881–888.
28. Hirose D, Schimizu S, Hirao K, Ogawa Y, Sato T, et al. (2019). Neuroimaging characteristics of frailty status in patients with Alzheimer's disease. *J Alzheimers Dis*. 67(4):1201–1208.
29. Sugimoto T, Ono R, Kimura A, Saji N, Niida S, et al. (2018). Physical frailty correlates with behavioural and psychological symptoms of dementia and caregiver burden in Alzheimer's disease. *J Clin Psychiatry*. Nov 13;79(6):17m11991.
30. Fick D, Agostini J, Inouye S. (2002). Delirium superiposed on dementia: A systematic review. *J Am Geriatr Soc*. Oct;50(10):1723–1732.

31. Sallim AB, Sayampanathan AA, Cuttilan A, et al. (2015). Prevalence of mental health disorders among caregivers of patients with Alzheimer disease. *J Am Med Dir Assoc*, 16:1034–1041.
32. Vandepitte S, Van Den Noortgate N, et al. (2016). Effectiveness of respite care in supporting informal caregivers of persons with dementia: A systematic review. *Int J Geriatr Psychiatry*, 1277–1288. doi: 10.1002/gps.4504.
33. Bhattacharyya S, Benbow SM. (2019). Assistive technologies and the carers of people with dementia: Empowerment and connection. In Management Association, I. (Ed.), *Chronic illness and long-term care: Breakthroughs in research and practice* (pp. 43–58). IGI Global, UK.
34. July J, Pranata R. (2021). Prevalence of dementia and its impact on mortality in patients with coronavirus disease 2019: A systematic review and meta-analysis. *Geriatr Gerontol Int*. Feb;21(2):172–177.
35. Liu N, Sun J, Wang X, Zhao M, Huang Q, et al. (2020). The impact of dementia on the clinical outcome of COVID-19: A systematic review and meta-analysis. *J Alzheimers Dis*. 78(4):1775–1782.
36. Hariyanto T, Putri C, Arisa J, Situmeang R, Kurniawan A. (2021). Dementia and outcomes from coronavirus disease 2019 (COVID-19) pneumonia: A systematic review and meta-analysis. *Arch Gerontol Geriatr*. Mar–Apr;93:104299.
37. Kuo CL, Pilling L, Atkins J, Masoli J, Delgado J, et al. (2020). APOE e4 genotype predicts severe COVID-19 in the UK biobank community cohort. *J Gerontol A Biol Sci Med Sci*. Nov;75(11):2231–2232.
38. Howard R, Burns A, Schneider L. (2020). Antipsychotic prescribing to people with dementia during COVID-19. *Lancet Neurol*. Nov;19(11):892.
39. Cagnin A, Lorenzo R, Marra C, Bonanni L, Cupidi C, et al. (2020). Behavioural and psychological effects of coronavirus disease-19 quarantine in patients with dementia. *Front Psychiatry*. Sep 9;11:578015.
40. Cohen G, Russo M, Campos J, Allegri R. (2020). COVID-19 epidemic in Argentina: Worsening of behavioural symptoms in elderly subjects with dementia living in the community. *Front Psychiatry*. Aug 28;11:866.
41. Simonetti A, Pais C, Jones M, Cipriani M, Janiri D, et al. (2020). Neuropsychiatric symptoms in elderly with dementia during COVID-19 pandemic: Definition, treatment, and future directions. *Front Psychiatry*. Sep 29;11:579842.
42. Rainero I, Bruni A, Marra C, Cagnin A, Bonanni L, et al. (2021). The impact of COVID-19 quarantine on patients with dementia and family caregivers: A nation-wide survey. *Front Aging Neurosci*. Jan 18;12:625781.
43. Keng A, Brown E, Rostas A, Rajji T, Pollock B, et al. (2020). Effectively caring for individuals with behavioural and psychological symptoms of dementia during the COVID-19 pandemic. *Front Psychiatry*. Oct 6;11:573367.
44. Giebel C, Pulford D, Cooper C, Lord K, Shenton J, et al. (2021). COVID-19-related social support service closures and mental well-being in older adults and hose affected by dementia: A UK longitudinal survey. *BMJ Open*. Jan 17;11(1):e045889.
45. Altieri M, Santangelo G (2021). The psychological impact of COVID-19 pandemic and lockdown on caregivers of people with dementia. *Am J Geriatr Psychiatry*. 27–34. doi: 10.1016/j.jagp.2020.10.009.

23
Optimizing Patient Care in Attenuated Psychosis Syndrome

Nikita Nalawade and Avinash De Sousa

Introduction	247
Historical Background and Current Understanding	247
Need for Optimization of Care in APS	248
Management Interventions	249
Risk Assessment	*249*
Aims of Treatment	*249*
Evidence-Based Interventions	250
Pharmacological Interventions	*250*
Psychosocial Interventions	*251*
Recommendations for Optimization of Treatment	252
Integrated Treatment	*254*
Conclusion and Future Implications	254

INTRODUCTION

Attenuated psychosis syndrome (APS) gained clinical interest after its inclusion in DSM-5 as a diagnosis for further research. It was proposed as a category to diagnose those individuals with psychotic symptoms who did not fit under another classification but still had significant impairment due to their symptoms which could also indicate an early sign of impending psychosis. One of the few reasons for the inclusion of this diagnosis in a formal classificatory system was to encourage early identification and intervention and to improve access to healthcare. This inclusion not only brought a new disorder into the clinical spotlight; it also came with its own share of conflicting views.

HISTORICAL BACKGROUND AND CURRENT UNDERSTANDING

Even if not formally brought under the classificatory perspective, both Kraeplin and Bleuler had spoken about their own descriptions of what was known as dementia praecox then and schizophrenias, which both begun with insidious changes and warning signs before the manifestation of overt psychosis. Harry Stack Sullivan had also spoken about the early signs of schizophrenia and how they might in time be key in possibly being able to stall the florid manifestation of the illness (1). Although 'early' mentions of symptoms of psychosis have been known, the term was formally introduced as 'prodromal' by Mayer-Gross in the early 1930s (2).

This opened a channel for a new outlook and encouraged research, with interventions and perspectives taking shape over time. Several studies were carried out, with a few notable ones by McGorry et al. (3,4), which attempted to recognize and define particular symptoms which could act as potential indicators as well breeding interventions.

With more understanding came more discord and contrarian views. Early identification and management can aid in decreasing the duration of untreated psychosis, but on the flip side, it also carries the risk of overdiagnosis and possible nonessential exposure to psychotropic agents. Prodromal features do pose an increased risk for developing a psychotic disorder, but conversion rates have varied between studies. Some studies claim the risk of transition is 30–40%, with declining risk in recent years (2,5), which again paradoxically could also be the result of the early interventions that have begun. Studies with longer follow-ups indicate a transition of psychosis, in those with a clinical and familial risk, being high within 3 years of presentation (6).

Particularly noteworthy in most of these statistics is that transition rates have been made for samples comprising help-seeking individuals, as compared to a general community sample, who sought help in proportion to their level of impairment and distress, which in itself may place them at a higher risk of psychosis.

Parallelly, the non-converting group in some studies did show an improvement in symptoms and functioning. However, this group also continued to remain on the lower edge of functioning in comparison to the non-psychiatric subjects (2,7).

This has led to the understanding that APS, apart from being a high-risk clinical state which could herald the onset of psychosis, is also an illness of its own. Symptoms, such as delusions, hallucinations, and disorganization, to name a few, albeit attenuated, can lead to functional impairment, additionally also adding to the caregiver distress.

This chapter focuses on the optimization of patient care in individuals with APS with an attempt to bring forth best care practices in the community.

NEED FOR OPTIMIZATION OF CARE IN APS

Psychiatric care has always emphasized a holistic approach that is not purely restricted to the alleviation of the symptoms but also based primarily on understanding the patient's subjective experience. This outlook is all the more necessary in APS considering the undefined nature of the illness.

Due to the pleiotropism of the symptoms, varied approaches to their management and care have been undertaken. Some vouch for the prescription of antipsychotics, while some rely on regular monitoring and non-pharmacological interventions. APS can also occur in the form of symptoms resembling depressive disorders, or anxiety disorders or comorbid with these and can be masked by substance use disorders as well (8–10). These disorders by themselves can be almost equally incapacitating.

Another cause for concern can be suicidality. APS, although occurring with subthreshold symptoms, can cause significant functional impairment and be quite distressing. According to a study with a small pilot sample, almost 60% of those who sought help had presented with at least mild suicidal ideation, and 47% had reported at least one suicide attempt before being accepted into the early intervention service (11).

Given that APS is commonly seen during the adolescent age group and in youth (12), optimization of care is key to ensure a more favorable pathway of care during this critical developmental period. Prevalence in this age group is associated with several inherent factors that need to be considered including developmental and social domains that play an essential role in the comprehensive functioning and wellbeing of the individual. A breach in the normal developmental timeline can lead to long-term residual impairments. Studies have suggested that identification of high-risk states in individuals coupled with adequate interventions during this phase before the development of florid psychosis can be instrumental in mitigating the long-term implications, potentially prevent or delay psychosis or even reduce the morbidity associated with developing a florid psychotic episode (13). The duration of untreated psychosis is also decreased in those who transition to psychosis after having sought early interventions, which has been known to have a better prognosis clinically.

A few other related crucial factors that need to be considered to ensure optimized care are regional sociocultural influences and explanatory models. These factors determine the expression of the illness as well as the pathway to care. In many countries, the manifestation of APS can often be interpreted as episodes of possession and trance or be colored by magicoreligious belief systems. The associated stigma of being 'labeled' with a psychiatric disorder as well as the alternative explanations can hinder access to care. Therefore, a 'clear and vast' understanding of the prevailing sociocultural ethos is essential in optimizing care not to avoid the 'cons' associated with overdiagnosis but also to relate to the patient and the family, which goes a long way in establishing a therapeutic alliance to ensure adequate long-term care.

MANAGEMENT INTERVENTIONS

Risk Assessment

A pivotal question that arises during the optimization of care in those with APS is how we can predict the risk of transition to a psychotic disorder based on symptoms that may or may not resemble defined criteria.

Apart from a detailed history, some interview measures have also been developed to augment the process for a more unified assessment. A few of the most commonly known ones are the Comprehensive Assessment of At-Risk Mental State (CAARMS) (14,2), the Structured Interview for Prodromal Symptoms (SIPS) (including the companion Scale of Prodromal Symptoms [SOPS]), the Early Recognition Inventory for the Retrospective Assessment of the Onset of Schizophrenia (ERIraos), and the Basel Screening Instrument for Psychosis (BSIP) (1,2). The Schizophrenia Proneness Instrument, adult version (SPI-A)59, and child and youth version (SPI-CY) have also been used (2).

Some indices can also be precautionary markers to delineate those with APS who may develop psychosis from those who may not. In APS, these have included features such as decline in social and vocational functioning, subthreshold positive and disorganized symptoms of psychosis, and new or worsening cognitive symptoms These clinical markers, in combination with a familial risk of psychosis, point towards increased risk (2).

The North American Prodrome Longitudinal Study (15) reported five clinical predictive variables in their sample of high risk participants: genetic risk with functional decline, high unusual thought content scores, high suspicion/paranoia scores, low social functioning, and history of substance abuse.

Another study reported that high risk individuals with higher scores in suspiciousness and high anhedonia/asociality scores had a higher transition risk at the end of a 7-year follow-up (16).

Aims of Treatment

The aim of the care provided needs to be primarily bifocal, with an immediate objective to not only reduce the individual's symptoms but also a more distal objective of attempting to prevent or mitigate these symptoms from progressing into psychosis. One of the pioneers in early interventions, the Personal Assessment and Crisis Evaluation (PACE) clinic, incorporated medical and psychological pathways of care based on the underlying stress vulnerability model (17). The patient and the families are equal role players in deciding the course of the management plan.

A multipronged approach, tailored to individual symptoms and needs, encompassing both pharmacological and psychological strategies, is needed.

Regular follow-up and monitoring of symptoms and functioning also need to be emphasized.

EVIDENCE-BASED INTERVENTIONS

Pharmacological Interventions

Antipsychotic Agents

A number of atypical antipsychotics have been tried, individually as well as in combination with psychotherapeutic and psychosocial interventions, in response to subthreshold psychotic symptoms with an aim of palliation of the prevailing symptoms as well as attempting to prevent or delay the onset of psychosis.

One of the first studies in this domain was by a randomized controlled trial conducted by McGorry et al., where in addition to a needs-based intervention, another arm of a specific preventive intervention comprising low-dose risperidone (mean dose of 1.3 mg per day) and cognitive behavioral therapy was tried. At the end of the 6-month follow-up period, although the difference between the two groups was no longer significant, it continued to remain effective in the risperidone-adherent subgroup of the trial, suggesting that a possible delay of psychosis was possible with specific interventions with antipsychotic agents. With reference to the long-term outcomes, both groups had experienced a decrease in the symptomatology in due course of the study (18). A consecutive study by the authors comparing low-dose risperidone with cognitive therapy as compared to cognitive therapy and placebo led to similar results (19). Both were found to be efficacious without a marked difference between pharmacological and psychotherapeutic interventions.

In another study conducted by McGlashan et al. (20) comparing the efficacy of olanzapine in a randomized double blind trial versus a placebo, a nearly significant difference of olanzapine over the placebo was found, demonstrating a potential for olanzapine to decrease the conversion to psychosis rate. Olanzapine nevertheless was efficacious in decreasing positive subthreshold symptoms.

A case report (21) of using low-dose Olanzapine at 7.5 to 10 mg per day has also been tried and reported to be effective up to a follow-up of 3 months.

Ruhrmann et al. (22) studied the effectiveness of low-dose Amisulpride (ranging from 50 to 800 mg with a mean daily dose of 118.7 mg/d) in addition to a needs-based intervention as compared to solely a needs-based intervention. Amisulpride appeared to provide symptomatic relief in terms of both positive and negative symptoms, albeit with an increase in prolactin levels in some.

Aripiprazole used in a small sample by Woods et al. (23) within the range of 5–30 mg per day also showed promising results in the improvement of symptoms over an 8-week follow-up period.

OTHER DRUGS

1. Omega 3 fatty acids: Omega-3 polyunsaturated fatty acids (PUFAs) has been shown to improve neuronal circuitry developmentally. A deficiency is also seen in a number of mental disorders including schizophrenia. This led to a hypothesis proposing their

use during critical developmental periods can aid in decreasing the progression to psychosis. An RCT conducted by Amminger et al. (24) compared the effectiveness and the long-term outcome with the use of omega-3 PUFAs in a 12-week intervention. This randomized, double blind, placebo-controlled trial showed a reduced risk of progression to psychosis.

A systematic review by Susai et al. (25), studying the effect of omega-3 fatty acids on functional outcome, involved four primary studies. Two of these were RCTs, the VHR study and the NEURAPRO study. Patients received 1.2 and 1.4 g per day of omega-3 FA, respectively, as compared to a placebo. Both studies measured a similar functional outcome but had contradictory results, with VHR showing a positive correlation between omega-3 FA use and better functional outcome, while the NEURAPRO study did not show a significant difference.

2. Galantine-memantine: A report by M. Koola (26) proposed the use of a combination of galantine-memantine in response to evidence suggesting attenuated mismatch negativity as a biomarker for prediction of transition to psychosis. Further studies are warranted to prove effectiveness.
3. Glycine: Keeping with the NMDA hypothesis of schizophrenia, Woods et al. (27) conducted two short-term pilot studies to evaluate the use of glycine in those with attenuated psychosis as well as to evaluate the effect on various other domains, including cognition. Though the two pilot studies showed positive results with respect to the symptoms as well as some neurocognitive domains, it also called for larger studies for more promising evidence.

Psychosocial Interventions

Given the subthreshold symptoms and the side effects associated with pharmacological agents, particularly antipsychotic agents, psychosocial interventions including psychotherapy have taken precedence. The use of pharmacological interventions in adolescents and youth, where APS is more commonly seen, has not been met with enough evidence of benefits outweighing the risk to warrant approval. Most studies that evaluated the efficacy of medications in APS have also used them in conjunction with various psychosocial interventions (1). Some commonly used interventions have been cognitive behavioral therapy/cognitive therapy, psychoeducation, family therapy, and others which aim to work around the socio-occupational deficits like cognitive remediation, social skills training, and supported education or employment, to name a few.

Cognitive Behavioral Therapy/Cognitive Therapy

Cognitive behavioral therapy and cognitive therapy (CBT/CT) have been the most commonly used non-pharmacological interventions. With the added benefit of avoiding the side effects associated with antipsychotic use, this intervention has been more often than not used as a first-line treatment. One of the earliest studies evaluating the effect of this intervention was conducted by McGorry et al. in conjunction with risperidone (18). Morrison et al. (28) then conducted a study evaluating the effect of CT through an early detection and intervention evaluation (EDIE) trial along with concurrent clinical monitoring and case management. Those in the group with received CT showed a significantly lower rate of transition to psychosis as well as a reduction in positive symptoms after a period of 12 months. A 3-year follow-up study also showed consistent benefits of CT (29). Addington et al. (30) also conducted an RCT comparing the effectiveness of CBT with supportive therapy in youth with APS over a period of 6 months with an additional 12-month follow-up. Though the difference in the transition rates was not significant, both groups of individuals noticed a decrease in anxious, depressive, and positive symptoms (30,1).

Most models of CBT/CT consist of similar components. For instance (13):

- Psychoeducation about the CBT model and the symptoms.
- Monitoring of cognitions, behavior and symptoms
- Testing beliefs or schema
- Behavioral activation
- Coping skills training
- Stress reduction

A modified CT model (28) that was used by Morrison et al. comprised methods that encouraged the normalization of symptoms, evaluation and development of alternative explanations, decatastrophizing, and testing alternative beliefs through behavioral changes. This model was also inclusive of treatment approaches for comorbid disorders.

Family Therapy

Family therapies have also been considered an effective part of the treatment protocol, with the onset of APS 'commonly' occurring in the adolescent age group during which familial influences are 'paramount'. Families act as caregivers and are also important buffers for stressors and triggers of psychosis. On the contrary, they can at times also be a crucial part of environmental triggers leading to an episode. Miklowitz et al. (31) conducted a randomized trial as a part of an eight-site intervention under the North American Prodrome Longitudinal Study (NAPLS) where adolescents and youth with APS and other clinically high-risk states were tried on family-focused therapy or family psychoeducation. Some methods implemented under the family-focused therapy arm were psychoeducation about the early signs of psychosis, problem solving, communication, and stress management. At the end of the follow-up at 6 months, those who received family-focused therapy showed a better improvement in symptoms, especially the attenuated positive symptoms.

Family therapy can take place with single and multifamily groups. It focuses on psychoeducation about the different domains of the symptoms, comorbid disorders, stressors, and their effect on the course of the illness. It also provides them with coping strategies, as environmental stressors are known to be triggers for psychosis.

Social Skills Training

Social skills training has been known to be effective in improving functioning in those with psychosis (1). Those individuals with APS who also have hints of impairment in the socio-occupational domain can also benefit from social skills training where skills can be practiced via role play and other methods which are usually conducted in groups to encourage interpersonal reciprocity.

Other psychosocial interventions like supported employment or education other community-based interventions like case management or assertive community treatment help in developing community skills and awareness by also using resources from the individual's proximal source of contact to ensure an overall as well as inclusive sense of wellbeing.

RECOMMENDATIONS FOR OPTIMIZATION OF TREATMENT

Some guidelines have been developed globally to help direct a general clinical practice in the management of attenuated symptoms. Most have been formed on similar grounds and recommend a substantially uniform pathway of care.

One of them, the European Psychiatric Association, recommends the following (32):

- Assessment and identification of APS by trained clinicians using evidence-based and uniform measures before the initiation of interventions.
- Broad outlook extending beyond symptoms and diagnosis with a focus on functional outcomes with interventions designed to address the functional and social deficits and not limited to preventing the transition to psychosis.
- A hierarchical intervention model graded in terms of merit suggesting the use of psychological interventions being used as first line and pharmacological interventions being used as augmenting agents in those who do not respond to first line or are severe enough to warrant use of medications. Low doses of second-generation antipsychotics are preferred to ameliorate symptoms enough for psychotherapeutic interventions to take effect.
- Risk stratification not only in terms of risk of conversion to psychosis but also in terms of functional impairment. Since a generalized treatment plan does not represent intra- and inter-individual heterogeneity, this will further refine the treatment protocol to suit individual needs.
- Continued monitoring of symptoms by trained, expert clinicians to ensure functioning and safety with long-term follow-ups.

Woodberry et al. (13) also proposed recommendations based on their review. They emphasized the importance of early signs and symptoms which could help in early identification, which in turn could affect the individual's clinical trajectory.

- A thorough assessment and evaluation by trained professionals according to guidelines is important before commencing an intervention with a specific psychosis prevention focus.
- A multidisciplinary approach with a team of professionals from various relevant fields. A multidimensional assessment will take into account not only the cross-sectional anomalies but also a longitudinal perspective of the individual's trajectory over a life span.
- They seconded the recommendation of offering psychosocial interventions and low-risk pharmacological agents such as omega-3 fatty acids prior to the more the more intensive psychotropic agents.
- These recommendations encouraged clinicians to provide appropriate feedback and to be mindful of the individual and family's cultural context and values while formulating a management plan.
- Cognitive and socio-occupational functioning should also be a center of focus of the treatment plan. They proposed the use of other strategies such as supported education or employment, social skills training, and cognitive remediation as well to help with functioning in these spheres.
- Diet and lifestyle were also emphasized as important targets. Lifestyle modifications to include regular sleep and exercise, among others, can positively influence overall wellbeing over and above the symptoms.

The British Association of Psychiatry proposed recommendations for clinical practice on similar lines. They recommended the use of low-dose antipsychotic medication in those seeking help for short-term relief. These dosages are usually lower than those prescribed for the first episode of psychosis as well (33).

Most guidelines have also highlighted the importance of treating comorbid disorders like anxiety, depressive disorders, and substance use disorders, which may have also masked the underlying symptoms. Anxiety and depressive disorders have been commonly noted to occur concurrently with attenuated psychosis (8). These disorders can affect the psychopathology, the functioning, harboring of self harm behaviors or suicidality, and the long-term outcome of the illness. Therefore, an important part of optimizing psychiatry care is also inclusive management of these comorbid disorders.

Integrated Treatment

An integrated treatment approach has also been tried to cater to the spectrum of symptoms and needs. Bechdolf et al. (34) compared integrated psychological intervention (IPI) with supportive therapy. The integrated psychological intervention including individual CBT, modified skills training, cognitive remediation, and multifamily psychoeducation. Individual CBT formed the core of the treatment module and was based on the principles of cognitive therapy as described by Beck. Skills training involved the scheduling and monitoring of mastery and pleasure activities, among others. Cognitive remediation used a computerized program consisting of cognitive exercises and focused on thought and perception deficits. These individuals were subsequently followed up over 24 months. They found that the conversion rates in those under the IPI arm were lower than those undertaking supportive therapy at both the 12-month and 24-month follow-ups, and those who did transition to psychosis transitioned faster under the supportive therapy arm.

CONCLUSION AND FUTURE IMPLICATIONS

With the evolution of the concept of psychosis from a chronically debilitating disorder from which recovery was nearly impossible as well as an evolving concept of recovery, newer interventions have begun to take shape. Given the multitude of expressions of illness models and the inability of 'fixed' criteria to adequately and justifiably represent attenuated psychosis, a wider approach to management is needed. A 'one size fits all' paradigm cannot be employed in such individuals.

Early intervention as a part of preemptive psychiatry plays an important role in delaying or possibly preventing the onset of psychosis, the effect of which also reverberates in other domains besides the individual's wellbeing, such as the economic as well as public health tier.

McGorry et al. (35) laid out some core components to optimize psychiatric care – community awareness, easy access to the service, home-based assessment and care, acute care, case management, medical and psychological interventions, and group programs, as well as family programs to provide suppose to the families of individuals.

Optimizing psychiatry care therefore cannot be limited to purely clinical or medical care and requires the collaboration of a multisectoral team ranging from mental health professionals to community members. Tailoring interventions according to the needs of the individual and the families, as well as setting up a base in the community to ensure access to healthcare, is key in ensuring more holistic care. At the same time, this also serves a greater purpose of generating awareness.

An anthropological outlook is also required when it comes to identifying and treating APS, an understanding of the cultural contexts, values, and explanations to distinguish between the 'normal' and 'abnormal'. Optimizing care, especially in psychiatry, which has been long associated with its own taboos and stigmas, requires a collaborative effort with the local faith healers as well to establish a point of contact for access to clinical healthcare while also respecting local beliefs. Most of the current evidence is based on those who seek help, while a large number of individuals go unrecognized and untreated. Integration with community members will help bridge this research gap and improve access to care.

Years of research have almost brought APS to the DSM. Most evidence for interventions with APS is currently based on relatively smaller samples and smaller duration of follow-up periods. Thus, more studies evaluating longer outcomes, especially in adolescents and youth, are needed for a wider understanding of this field.

Novel technologies of predicting the degree of an inherent risk of transitioning from a high risk state to psychosis, genetically using psychobiological approaches to increase sensitivity and specificity, can help streamline the treatment pathway.

A more malleable approach is needed to mirror the nature of the disorder itself. We have come a long way from viewing psychosis as having a future of despondency to the present, where interventions to possibly prevent psychosis have taken root. With further research and understanding, there may be further unfolding of perspectives that are currently unheard of.

References

1. Li H, Shapiro DI, Seidman LJ, editors. *Handbook of attenuated psychosis syndrome across cultures: International perspectives on early identification and intervention.* Springer Nature, UK; 2019 Aug 23.
2. Fusar-Poli P, Borgwardt S, Bechdolf A, Addington J, Riecher-Rössler A, Schultze-Lutter F, Keshavan M, Wood S, Ruhrmann S, Seidman LJ, Valmaggia L. The psychosis high-risk state: A comprehensive state-of-the-art review. *JAMA Psychiatry.* 2013 Jan 1;70(1):107–120.
3. Yung AR, McGorry PD. The prodromal phase of first-episode psychosis: Past and current conceptualizations. *Schizophrenia Bulletin.* 1996 Jan 1;22(2):353–370.
4. McGorry PD, Yung AR, Phillips LJ. The "close-in" or ultra high-risk model: A safe and effective strategy for research and clinical intervention in prepsychotic mental disorder. *Schizophrenia Bulletin.* 2003 Jan 1;29(4):771–790.
5. Yung AR, Stanford C, Cosgrave E, Killackey E, Phillips L, Nelson B, McGorry PD. Testing the ultra high risk (prodromal) criteria for the prediction of psychosis in a clinical sample of young people. *Schizophrenia Research.* 2006 May 1;84(1):57–66.
6. Fusar-Poli P, Bonoldi I, Yung AR, Borgwardt S, Kempton MJ, Valmaggia L, Barale F, Caverzasi E, McGuire P. Predicting psychosis: Meta-analysis of transition outcomes in individuals at high clinical risk. *Archives of General Psychiatry.* 2012 Mar 5;69(3):220–229.
7. Schultze-Lutter F, Ruhrmann S, Berning J, Maier W, Klosterkötter J. Basic symptoms and ultra-high risk criteria: Symptom development in the initial prodromal state. *Schizophrenia Bulletin.* 2010 Jan 1;36(1):182–191.
8. Fusar-Poli P, Nelson B, Valmaggia L, Yung AR, McGuire PK. Comorbid depressive and anxiety disorders in 509 individuals with an at-risk mental state: Impact on psychopathology and transition to psychosis. *Schizophrenia Bulletin.* 2014 Jan 1;40(1):120–131.
9. Addington J, Case N, Saleem MM, Auther AM, Cornblatt BA, Cadenhead KS. Substance use in clinical high risk for psychosis: A review of the literature. *Early Intervention in Psychiatry.* 2014 May;8(2):104–112.
10. Addington J, Piskulic D, Liu L, Lockwood J, Cadenhead KS, Cannon TD, Cornblatt BA, McGlashan TH, Perkins DO, Seidman LJ, Tsuang MT. Comorbid diagnoses for youth at clinical high risk of psychosis. *Schizophrenia Research.* 2017 Dec 1;190:90–95.
11. Hutton P, Bowe S, Parker S, Ford S. Prevalence of suicide risk factors in people at ultra-high risk of developing psychosis: A service audit. [Abstract] *Early Intervention in Psychiatry.* 2011 Nov;5(4):375–380.
12. Devoe DJ, Farris MS, Townes P, Addington J. Attenuated psychotic symptom interventions in youth at risk of psychosis: A systematic review and meta-analysis. *Early Intervention in Psychiatry.* 2019 Feb;13(1):3–17.
13. Woodberry KA, Shapiro DI, Bryant C, Seidman LJ. Progress and future directions in research on the psychosis prodrome: A review for clinicians. *Harvard Review of Psychiatry.* 2016 Mar;24(2):87.
14. Nelson B. The CAARMS: Assessing young people at ultra high risk of psychosis. Orygen Youth Health Research Centre; 2014.
15. Seidman LJ, Giuliano AJ, Meyer EC, Addington J, Cadenhead KS, Cannon TD, McGlashan TH, Perkins DO, Tsuang MT, Walker EF, Woods SW. Neuropsychology of the prodrome to psychosis in the NAPLS consortium: relationship to family history and conversion to psychosis. *Archives of General Psychiatry.* 2010 Jun 1;67(6):578–588.

16. Riecher-Rössler A, Gschwandtner U, Aston J, Borgwardt S, Drewe M, Fuhr P, Pflüger M, Radü W, Schindler C, Stieglitz RD. The Basel early-detection-of-psychosis (FEPSY)-study: Design and preliminary results. *Acta Psychiatrica Scandinavica.* 2007 Feb;115(2):114–125.
17. Yung AR, McGorry PD, Francey SM, Nelson B, Baker K, Phillips LJ, Berger G, Amminger GP. PACE: A specialised service for young people at risk of psychotic disorders. *Medical Journal of Australia.* 2007 Oct;187(S7):S43–S46.
18. McGorry PD, Yung AR, Phillips LJ, Yuen HP, Francey S, Cosgrave EM, Germano D, Bravin J, McDonald T, Blair A, Adlard S. Randomized controlled trial of interventions designed to reduce the risk of progression to first-episode psychosis in a clinical sample with subthreshold symptoms. *Archives of General Psychiatry.* 2002 Oct 1;59(10):921–928.
19. McGorry PD, Nelson B, Phillips LJ, Yuen HP, Francey SM, Thampi A, Berger GE, Amminger GP, Simmons MB, Kelly D, Dip G, Thompson AD, Yung AR. Randomized controlled trial of interventions for young people at ultra-high risk of psychosis: Twelve-month outcome. [Abstract] *Journal of Clinical Psychiattry.* 2013 Apr;74(4):349–356.
20. McGlashan TH, Zipursky RB, Perkins D, Addington J, Miller T, Woods SW, Hawkins AK, Hoffman ER, Preda A, Epstein I, Addington D. Randomized, double-blind trial of olanzapine versus placebo in patients prodromally symptomatic for psychosis. *American Journal of Psychiatry.* 2006 May;163(5):790–799.
21. Arora S, Bhagabati D, Das S, Phookun HR, Hazarika M, Talukdar SK. 'White handkerchief': A patient of attenuated psychosis syndrome. *Journal of Rural and Community Psychiatry.* 2014 Jul;1(2):88.
22. Ruhrmann S, Bechdolf A, Kühn KU, Wagner M, Schultze-Lutter F, Janssen B, Maurer K, Häfner H, Gaebel W, Möller HJ, Maier W. Acute effects of treatment for prodromal symptoms for people putatively in a late initial prodromal state of psychosis. *The British Journal of Psychiatry.* 2007 Dec;191(S51):s88–s95.
23. Woods SW, Tully EM, Walsh BC, Hawkins KA, Callahan JL, Cohen SJ, Mathalon DH, Miller TJ, McGlashan TH. Aripiprazole in the treatment of the psychosis prodrome: An open-label pilot study. *The British Journal of Psychiatry.* 2007 Dec;191(S51):s96–s101.
24. Amminger GP, Schäfer MR, Schlögelhofer M, Klier CM, McGorry PD. Longer-term outcome in the prevention of psychotic disorders by the Vienna omega-3 study. *Nature Communications.* 2015 Aug 11;6(1):1–7.
25. Susai SR, Sabherwal S, Mongan D, Föcking M, Cotter DR. Omega-3 fatty acid in ultra-high-risk psychosis: A systematic review based on functional outcome. *Early Intervention in Psychiatry.* 2021 Mar 2.
26. Koola MM. Attenuated mismatch negativity in attenuated psychosis syndrome predicts psychosis: Can galantamine-memantine combination prevent psychosis? *Molecular Neuropsychiatry.* 2018;4(2):71–74.
27. Woods SW, Walsh BC, Hawkins KA, Miller TJ, Saksa JR, D'Souza DC, Pearlson GD, Javitt DC, McGlashan TH, Krystal JH. Glycine treatment of the risk syndrome for psychosis: Report of two pilot studies. *European Neuropsychopharmacology.* 2013 Aug 1;23(8):931–940.
28. Morrison AP, French P, Walford L, Lewis SW, Kilcommons A, Green J, Parker S, Bentall RP. Cognitive therapy for the prevention of psychosis in people at ultra-high risk: Randomised controlled trial. *The British Journal of Psychiatry.* 2004 Oct;185(4):291–297.
29. Morrison AP, French P, Parker S, Roberts M, Stevens H, Bentall RP, Lewis SW. Three-year follow-up of a randomized controlled trial of cognitive therapy for the prevention of psychosis in people at ultrahigh risk. *Schizophrenia Bulletin.* 2007 May 1;33(3):682–687.
30. Addington J, Epstein I, Liu L, French P, Boydell KM, Zipursky RB. A randomized controlled trial of cognitive behavioral therapy for individuals at clinical high risk of psychosis. *Schizophrenia Research.* 2011 Jan 1;125(1):54–61.
31. Miklowitz DJ, O'Brien MP, Schlosser DA, Addington J, Candan KA, Marshall C, Domingues I, Walsh BC, Zinberg JL, De Silva SD, Friedman-Yakoobian M. Family-focused treatment for adolescents and young adults at high risk for psychosis: Results of a randomized trial. *Journal of the American Academy of Child & Adolescent Psychiatry.* 2014 Aug 1;53(8):848–858.
32. Schmidt SJ, Schultze-Lutter F, Schimmelmann BG, Maric NP, Salokangas RK, Riecher-Rössler A, van der Gaag M, Meneghelli A, Nordentoft M, Marshall M, Morrison A. EPA guidance on the early intervention in clinical high risk states of psychoses. *European Psychiatry.* 2015 Mar;30(3):388–404.
33. Barnes TR, Drake R, Paton C, Cooper SJ, Deakin B, Ferrier IN, Gregory CJ, Haddad PM, Howes OD, Jones I, Joyce EM. Evidence-based guidelines for the pharmacological treatment of schizophrenia:

Updated recommendations from the British Association for Psychopharmacology. *Journal of Psychopharmacology.* 2020 Jan;34(1):3–78.
34. Bechdolf A, Wagner M, Ruhrmann S, Harrigan S, Putzfeld V, Pukrop R, Brockhaus-Dumke A, Berning J, Janssen B, Decker P, Bottlender R. Preventing progression to first-episode psychosis in early initial prodromal states. *The British Journal of Psychiatry.* 2012 Jan;200(1):22–29.
35. McGorry PD. Early intervention in psychosis: Obvious, effective, overdue. *The Journal of Nervous and Mental Disease.* 2015 May;203(5):310.

24
Optimising Patient Care in Psychiatry – Anxiety Disorders

Prerna Khar, Vinyas Nisarga and Prajakta Patkar

Introduction	259
Concepts of Anxiety Disorder	259
Panic Disorder	260
A Single Panic Attack Is Not Necessarily Indicative of a Psychiatric Disorder	260
Epidemiology	260
Aetiology	261
Clinical Features	261
Differential Diagnosis	261
Comorbidities	262
Course and Prognosis	262
Treatment	262
Agoraphobia	262
Diagnostic Criteria	263
Epidemiology	263
Aetiology	263
Clinical Features	263
Comorbidities	263
Differential Diagnosis	263
Course and Prognosis	264
Treatment	264
Social Anxiety Disorder	264
Definition	264
Epidemiology	264
Aetiology and Risk Factors	264
Clinical Features	265
Course and Prognosis	265
Comorbidities	266
Generalized Anxiety Disorder	267
Definition	267
Clinical Features	267
Epidemiology	268
Comorbidities	268
Aetiology	268

Prognosis	269
Treatment	270
Specific Phobias	270
Epidemiology	270
Aetiology	270
Differential Diagnosis	271
Prognosis	271
Treatment	271

INTRODUCTION

Anxiety disorders are one of the most common psychiatric disorders, and they begin in childhood. The worldwide prevalence of anxiety disorders ranges from 0.9–28.3%, and among children, it is 6.5%. When abnormal anxiety causes clinically significant distress, impairment of daily activities or disruption in normal functioning, it becomes clinically relevant.

Anxiety disorders can be further classified based on symptoms into episodic (panic, phobias) and continuous (general anxiety disorders).

They are classified into:

1. General anxiety disorder
2. Panic disorder
3. Separation anxiety disorder
4. Specific phobias
5. Post-traumatic stress disorder
6. Social anxiety disorder

They can be differentiated from one another by the types of objects or situations that induce fear, anxiety or avoidance of a particular situation and the associated cognitive ideation. They are highly comorbid with each other.

CONCEPTS OF ANXIETY DISORDER

Fear is a primitive automatic neurophysiological state of alarm involving the *cognitive appraisal* of imminent threat or danger to the safety and security of an individual.

In other words, fear is an alarm response to real danger.

Anxiety is a complex cognitive, affective, physiological and behavioural response system (i.e., *threat mode*) that is activated when anticipated events or circumstances are deemed highly aversive because they are perceived as unpredictable, uncontrollable events that could potentially threaten the vital interests of an individual. In other words, *normal anxiety* is a response to threatening situations, an anticipation of future threat.

Abnormal anxiety is out of proportion to the threat, occurs when there is no threat and/or is more prolonged. Here the focus of attention is to the physiological response and not the external threat.

Physiological responses include increase in heart rate, blood pressure, breathing and muscle tension and increased sympathetic system activity in the form of increased tremors, sweating, polyuria and diarrhoea. These prepare for defence or escape ('fight or flight').

Cognitive changes noticed are increased attention to and concentration on the threatening situation and dysfunctional cognition. Affective changes are feelings of nervousness and agitation. Behavioral changes represents early defensive behaviours: mobilization, immobility, escape and avoidance.

PANIC DISORDER

A *panic attack* is a period of intense fear or apprehension that may last from minutes to hours. The important features of a panic attack are:

- anxiety builds up quickly
- the symptoms are severe
- the person fears a catastrophic outcome.

Per the DSM 5 criteria, it is associated with minimum of four of the following symptoms:

1. Palpitations
2. Sweating
3. Trembling or shaking
4. Sensations of shortness of breath
5. Feelings of choking
6. Chest pain or discomfort
7. Nausea or abdominal distress
8. Feeling dizzy or light-headed
9. PChills or heat sensations
10. Paresthesia (numbness or tingling sensations)
11. Derealization (feelings of unreality) or depersonalization (being detached from oneself)
12. Fear of losing control/'going crazy'
13. Fear of dying (sense of impending doom)

A Single Panic Attack Is Not Necessarily Indicative of a Psychiatric Disorder

According to DSM 5, a *panic disorder* is characterised by:

A. Recurrent panic attacks
B. *At least one of the attacks* has been followed by *1 month (or more)* of one or both of the following:
   1. Persistent concern about additional panic attacks or their consequences (e.g., losing control, having a heart attack, 'going crazy').
   2. A significant maladaptive change in behaviour related to the attacks (e.g., behaviours designed to avoid having panic attacks, such as avoidance of exercise or unfamiliar situations).
C. The disturbance is not attributable to the physiologic effects of a substance (e.g., a drug of abuse, a medication) or another medical condition (e.g., hyperthyroidism, cardiopulmonary disorders).
D. The disturbance is not better explained by another mental disorder (e.g., social anxiety/ separation anxiety, phobic objects)

Epidemiology

The lifetime prevalence is 1–4%. It is two to three times more common in women than in men. The mean age of onset is 25 years, and the disorder peaks in the late teens and early 20s.

Aetiology

A. *Neuroanatomical changes:* Abnormal interactions between hippocampus, amygdala and para-hippocampal cortex, with amygdala hypersensitivity to environmental cues.
B. *Neurochemistry:*
   1. Dysfunction of the norepinephrine (NE) system – unrestrained and excessive system activation
   2. Hypothalamo-pituiatry axis (HPA) dysfunction – excessive cortisol release
   3. Persistently increased corticotropin-releasing hormone (CRH) concentration
   4. Dopaminergic system – high levels of dopamine in prefrontal cortex
   5. Serotonergic system – low activity of postsynaptic 5-HT1A receptors
C. *Panicogens:* Panic-inducing substances (sometimes called panicogens) induce panic attacks in most patients with panic disorder. They act by causing respiratory stimulation and a shift in the acid–base balance. Carbon dioxide (5–35% mixtures), sodium lactate and bicarbonate as considered panicogens. Consumption of coffee, nicotine, alcohol and other substances can also precipitate a panic attack.
D. *Genetic factors:* Panic disorder is familial, with approximately a five-time increased risk in first-degree relatives. The heritability rate is around 40%.
E. *Psychosocial factors:* Psychoanalytic theories consider panic attacks to arise from an unsuccessful defence against anxiety-provoking impulses. A mild signal anxiety becomes an overwhelming feeling of apprehension, complete with somatic symptoms. Experiencing loss in childhood and a history of child sexual/physical abuse are some of the risk factors.

Typical defence mechanisms seen in individuals with panic disorder are reaction formation, undoing, externalization and somatization.

Clinical Features

The first panic attack is generally completely spontaneous, although some may follow periods of excitement, physical exertion, sexual activity or moderate emotional trauma. Hence, a detailed history taking is imperative. The attack usually begins with a 10-minute period of rapidly escalating symptoms reaching a peak. The major symptoms are extreme fear and a sense of impending death and doom. The physical signs are tachycardia, palpitations, dyspnoea and sweating. The attack generally lasts 20 to 30 minutes and rarely exceeds an hour.

Differential Diagnosis

A. *Medical conditions which can mimic a panic attack are as follows:*
   1. Cardiovascular diseases: Anaemia, hypertension, mitral valve prolapse
   2. Endocrine disorders: Hyperthyroidism, pheochromocytoma, hypoparathyroidism, hypoglycaemia
   3. Respiratory disorders: Pulmonary embolism, asthma, hyperventilation
   4. Neurological disorders: Epilepsy, migraine
B. *Psychiatric conditions:*
   1. Specific phobias: The panic attack is in the presence of a specific stimulus (e.g., elevators in the case of claustrophobia, a building terrace in the case of acrophobia)

2. Substance intoxication: Amphetamines, cannabis, cocaine, hallucinogens
   3. Substance withdrawal: Alcohol, opioids, sedatives-hypnotics
   4. PTSD may be associated with panic attacks
   5. OCD may be associated with panic attacks

Comorbidities

Depression, specific phobias, obsessive-compulsive disorder and generalized anxiety disorder are the common comorbidities associated with panic disorder.

Course and Prognosis

The disorder is usually a chronic condition with variable outcome among patients. On long-term follow-up, around 50% of patients have mild symptoms, 10–20% have significant symptoms and 30–40% are symptom free. The disorder has a negative impact on the personal and professional life of the individual – work absenteeism and marital discord are often witnessed. Patients with good pre-morbid functioning, absence of comorbid conditions and a shorter duration of symptoms have a better prognosis.

Treatment

A. *Pharmacotherapy:*
   1. SSRIs: Considered the first-line treatment. Paroxetine, sertraline, fluoxetine and escitalopram are commonly used.
   2. Benzodiazepines: Clonazepam and alprazolam are used during the initial phases of the treatment and later on an SOS basis during an attack.
   3. Serotonin-norepinephrine reuptake inhibitors (SNRIs): Venlafaxine, desvenlafaxine, in case SSRIs prove ineffective.
   4. TCAs: Clomipramine, imipramine are considered very effective.

B. *Psychotherapy:*
   1. *Psycho-education:* This goes a long way in reducing the morbidity of the disorder. It entails explaining to the patient that the physical symptoms are caused by anxiety and, though frightening, are harmless. Relaxation, grounding techniques and minimizing avoidance (safety) behaviours should be explained to the patient. Progressive muscle relaxation is very useful in the initial phase of the treatment. Gathering support of family members is also essential in the management.
   2. *Cognitive behaviour therapy*: Works at reducing the fears of the physical effects of anxiety, which are considered to provoke and maintain the panic attacks. Common fears seen are that palpitations indicate an impending heart attack or that dizziness indicates impending loss of consciousness. In treatment, the physical symptoms that the patient fears are induced by hyperventilation or exercise. The therapist then points out the sequence of physical symptoms that leads to fear and explains that a similar sequence occurs in the early stages of a panic attack.

AGORAPHOBIA

Agoraphobia is a condition wherein the person experiences anxiety in unfamiliar situations from which they feel they cannot escape or in which they perceive they have little control. This anxiety leads to avoidance of those situations. It is derived from the Greek word 'agora,' which means marketplace. The anxiety and avoidance behaviour persist for more than 6 months.

Diagnostic Criteria

The DSM-5 diagnostic criteria for agoraphobia are as follows: marked fear or anxiety about *at least one situation from two or more of five situation* groups: (1) using public transportation (e.g., bus, train, cars, planes), (2) in an open space (e.g., park, shopping centre, parking lot), (3) in an enclosed space (e.g., stores, elevators, theatres), (4) in a crowd or standing in line, or (5) alone outside of the home. The fear or anxiety must be *persistent and last for a minimum of 6 months*

Epidemiology

The mean age of onset is 20 years, with the disorder peaking in the late teens and early 20s. Agoraphobia without panic is a rarer entity than with co-existing panic disorder.

Aetiology

1. *Biological:* Excessive activation of the NE system and dysfunctional HPA axis are the mechanisms involved.
2. *Psychosocial:* Individuals are generally described as having dependent traits. A childhood characterised by overprotective parents could also contribute.

Clinical Features

These individuals usually avoid markets, public transport, crowded shops and empty streets. Anticipatory anxiety may occur several hours before the person has to enter the feared place/situation. Anxious thoughts are common, with the predominant themes being loss of control and fainting.

Comorbidities

Panic disorder is the most common comorbidity. Depressive disorders are seen in approximately 33 to 52% of cases. Social phobias are also found in around 50% of the patients. Other anxiety disorders and substance use disorders are also seen as comorbidities.

Differential Diagnosis

1. Specific phobias: The anxiety pertains to a specific situation only (e.g., fear of heights – avoidance of only those places).
2. Social anxiety disorder: The person avoids going outside out of fear of being judged/being embarrassed and not because of fear of being unable to escape from the situation.
3. Separation anxiety disorder: The fear is of being away from the attachment figure.
4. PTSD: The avoidance is for specific situations which trigger the traumatic memories.
5. OCD: Avoidance is due to fear of contamination.
6. Generalized anxiety disorder: The worries are usually regarding all aspects of life and not confined to travel/being in unfamiliar situations.

Course and Prognosis

As the disorder progresses, the avoidance increases, and eventually the person may be confined to their home. The anxiety is often reduced by the presence of a trusted friend/companion or a reassuring object such as a few anxiolytic tablets which are carried but may not be consumed. The individual may become heavily dependent on friends/spouse/relatives for activities such as shopping, which can later lead to interpersonal issues. In severe cases, the person may eventually be confined to their home.

The disorder generally has a chronic course. It may be one of the most disabling phobias, as it leads to interference at work and in social settings.

Treatment

1. *Psycho-education:* The patients can be told that the panic symptoms that often occur are akin to a false alarm (can be compared to a oversensitive smoke sensor) activated as a result of chronic stress. The avoidance symptoms can be compared to anxiety from driving a car after an accident. These analogies help the patient and family member to understand the basis of the illness. Family support goes a long way, but at the same time they should be warned about over-involvement, which can impede the treatment.
2. *Cognitive behaviour therapy:* This involves exposure to the provoking situations in a graded manner and cognitive restructuring for the anxiety/panic symptoms that follow. Prior to this, basic relaxation techniques must be taught to the patient, to be practised on a regular basis before exposure is tried.
3. *Virtual therapy*: Recently, computer programs have been developed that allow patients to see themselves as avatars who are then placed in open or crowded spaces (parking lots, bridges, markets, fields). As the sessions progress, they are able to overcome their anxiety via deconditioning.
4. *Pharmacotherapy:* Must be offered at the outset, especially in case of panic attacks. SSRIs are generally preferred along with short-term usage of benzodiazepines to overcome the panic attacks.

SOCIAL ANXIETY DISORDER

Definition

Social anxiety disorder is defined as marked fear or anxiety about one or more social situations in which the individual is exposed to possible scrutiny by others. They are concerned about being negatively evaluated for their performance or interpersonal interactions. It is also called social phobia.

Epidemiology

Epidemiological studies have shown a current worldwide prevalence of 5 to 10% and a lifetime prevalence of 8.4 to 15%. Age of onset is usually during adolescence, the average being 10–16 years of age. It is more common in females.

Aetiology and Risk Factors

Genetics: First-degree relatives of the individuals with the disorder have a greater risk of developing it than the general population. Concordance rates are higher for monozygotic twins than dizygotic twins (34 vs 17).

Neurochemicals: Imbalance in the neurotransmitter system, that is, dopaminergic, serotonergic, GABAnergic and glutamate system. Dysregulation of hypothalamic pituitary axis function with elevated levels of corticotropin-releasing hormone.
Neuroimaging: Increased involvement of limbic and paralimbic system.
Psychosocial factors:
- *Parents:* Overprotective parents, insecure attachments with parents.
- Early childhood experiences such as childhood maltreatment and adversity.
- *Temperament:* Behavioural inhibition temperament in children, which is characterized by avoidance behaviour and increased physiological reactivity during a challenging situation.
- Non-face-to-face communication such as greater social media usage and increased digital connectivity.
- Less education.
- Low socioeconomic status.

Clinical Features

It is characterized by fear or anxiety out of proportion to the actual threat posed by the social situations. It is persistent and lasting for more than 6 months. It can cause clinically significant distress or impairment in social, occupational or other important areas of functioning.

Situations: Places that provoke anxiety include restaurants, canteens, dinner parties, seminars and board meetings. Situations that provoke anxiety include whenever it is necessary to speak in public; meeting unfamiliar people; performing in front of others; and actions that are being observed and open to scrutiny, for example, writing, eating or drinking in front of another person. Anticipatory anxiety is present when the person anticipates entering anxiety-provoking social situations.

Avoidance: Complete or partial avoidance of social situations in the form of failing to initiate or maintain conversation or sitting in an inconspicuous place in a social event. Presentation in children and adolescents: Anxiety must occur during interaction with peers as well as adults. It may be expressed by crying, tantrums, freezing, clinging, shrinking or failing to speak (mutism) in social situations and school refusal. They are often more emotionally sensitive than peers and more easily brought to tears and frequently present with somatic complaints such as nausea, vomiting, stomach aches, unexplained pain in various parts of the body, sore throat and flu-like symptoms.

Adolescents and adults complain of classical somatic experiences such as cardiovascular and respiratory symptoms – palpitations, dizziness, faintness, hyperventilation and feelings of strangulation.

Physical signs: Avoiding gaze, trembling of the hands, low tone of voice, stuttering, autonomic hyperactivity.

Some people use alcohol to relieve anxiety. Hence, alcohol abuse is more common in them compared to people with other phobias. They commonly have low self-esteem and perfectionism traits.

Course and Prognosis

It emerges in early adolescent years. In late adolescence, it has a waxing and waning course with progressive worsening or persistence of symptoms in adulthood. The factors responsible for persistence are early onset, behavioural inhibition and harm avoidance temperament, parental social anxiety and depression, severe impairment and avoidance, co-occurrence of panic and increased anxiety cognitions. If left untreated, it can result in lower educational and occupational achievement, low socioeconomic status and financial problems, poor development of social skills, development of substance use, development of depression and suicidal ideas/attempts, difficulty in maintaining relationships and remaining unmarried.

Comorbidities

Other anxiety disorders, mood disorders, post-traumatic stress disorder, selective mutism, autism, substance use disorders and body dysmorphic disorder.

DIFFERENTIAL DIAGNOSIS

- Separation anxiety disorder: Concerns about being apart from caregiver not associated with fear of possible potential scrutiny by others and being embarrassed.
- Generalized anxiety disorder: Presence of global worry not associated with fear of potential scrutiny by others and being embarrassed.
- Depressive disorder: Presence of the core symptoms low mood, anhedonia and loss of energy.
- Schizophrenia: Presentations can be similar during premorbid symptoms of schizophrenia and when paranoid delusions are present.
- Anxious/avoidant personality disorder: it develops more gradually and is characterized by lifelong shyness and lack of self-confidence.
- Panic disorder with agoraphobia: Here panic attacks are typically unexpected and are not associated with anticipation of negative evaluation by others.
- Autism: Distinguished by other features such as difficulty in verbal and non-verbal communication, difficulty maintaining relationships, language delay, stereotypy and repetitive and restricted behaviours.
- Substance use disorder: Similarities during intoxication or during withdrawal.
- Medical: Parkinson's, medication induced tremors.

MANAGEMENT

Assessment instruments: Social Phobia Inventory (SPIN), Mini-SPIN, Liebowitz Social Anxiety Scale (LSAS), Liebowitz Self-Rated Disability Scale, Brief Social Phobia Scale (BSPS), Social Phobia Safety Behaviors Scale and Self Statements During Public Speaking Scale

Diagnostic criteria: Diagnosis is made with DSM-5 criteria and ICD 11 criteria.

Treatment

GENERAL MEASURES

- Psychoeducation of patient and family members about the disorder, treatment options and duration of treatment, side effects of medications, course and prognosis.
- Problem-solving techniques.
- Relaxation techniques: Jacobson's progressive muscle relaxation, breathing retraining to manage hyperventilation episodes.

PSYCHOTHERAPY

- Self-help books can be suggested based on cognitive behavioural techniques
- Group/computerized and individual cognitive behavioural therapy
- Graded-exposure therapy – systemic desensitization
- Social effectiveness therapy for children – enhancing social skills

- Coping CBT for children
- Teaching alternative coping techniques

PHARMACOTHERAPY

- Antidepressants: SSRIs – paroxetine, fluvoxamine, escitalopram and sertraline; SNRIs – venlafaxine, buspirone.
- Anxiolytics: Short-term benzodiazepines such as alprazolam, clonazepam.
- Beta blockers: Propranolol.

GENERALIZED ANXIETY DISORDER

Definition

This disorder is characterised by excessive anxiety and worry about several events or activities for most days during at least a 6-month period. Usually the worry that the patient feels is difficult to control and is often associated with somatic symptoms, such as muscle tension, irritability, difficulty sleeping and restlessness. The anxiety caused during this is not secondary to another disorder, is not caused by substance use or a general medical condition and does not occur only during a mood or psychiatric disorder. The anxiety is difficult to control and is subjectively distressing. Its presence produces impairment in important areas of a person's life.

Clinical Features

All of the symptoms of anxiety can occur in generalized anxiety Disorder (GAD), but there is a characteristic pattern, which consists of the following features:

1. *Worry and apprehension:* These are more prolonged than in healthy people. The worries are not focused on a specific issue as they are in panic disorder (i.e., on having a panic attack), social phobia (i.e., on being embarrassed) or OCD (i.e., on contamination). The person feels that these widespread worries are difficult to control.
2. *Psychological arousal:* Manifested as irritability, poor concentration and/or sensitivity to noise. Some patients complain of poor memory, but this is because of poor concentration. If true memory impairment is found, a careful search should be made for a cause other than anxiety.
3. *Autonomic overactivity:* Most often experienced as sweating, palpitations, dry mouth, epigastric discomfort and dizziness.
4. *Muscle tension:* Experienced as restlessness, trembling, inability to relax, headache (usually bilateral and frontal or occipital) and aching of the shoulders and back.
5. *Hyperventilation:* May lead to dizziness, tingling in the extremities and, paradoxically, a feeling of shortness of breath.
6. *Sleep disturbances:* Include difficulty in falling asleep and persistent worrying thoughts. Sleep is often intermittent, unrefreshing and accompanied by unpleasant dreams. Some patients have night terrors and wake suddenly feeling extremely anxious. Early-morning waking is not a feature of GAD, and its presence strongly suggests a depressive disorder.
7. Other features, which include tiredness, depressive symptoms, obsessional symptoms and depersonalization. These symptoms are never the most prominent feature of GAD. If they are prominent, another diagnosis should be considered (see the section on differential diagnosis).

Epidemiology

GAD prevalence rates range from 3–8% in 1 year. The ratio of women to men with the disorder is about 2 to 1, but the ratio of women to men who are receiving inpatient treatment for the disorder is about 1 to 1. This disorder usually has its onset in late adolescence or early adulthood, but cases are commonly seen in older adults. GAD is associated with several indices of social disadvantage, including lower household income and unemployment, as well as divorce and separation.

Comorbidities

Often coexists with another mental disorder, usually social phobia, specific phobia, panic disorder or a depressive disorder. As many as 50 to 90% of patients with generalized anxiety disorder have another coexisting mental disorder. About 25% of patients eventually experience panic disorder.

A high percentage of patients are likely to have major depressive disorder, dysthymic disorder and substance-related disorders.

Aetiology

Neurobiological Basis

- The neurobiological mechanisms involved in GAD are mostly those that mediate normal anxiety.
- The amygdala plays a key role, which receives sensory information both directly from the thalamus and from a longer pathway involving the somatosensory cortex and anterior cingulate cortex.
- The hippocampus is also believed to have an important role in the regulation of anxiety, because it relates fearful memories to relevant present contexts.
- Noradrenergic neurons which originate in the locus coeruleus increase arousal and anxiety, whereas 5-HT neurons that arise in the raphe nuclei have much more complex effects and serve both to signal the presence of anxiety-producing stimuli in the environment and also to restrain the associated behavioural responses.
- Gamma-aminobutyric acid (GABA) receptors, which are widely distributed in the brain, are inhibitory and reduce anxiety, as do the associated benzodiazepine-binding sites.
- There is probably also an important role for corticotropin-releasing hormone, which increases anxiety-related behaviours and is found in high concentration in the amygdala.
- However, although pharmacological manipulation of 5-HT and GABA mechanisms can be helpful in the treatment of generalized anxiety, there is no firm evidence that changes in these neurotransmitters are fundamentally involved in the pathophysiology of the disorder.

Personality

GAD is associated with neuroticism, and twin studies have shown an overlap between the genetic factors related to neuroticism and those related to GAD. GAD occurs in people with anxious–avoidant personality disorders but also in individuals with other personality disorders.

Cognitive Behavioral Theory

Particular coping and cognitive styles may also predispose individuals to the development of GAD, although it is not always easy to distinguish predisposition from the abnormal cognitions that are seen in the illness itself. Studies show it's likely that people who lack a sense of control of events and of personal effectiveness, perhaps because of early life experiences, are more prone to anxiety disorders. Such individuals may also demonstrate trait-like cognitive biases in the form of increased attention to potentially threatening stimuli, overestimation of environmental threat and enhanced memory of threatening material. This has been referred to as the looming cognitive style, which appears to be a general psychological vulnerability factor for a number of anxiety disorders. However, this can lead to 'worry about worry', when a person comes to believe, for example, that worrying in this way, although necessary for them, is also uncontrollable and harmful. This 'metacognitive belief' may form a transition between excessive but normal worrying and GAD.

Stressful Events

Clinical observations indicate that GADs often begin in relation to stressful events, and some become chronic when stressful problems persist.

Genetic Factors

Overall, the findings suggest that genes play a significant although moderate role in the aetiology of GAD but that the genes involved predispose one to a range of anxiety and depressive disorders rather than GAD specifically.

Early Experiences

Studies suggest that there is a strong relationship with adverse events in childhood and anxiety disorders. Parenting styles characterized by overprotection and lack of emotional warmth may also be a risk factor for GAD, as well as for other anxiety and depressive disorders in offspring.

Psychoanalytic Theory

Studies suggest that anxiety arises from an intrapsychic conflict in the mind. In GADs, the ego is readily overwhelmed because it has been weakened by a development failure in childhood. Normally, children overcome this anxiety through secure relationships with loving parents. However, if they do not achieve this security, as adults they will be vulnerable to anxiety when experiencing separation or potentially threatening events. Thus both psychoanalytic ideas and objective studies suggest that good parenting can protect against anxiety by giving the child a secure emotional base from which to explore an uncertain world.

Prognosis

The high incidence of comorbid mental disorders in these patients makes the clinical course and prognosis of the disorder difficult to predict. The occurrence of several negative life events greatly increases the likelihood that the disorder will develop. Overall, generalized anxiety disorder is a chronic condition that may well be lifelong.

Treatment

The most effective treatment of generalized anxiety disorder is probably one that combines psychotherapeutic, pharmacotherapeutic and supportive approaches. The treatment may take a significant amount of time for the involved clinician, whether the clinician is a psychiatrist, a family practitioner or another specialist.

SPECIFIC PHOBIAS

Phobia refers to an excessive fear of a specific object, circumstance or situation.

A person with a specific phobia is inappropriately anxious in the presence of a particular object or situation. In the presence of that object or situation, the person experiences intense symptoms of anxiety.

CLINICAL FEATURES

1. Anticipatory anxiety is common.
2. Avoidance behaviour: patient usually seeks to escape from and avoid the feared situation.
3. Presence of severe anxiety on exposure to the phobic stimulus.
4. Perhaps as another way to avoid the stress of the phobic stimulus, many patients have substance-related disorders, particularly alcohol use disorders.
5. Almost one-third of patients with social phobia have major depressive disorder.
6. On the mental status examination, there is the presence of an irrational and ego-dystonic fear of a specific situation, activity or object; patients are able to describe how they avoid contact with the phobia. Depression is commonly found in the mental status examination and may be present in as many as one-third of all patients with phobia.
7. Specific phobias can be characterized further by adding the name of the stimulus (e.g., spider phobia).
   - Acrophobia: fear of heights
   - Agoraphobia: fear of open spaces
   - Ailurophobia: fear of cats
   - Claustrophobia: fear of closed spaces
   - Cynophobia: fear of dogs
   - Hydrophobia: fear of water
   - Mysophobia: fear of dirt and germs
   - Pyrophobia: fear of fire
   - Xenophobia: fear of strangers
   - Zoophobia: fear of animals

Epidemiology

The lifetime prevalence of specific phobia is about 10%.

Specific phobia is the most common mental disorder among women and the second most common among men, second only to substance-related disorders.

The age of onset of most specific phobias is in childhood.

Aetiology

1. *Persistence of childhood fears:* Most specific phobias in adulthood are a continuation of childhood phobias. Specific phobias are common in childhood.

2. *Genetic factors:* In one study, 31% of first-degree relatives of people with specific phobia also had the condition. Genetic vulnerability may involve differences in the strength of fear conditioning, which has a heritability of around 40%. The blood-injection-injury type has a particularly high familial tendency. Two-thirds to three-fourths of affected patients have at least one first-degree relative with specific phobia of the same type, although there is no statistical data stating the same.
3. *Psychoanalytical theories:* They suggest that phobias are not related to the obvious external stimulus but to an internal source of anxiety. The internal source is excluded from consciousness by repression and attached to the external object by displacement.
4. *Cognitive theories:* according to this, specific phobias arise through association learning. A minority of specific phobias appear to begin in this way in adulthood in relation to a highly stressful experience. Some specific phobias may be acquired by observational learning, as the child observes another person's fear responses and learns to fear the same stimuli.
5. *Prepared learning*: This term refers to an innate predisposition to develop persistent fear responses to certain stimuli. Some young primates seem to be prepared to develop fears of snakes, but it is not certain whether the same process accounts for some of the specific phobias of human children.
6. *Neural mechanisms*: There is significant hyperactivity of the amygdala upon presentation of the feared stimulus, which appears to diminish with successful treatment. Anticipation of a phobic stimulus activates the anterior cingulate cortex and the insular cortex. Imaging studies show that specific phobias are characterized by increased activation in the regions linked to emotional appraisal and fear (amygdala, insula, anterior cingulate)

Differential Diagnosis

1. Depression: the possibility of an underlying depressive disorder should always be kept in mind, since some patients seek help for long-standing specific phobias when a depressive disorder makes them less able to tolerate their phobic symptoms.
2. Obsessional disorders: present with fear and avoidance of certain objects (e.g., knives). In such cases a systematic history and mental state examination will reveal the associated obsessional thoughts (e.g., thoughts of harming a person with a knife).
3. Nonpsychiatric medical conditions that can result in the development of a phobia include the use of substances (particularly hallucinogens and sympathomimetics), CNS tumours and cerebrovascular diseases.
4. Schizophrenia: phobic symptoms can occur as a part of psychosis.

Prognosis

Specific phobias that originate in childhood continue for many years, whereas those that start after stressful events in adulthood have a better prognosis.

Treatment

1. Behavioral therapy: The main mode of treatment is the exposure form of behaviour therapy. The phobia is usually reduced considerably in intensity, and so is the social disability. But the phobia might not go away completely. The outcome depends importantly on repeated and prolonged exposure.

2. B-adrenergic receptor antagonists: These are useful in the treatment of specific phobia, especially when the phobia is associated with panic attacks. Pharmacotherapy (e.g., benzodiazepines), psychotherapy or combined therapy directed to the attacks may also be of benefit.

Bibliography

1. Baxter A, Scott JM, Vos T, Whiteford H. Global prevalence of anxiety disorders: A systematic review and meta-regression. *Psychological Medicine.* 2013;43:897–910.
2. Polanczyk GV, Salum GA, Sugaya LS, Caye A, Rohde LA. Annual research review: A meta-analysis of the worldwide prevalence of mental disorders in children and adolescents. *J Child Psychol Psychiatry.* 2015;56(3):345–365.
3. American Psychiatric Association. *Diagnostic and statistical manual of mental disorders (DSM-5 (R)).* 5th ed. Arlington, TX: American Psychiatric Association Publishing; 2013.
4. Boland R, Verduin M, Ruiz P. *Kaplan & Sadock's synopsis of psychiatry.* 12th ed. Baltimore, MD: Wolters Kluwer Health; 2021.
5. Geddes JR, Andreasen NC. *New Oxford textbook of psychiatry.* Oxford, USA: Oxford University Press; 2020 Feb 20.
6. Clark DA, Beck AT. *Cognitive therapy of anxiety disorders: Science and practice.* UK: Guilford Press; 2011 Aug 10.
7. Sadock B, Sadock V, Ruiz P. *Kaplan and Sadock's comprehensive textbook of psychiatry.* UK: Wolters Kluwer Health. 2017.
8. Harrison P, Cowen P, Burns T, Fazel M. *Shorter Oxford textbook of psychiatry.* New York, NY: Oxford University Press. 2018.
9. Rose GM, Tadi P. Social anxiety disorder. StatPearls [Internet]. 2021.
10. Norris LA, Kendall PC. A close look into coping cat: Strategies within an empirically supported treatment for anxiety in youth. *Journal of Cognitive Psychotherapy.* 2020 Jan 9;34(1):4–20.

25
Optimizing Patient Care in Sleep Disorders

Karishma Rupani and Shilpa Adarkar

Introduction	273
Functions of Sleep	273
Sleep Requirements	274
Sleep–Wake Rhythm	274
Sleep Disorder Classification	275
Conclusion	283

INTRODUCTION

Sleep is one of the most significant of human behaviors, occupying roughly one-third of human life. Sleep is a complex biological process. It is a reversible state of unconsciousness in which there is reduced metabolism and motor activity. Sleep disorders are one of the most common clinical problems encountered in outpatient settings and inpatient settings. Sleep is an essential process for proper brain functioning and serves a restorative and homeostatic function and appears to be crucial for normal thermoregulation and energy conservation. Approximately 10% to 30% of adults experience a sleep disorder during their lifetime, and over half do not seek treatment. Lack of sleep can lead to the inability to concentrate, memory complaints, and deficits in neuropsychological testing. Additionally, sleep disorders can have serious consequences, including fatal accidents related to sleepiness. Disturbed sleep can be a primary diagnosis itself or a component of another medical or psychiatric disorder. Careful diagnosis and specific treatment are essential. Female sex, advanced age, medical and mental disorders, and substance abuse are associated with an increased prevalence of sleep disorders. (1)

FUNCTIONS OF SLEEP

It has been observed that there is a 5–25% decrease in metabolic rate during night sleep. Conservation of energy therefore appears to be one of the important functions of sleep. It also has a restorative function for the whole body (particularly during NREM-sleep) and for the brain (cognitive functions; especially during REM-sleep). On the other hand, those with sleep disorders carry a higher mortality, for example, coronary artery disease, nocturnal asthma, and sudden nocturnal death. Additionally, sleep deprivation may lead to ego disorganization, hallucinations, and delusions.

Sleep Requirements

Short sleepers require fewer than 6 hours of sleep, while long sleepers need more than 9 hours each night to function adequately. Short sleepers are generally efficient, ambitious, socially adept, and content. Long sleepers tend to be mildly depressed, anxious, and socially withdrawn. (2)

Sleep–Wake Rhythm

Sleep–wake cycles are governed by a complex group of biological processes that serve as internal clocks. The suprachiasmatic nucleus, located in the hypothalamus, is thought to be the body's anatomic timekeeper, responsible for the release of melatonin on a 24.8-hour cycle. The pineal gland secretes less melatonin when exposed to bright light; therefore, the level of this chemical is lowest during the daytime hours of wakefulness.

Multiple neurotransmitters are also thought to play a role in sleep. These include serotonin from the dorsal raphe nucleus, norepinephrine contained in the neurons with cell bodies in the locus ceruleus, and acetylcholine from the pontine reticular formation and gamma aminobutyric acid (GABA). Dopamine, on the other hand, is associated with wakefulness. (2)

Abnormalities in the delicate balance of all of these chemical messenger systems may disrupt various phases of sleep. The circadian rhythm develops over the first 2 years of life. Sleep patterns are not physiologically the same when a person sleeps in the daytime or during the time when they are accustomed to being awake; the psychological and behavioral effects of sleep differ as well.

Stages of Sleep

NREM Sleep Stages

Sleep consists of two physiologic states: rapid eye movement (REM) sleep and non-rapid eye movement (NREM) sleep. NREM sleep consists of four sleep stages, named stage I through stage IV. Dreaming occurs mostly in REM sleep, but additionally, some dreaming occurs in stage III and IV sleep. Sleep is measured with a polysomnograph, which simultaneously measures brain activity (electroencephalogram [EEG]), eye movement (electro-oculogram), and muscle tone (electromyogram). Other physiologic tests can be applied during sleep and measured along with the previous. (2)

EEG findings are used to describe sleep stages as follows:

1. Awake: Low voltage, random, very fast EEG waves.

NREM Sleep

- Stage I: Theta waves (3–7 CPS), slight slowing.
- Stage II: Further slowing, K complex (triphasic complexes), sleep spindles, true sleep onset.
- Stage III: Delta waves (0.5–2 CPS), high-amplitude slow waves.
- Stage IV: At least 50% delta waves. Stages III and IV constitute delta sleep.

REM Sleep

Sawtooth waves, similar to drowsy sleep on EEG.
Characteristics of REM sleep (also called paradoxical sleep)

1. Autonomic instability
    a. Increased heart rate (HR), blood pressure (BP), and respiratory rate (RR).
    b. EEG appears similar to that of a patient who is awake.
2. Tonic inhibition of skeletal muscle tone leading to paralysis.
3. Rapid eye movements.
4. Dreaming.
6. Relative poikilothermia (cold-bloodedness).
7. Penile tumescence or vaginal lubrication.

Sleep Disorder Classification

The DSM-5 classifies sleep disorders on the basis of clinical diagnostic criteria and presumed etiology. The sleep–wake disorders described in DSM-5 provide a framework for clinical assessment. The current classification includes the following sleep disorders each of which is described in detail in the following.

Insomnia Disorder

DSM-5 defines insomnia disorder as dissatisfaction with sleep quantity or quality associated with one or more of the following symptoms:

A. Difficulty in initiating sleep; difficulty in maintaining sleep, with frequent awakenings or problems returning to sleep; and early morning awakening with inability to return to sleep.
B. Insomnia can be categorized in terms of how it affects sleep (e.g., sleep-onset insomnia, sleep-maintenance insomnia, or early-morning awakening). Insomnia can also be classified according to its duration (e.g., transient, short term, and long term).

Primary insomnia is diagnosed by nonrestorative sleep or difficulty in initiating or maintaining sleep, and the complaint continues for at least a month (according to ICD-10, the disturbance must occur at least three times a week for a month). Insomnia is the most common type of sleep disorder. (3)

Approach to Sleep Disorders

HISTORY AND PHYSICAL EXAMINATION

An accurate and detailed history from the patient, bed partner, or family member combined with a sleep questionnaire can elicit critical information. Most sleep complaints fall into three categories: insomnia (sleep onset, maintenance, or early morning awakening); excessive sleepiness; or abnormal behaviors during sleep. The procedure is as follows.

- Inquire into the chief complaint, when symptom(s) started; the pattern since onset; and associated factors (medical, environmental, occupational, psychological/stress, lifestyle choices) that may have predisposed to or precipitated the illness, perpetuated the condition, and improved or worsened symptoms.
- Assess the impact of the sleep complaint on the patient's life and inquire about meal and sleep schedules, sleep hygiene, restless leg sensation, snoring, witnessed apnoeic episodes, sweating, coughing, gasping/choking/snorting, dryness of the mouth, bruxism, excessive movements during sleep, periodic limb movements, any abnormal behaviors during sleep, daytime sleepiness. Ask about caffeine intake, alcohol and nicotine use, as well as use of illicit drugs.

- Review the medical/surgical/psychiatric history and past treatments and their efficacy or lack thereof.
- Determine if there is any family history of sleep disorders (snoring, narcolepsy, restless leg syndrome).
- A completed 2-week sleep log or sleep diary can be utilized to compute sleep efficiency, total sleep time, and number of awakenings during the night and can be used to diagnose sleep disorders and monitor efficacy of treatment. On the basis of the information from questionnaires and sleep diaries, the chief complaint, and the history, a working diagnosis is outlined.

There are non-pharmacological and pharmacological treatment modalities for insomnia.

SLEEP HYGIENE MEASURES (NON-PHARMACOLOGICAL)

1. Arise at the same time daily.
2. Limit daily in-bed time to the usual amount before the sleep disturbance.
3. Discontinue CNS-acting drugs (caffeine, nicotine, alcohol, stimulants).
4. Avoid daytime naps (except when a sleep chart shows they induce better night sleep).
5. Establish physical fitness by means of a graded program of vigorous exercise early in the day.
6. Avoid evening stimulation; substitute radio or relaxed reading for television.
7. Eat at regular times daily; avoid large meals near bedtime.
8. Practice evening relaxation routines, such as progressive muscle relaxation or meditation.
9. Maintain comfortable sleeping conditions.

COGNITIVE RESTRUCTURING

Paradoxical intention is a form of cognitive restructuring to alleviate performance anxiety and is based on the premise that performance anxiety hinders sleep onset.

It is a method that consists of persuading a patient to engage in his most feared behavior, that is, staying awake.

Relaxation treatments include progressive muscle relaxation (PMR), imagery training, meditation, and biofeedback. (4)

If the difficulty in initiating sleep is the main symptom, then a benzodiazepine with a shorter half-life should be used, such as temazepam, oxazepam, or lorazepam. If the difficulty in maintaining sleep is the predominant symptom, then a longer-acting benzodiazepine, such as nitrazepam, lorazepam, or even diazepam, should be used. Physicians should be careful to avoid benzodiazepine abuse or dependence in patients presenting with insomnia. Non-benzodiazepine hypnotics such as zolpidem and trazodone are useful alternatives. (5)

PHARMACOLOGICAL TREATMENT

Table 25.1 Common drugs used in the management of insomnia.

Class of drugs	Drugs	Commonly used dosages
Benzodiazepines	Lorazepam	1 mg to 3 mg
	Chlordiazepoxide	10 mg to 30 mg
	Oxazepam	10 mg to 30 mg
Non-benzodiazepine GABA agonists	Zolpidem	5 mg to 10 mg
Antidepressant	Trazodone	50 mg to 100 mg

Hypersomnolence Disorders

This is diagnosed when there is no other cause found for greater than 1 month of excessive somnolence (daytime sleepiness) or excessive amounts of daytime sleep. Usually begins in childhood. Can be a consequence of (1) insufficient sleep, (2) basic neurologic dysfunction in brain systems regulating sleep, (3) disrupted sleep, or (4) the phase of an individual's circadian rhythm. Treatment consists of stimulant drugs. Also, drugs such as modafinal and armodafinal are used. (6), (7), (8)

1. **Types of hypersomnia**
   a. Kleine–Levin syndrome. Rare condition consisting of recurrent periods of prolonged sleep (from which patients may be aroused) with intervening periods of normal sleep and alert waking.
      1. It is a periodic disorder of episodic hypersomnolence.
      2. Usually affects young men, ages 10 to 21.
      3. May sleep excessively for several weeks and awaken only to eat (voraciously).
      4. Associated with hypersexuality, extreme hostility, irritability, and occasionally hallucinations during episodes.
      5. Amnesia follows attacks.
      6. May resolve spontaneously after several years.
      7. Patients are normal between episodes.
      8. Treatment consists of stimulants (amphetamines, methylphenidate) for hypersomnia and preventive measures for other symptoms. Lithium also has been used successfully.
   b. Menstrual-related hypersomnia
      Recurrent episodes of hypersomnia related to the menstrual cycle, experiencing intermittent episodes of marked hypersomnia at, or shortly before, the onset of their menses.
   c. Idiopathic hypersomnia
      Disorder of excessive sleepiness in which patients do not have the symptoms associated with narcolepsy. It is associated with long non-refreshing naps, difficulty awakening, sleep drunkenness, and automatic behaviors with amnesia. Other symptoms include migraine-like headaches, fainting spells, syncope, and orthostatic hypotension.
   d. Hypersomnia due to a medical condition.
   e. Hypersomnia due to drug or substance abuse.

Treatment

Regularizing sleep periods and wakefulness-promoting drugs like modafinil can be used.

Narcolepsy

1. *Narcolepsy* consists of the following characteristics:
   a. Excessive daytime somnolence (sleep attacks) is the primary symptom of narcolepsy; this is distinguished from fatigue by irresistible sleep attacks of short duration (less than 15 minutes).
      The sleep attacks may be precipitated by monotonous or sedentary activity. The naps are highly refreshing.
2. *Cataplexy*
   This is reported by over 50% of narcoleptic patients. There are brief (seconds to minutes) episodes of muscle weakness or paralysis, without loss of consciousness if

the episode is brief. When the attack is over, the patient is completely normal. They may manifest as partial loss of muscle tone (weakness, slurred speech, buckled knees, dropped jaw) and are often triggered by laughter (common), anger (common), athletic activity, excitement, fear, or embarrassment. A diagnosis of cataplexy automatically results in a diagnosis of narcolepsy. If cataplexy does not occur, multiple other characteristics are necessary for the diagnosis of narcolepsy. (9)

3. *Sleep paralysis*
This is a temporary, partial, or complete paralysis in sleep–wake transitions. The patient remains conscious but is unable to move or their open eyes. This most commonly occurs on awakening and is very often described as an anxiety-provoking, 'scary' event. It generally lasts less than 1 minute.

4. *Hypnagogic and hypnopompic hallucinations*
These are dreamlike experiences during transition from wakefulness to sleep and vice versa. Vivid auditory or visual hallucinations occur either while falling asleep (hypnagogic) or on waking up (hypnopompic).

5. *Sleep-onset REM latency*
This is reduced considerably and is defined as the appearance of REM sleep within 15 minutes of sleep onset (normally it takes approximately 70 to 90 minutes for REM sleep to begin).

Tests Used

Polysomnography and a multiple sleep latency test (MSLT), which measures excessive sleepiness. An MSLT consists of at least four recorded naps at 2-hour intervals. More than two such episodes are considered diagnostic of narcolepsy (seen in 70% of patients with narcolepsy, in fewer than 10% of patients with other hypersomnias).

Etiology

Narcolepsy is plausibly caused by an abnormality of REM-inhibiting mechanisms, and recent research involving hypocretin, a neurotransmitter, suggests that hypocretin is significantly reduced in narcolepsy patients.

Treatment

a. Regular bedtime.
b. Daytime naps scheduled at a regular time of day.
c. Safety considerations, such as caution while driving and avoiding furniture with sharp edges.
d. Stimulants (e.g., modafinil) for daytime sleepiness.
e. High-dose propranolol may be effective.
f. Tricyclics and selective serotonin reuptake inhibitors (SSRIs) are useful for REM-related symptoms, especially cataplexy.

Breathing-Related Sleep Disorders (10)

These disorders are characterized by sleep disruption that is caused by a sleep-related breathing disturbance, leading to excessive sleepiness, insomnia, or hypersomnia. Breathing disturbances include apneas, hypoapneas, and oxygen desaturation.

Apnea

The two types of sleep apnea are obstructive sleep apnea and central sleep apnea (CSA).

More than 40% of patients evaluated for somnolence using polysomnography are found to have sleep apnea. Sleep apnea may account for a number of unexplained deaths.

A. OBSTRUCTIVE SLEEP APNEA (OSA)

This is caused by cessation of air flow through the nose or mouth in the presence of continuing thoracic breathing movements, resulting in a decrease in arterial oxygen saturation and a transient arousal, after which respiration resumes normally.

This is typically seen in middle-aged, overweight men (Pickwickian syndrome) and also tends to occur more frequently in patients with smaller jaws or micrognathia, acromegaly, and hypothyroidism.

The main symptoms are loud snoring with intervals of apnea, extreme daytime sleepiness with long and unrefreshing daytime sleep attacks. Other symptoms include severe morning headaches, morning confusion, depression, and anxiety. Medical consequences include cardiac arrhythmias, systemic and pulmonary hypertension, and decreased sexual drive or function with progressive worsening without treatment.

The episodes of apnea occur in both REM and NREM sleep, and each event lasts 10 to 20 seconds. There are usually 5 to 10 events per hour of sleep. Patients are unaware of episodes of apnea.

Treatment consists of nasal continuous positive airway pressure (CPAP), uvulopharyngopalatoplasty, weight loss, buspirone, SSRIs, and tricyclic drugs. If a specific abnormality of the upper airway is found, surgical intervention is indicated, such as in those with inflamed adenoids.

PRECAUTIONS

Sedatives and alcohol should be avoided because they can considerably exacerbate the condition, which may then become life threatening.

B. CENTRAL SLEEP APNEA (CSA)

This is defined as the absence of breathing due to lack of respiratory effort. It is a disorder of ventilatory control, with repeated episodes of apneas and hypopneas occurring in a periodic or intermittent pattern during sleep caused by variability in respiratory effort. This is usually seen in the elderly.

TREATMENT

Consists of mechanical ventilation.

1. There are three subtypes of CSA:
   - Idiopathic CSA: They present with daytime sleepiness, insomnia, or awakening with shortness of breath.
   - Cheyne–Stokes breathing: Prolonged hyper-apneas alternate with apnea and hypopnea episodes that are associated with reduced ventilatory effort.

CSA could also be comorbid with opioid use: chronic use of long-acting opioid medications and impairment of neuromuscular respiratory control.

Circadian Rhythm Sleep Disorders (11)

This includes a wide range of conditions involving a misalignment between desired and actual sleep periods.

The six types are

1. delayed sleep phase,
2. advanced sleep phase type,
3. irregular sleep–wake type,
4. non–24-hour sleep–wake type,
5. shift work type, and
6. jet lag type.

Very often self-limited. Resolves as the body readjusts to new sleep–wake schedule.

Patients with delayed and advanced sleep phase insomnia can be treated with proper timing of bright light and behavioral changes. The goal of light therapy is to entrain the endogenous sleep–wake rhythm to coincide with the patient's social and occupational schedule. Melatonin administration can be utilized to entrain the circadian rhythm and may also be helpful in blind subjects.

Parasomnias (12)

This class of disorders are characterized by physiological or behavioral phenomena that occur during or are potentiated by sleep.

NREM Sleep Arousal Disorders

A. SLEEPWALKING DISORDER (SOMNAMBULISM)

This is characterized by a complex activity wherein there are brief episodes of leaving bed while asleep and walking about without full consciousness.

They often begin between the ages of 4 and 8 years, with peak prevalence at about 12 years of age; they generally disappear spontaneously with age. About 15% of children have an occasional episode and it is more common in boys. The patients often have a familial history of other parasomnias.

There is amnesia for the event, wherein the patient does not remember the episode. It usually occurs during deep NREM sleep (stage III and IV sleep). The patient can usually be guided back to bed. In adults and elderly persons, these episodes may reflect psychopathology of the central nervous system (CNS),

TREATMENT

Drugs that suppress stage IV sleep, such as benzodiazepines, can be used to treat somnambulism.

B. SLEEP TERROR DISORDER

This is characterized by sudden awakening with intense anxiety.

There is autonomic overstimulation, movement, crying out, increased heart rate, and diaphoresis. It is especially common in children (about 1% to 6%), more common in boys, and tends to run in families. The patient does not remember the event in the morning.

It occurs during deep, non-REM sleep, usually stage III or IV sleep, often within the first few hours of sleep. Occurrence starting in adolescence or later may be the first symptom of temporal lobe epilepsy. Treatment rarely needed in childhood. Awakening a child before night terror for several days may eliminate terrors for extended periods. In rare cases, when medication is required, diazepam in small doses at bedtime may be beneficial.

Parasomnias Usually Associated With REM Sleep (13)

a. *REM sleep behavior disorder* (including parasomnia overlap disorder and status dissociatus)
   1. Loss of atonia during REM sleep, with emergence of complex, often violent behaviors (acting out dreams). It is chronic and progressive, seen chiefly in elderly men. There is a potential for serious injury. Neurologic cause in many cases, such as small stroke or early Parkinson's disease, should be ruled out.
   Treatment is with 0.5 to 2.0 mg of clonazepam daily, or 100 mg of carbamazepine three times daily.
b. *Recurrent isolated sleep paralysis*
   1. Isolated symptom.
   2. Hypnagogic hallucinations.
   3. Last one to several minutes.
   4. Episode terminates with touch, noise (some external stimulus), or voluntary repetitive eye movements.

Nightmare Disorder

a. Nightmares are vivid dreams in which one awakens frightened.
b. About 50% of the adult population may report occasional nightmares.
c. Almost always occur during REM sleep.
d. Good recall (quite detailed) and less anxiety, vocalization, motility, and autonomic discharge than in sleep terrors.

No specific treatment is required unless severe, in which case benzodiazepines, tricyclic antidepressants, and SSRIs may be of help.

Other Parasomnias

a. *Sleep enuresis*
   Primary
   The patient urinates during sleep while in bed; if there is continuance of bed-wetting since infancy, it is called primary enuresis, whereas in secondary enuresis, there is a relapse after toilet training is complete and there was a period during which the child remained dry.
   Rule out nocturnal seizures and urologic anomalies.
   Treatment modalities include medicines (imipramine, synthetic vasopressin), behavioral treatments such as bladder training, using conditioning devices (bell and pad), and fluid restriction.
b. *Sleep-related hallucinations*
   1. At sleep onset (hypnagogic) or on awakening (hypnopompic).
   2. Common in narcolepsy.
   3. Vivid and frightening images.
c. *Sleep-related eating disorder*
   1. Inability to get back to sleep after awakening unless the individual eats or drinks.
   2. Mostly in infants and children.
5. **Parasomnias** due to drug or substance use and parasomnia due to medical conditions. Many drugs, including alcohol, trigger parasomnias that can lead to sleepwalking. Other drugs include tricyclic antidepressants, monoamine oxidase inhibitors (MAOIs), caffeine, venlafaxine, selegiline, and serotonin agonists. Sleep-related breathing disorders

trigger sleepwalking, enuresis, sleep terror, confusional arousal, and nightmares. Neurologic conditions include Parkinson's disease, dementia, and progressive supranuclear palsy, among others.

Sleep-Related Movement Disorders (14)

1. **Restless legs syndrome** (Ekbom syndrome)
   In which there is an uncomfortable sensation in legs at rest and relieved by movement. This condition peaks in middle age; it occurs in 5% of the population. It can interfere with falling asleep, though symptoms are not only limited to sleep. It is associated with pregnancy, renal disease, iron deficiency, and vitamin B12 deficiency.
   Treatment includes benzodiazepines, levodopa, quinine, opioids, propranolol, valproate, carbamazepine, and carbidopa. A new drug, ropinirole, has been reported to be effective.
2. **Periodic leg movement disorder** (formerly called nocturnal myoclonus) consists of
   a. Stereotypic, periodic leg movements (every 20 to 60 seconds) during NREM sleep (at least five leg movements per hour).
   b. Most prevalent in patients over age 55.
   c. Frequent awakenings.
   d. Unrefreshing sleep.
   e. Daytime sleepiness is a major symptom.
   f. Associated with renal disease, iron deficiency, and vitamin B12 deficiency.
   g. Various drugs have been reported to help. These include clonazepam, quinine, and levodopa.
   h. Other treatments include stress management and anxiety-relieving programs.
3. **Sleep-related leg cramps**
   a. Occur during wakefulness
   b. Painful and affect calf muscles.
   c. Precipitated by metabolic disorders, mineral deficiencies, diabetes and pregnancy.
4. **Sleep bruxism (tooth grinding)**
   a. Occurs throughout the night, though primarily occurs in stage I and II sleep or during partial arousals or transitions.
   b. Occurs in greater than 5% of the population.
   c. Treatment consists of bite plates to prevent dental damage.
5. **Sleep rhythmic movement disorder** (jactatio capitis nocturna)
   a. Rhythmic head or body rocking just before or during sleep; may extend into light sleep.
   b. Usually limited to childhood.
   c. No treatment required in most infants and young children. Crib padding or helmets may be used. Behavior modification, benzodiazepines, and tricyclic drugs may be effective.

Sleep-Related Movement Disorder Due to Drug or Substance Use and Sleep-Related Movement Disorder Due to Medical Condition

A variety of drugs, substances, and comorbid conditions can produce or exacerbate sleep-related movement disorders. Stimulants can produce rhythmic movement disorders and bruxism. Antidepressants (including most tricyclics and SSRIs), antiemetics, lithium, calcium-channel blockers, antihistamines, and neuroleptics can provoke restless leg symptoms and periodic limb movement disorder.

Significance of Sleep Disorders in Clinical Practice

One who complains of insomnia for more than 1 year is 40 times more likely than the general population to have a diagnosable psychiatric disorder. In 35% of patients who present to sleep disorder centers with a complaint of insomnia, the underlying cause is a psychiatric disorder. Half of these patients have major depression. Roughly 80% of patients with major depression complain of insomnia. In patients with major depression, sleep involves relatively normal onset but repeated awakenings in the second half of the night, premature morning awakening, decreased stage III and IV sleep, a short REM latency, and a long first REM period are seen. Treatment for insomnia in a depressed patient may include use of a sedating antidepressant, for example, treating with amitriptyline.

Posttraumatic stress disorder patients typically describe insomnia and nightmares.

Hypersomnia related to a mental disorder is usually found in a variety of conditions such as the early stages of mild depressive disorder, grief, personality disorders, dissociative disorders, and somatoform disorders. Treatment of the primary disorder should resolve the hypersomnia. For sleep disorder resulting from a general medical condition, though not listed as a category in DSM-5, clinicians should be aware of the following medical disorders associated with sleep disorders. (15)

1. Sleep-related epileptic seizures. Seizures occur almost exclusively during sleep (sleep epilepsy).
2. Sleep-related cluster headaches. Sleep-related cluster headaches are severe and unilateral, appear often during sleep, and are marked by an on–off pattern of attacks.
3. Chronic paroxysmal hemicrania. Chronic paroxysmal hemicrania is a unilateral headache that occurs frequently and has a sudden onset (only occurs during REM).
4. Sleep-related abnormal swallowing syndrome. A condition during sleep in which inadequate swallowing results in aspiration of saliva, coughing, and choking. It is intermittently associated with brief arousals or awakenings.
5. Sleep-related asthma. Asthma that is exacerbated by sleep. In some people, it may result in significant sleep disturbances.
6. Sleep-related cardiovascular symptoms. Associated with disorders of cardiac rhythm, congestive heart failure, valvular disease, and blood pressure variability that may be induced or exacerbated by alterations in cardiovascular physiology during sleep.
7. Sleep-related gastroesophageal reflux. Patient wakes from sleep with burning substernal pain, a feeling of tightness or pain in the chest, or a sour taste in the mouth. Often associated with hiatal hernia. Gastroesophageal reflux disorder (GERD) can also lead to sleep-related asthma due to reflux into the lungs.
8. Sleep-related hemolysis (paroxysmal nocturnal hemoglobinuria). Rare, acquired, chronic hemolytic anemia. The hemolysis and consequent hemoglobinuria are accelerated during sleep so that the morning urine appears brownish red.
9. Painful conditions, such as arthritis, may lead to insomnia. Treatment, whenever possible, should be of the underlying medical condition.

CONCLUSION

Sleep disorders are very common and, if untreated, can cause great socio-occupational dysfunction. A prompt diagnosis and treatment are essential. Table 25.2 summarizes all the sleep disorders.

Table 25.2 Various types of sleep difficulties seen in clinical practice.

Symptom	Insomnia secondary to medical conditions	Insomnia secondary to psychiatric or environmental conditions
Difficulty in falling asleep	Any painful or uncomfortable condition CNS lesions Conditions listed subsequently	Anxiety Tension anxiety, muscular Environmental changes Circadian rhythm sleep disorder
Difficulty in remaining asleep	Sleep apnea syndromes Nocturnal myoclonus and restless leg syndrome Dietary factors (probably) Episodic events (parasomnias) Direct substance effects (including alcohol) Substance withdrawal effects (including alcohol) Substance interactions Endocrine or metabolic diseases Infectious, neoplastic, or other diseases Painful or uncomfortable conditions Brainstem or hypothalamic lesions or diseases Aging	Depression, especially primary depression Environmental changes Circadian rhythm sleep disorder Posttraumatic stress disorder Schizophrenia

References

1. American Academy of Sleep Medicine. *The International Classification of Sleep Disorders, Revised: Diagnostic and Coding Manual.* Rochester, MN: American Academy of Sleep Medicine. 2000.
2. Zee P., Harsanyi K. Highlights of sleep neuroscience. In: Bowman T, ed. *Review of Sleep Medicine.* Burlington, MA: Butterworth Heinemann. 2003:19–39.
3. The Clinical Use of the Multiple Sleep Latency Test. The standards of practice committee of the American sleep disorders association. *Thorpy MJSleep.* 1992 Jun;15(3):268–276.
4. Petit L, Azad N, Byszewski A, Sarazan FF. Non-pharmacological management of primary and secondary insomnia among older people: Review of assessment tools and treatments. *Power B Age Ageing.* 2003 Jan;32(1):19–25.
5. Shorr R, Robin DW. Rational use of benzodiazepines in the elderly. *Drugs Aging.* 1994;4:9–20.
6. Guilleminault C, Stoohs R, Clerk A, Cetel M, Maistros P. A cause of excessive daytime sleepiness: The upper airway resistance syndrome. *Chest.* 1993;104:781–787.
7. Meoli AL, Casey KR, Clark RW, Coleman JA Jr, Fayle RW, Troell RJ, Iber C. Clinical practice review committee. *Sleep.* 2001 Jun 15;24(4):469–470.

8. Guilleminault C, Kim YD, Palombini L, Li K, Powell N. Upper airway resistance syndrome and its treatment. *Sleep*. 2000;23(suppl 4):S197–S200.
9. Black J. Narcolepsy: Evaluation and management. *CNS News Special Ed*. 2001:25–29.
10. Sforza E, Lugaresi E. Daytime sleepiness and nasal continuous positive airway pressure therapy in obstructive sleep apnea syndrome patients; effects of chronic treatment and 1-night therapy withdrawal. *Sleep*. 1995;18:195–201.
11. Turek F, Dugovic C, Zee P. Current understanding of the circadian clock and the clinical implications for neurological disorders. *Arch Neurol*. 2001;58:1781–1787.
12. Broughton R. NREM arousal parasomnias. In: Kryger MH, Roth T, Dement WC, eds. *Principles and Practice of Sleep Medicine*. 3rd ed. Philadelphia, PA: WB Saunders. 2000:687–692.
13. Olson E, Boeve B, Silbert M. Rapid eye movement sleep behaviour disorder: Demographic, clinical and laboratory findings in 93 cases. *Brain*. 2000;123:331–339.
14. Chokroverty S, Jankovic J. Restless legs syndrome. *Neurology*. 1999;52:907.
15. Chokroverty S. Diagnosis and treatment of sleep disorders caused by comorbid disease. *Neurology*. 2000;54(5 suppl 1):S8–S15.

26
Optimizing Patient Care in Psychiatry – OCD and Habit Disorders

Javed Ather Siddiqui and Shazia Farheen Qureshi

Introduction 286

INTRODUCTION

Obsessive-compulsive disorder (OCD) is a common, disabling, relapsing chronic psychiatric illness with a waxing and waning course [1]. It is a mental illness that causes repeated unwanted thoughts or ideas (obsessions) or the urge to do something over and over again (compulsions). OCD isn't about habits or thinking negative thoughts but habit-disorder behavior which causes impairment and results in negative physical and social consequences [2]. Individuals with habit disorders report an uncomfortable urge that is satisfied by doing a particular behavior. They get relief from doing the particular behavior, which reinforces them, and they are more likely to do the behavior again. It is like positive reinforcement.

There is a specific need to increase the efficiency of service provision in the care of OCD patients. This is recognized by guidelines which recommend management of these patients using a stepped care approach [3]. A stepped care approach refers to treatment at different levels [3]. Within a stepped care approach, the treatment must be the least restrictive but still provide significant improvements to health. With this concept in mind, if the treatment is provided at a lower level or step, and the client is not improving post-treatment, the client needs to be evaluated and an appropriate step taken for treatment. While referring the patient to a therapist, the availability of the therapist and the amount of time required by a specialist therapist would be considered [4]. The National Institute for Health and Clinical Excellence (NICE) Guidelines for Obsessive Compulsive Disorder [5] is a world-renowned document outlining evidence-based approaches to treating the disorder. The NICE Guidelines outline six levels of intervention, as follows.

Step 1: to maintain awareness and recognition; Step 2: recognition and assessment (including referral to appropriate services) of the patient; Step 3: get initial treatment by guided self-help and cognitive behaviour therapy (CBT) via group or individual format; Step 4: for OCD with comorbidity or a poor response to initial treatment – treatment via CBT within a multidisciplinary team, possible medication; Step 5: for OCD with significant comorbidity, severe impairment or limited treatment response – specialist treatment services with expertise in CBT, possible medication; Step 6: inpatient or intensive treatment programs, including medication and CBT to reduce the risk to life, severe self-neglect or severe distress or disability.

Higher-level steps within this healthcare model indicate the need for exposure and response prevention (ERP)-based psychotherapy on an individual basis, where there is scope for exploring less intensive, less costly and more accessible formats for the delivery of these programs. Studies reveal up to 25% of patients refuse ERP treatment due to time commitments, a fear that the exposure exercises will bring overwhelming anxiety or a fear of a dreaded outcome related to the individual failing to complete their rituals [6]. We should continue to explore new psychological treatment approaches and can offer hope to those who refuse or do not respond to the current standard treatment approaches.

Psychiatric care and management of OCD are indicated when signs and symptoms interfere with functioning or cause significant distress. Psychiatric care should be offered throughout the course of illness consistent with the patient's needs, capacities and desires. The components of psychiatric management across the stages of illness are described in more detail in the following.

1. Establish a therapeutic alliance
   Patient care is a joint endeavor, as the physician's first attempt is to establish and maintain a therapeutic alliance. This alliance allows the psychiatrist to obtain the information needed to plan effective treatment. The alliance allows the patient to trust the physician to motivate adherence to collaboratively planned treatments. Explaining the signs and symptoms in understandable forms is encouraging to the patient. In building the alliance, the psychiatrist should consider the patient's feelings and actions toward him or her, as well as why the patient came to him or her specifically and why at this point in time.
2. Assess the patient's symptoms
   The psychiatrist should assess the patient for signs and symptoms of OCD, guided by Diagnostic and Statistical Manual of Mental Disorders, 5th edition (DSM-5) criteria. OCD is usually underdiagnosed unless specific screening is done [7]. Some of screening questions include: Do you have unpleasant thoughts that you can't get rid of? Do you worry that you might harm someone impulsively? Do you have to count things, or wash your hands, or check things over and over? Do you worry a lot about whether you performed religious rituals correctly or are immoral? Do you have troubling thoughts about sexual matters? Do you need things arranged symmetrically or in exact order? Do you have trouble discarding things? Do these worries interfere with your functioning at work, with your family or in social activities? As a part of the assessment, the psychiatrist must differentiate between the obsessions, compulsions and rituals and other similar signs and symptoms found in other disorders.
3. Consider rating the severity of OCD and co-occurring symptoms and their effects on the patient's functioning
   The Y-BOCS Symptom Checklist [8] includes current and past symptoms, or the 18-item Obsessive-Compulsive Inventory [9] may be helpful. These scales may help to document variety and the clustering of the patient's symptoms. There should be consideration of co-occurring conditions and their effects on the patient's functioning by the psychiatrist.
4. Evaluate the safety of the patient and others
   As with all psychiatric patients and individuals with OCD, assessing the risk for suicide and self-injurious behavior is crucial. In assessing and evaluating the patient's potential for self-injury or suicide, a number of factors should be taken into consideration. Individuals with OCD alone or with a lifetime history of any co-occurring disorder have a higher suicide attempt rate than individuals without any psychiatric problem in the general population [10].

5. Complete the psychiatric assessment
   During completion of psychiatric assessment, the psychiatrist should be alert for signs, symptoms and history of co-occurring conditions like depressive disorders and bipolar disorder, which are commonly seen in patients with OCD, then others such as generalized anxiety disorder, panic disorder, social phobia, anorexia nervosa and bulimia nervosa, which are more common in patients with OCD. Evaluation should include screening for alcohol or substance abuse, such as dependence or depression. Other disorders with elevated prevalence in OCD include impulse-control disorders, such as skin picking and trichotillomania. Regarding past psychiatric history, a chronological history should be obtained of past psychiatric illnesses, including substance use disorders and treatment and history of hospitalizations.
6. Establish goals for treatment
7. Establish the appropriate setting for treatment
8. Enhance treatment adherence
   Treatment side effects can influence adherence. The psychiatrist plays a crucial role to consider the role of patient's family and social support system in treatment adherence. Psycho-educate the family members so that they may be important associates in the treatment efforts [11, 12].

In OCD, established treatments include selective serotonin reuptake inhibitors (SSRIs) and cognitive behavior therapy with exposure and response prevention. Though many cases are improved with these treatments, the rates of incomplete recovery and treatment resistance to standard therapies are high. Approximately 40% of patients fail to respond, and 50% need further assessment [12].

According to the American Psychiatric Association's (2013) DSM-5 criteria, disorders like OCD and habit disorders have been classified under the obsessive compulsive related disorders (OCRDs) [13]. These include nail-biting (onychophagia), body dysmorphic disorder (BDD), hoarding disorder, trichotillomania (hair-pulling disorder) and excoriation disorder. As compared with OCD, these OCRDs have received less interventional analysis. The main aim of the management of these disorders is to motivate the patient, provide emotional support and relieve stress by educating them, create good habits and develop conscious awareness, which will give effective results [14]. Emotional support and encouragement is the one of the best methods, and it should be given during treatment. Behavioral modification techniques, positive reinforcement and regular consistent follow-ups are important key factors for the treatment. Punishment, ridicule, nagging, threats and application of bitter-tasting substances are not appropriate approaches to manage the patient.

As compared to all the different modalities of non-pharmacologic treatment of nail biting (NB), behavioral therapy [15] is the first-line gold standard treatment. Psychotherapies in both OCD and habit disorders play an important role along with pharmacotherapy; these are as follows.

Cognitive behavioral therapy: It is based on cognitive, behavioral and learning principles. It is a commonly used psychotherapy and is beneficial when simpler measures are not effective. It helps patients to understand their beliefs and how to correct behavior which might be incorrect. This helps to change behavior by becoming aware of negative emotions and related habits so that they can be handled in more effective ways. It can be combined with one of the following methods, like competing response. The individual engages in compulsions to reduce obsessional distress. Exposure and response prevention is a behavioral component of CBT that directs the individual to confront the aversive stimulus such as a thought, item or situation and experience the associated distress without engaging in rituals. Such distress will naturally habituate over time in the absence of ritual engagement. CBT for

OCD is a multi-component approach, conducted in a sequential manner. Initially, individuals are provided with psychoeducation regarding OCD; its behavioral, cognitive and neurobiological underpinnings; and the treatment regimen. Obsessive-compulsive disorder may be described to patients as a brain hiccup or odd wiring that causes individuals to experience anxiety when certain thoughts or actions arise. It is then explained that engaging in compulsions triggered by obsessions reinforces this relationship by reducing distress, thereby increasing the likelihood of engaging in rituals whenever an anxiety-inducing stimulus is encountered. Thus, this treatment focuses on eliciting anxiety by presenting an obsessional trigger and prohibiting compulsions. By doing so, the obsessive-compulsive cycle is broken and eventually extinguished, as the person learns that the feared event does not occur if the compulsion is not performed. In turn, the aversive trigger no longer elicits distress at the original levels. Later, a stimulus hierarchy is created to rank the degree of distress experienced by patient with exposure to an obsessional trigger while refraining from ritual engagement. The exposure itself consists of having an individual confront the trigger, starting with less anxiety-provoking stimuli first without engaging in compulsions.

Exposure therapy (ET): Allowing an individual to confront their fears in an environment that is both safe and controlled can be useful when it comes to reducing the impact of OCD. Engaging in this type of therapy may encourage individuals to become more desensitized to specific situations that usually trigger their anxiety. Studies show that a combination of medication, CBT and ET is the best remedy for OCD, which is recommended by psychiatrists for quick and effective results.

Interpersonal psychotherapy (IPT): This type of psychotherapy focuses on interpersonal issues within a family. It targets improving interpersonal communication and increased social support among family members to make them understand the problem of the person suffering from OCD and habit disorders.

Habit reversal therapy (HRT): It is based on changing the habit of nail biting and possibly replacing it with a more productive habit. This behavioral therapy uses similar or dissimilar competing responses competing with each other to improve oral-digital behavior. It is best addressed when the automatic response is still weak. It is four-step process which teaches a person how to breathe and feel grounded, achieve relaxation and to complete muscle-response exercises. In this therapy, self-control intervention builds self-confidence and self-esteem [16, 17]. HRT consists of many components such as awareness training, bringing the habit into consciousness and relaxation training. Competent response training is engaging in an opposing behavior that makes it impossible to pick or bite until the urge subsides. In an awareness training program, the patient should explain the act of biting and negative consequences. Social support includes loved ones or a friend who is also trying to break a bad habit by praising and encouraging the nail biter. They advise the patient to stop picking or biting and offer encouragement when the patient engages in competing responses. The principle behind habit reversal is the belief that the less the behavior is enacted, the weaker the habitual response becomes, eliminating the destructive habit completely.

Stimulus control: This therapy is based on the principle of identifying and then eliminating the stimulus that often triggers biting urges. This type of behavioral treatment helps to identify, get rid of and transform the environmental circumstances or emotions that trigger nail biting. The main goal of this therapy is to control triggers through conscious behavior modification. It is self-monitoring, converting unhealthy urges into behaviors which are nondestructive. It is an unconscious act, and taking notes can create more awareness of the behavior.

Nail cosmetics: It can help to enhance nail-biting social effects [18].

Aversion stimulus: In this method, an aversive stimulus such as a bitter substance is placed on the nail biter's nail so they will think twice before putting the nail in their mouth [19].

This technique is based on reinforcement learning and consists of a reminder, which is self-terminating.

Self-help techniques: This behavioral method has shown preliminary positive results. Wrist bands should be used as non-removable reminders. This self-help technique is performed in a number of steps. Initially, the nail biter is taught that the affected behavior is a problem, which needs to be changed. Then, the nail biter is asked to find the cause of NB and possible thoughts and feelings related to the behavior. Third, the person is advised to do self-monitoring, as it can increase their awareness of the behavior. Fourth, children are educated to use some learned skills such as self-talk and self-reward to change the automated behavior. Finally, the nail biter is trained to use the learned skills to manage and change other similar pathologic behaviors [20]. When they reach a milestone such as no picking for 2 weeks, a reward is given to the patient, such as going out for a celebration dinner.

Emotional freedom technique (EFT): This is a powerful self-help technique using energy therapy used to prevent NB. It has been proved highly effective when used in dealing with addictive habitual behavioral actions to overcome unwanted habitual patterns. EFT can help a patient stop biting their nails by working on the underlying triggers such as stress and others. It is used to install new behavior in response to stress, strain or boredom. This type of therapy is routinely used in sports psychology by relieving the stress and boosting sports performance. It is one of the forms of psychological acupressure. It is based on the same energy meridians used in traditional acupuncture to treat physical and emotional ailments. It is also called the tapping method, where the psychotherapist taps different parts of the body with their fingertips using kinetic energy to specific meridians on your head and chest while you think about your specific problem, either a traumatic event or an addiction, like NB. Tapping sites are the top of the head, eyebrow, sides of eyes, below the nose, chin, collar bone, and under the arm. EFT doesn't work on the nail biting problem; it works on the underlying emotional pattern that precedes each bout of nail biting

Hypnosis: is sometimes utilized to make the person aware of the habit and find other methods of relaxation.

References

1. Skoog G, Skoog I. A 40-year follow-up of patients with obsessive-compulsive disorder. *Arch Gen Psychiatry*. 1999;56:121–127.
2. Woods D, Flessner C, Conelea C. Habit disorders. In M. Hersen (Series Ed.) & D. Reitman (Vol. Ed.) Handbook of psychological assessment, case conceptualization, and treatment. *Children and Adolescents*. 2008;7:542–570.
3. NICE. *Obsessive-compulsive disorder: Core interventions in the treatment of obsessive-compulsive disorder and body dysmorphic disorder*. Leicester, UK: British Psychological Society.2006.
4. Bower P, Gilbody S. Stepped care in psychological therapies: Access, effectiveness and efficiency. *British Journal of Psychiatry*. 2005;186:11–17.
5. National Collaborating Centre for Mental Health. *Obsessive compulsive dis-order: Core interventions in the treatment of obsessive compulsive disorder and body dysmorphic disorder*. Leicester: British Psychological Society.2005.
6. Greist J. The comparative effectiveness of treatments for obsessive-compulsive disorder. *Bulletin of the Meninger Clinic*. 1998;62:A65–A81.
7. Fireman B, Koran LM, Leventhal JL, Jacobson A. The prevalence of clinically recognized obsessive-compulsive disorder in a large health maintenance organization. *Am J Psychiatry*. 2001;158:1904–1910.
8. Goodman WK, Price LH, Rasmussen SA, Mazure C, Fleischmann RL, Hill CL, Heninger GR, Charney DS. The yale-brown obsessive compulsive scale, I: Development, use, and reliability. *Arch Gen Psychiatry*. 1989;46:1006–1011.
9. Foa EB, Huppert JD, Leiberg S, Langner R, Kichic R, Hajcak G, Salkovskis PM. The obsessive-compulsive inventory: Development and validation of a short version. *Psychol Assess*. 2002;14:485–496.

10. Hollander E, Greenwald S, Neville D, Johnson J, Hornig CD, Weissman MM. Uncomplicated and comorbid obsessive-compulsive disorder in an epidemiologic sample. *Depress Anxiety.* 1996;4:111–119.
11. Renshaw KD, Steketee G, Chambless DL. Involving family members in the treatment of OCD. *Cogn Behav Ther.* 2005;34:164–175.
12. Fineberg N, Reghunandanan S, Simpson HB, Phillips KA, Richter MA, Matthews K. Obsessive-compulsive disorder (OCD): Practical strategies for pharmacological and somatic treatment in adults. *Psychiatry Res.* 2015;227:114–125.
13. American Psychiatric Association. *Diagnostic and statistical manual of mental disorders*, 5th Edn. Washington, DC: American Psychiatric Association.2013.
14. Siddiqui JA, Qureshi SF, Marei WM, Mahfouz TA. Onychophagia (Nail Biting): A body focused Repetitive behavior due to psychiatric co-morbidity. *J Mood Disorders.* 2017;7:47–49.
15. Ravindran AV, da Silva TL, Ravindran LN, Richter MA, Rector NA. Obsessive-compulsive spectrum disorders: A review of the evidence-based treatments. *Can J Psychiatry.* 2009;54:331–343.
16. Bate KS, Malouff JM, Thorsteinsson ET. The efficacy of habit reversal therapy for tics, habit disorders, and stuttering: A meta-analytic review. *Clinical Psychology Review.* 2011;31 (5):865–871.
17. Ghanizadeh A, Bazrafshan A, Firoozabadi A, Dehbozorgi G. Habit reversal versus object manipulation training for treating nail biting: A randomized controlled clinical trial. *Iranian Journal of Psychiatry.* 2013;8(2):61–67.
18. Lorizzo M, Piraccini BM, Tosti A. Nail cosmetics in nail disorders. *J CosmetDermatol.* 2007;6 (1):53–58.
19. Silber KP, Haynes CE. Treating nail-biting: A comparative analysis of mild aversion and competing response therapies. *Behav Res Ther.* 1992;30:15–22.
20. Ronen T, Rosenbaum M. Helping children to help themselves: A case study of enuresis and nail biting. *Research on Social Work Practice.* 2001;11:338–356.

27
Optimizing Patient Care in Alcohol Dependence Using Disulfiram Therapy

Pooja Kapri, Avinash De Sousa

Introduction	292
History	293
Mode of Action	293
Drug Interactions	294
Use	295
Side Effects and Precautions	295
Usage in Special Groups	296
Consent	297
Psycho-Education	297

INTRODUCTION

Disulfiram is a drug used to support the treatment of alcohol use disorder by producing an acute sensitivity to ethanol. Disulfiram works by inhibiting the enzyme acetaldehyde dehydrogenase. The chemical compound is tetra-ethyl-thiuram-disulfide, a grey-colored crystalline powder which is a sulfur compound.[1] It is a nearly tasteless and odorless drug.

Alcoholism is defined as any drinking of alcohol that can result in significant mental or physical health problems. In 1979, the World Health Organization (WHO) discouraged the use of "alcoholism" due to its inexact meaning, preferring to use "alcohol dependence syndrome".[4] Furthermore, the diagnostic classification given by DSM-5[2] is "Alcohol use disorder" and "Alcohol dependence" as given by ICD-11.[3] The World Health Organization has estimated that as of 2016, there were 380 million people with alcohol use disorder worldwide (5.1% of the population over 15 years of age).[5,6]

Although the intake of small quantities of alcohol occasionally (like red wine) has been shown to have certain health benefits like improving cardiovascular health and bone density as a result of the presence of good amounts of antioxidants and polyphenols, most people are addicted to liquor in amounts and frequencies that are detrimental to their physical and mental health. The deleterious effects of alcohol on our body include gastritis, increased risk of upper gastro-intestinal cancers, fatty liver and cirrhosis, pancreatitis, alcoholic cardio-myopathy, bleeding from gastro-intestinal lining leading to anemia, ascitis, increased risk of Type 2 diabetes mellitus and hypertension, decreased immunity, sexual dysfunctions, peripheral neuropathy and retinopathy (especially with drinks spuriously mixed with methanol). Pernicious effects on our brain include permanent brain damage, leading to memory

DOI: 10.4324/9780429030260-30

and gait disturbances; Wernicke's disorder and Korsakoff syndrome; increased risk of stroke and seizure disorders; psychosis; depression; anxiety disorders; delirium tremens; alcohol withdrawal; and other psychiatric illnesses. Alcohol use not only affects the person ingesting it but also destroys the entire family as result of strained relationships, loss of work and financial constraints. Moreover, intake of alcohol by pregnant women may pose an increased risk of miscarriages and fetal alcohol syndrome – a child born with stunted growth, low birth weight and behavioral and learning difficulties. As a result of these grave dangers posed by heavy and long-term alcohol use, it is of the utmost importance to develop a management plan that not only includes pharmacology but also psycho-education and psychotherapy, along with strong family and socio-vocational support.

Pharmacotherapy includes the use of anti-craving drugs like acamprosate, naltrexone and baclofen and the use of deterrents like disulfiram, along with supporting treatment to treat psychotic and depressive features, withdrawal complaints and vitamin deficiencies (vitamin B1 – thiamine)

In this chapter we will specifically consider the use of disulfiram to treat alcohol dependence and pointers to be kept in mind while using it in special groups and in the presence of certain health conditions.

History

Disulfiram has been in use in the rubber industry since the late 1800s. It wasn't until 1937 that its interaction with alcohol became prominent, when it was reported by physician E. E. Williams that rubber industry workers who were using a sulfur compound for vulcanization of rubber suffered from distressing reactions on consuming alcohol.[7] By 1940, some dermatologists were already using disulfiram to treat human and animal scabies, and it was being used by physicians to treat intestinal worms.[8] A pharmacologist, Erik Jacobson, who had ingested disulfiram for intestinal worms, reported complaints of flushing, dizziness, nausea and anxiety on consuming a small quantity of alcohol at a dinner party.[9] He and his fellow researchers carried out further studies, and this was the inception of the ethanol–disulfiram reaction.[10] Treatment of alcohol use with disulfiram was introduced first in the Scandinavian countries Sweden and Denmark in 1949.

The commonly used marketed name for disulfiram, Antabuse, has a Danish origin, which is now used worldwide. Meanwhile in the United States, disulfiram (Antabuse) was approved by the Federal Drug Administration (FDA) in 1951. Disulfiram was the primary drug used in alcohol abuse, as it wasn't until the early 1900s and early 2000s that naltrexone and acamprosate were respectively approved by the Federal Drug Administration.

Mode of Action

Once alcohol in ingested, it is converted by alcohol dehydrogenase (ADH) to acetaldehyde in the liver, and acetaldehyde is acted upon by acetaldehyde dehydrogenase (ALDH), leading to formation of acetate. This acetic acid is eventually converted at cellular level to carbon dioxide and water in our body.

Disulfiram belongs to a class of drugs called acetaldehyde dehydrogenase (ALDH) inhibitors and is used clinically as an alcohol-deterrent agent.[11] These drugs are known to convert the effect of alcohol from a pleasant to an unpleasant one. They lead to accumulation of acetaldehyde at levels that become distressing even on ingesting small amounts of alcohol and thereby force the person not to drink any alcohol at all, promoting a forced abstinence.[12] The release of acetaldehyde produces flushing of the skin as a result of cutaneous vasodilatation and hypotension due to a fall in diastolic blood pressure with reflex tachycardia, breathlessness, tachypnoea (increased respiratory rate), uneasiness and tightness in chest, palpitations, anxiety, panic, throbbing headache, nausea and vomiting.

After oral ingestion, disulfiram is metabolized to diethyl-dithiocarbamic acid (DDC) in the strong acidic conditions of the stomach.[13] Oral absorption of disulfiram ranges from 75–85%. After its distribution across the gastrointestinal mucosa into blood, disulfiram is rapidly reduced to its monomer DDC[14] and distributed throughout various body tissues. Cytochrome P450 plays an important role in metabolism and is especially to be carefully used with other drugs that act through a similar pathway. The metabolites of disulfiram are mainly excreted via the kidney (60–80%), feces (10–30%) and lungs.[15] This way, breath analyzers and urine estimation techniques can be used in assessment of compliance with disulfiram therapy.

Higher doses of disulfiram have also been reported to inhibit cerebrospinal (CSF) levels of the enzyme dopamine β-hydroxylase (DBH) in animal models and human studies as well.[16] This reaction leads to an increased level of dopamine and decreasing nor adrenaline levels in the brain, leading to transient and reversible psychotic features.[17] As result of this side effect, disulfiram needs to be cautiously used in patients with underlying psychotic complaints. This has now been recognized as one of the mechanisms of disulfiram for reducing the effect of cocaine via dopamine, and thus it is currently being used as a drug of choice for cocaine dependence.[18]

Drug Interactions

Disulfiram can lead to many drug-to-drug interactions, provoking mild to severe complaints; hence, the utmost care should be undertaken while prescribing medications while on disulfiram therapy. Dose reduction may be advised if needed by the treating physician for medications that the patient might already be on.

There are many over-the-counter cough syrups, fermented vinegars, deodorants, perfumes (*attar*), after shaves, body washes and lotions in the market that contain alcohol in various strengths, so their use needs to limited while on disulfiram therapy. Use of traditional medicines also needs to be undertaken carefully. Clearance of caffeine is delayed in some individuals, leading to prolonged coffee attentiveness.[25]

A large variety of drugs like cephalosporin antibiotics[19] (cefoperazone), amitriptyline[20] (tricyclic anti-depressant), sulphonylurea hypoglycemic agents[21] (tolbutamide, glipizide, glimepiride) and metronidazole[22] (antibiotic and anti-protozoal agent) have been reported to produce disulfiram-ethanol reaction (DER)–like side effects in combination with alcohol. Most of those drugs exert their action by inhibiting ALDH activity but generally to a lesser degree as compared to disulfiram. However, it might pose a problem in patients who are concomitantly also advised disulfiram.

When combined with ethanol, tacrolimus and pimecrolimus ointment (indicated in atopic dermatitis) may cause erythematous flushing of skin locally even on consumption of a small amount of alcohol.[23]

Disulfiram-like reactions have been reported in patients who consume alcoholic beverages while being treated with furazolidone (indicated in diarrhea).[24]

With its use via the cytochrome P450 system, disulfiram has a high propensity to raise levels of phenytoin (anti-epileptic) when both are administered simultaneously, and phenytoin toxicity has been reported in these patients.[26]

Benzodiazepines like chlordiazepoxide and diazepam, which mainly get metabolized via hepatic oxidation, show reduced clearance. Meanwhile, lorazepam, which is metabolized via glucuronidation, shows no effect in its clearance.[27] These drugs play a major role in alcohol withdrawal management, so one needs to be aware regarding any harmful drug reaction.

Bronchodilators like aminophylline and theophylline, recommended in asthma, also show a reduction in metabolism when used concurrently with disulfiram and hence might require dose reduction.[28]

Use

Disulfiram has been used successfully for over seven decades now in the long-term management of alcohol dependence. Oral use in India is generally given at two strengths, 250 and 500 mg. It is always preferable to start disulfiram therapy in an inpatient setup so as to observe the patient for any side effects. Disulfiram has also been used for over four decades as a subcutaneous implantation, which was first introduced in 1968. The origin of disulfiram implants was to overcome adherence problems.

Patients are advised not to take disulfiram if they have consumed alcohol within the past 12 hours, and they need to be told that the disulfiram-ethanol reaction can occur up to 14 days after one stops taking this medicine. It is advisable to take disulfiram in the morning after breakfast; however, some patients do report drowsiness following its intake. In such individuals, night-time shifting of medications can be done to avoid daytime sedation. Disulfiram therapy is usually continued for months and sometimes years. Some doctors ask their patients to wear a medical alert tag or carry an ID card stating that they are on disulfiram therapy. Any medical care provider who treats such a patient during an emergency situation can thus easily be aware of any potential adverse drug reactions.

Cocaine dependence is another indication for disulfiram therapy. Disulfiram reduces cocaine craving by increasing neurotransmitter dopamine levels and decreasing the norepinephrine levels by blocking the activity of the enzyme dopamine beta hydroxylase (DBH).

Pathological gambling (PG) is a disorder characterized by recurrent patterns of gambling and associated multiple socio-psychological problems like high rates of bankruptcy, divorce and suicide. A similar neurochemical disturbance has been reported in PG; therefore, disulfiram might not only be effective in the treatment of cocaine addiction but also in the treatment of PG.[29,30]

Research has shown that disulfiram therapy is superior to naltrexone, acamprosate, baclofen (anti-craving drugs) and Topiramate in the management of alcohol dependence. The various combinations of these drugs bring the best results in the management of polysubstance use disorder.

Side Effects and Precautions

As disulfiram undergoes metabolism through the liver, one needs to be cautious when using the drug in patients with alcohol use disorder who have underlying deranged liver functions. Although not common, chances of disulfiram-induced hepatitis, both cholestatic and fulminant, can occur. It has been suggested that the mechanism of hepatotoxicity is dosage independent and is an allergic or hypersensitivity reaction.[31] As a routine, baseline liver function tests (LFTs) must be carried out prior to starting disulfiram, and repeat testing as advised for the clinician from time to time.

Uncommonly, occurrences of polyneuropathy and toxic optic neuropathy are reported with disulfiram therapy, and these complaints reverse completely with withdrawal of the drug. This reaction is dose dependent, and the pathology is due to an accumulation of carbon disulfide, which is a by-product of the metabolism of disulfiram in the liver.[32] Clinically, it is difficult to distinguish disulfiram-induced neuropathy and alcoholic neuropathy, as in both cases, patients report complaints of tingling numbness over limb extremities.

Disulfiram-induced psychosis can occur in patients without any previous history of psychosis, although it is more common if there is a predisposition in the individual, such as a positive family history of psychosis, past history of psychosis or schizophrenia in the individual, past history of drug-induced psychosis or disulfiram-induced psychosis, usage of higher than recommended dosing of disulfiram, older age bracket, deranged liver function tests and simultaneous use of dopaminergic medications (commonly used in Parkinson's and related disorders).[33,34]

Disulfiram-induced reversible hypertension can arise in some individuals, but this condition resolves completely on withdrawal of the offending medication.

Newer studies have outlined sexual dysfunction as a side effect in about 10% of patients receiving disulfiram. These complaints can range from arousal deficits and erectile dysfunction to orgasmic difficulties. It is, however, difficult to ascertain whether these dysfunctions are purely disulfiram induced or related to alcohol use as well.[35,36]

Common but mild side effects that can occur with disulfiram include skin rash, acne, skin flushing (warmth, redness or prickly tingly feeling), sweating, mild headache, fatigability, metallic or garlic-like aftertaste in the mouth, nausea and giddiness. These side effects do not necessarily require stoppage of the drug or specific management. They are usually experienced during the first couple of weeks of disulfiram therapy, resolving spontaneously or in some cases requiring dose reduction. Skin eruptions or rash can be managed by administering oral antihistamines as disulfiram is continued.

Due to the DER, drinking even small amounts of alcohol produces flushing, throbbing headache, orbital pain, sudden loss of vision or blurred vision, nausea, copious vomiting, sweating, excessive thirst, chest pain, palpitation, respiratory difficulty (dyspnea), hyperventilation, tachycardia, hypotension, syncopal attack, marked uneasiness, weakness, vertigo and yellowish discoloration of skin (jaundice), along with dark-colored urine, clay-colored stools and confusion or altered behavior. In severe reactions, there may be respiratory depression, cardiovascular collapse, arrhythmias, myocardial infarction, acute congestive heart failure, unconsciousness, convulsions and a comatose state, eventually leading to death. The intensity of this reaction varies with each individual but is generally proportional to the amounts of disulfiram and alcohol ingested. Mild reactions may occur in a sensitive individual on disulfiram therapy when the blood alcohol concentration is increased to as little as 5 to 10 mg per 100 mL. Symptoms are fully developed at 50 mg per 100 mL, and unconsciousness usually results when the blood alcohol level reaches 125 to 150 mg per 100 mL of blood. The duration of the disulfiram–ethanol reaction varies from 30 to 60 minutes, to several hours in the more severe cases, or as long as there is the presence of alcohol in the blood. In case of onset of any of these symptoms, one needs to inform their doctor urgently, and the patient needs to be brought to the emergency room as soon as possible.

Usage in Special Groups

Usage in pregnancy: Safe use of this drug in pregnancy has not been confirmed. Therefore, disulfiram should be used during pregnancy only when, in the judgment of the treating physician, the probable benefits outweigh the possible risks.

Nursing mothers: It is not clearly known to what extent this drug is excreted in human milk; hence, it is prudent to avoid disulfiram therapy in lactating mothers.

Pediatric use: Safety and effectiveness in the pediatric age group (under 18 years) have not yet been established.

Geriatric use: A determination has not been made whether controlled clinical studies of disulfiram included sufficient numbers of subjects aged 65 years and above to define a clear-cut difference in response from younger subjects. Meanwhile, other reported clinical experiences have not identified any differences in responses between elderly and younger patients. In general, dose selection for an elderly individual should be cautious, usually starting at the lower end of the dosing range, reflecting the greater frequency of decreased hepatic, renal or cardiac function and of concomitant disorders or other drug therapy.

Care should be taken in starting disulfiram therapy in individuals with underlying liver disease, heart disorder, seizure disorder, organic brain disorders and thyroid illness.

Consent

One of the most important things determining success when advising disulfiram therapy is that the patient himself/herself needs to be motivated to adhere to the treatment plan and to quit drinking. It has been noted that, many times, disulfiram is surreptitiously added to patients' food or beverages by relatives when they want their family member to quit alcohol, but this also has been a matter of grave concern.[37] Many wives of alcohol-dependent patients give disulfiram to their husbands without their knowledge, and, as the patient is clueless, following intake of drinks, it precipitates a disulfiram-ethanol reaction. This can cause severe to fatal consequences. In some corners of India, the self proclaimed God men – *sadhu babas* and *fakirs* – often provide distraught family members with 'medicines' to be given mixed in meals to help the patient quit alcohol. These usually contain disulfiram, and as the patient ingests alcohol, oblivious, it leads to distressing and harmful repercussions. Ethical points are raised when disulfiram therapy is administered to unaware individuals, and relatives/pharmacists/doctors are advised to refrain from such practices.

Whenever the patient and their family members are given the option of disulfiram therapy, it is very important to have an informed consent duly signed by both the patient and their relative, who will be supervising tablet intake. This consent form should mention details of potential side effects or allergic reactions, symptoms of disulfiram-ethanol reaction, certain pre-existing health conditions that need special care in this therapy and all the drugs/common items like perfumes and sauces that can precipitate DER. Patients and relatives need to be told every detail in the language best understood by them to avoid any unfavorable consequences.

Psycho-Education

An integrative holistic treatment plan that not only includes pharmacological interventional but also psychotherapy for disulfiram abidance acts like a double-pronged attack on alcohol dependence. Psychotherapy acts like a roadmap that guides clinicians in understanding the patient's thoughts, emotions and problems better and developing solutions. Talk therapy can either be one on one, family or group therapy.

Cognitive behavior therapy (CBT) is a solutions-oriented approach that helps patients focus on constructive thoughts and actions like challenging harmful beliefs, confronting fears and crafting strategies to overcome cravings.

Motivational interviewing (MI) is a method used to overcome ambivalence, set goals for self improvement and develop willpower for better adherence to intake of alcohol deterrents.

Attending recovery support groups like Alcoholics Anonymous (AA), which is a 12-step program that helps in supplementing long-term sobriety, carried out jointly with psychologists and individuals in remission by sharing their experiences regarding medication compliance.

Other methods include yoga and meditation, which help patient manage cravings and stay focused on the recovery path. Many rehab centers offer art and music therapy that helps individuals tap into their deeper emotions and alleviate depressive and anxiety complaints.

It cannot be emphasized enough that medication adherence and compliance with disulfiram can be improved with good psycho-education, family support and supervised disulfiram therapy when administered by a family member.[38] Research also suggests that the effective mode of action of disulfiram is a combined psychological deterrent action and a physiological deterrent action.[39] However, experiencing the disulfiram-ethanol reaction is not a prerequisite for disulfiram's action and does not lead to any better treatment outcomes.[40]

References

1. Suh JJ, Pettinati HM, Kampman KM, O'Brien CP. The status of disulfiram: A half of a century later. *J Clin Psychopharmacol*. 2006;26(3):290–302.
2. American Psychiatric Association. *Diagnostic and statistical manual of mental disorders: DSM-5* (5th ed.). Washington, DC: American Psychiatric Association. 2013.
3. "Diagnostic Criteria for Alcohol Abuse and Dependence – Alcohol Alert No. 30–1995." Archived from the original on 27 March 2010. Retrieved 17 April 2010.
4. WHO. "Lexicon of alcohol and drug terms published by the World Health Organization." World Health Organization. Archived from the original on 5 February 2013.
5. World Health Organization. *Global status report on alcohol and health 2018(PDF)*. World Health Organization; 2018. pp. 72, 80. ISBN 978-92-4-156563-9
6. *World Population Prospects – Population Division – United Nations*. population.un.org.
7. Billet SL. *Antabuse therapy: Alcoholism: The total treatment approach*. Springfield, IL: Charles C. Thomas; 1968.
8. Landegren J, Borglund E, Storgårds K. Treatment of scabies with disulfiram and benzyl benzoate emulsion: A controlled study. *Acta Derm Venereol*. 1978;59(3):274–276.
9. Jacobsen E. The pharmacology of antabuse (tetraethylthiuramdisulphide). *Addiction*. 1950;47(1):26–40.
10. Hald J, Jacobsen E, Larsen V. The sensitizing effect of tetraethylthiuramdisulphide (antabuse) to ethylalcohol. *Basic Clin Pharmacol Toxicol*. 1948;4(3–4):285–296.
11. Petersen EN. The pharmacology and toxicology of disulfiram and its metabolites. *Acta Psychiatr Scand*. 1992;86(S369):7–13.
12. Peachey JE, Brien JF, Roach CA, Loomis CW. A comparative review of the pharmacological and toxicological properties of disulfiram and calcium carbimide. *J Clin Psychopharmacol*. 1981;1(1):21–26.
13. Yourick JJ, Faiman MD. Disulfiram metabolism as a requirement for the inhibition of rat liver mitochondrial low Km aldehyde dehydrogenase. *Biochem. Pharmacol*. 1991;42(7):1361–1366.
14. Brien JF, Loomis CW. Disposition and pharmacokinetics of disulfiram and calcium carbimide (calcium cyanamide). *Drug Metab Rev*. 1983;14(1):113–126.
15. Yourick JJ, Faiman MD. Diethyldithiocarbamic acid-methyl ester: A metabolite of disulfiram and its alcohol sensitizing properties in the disulfiram-ethanol reaction. *Alcohol*. 1987;4(6):463–467.
16. Ewing JA, Rouse BA, Mueller RA, Silver D. Can dopamine beta-hydroxylase levels predict adverse reactions to disulfiram? *Alcohol Clin Exp Res*. 1978;2(1):93–94.
17. Ewing JA, Mueller RA, Rouse BA, Silver D. Low levels of dopamine beta-hydroxylase and psychosis. *Am J Psychiatry*. 1977;134(8):927–933.
18. Kosten TR, Wu G, Huang W, Harding MJ, Hamon SC, Lappalainen J, Nielsen DA. Pharmacogenetic randomized trial for cocaine abuse: Disulfiram and dopamine β-hydroxylase. *Biol Psychiatry*. 2013;73(3):219–224.
19. Uri JV, Parks DB. Disulfiram-like reaction to certain cephalosporins. *Ther Drug Monit*. 1983;5(2):219–224.
20. Weathermon R, Crabb DW. Alcohol and medication interactions. *Alcohol Res Health*. 1999;23(1):40–54.
21. Towell J, Garthwaite T, Wang R. Erythrocyte aldehyde dehydrogenase and disulfiramlike side effects of hypoglycemics and antianginals. *Alcohol Clin Exp Res*. 1985;9(5): 438–442.
22. Visapää JP, Tillonen JS, Kaihovaara PS, Salaspuro MP. Lack of disulfiram-like reaction with metronidazole and ethanol. *Ann Pharmacother*. 2002;36(6):971–974.
23. Wilkin JK. Flushing reactions: Consequences and mechanisms. *Ann Intern Med*. 1981;95(4):468–476.
24. Vasiliou V, Malamas M, Marselos M. The mechanism of alcohol intolerance produced by various therapeutic agents. *Basic Clin Pharmacol Toxicol*. 1986;58(5):305–310.

25. Beach CA, Mays DC, Guiler RC, Jacober CH, Gerber N. Inhibition of elimination of caffeine by disulfiram in normal subjects and recovering alcoholics. *Clin Pharmacol Ther*. 1986;39(3):265–270.
26. MacLeod SM, Sellers EM, Giles HG, Billings BJ, Martin PR, Greenblatt DJ, Marshman JA. Interaction of disulfiram with benzodiazepines. *Clin Pharmacol Ther*. 1978;24(5):583–589.
27. Abernethy DR, Greenblatt DJ, Ochs HR, Shader RI. Benzodiazepine drug-drug interactions commonly occurring in clinical practice. *Curr Med Res Opin*. 1984;8(Suppl 4):80–93.
28. Loi CM, Day JD, Jue SG, Bush ED, Costello P, Dewey LV, Vestal RE. Dose-dependent inhibition of theophylline metabolism by disulfiram in recovering alcoholics. *Clin Pharmacol Ther*. 1989;45(5):476–486.
29. Mutschler J, Grosshans M, Bühler M, Diehl A, Kiefer F. Disulfiram in the treatment of pathological gambling? *Pharmacopsychiatry*. 2009;42(5):110.
30. Mutschler J, Bühler M, Diehl A, Mann K, Kiefer F. Disulfiram, an old drug with new potential in the treatment of pathological gambling? *Med Hypotheses*. 2010;74(1):209–210.
31. Petersen EN. The pharmacology and toxicology of disulfiram and its metabolites. *Acta Psychiatr Scand*. 1992;86(S369):7–13.
32. Mohapatra S, Sahoo MR, Rath N. Disulfiram-induced neuropathy: a case report. *Gen Hosp Psychiatry*. 2015;37(1):97–99.
33. Melo RC, Lopes R, Alves JC. A case of psychosis in disulfiram treatment for alcoholism. *Case Rep Psychiatry*. 2014;2014:561092.
34. Malcolm R, Olive MF, Lechner W. The safety of disulfiram for the treatment of alcohol and cocaine dependence in randomized clinical trials: Guidance for clinical practice. *Expert Opin Drug Saf*. 2008;7(4):459–472.
35. Grover S, Mattoo SK, Pendharkar S, Kandappan V. Sexual dysfunction in patients with alcohol and opioid dependence. *Indian J Psychol Med*. 2014;36(4):355–365.
36. Jensen SB. Sexual function and dysfunction in younger married alcoholics: A comparative study. *Acta Psychiatr Scand*. 1984;69(6):543–549.
37. Sarkar S. Surreptitious use of disulfiram. *Indian J Med Ethics*. 2013;10:71–72.
38. Brewer C, Meyers RJ, Johnsen J. Does disulfiram help to prevent relapse in alcohol abuse? *CNS Drugs*. 2000;14(5):329–341.
39. Brewer C. Long-term, high-dose disulfiram in the treatment of alcohol abuse. *Br J Psychiatry*. 1993;163(5):687–689.
40. Mutschler J, Dirican G, Funke S, Obermann C, Grosshans M, Mann K, Kiefer F, Diehl A. Experienced acetaldehyde reaction does not improve treatment response in outpatients treated with supervised disulfiram. *Clin Neuropharmacol*. 2011;34(4):161–165.

28
Optimising Patient Care Using Naltrexone for Opioid Use Disorders

Colin Brewer

Introduction	300
Background	300
Naltrexone Is Not Just a Drug: Psychological, Pharmacological and Educational Components of Naltrexone Treatment	303
Some Problems of NTX Treatment	308
Confirming the Blockade	308
Regular Challenges	309
Overcoming the Blockade	309
Pseudo-Breakthrough	309
Case History	310
Opiate Overdose Prevention	310
Naltrexone and Sexual Function	310
Initiating NTX Treatment	311
Future Developments	313

INTRODUCTION

This chapter discusses the use of the opiate antagonist naltrexone (NTX) in opiate abuse. It does not discuss – or mentions only briefly – the use of NTX in alcohol abuse, stimulant abuse or non-chemical addictive behaviours such as compulsive gambling or excessive eating or other compulsive behaviour. The main reason for the distinction is that while NTX, when logically, consistently and appropriately prescribed and administered, can have a large impact on opiate abuse, its effectiveness in alcoholism, compared with placebo, is modest, and for those other addictions, it is marginal.

BACKGROUND

Among the small range of effective medications for the treatment of opiate abuse, naltrexone (NTX) has several useful and desirable features. Unlike prescribed opiate agonists, it involves no problems of abuse, withdrawal syndromes, respiratory depression, legislative restriction or diversion. Over 40 years of clinical experience have shown that it is remarkably safe in overdose and apparently completely lacking in serious, clinically important organ toxicity. In particular – and contrary to many claims and warnings in scientific papers and product information leaflets – it has *no clinically significant hepatotoxicity*, as will shortly be documented. When adequate blood levels are maintained, NTX can also be more effective than opiate agonist maintenance (OAM) with methadone, buprenorphine or morphine at preventing relapse to regular illicit opiate use. Indeed, there are few other drugs in any field that will so obligingly 'do what it says on the packet' with so few adverse effects.

The pharmacokinetics and relatively low daily dose-requirement of parenteral NTX (avoiding first-pass metabolism) make it suitable for clinically useful long-acting depot or implanted NTX (DINTX) preparations, also categorised as 'extended-release'. Poor compliance with oral NTX seriously undermined its potential use and effectiveness in most settings until DINTX preparations started to become licensed for treating opiate abuse some 10 years ago – and about 40 years after the first animal studies of NTX implants indicated their potential.[1] They are now widely and increasingly used but many clinicians showed a depressing lack of imagination and awareness of the several validated and common-sense techniques for improving oral compliance. An early example of imaginative prescribing was Brahen et al.'s 1984 study of prisoners – previously addicted to heroin and mostly jailed for drug-related offences – who were allowed day-release employment if they took oral NTX daily under supervision before leaving prison for work. Despite their unpromising demographics and reputation as a group, compliance was high, and they soon became among the most trusted inmates.[2] This chapter will review the evolution of treatment with NTX (and, by implication at least, with other existing and future opioid antagonists) in the management of opiate abuse. It will also discuss some conceptual, psychological and medico-political aspects of NTX treatment and describe some clinical techniques that the author has found helpful since first treating patients with oral NTX in 1985 and with DINTX in 1997.

From the steadily increasing number of randomised controlled trials (RCTs), it is clear that DINTX is superior to depot or implanted placebo preparations in terms of abstinence or large reductions in opiate use. Not all these trials will be discussed in detail, but in a large 24-week RCT in Russia of monthly depot NTX injections, urine-confirmed abstinence was 90% for NTX vs 35% for placebo and median treatment retention was 168 vs 96 days.[3] These results have been broadly repeated in subsequent trials, though, as always, outcomes are better or worse depending, in part, on whether patients are recruited from higher or lower socio-educational classes or from offenders. In another Russian study, implanted NTX (duration approximately 8 weeks) was – perhaps unsurprisingly – also superior to placebo implant plus oral NTX (53% vs 16% treatment retention) and to double placebo (11%).[4] The Russian studies received some criticism on the grounds that the illegality of opiate agonist maintenance (OAM) gave patients little choice in medical treatments, but most RCTs have been done in countries where OAM is available for patients who, for various reasons, are not ready or willing to try what one might call 'antagonist-assisted abstinence' (or who prefer the unassisted variety). In one such country – Australia – a large record-linked study comparing the 6-month Perth implant with OAM programmes using buprenorphine or methadone, found that

> Crude mortality rates are comparable in patients with an opioid use disorder treated with implant naltrexone, methadone, and buprenorphine. However, implant naltrexone may be associated with benefits during the first 28 days of treatment and in female patients compared to methadone.[5]

In 2014, a qualitative literature review concluded that

> The majority of studies indicate that [DINTX] is effective in reducing heroin use, and the most frequently studied [DINTX] formulations have acceptable adverse events

profiles. Registry data indicate a protective effect of [DINTX] on mortality and morbidity. In some studies, [DINTX] also seems to affect other outcomes, such as concomitant substance use, vocational training attendance, needle use, and risk behaviour for blood-borne diseases such as hepatitis or human immunodeficiency virus.[6]

NTX was the result of a US government-backed project in the 1960s to develop opiate antagonists specifically for their possible use in treating heroin addicts. Dole and Nyswander's promotion of methadone maintenance therapy (MMT) in the same decade[7] was not universally welcomed at the time and is still deplored by some people (and some countries, most notably Russia), who regard it as simply 'giving drugs to addicts'. In reality, the closest comparison of OAM is with nicotine replacement therapy – including informal replacement by vaping – for tobacco addiction. Both politically and pharmacologically, NTX is as different from OAM as it is possible to be but it is important to understand that NTX is not 'better' (or 'worse') than OAM. Each treatment has advantages and disadvantages and both may be indicated at different stages of the same patient's addiction career. In particular, it is much easier to initiate OAM than NTX, and since treatment strategy – as opposed to short-term interventions – should not usually be decided in a hurry, a short period of OAM (where legislation permits) is often both appropriate and helpful before a decision to aim for antagonist-assisted abstinence. It also gives lungs, veins and other organs damaged by the addiction a chance to recover before a NTX induction process that sometimes needs high levels of sedation to ensure success, as discussed later. A good addiction clinic should resemble a good family-planning clinic in that it should offer – or at least discuss – the whole menu of evidence-based interventions, honestly explain the advantages and disadvantages of each item on the menu, allow the patient an important voice in treatment decisions and be willing to change the treatment if it does not seem to be working or has unacceptable side effects.[8] It should certainly not base treatment recommendations on what is most profitable for the clinic. Private residential clinics that offer only one type of treatment (and often proclaim that only one type of addiction treatment is appropriate, usually based on '12-step' principles or adherence to a particular religion) are unlikely to provide honest and independent advice about all evidence-based treatments.[9] It is unfortunate that in some countries where methadone and buprenorphine maintenance had become available only after overcoming public and governmental opposition, NTX programmes were seen by some physicians as a threat – both ideological and financial. Conversely, some political and medical enthusiasts regarded NTX as an argument for reducing support for OAM programmes or even abolishing them. Neither of these positions can be described as 'patient-centred'.

After a few false starts, the antagonist programme's first useful product was naloxone. Poorly absorbed by mouth and with a short half-life, it was unsuitable for addiction treatment but soon became an invaluable drug for opiate overdoses and the therapeutic reversal of opiates in other situations, notably in recovery from anaesthesia and in childbirth. Naltrexone was synthesised in the late 1960s when many US soldiers fighting in Vietnam became addicted to locally produced opium and heroin. According to former US deputy drug czar Prof Herb Kleber, clearance for its experimental use was therefore expedited. The first clinical trials started in 1972, though, as is abundantly documented, when the addicted veterans returned to the United States, a large majority – to the surprise of most clinicians and academics – stopped using heroin with little or no treatment. (The 12-step movement, for whom overcoming addiction requires daily and lifelong exertions, were particularly surprised.) However, because there was still some uncertainty about its effects on the liver, the FDA required a 'black box' warning about possible hepatotoxicity.[10] The caution has never been withdrawn, even though no evidence of clinically significant disturbance of liver functions has been reported. Indeed, the most convincing proof of NTX's lack of hepatotoxicity is that NTX, in oral doses at or above the normal 50 mg daily, is routinely and safely used 'off label' to relieve the intolerable itching of severe jaundice caused by a range of severe liver diseases – some of them so severe that liver transplantation was being actively considered. This has been known since the 1990s[11] and should have influenced prescribing advice. In one case report, a patient who had received a NTX implant became jaundiced from hepatitis B, acquired when he shared injecting equipment on a single occasion four weeks before implantation. The implant was not removed, and the hepatitis resolved completely in the usual time-scale with no more than typical elevations of liver function tests. There is no evidence that NTX has any clinically significant hepatotoxicity and much evidence that it has none. In short: *naltrexone is not hepatotoxic.*[12] Since NTX is a thebaine derivative and structurally similar to morphine – a drug notably lacking in organ toxicity – perhaps that should not be surprising.

NALTREXONE IS NOT JUST A DRUG: PSYCHOLOGICAL, PHARMACOLOGICAL AND EDUCATIONAL COMPONENTS OF NALTREXONE TREATMENT

One of the hopes and theories behind the antagonist development programme was that if addicts continued to smoke, sniff or inject heroin while its desirable effects were blocked by an antagonist, a process of Pavlovian conditioned extinction would soon change the patient's habits.[13] It quickly became clear that early extinction did not occur, though the debate has not entirely disappeared,[14,15,16] Compliance with oral medication is poor in many conditions, and addicts are naturally ambivalent about taking a medication that is designed to reduce or prevent an activity that a part of them still finds attractive. (If they were not ambivalent, they would either decline all treatment or not need any treatment, except for withdrawal.) Consequently, very few patients took oral NTX for long enough for the purported extinction process to occur. Those patients were often unusually well motivated or obliged by professional or legal undertakings to comply with treatment, although strong family bonds in some cultures sometimes translated to good medium-term outcomes from family-supervised oral NTX. At the time of writing, there have only been few studies of NTX in opiate abuse lasting for at least a year and only one without significant levels of drop-out that might invalidate or modify conclusions.[17] It involved supervised oral NTX as one condition of parole for heroin-related offenders, together with counselling, and its 2-year follow-up period[18] may still be the longest for NTX in opiate abuse. The 75% 12-month success rate (no opiate use on thrice-weekly supervised urine testing, no further offences) vs 25% without NTX proved it to be very effective. The absence of an immediate increase in relapse when the NTX component was discontinued at 12 months also indicates that achieving a lengthy period of consistent abstinence while patients live in their ordinary temptation-filled environments can cause lasting and positive changes in addictive behaviour – an important clinical and theoretical point that will be discussed in more detail later. However, while this Singaporean study and a later US one[19] are particularly important within a judicial context, the impressive short- and medium-term outcomes were not representative of the essentially voluntary treatment programmes that are typical of ordinary practice in most countries. Nevertheless, because there are many similarities between the psychological principles of alcoholism treatment with supervised oral disulfiram (DSF, Antabuse) and those of opiate abuse treatment with supervised oral NTX and DINTX formulations, it is both legitimate and clinically useful to draw on the much larger evidence base for supervised disulfiram treatment. In contrast to NTX studies in opiate dependence, there are several studies of DSF treatment for alcoholism in which patients were followed for periods of up to several years,[20,21] the longest by far being the 9 years of the most convincing, successful and informative study of supervised DSF by Krampe et al.[22]

To understand this similarity with DSF treatment and the implications that flow from it, it is first necessary to understand the relationship between the psychological and pharmacological components of both NTX treatment and DSF treatment. NTX is a pure, competitive opiate antagonist, and at adequate blood levels, it has been shown to block the euphoriant and other typical opiate effects (including respiratory depression) of up to 500 mg of intranasal diamorphine[23] and 1000 mcg of intravenous (i/v) fentanyl[24] – opiate amounts or equivalents greater than most addicts would use in a single dose even if they were planning suicide. That is the pharmacological component. NTX does not, however, directly *prevent* the use of opiates, and a significant proportion of patients use opiates at least once while taking oral or DINTX, even though most of them will not experience any genuine opiate effects. The reasons for continued opiate use will be discussed later, but some NTX patients use opiates only once or twice, just to confirm that NTX really does block them. For others, repeated testing of the blockade indicates varying degrees of ambivalence about treatment and may be a prelude to the abandonment of antagonist treatment in favour of OAM or to abandoning treatment altogether. In placebo-controlled studies (which now mainly involve DINTX) the often-claimed specific anti-craving effects of NTX are hard to discern in terms of time to first use of opiates[25] – an important finding discussed in more detail below. Furthermore, in a comparison of DSF and oral NTX for alcohol abuse, although craving was lower in the NTX group, DSF was significantly – and considerably – more effective in terms of abstinence and time to first relapse.[26]

Depending on patient selection, many NTX patients never challenge the blockade even once, whether they are in the active or placebo wing. They are *deterred* from doing so by the knowledge or belief that if they use opiates, they will experience disappointment but no opiate effects and will have wasted their money. In this respect, they resemble the large proportion of supervised DSF patients – a sizeable majority in most studies – who never risk drinking even once while taking DSF and also, in placebo-controlled trials, regardless of whether the medication is active or placebo. They, too, are *deterred* from using their drug of choice. The main difference is that instead of being deterred, in NTX treatment, by the prospect of *psychological* unpleasantness – disappointment and frustration – instead of the expected pleasant effects of opiates, DSF patients are deterred from drinking by the prospect of an unpleasant *physical* experience – the disulfiram-ethanol reaction – instead of alcohol's desired effects. When NTX and DSF patients consistently maintain abstinence without challenging the blockade or risking a DER, the mechanism must therefore be entirely psychological, since the pharmacologies of NTX and DSF are never required to come into play, and similar findings occur with placebo NTX and placebo DSF; and also with DSF implants that do not produce pharmacologically effective – or even detectable – levels of DSF and its active metabolite.[27] (As Skinner et al.[28] have pointed out, that is why DSF – almost uniquely for a medication – is not suited to placebo-controlled trials, since most blinded placebo patients are also reluctant to risk a DER.) The psychological components of this variety of abstinence are a mixture of placebo and non-specific effects and deterrence, the latter caused by the patient's *perception* of and belief in the pharmacological effects but not directly by those effects.

With NTX, deterrence and pharmacology combine to become the main mechanisms of abstinence if patients do use opiates but cooperate with taking NTX as prescribed. Most of these patients do not continue to use opiates in significant quantities because they are deterred not by the prospect but by the actual experience of opiate blockade. That mechanism is more clearly based on pharmacology, since placebo patients who take opiates find that they are not blocked and are, unsurprisingly, more likely to continue to use them – though not all do.

Similar considerations apply to DSF which, like NTX, does not directly *prevent* patients from using their drug of choice. A minority of patients do test out DSF's ability to produce a DER by drinking and are then deterred from further drinking by the actual experience of the DER, provided that the DSF dose is adequate. If it is not sufficient to produce a DER with no more than one unit of alcohol, the dose of DSF should be increased.,[29,30] Similarly, if the standard dose of oral or depot NTX does not provide complete opiate blockade (as may occasionally happen, especially in very overweight patients), the dose should be increased unless physical dependence and tolerance have recurred, in which case detoxification and re-induction of NTX may be needed.

With both NTX and DSF, continued taking of medication is nearly always associated with continued abstinence or with very large reductions in the amount and frequency of target drug intake. Although for some patients, this reduction has a significant pharmacological basis, the deterrent effect is primarily – and increasingly – a psychological process. That becomes more obvious as a steadily increasing period passes with no opiate or alcohol use. However, part of the improvement is due to the 'healthy complier' effect, which tells us a lot about both placebos and compliance. While good compliance with effective treatment (i.e., diligently following 'doctor's orders') leads to better outcomes than half-hearted compliance or leaving treatment, compliance itself, *even to placebos*, is a very important predictor of good outcomes. In other words, and particularly where well-motivated patients are concerned, the nature of the treatment complied with may be much less important than whether the level of compliance with treatment is high or low, probably because good compliers tend to be diligent, health-conscious and well-organised people. These personality traits are useful in most areas of life and are likely to facilitate recovery from any illness, condition or misfortune. In contrast, poor compliers are more likely to be disorganised and short on self-discipline – traits that are not helpful if they are trying to lose old and maladaptive habits and to acquire, perfect and make routine new and better ones, which is the aim of all addiction treatment.[31]

As with alcohol, persistently abstaining from opiates even when they are easily available involves changing a well-established drug habit and the several additional habits that usually go with it – mostly involving association with like-minded people in particular environments and using drugs to avoid or palliate unpleasant feelings (including withdrawal symptoms) or to facilitate pleasant ones. Since opiate abuse usually starts in adolescence and may be commoner in families with low 'social capital', some patients may never have acquired the habits of mind and behaviour (and the education) that make people attractive to employers. These patients may need help to acquire those habits from scratch, often along with important social skills. In other patients, important habits and skills may have atrophied following significant periods of unemployment, imprisonment or inability to work because of blood-borne virus infections such as hepatitis. These learned and – by definition – maladaptive habits need to be not just unlearned but replaced with habits that are ideally and typically agreed by both patient and therapist to be more adaptive and desirable. That takes time, and while avoiding relapse to opiate use is an important goal (and often a primary goal at this stage), it is particularly important to avoid relapse early in treatment when the patient's confidence in his ability to change may be low. A relapse at this stage can be very damaging to the patient's morale and does not exactly foster enthusiasm and optimism in the therapist or therapeutic team. Both DSF and NTX can make it much easier for patients to avoid relapse during those crucial first weeks and months of treatment and they do so, as we have seen, by very similar mechanisms.

That first stage typically lasts for at least 3 months, by which time most patients will have recovered from the pharmacological withdrawal syndrome and their sleep, appetite, mood and libido will be much improved without the need for continuing additional medication. However, a small but significant proportion of patients suffer prolonged opiate withdrawal symptoms – notably persistent insomnia, which can be very demoralising and is a common cause of relapse. Despite the risks of dependence, it is the author's view that when insomnia is prolonged and clearly distressing, chemical sleep is better than no sleep. Even an opiate withdrawal syndrome that lasts no more than the usual 3 to 4 weeks may need energetic and targeted symptomatic relief with non-sedative drugs such as clonidine or lofexidine (for persistent sweating) non-opiate analgesics (for arthralgia or persistent pain from old injuries) and octreotide (for severe and persistent diarrhoea). Some unfortunate patients with prolonged withdrawal symptoms may need to consider whether a change to opiate agonist maintenance might be more helpful, even if they do not like the idea of resuming indefinite opiate dependence. The existence of prolonged withdrawal symptoms has been known for many decades,[32] and an OAM programme that enables a patient to work and thrive is better than a NTX programme that doesn't. Naturally, some patients will drop out of treatment during the first stage. Effective treatment of withdrawal symptoms and simple 'supportive therapy' seem likely to reduce drop-out. So does rapid-readmission and the resumption of NTX treatment if a short lapse in treatment — such as between DINTX doses — leads to the return of physical dependence. Evidence from a unique study indicates, as one might expect, that longer-acting depot preparations give better continuity of treatment than shorter-acting ones, presumably because fewer decisions to continue treatment need to be made, especially in the first 4 weeks when ambivalence (and withdrawal symptoms) may still be prominent. De Jong, a Dutch physician, normally inserted 6-month implants produced by Go-Medical in Perth after rapid opiate withdrawal under anaesthesia (see below) but used 2-month implants when the Perth ones were unavailable. Although this was a 'natural experiment' rather than a controlled or prospective study, there were significantly fewer relapses and more sustained abstinences with the longer-acting implants.[33]

As well as complete recovery from the withdrawal syndrome, the end of the first stage of treatment is marked by consistent abstinence from opiates or only very occasional use, as admitted by the patient or detected by testing. Testing hair as well as urine can both detect and deter occasional opiate use and is particularly helpful when patients have returned to work and may not easily be able to appear for regular urine testing.[34] Since most drop-out occurs early in treatment, the patients who are still complying with medication at 3 months are likely to be those who are better motivated and therefore have a better prognosis. However, motivation is not static and is likely to be improved if brief lapses are prevented from becoming relapses (i.e., involving repeated use and the return of physical dependence), thus enabling the patient to feel some optimism about the future.

After that first stage, pharmacology and deterrence are gradually replaced in importance by specific cognitive-behavioural psychological processes that are similar to those that mediate the learning of skills relevant to professional training or sporting activities and education more generally. In many ways, successfully learning to abstain resembles the processes that mediate the learning of a second language — a subject about which a great deal is known.[35] Common sense and universal experience, as well as numerous studies, indicate that one of the simplest and quickest ways to become fluent in a second language is to live for at least a few months in a country where almost everyone speaks the second language. One should also spend as much time as possible mixing with the locals and as little time as possible with people who speak only your first language. This process is known as 'immersion', and all good language schools use it, but it also involves deterrence. The student is *deterred* from speaking his first language, partly because he has been instructed to avoid doing so but also because the locals may not understand him if he does, and it therefore becomes pointless — rather like using opiates while taking NTX. In a language school, the teachers will not respond unless the student speaks in the second language, however imperfectly and hesitantly. This is a variety of exposure and response prevention — a well-researched cognitive-behavioural technique for changing behaviours. Eventually, speaking the second language (exposure) and resisting the strong temptation to continue speaking the first language (response-prevention) become progressively easier and more normal. With NTX and DSF, deterrence similarly combines with following the agreed treatment programme to make abstaining from the target drugs progressively easier and more normal. As patients become increasingly fluent in the language of abstinence, that, in turn, enables them to devote more time and attention to learning – if necessary – what to do instead of using opiates or alcohol.

This second stage of treatment may need anything from 6 to 24 months. In most cases, once the withdrawal syndrome has faded, the patient's mood will have improved considerably without any specific treatment. The same will be true for other psychiatric symptoms. 'Dual diagnoses' do exist, but unless there is clear evidence that psychiatric diagnosis was merited well before serious addiction problems began, the confident diagnosis of allegedly underlying or co-morbid conditions should generally be delayed until withdrawal is complete, abstinence is well established and patients can reasonably begin to feel that they are making steady and significant progress towards the agreed treatment goals. The evidence from the OLITA study is that with continued abstinence, steady and spontaneous improvement in depression ratings is to be expected. Most treatment-seeking patients would have to have very unusual personalities and attitudes not to feel unhappy about what their addiction has been doing to them, and 'understandable misery' is often a more appropriate description of their condition than 'depression' or 'bipolar disorder'. Conversely, where a genuinely separate psychiatric condition does seem to exist, it is much easier to be sure of the diagnosis and optimise treatment when it is not complicated by withdrawal symptoms, acute regret or awareness of the amount and duration of rehabilitation that is needed, not to mention the ordinary processes of maturing out of common adolescent habits of thought and behaviour. During the second stage, patients who have jobs or are easily employable should ideally be working. If they lack important employment skills, they should receive appropriate training and education. If possible, important relationships should be repaired. Clearly, the whole range of individual, family and social therapies should be available, particularly those categorised as community reinforcement or network therapies. However, patients who have been on OAM for many years and are already 'rehabilitated' may need little more than support and appropriate medication to get through withdrawal. These people often have steady jobs and relationships and have stopped associating with other drug abusers. They will also generally be in their 30s or older and should thus have largely left adolescence and its discontents behind.

The third stage of treatment involves cautious trials of maintaining abstinence without NTX (or DSF) on the understanding that any lapse should be detected and terminated as soon as possible, together with the resumption, at least temporarily, of medication. Since evidence from the OLITA study and elsewhere suggests that some 18 months are often needed before these cautious trials can be made[36] and since very few NTX trials have lasted, or maintained a sufficient proportion of patients in treatment, for more than a year, much still remains to be learned about the optimal minimum period of NTX treatment. However, as a general rule, for all addiction treatments, greater length in treatment correlates with better outcomes – though that may also reflect the 'healthy complier effect'. The very encouraging lesson of the OLITA study is that when patients have been relapse-free on DSF for between 18 and 24 months, most of them are able to stop DSF in the next year or two without relapsing. Even of those who only took DSF for 12–20 months, 50% – on an intention-to-treat basis – were still abstinent 9 years after starting the OLITA programme. For those who took it for more than 20 months, the figure was 75%. After 18–24 months of consistent abstinence, patients tend to have changed their self-perception from 'I'm an alcoholic and always at risk of relapse' to 'I used to be an alcoholic but now alcohol is not important to me. I've leaned to live happily without it'. This is, of course, rather different from the 12-step philosophy, which encourages abstinent alcoholics to fear the possibility of relapse every day for the rest of their lives.

What applies to alcoholics treated with DSF in the OLITA programme might well apply to opiate addicts treated with NTX in a similar programme. Some patients would reach Stage 3 sooner (or later) than the average, but the OLITA study tells us that we should not be pessimistic about patients with a previous history of many relapses. The OLITA patients all had long histories of numerous unsuccessful treatments and had experienced an average of over seven in-patient detoxifications. Their average daily alcohol consumption, equal to well over a bottle of spirits daily, was high and their employment status poor. Yet most of them were treated for most of the time as out-patients or day-patients, which greatly reduces the staffing, administration and infrastructure costs compared with residential treatment. Initial intensive treatment became gradually less intensive but patients could easily access the service – including short-term admissions – if problems arose.

The final important similarity between DSF and NTX treatment is the way in which both drugs effectively remove one of the most annoying features of both alcoholism and opiate dependence – the endless internal arguments and conversations that patients have with themselves almost every minute of the day (especially early in treatment) about whether they should or shouldn't drink – or use opiates – when they are supposed to be abstaining. In one study,[37] alcoholic patients described it "in terms of an incessant internal homunculus that demanded alcohol". Disulfiram replaced those endless ruminations and temptations with "a life-world where alcohol is simply no longer an option", and NTX does much the same for opiates. One patient described how, when he wasn't taking disulfiram, he was "always tossing up whether I should drink or not. And I list all the pros, all the cons, but at the end of it, I just go 'fuck it, fuck it'. . . . When I'm on Antabuse, it's just like. Well, I can't". There has been little systematic study of equivalent changes in attitude by opiate-dependent patients treated with depot NTX. However, it is difficult not to be impressed by the number of patients who – as soon as a NTX implant is inserted – say things like: 'what a relief! . . . there's no point in using heroin now because I know that it won't have any effect!' This change is clearly a psychological rather than a psychopharmacological process because it occurs before any NTX has entered the bloodstream, but – like DSF – the change is based on the patient's accurate perception of a pharmacological reality.

SOME PROBLEMS OF NTX TREATMENT

Novel treatments commonly generate novel problems. NTX is not a new drug, but the widespread use of DINTX preparations is comparatively recent. With oral NTX treatment, an abstinent patient who very strongly wished to experience opiate effects again merely had to stop taking the tablets, and within 24–72 hours, depending on dose and metabolism, the blockade would have ended. With DINTX preparations, the gap between a determination to experience opiate effects and actually being able to experience them can be anything from 4–5 weeks, in the case of Vivitrol injections, to 6 months or more with the long-acting Perth implants. Most patients who are determined to resume opiate use probably wait until near the expected disappearance of the blockade before challenging it regularly in the hope of breakthrough, because to do so much before that stage would be a waste of money. Nevertheless, some patients do challenge it repeatedly – though usually infrequently – from the start of treatment. There are several reasons they do so.

CONFIRMING THE BLOCKADE

As already mentioned, some patients use opiates once or twice after initiating DINTX treatment merely to confirm that it really does 'do what it says on the can'. They do not want or intend to relapse but are worried that DINTX may not actually block opiates if they are temped to use them. Once reassured, they do not challenge the blockade again and will probably continue with uninterrupted DINTX treatment if it is recommended.

REGULAR CHALLENGES

Particularly with Vivitrol, where the short pharmacological 'tail' means a period of only a week or two between full blockade and no blockade at all, the duration of blockade may be significantly less than the duration of a strong desire to use opiates, especially if distressing withdrawal symptoms are still present at 4–5 weeks. Such patients may be impatient for the blockade to wear off and despite warnings about the risk of accidental overdose (see subsequently) challenge the blockade regularly and frequently at 4–5 weeks, resuming daily use (and/or agonist maintenance) as soon as pharmacologically possible.

Following a few individual case histories[38] and small uncontrolled series[39] of patients who use opiates despite adequate blockade, larger placebo-controlled studies have shed some useful light on this behaviour, which has both theoretical and practical implications. The first to examine the problem specifically concluded that

> Challenging naltrexone blockade with heroin on at least one occasion is common among sustained-release naltrexone patients, but only a minority of patients use opioids regularly. Challenges represent a warning sign for poor outcomes and often occur in the context of polydrug use and social adjustment problems.[40]

The most recent study[41] confirmed previous findings (and the intuitive expectation) that while many patients in both placebo and active wings never challenged the blockade, those who did so were significantly more likely to use opiates again if they were in the placebo wing. It also found that "Just under a third of patients (31%) on XR-NTX had no opioid-positive urine tests across the trial, but the hypothesis that this would differ from placebo (20%) was not confirmed". Although the difference was almost at the significant level, the finding added to the considerable evidence that the often-claimed specific anti-craving effects of NTX are rather modest in practice and that cognitive and learning effects of the real or perceived opiate blockade are more important than conditioned extinction as mechanisms for lasting abstinence.[42,43]

OVERCOMING THE BLOCKADE

Because of individual variations in drug absorption, drug metabolism and receptor sensitivity, some patients may not have adequate blockade from the standard doses of oral or DINTX. In some cases, serum NTX levels will be sub-optimum; in others, the levels are supposedly optimal but insufficient in practice. Since NTX is a competitive antagonist, this means that if patients challenge the blockade, they may experience opiate breakthrough. In that event, well-motivated patients – like well-motivated DSF patients – will accept or even request a dose increase, because they want the protection that NTX gives.

PSEUDO-BREAKTHROUGH

Some essentially well-motivated patients test the blockade early in treatment either to confirm its existence or in the hope of at least an occasional opiate experience and are worried when they think they actually experienced breakthrough. Although they may still be ambivalent about abstinence, on balance they want treatment to succeed. It may be obvious from their description that what they are experiencing is not actually breakthrough and may reflect opiate-related histamine release (which is not blocked by NTX) suggestion or high anxiety. If there is doubt or if reassurance fails, test-dosing with a short-acting opiate such as morphine or fentanyl will instantly clarify the situation.

Case History

A young woman with a history of anxiety preceding the onset of i/v heroin abuse and of much failed addiction treatment, received an implant expected to block opiates for at least 8 weeks. She resumed injecting heroin occasionally during the first month after implantation but, following a third consecutive implant, started to inject almost daily. She insisted that she was getting typical heroin effects, but there was no objective opiate response to a large test dose of i/v diamorphine (legally possible in Britain) and no reaction to high doses of i/v naloxone either, proving that she had not developed physical dependence. On two occasions, NTX and 6-beta-NTX levels were well above conventional minimally effective antagonist levels. Fortunately, with appropriate counselling and support, she was able to abandon this behaviour. Six years later, she had remained opiate-free and was leading a full and fairly conventional life.

OPIATE OVERDOSE PREVENTION

The current epidemic of fatal opiate overdose deaths (OOD) in the United States has focused attention on the ability of DINTX to prevent or reduce them. Early fears that NTX might up-regulate mu-opiate receptors, making patients more at risk of OOD after stopping NTX, do not appear to have been supported but all patients who leave treatment prematurely, and all drug-free abstinence programmes have an increased risk of OOD compared with consistent opiate agonist or antagonist treatment. What is clear is that the long-acting Perth (GO-Medical) implants can not only provide complete blockade against opiate-induced euphoria for about 6 months but can also prevent opiate-induced respiratory depression – the main mechanism of OOD – for another 3 to 6 months because of their long pharmacological 'tail'.[44]

In addition to the previously-noted ability of NTX to block very large known amounts of opiates, one remarkable case report describes a Russian man with a history of heroin addiction who was employed as a heroin courier precisely because his NTX implant was thought to have made him impervious to temptation. For some non-suicidal reason, he decided to inject most of the large but unknown amount of heroin that he carried. He became briefly unconscious (and apnoeic) but recovered both consciousness and normal respiration without treatment before he could suffer significant anoxic brain damage. Presumably his peak heroin blood level was high enough to overcome the blockade for a minute or two, but as it quickly declined, the lower but still very high levels were adequately antagonised.[45] Oral NTX also prevented a fatal outcome in a Russian patient who attempted suicide with heroin after learning that he was HIV-positive.[46]

NALTREXONE AND SEXUAL FUNCTION

Since drop-out and relapse rates in most NTX follow-up studies are high, it has been difficult to do post-detox studies that can distinguish between the changes in sexual function after a completed detox followed by lasting abstinence and those that may relate specifically to the NTX component of treatment. Only one study – yet to be submitted for publication[47] – has had a long enough course and a low enough drop-out rate to provide reasonably robust indications. It was not possible, for practical and ethical reasons, to have a placebo control group, but it did not appear that NTX had adverse effects on sexual function that were significant in incidence or degree.

INITIATING NTX TREATMENT

NTX treatment, whether oral or DINTX, is normally initiated (and advised, in many publications) only when patients have been opiate free for a week or more and after a negative naloxone challenge, because of the risk of aggravating or precipitating opiate withdrawal symptoms. One of the main obstacles to expanding NTX treatment – and the most easily avoidable one apart from its cost – is the high dropout and low completion rate of conventional opiate withdrawal ('detox/detoxification') techniques. Even among well-motivated patients who were admitted after remaining on the waiting list for many months, the completion rate at a major British 'Centre of Excellence' attached to the famous Maudsley Psychiatric Hospital in London was remarkably low. Only 27% of patients stayed for the whole 28-day in-patient programme. Most discharged themselves a day or two after receiving the last dose of a 12-day methadone reduction. The programme did not include NTX initiation, but it is noteworthy that of this successful minority of patients, nearly half had resumed heroin use within a month and 10% died of opiate overdose or other heroin-related conditions in the following year.[48]

As with alcoholism, where the incidence of severe symptoms (including delirium tremens and seizures) during admission was under 10% in a large predictive meta-analysis,[49] most opiate addicts do not experience very severe withdrawal symptoms, but the symptoms usually persist for much longer than with alcohol. Even modest levels of discomfort can undermine motivation and resolve when continued for several days. Persistent insomnia, combined with the inadequate symptomatic relief that is so often the experience of heroin addicts due to punitive or merely unsympathetic attitudes among medical and nursing staff, add to the cumulative demoralisation caused by several days of diarrhoea, nausea, sweating, shivering, painful muscle spasms, fatigue and arthralgia. Outside of prison settings or geographically isolated clinics, patients often withdraw from treatment rather than from opiates. Self-discharge on the day of admission or failure to appear are common but often omitted from reported completion rates that are not calculated on a strict 'intention to treat' basis. Even when appropriate medication and support are offered, very few clinics report completion rates of more than 60% for conventional methods. Furthermore, when NTX or naloxone are administered a week after the last opiate dose, they may still cause a brief exacerbation of withdrawal that, unsurprisingly, deters some patients from accepting long-term NTX treatment. Even among patients with no history of recent opiate use or dependence and receiving NTX for alcohol abuse, some 10–15% experience transient but unpleasant symptoms after the first dose that are very similar to those of opiate withdrawal. They may represent the acute blockade of endorphins in a susceptible minority of patients.

For these reasons and to maximise the rates of withdrawal completion and NTX induction, techniques that used the ability of NTX (or naloxone – NLX) both to precipitate and to shorten opiate withdrawal were devised and published in the late 1970s[50] and early 1980s.[51] These techniques, broadly categorised as rapid opiate detoxification (ROD) – though rapid naltrexone induction would be equally accurate – mostly involved giving small but increasing doses of NTX or NLX while buffering the precipitated withdrawal symptoms with generous doses of sedatives and non-opiate analgesics and – once their theoretically predicted antiwithdrawal effects had been confirmed – alpha-adrenergic agonists such as clonidine. These simple out-patient or day-patient techniques, usually spread over 3–4 days, obtained rates of completion and oral NTX induction of around 80%. In-patient versions using higher levels of sedation achieved almost 100%.[52] By the late 1980s, Loimer et al. – whose psychiatric department in Vienna had, for some reason, a small but conventional intensive treatment unit (ITU) attached to it – showed that under general anaesthesia, a high-dose infusion of NLX could be safely given. When patients woke after around 6 hours of anaesthesia, most of them experienced only mild and diminishing withdrawal symptoms that were not exacerbated by continuing the NLX infusion for 48 hours.[53] (NTX was not then available in Austria.) After visiting Loimer's unit, I and an anaesthetist colleague were the first to use the technique outside Vienna – slightly modified to include both clonidine and the administration of NTX via naso-gastric tube.[54] However, because most addiction units had neither the facilities nor the expertise to use this humane development and similar ones involving lower levels of sedation (it is not inappropriate to compare it with anaesthesia or good analgesia in childbirth and dentistry) it went largely un-noticed, except in Israel and Spain, where family links that involved an intensive-care anaesthetist, a psychologist with an interest in addiction and an ambitious general physician led to the commercialisation and international promotion of what was called (and trademarked as) UROD – Ultra-Rapid Opiate Detoxification. In reality, the term 'Ultra Rapid', which soon became synonymous with the use of anaesthesia, is inappropriate. It is no more rapid than other ROD techniques that involve the administration of a full oral dose of NTX (or a depot/implant preparation) within a few hours and without full anaesthesia. One of these – the 'Asturian' technique, developed and widely used in Northern Spain – is so simple and safe that it involves no supervision by medical or nursing staff. Suitably instructed family members administer the medications at home according to a fixed protocol, and the patient returns to the clinic the following day for assessment, symptomatic relief and the continuation of oral NTX treatment under family supervision or the insertion of a NTX implant.[55]

Unfortunately, the commercialisation, combined with excessive and unjustified claims of both short-term and long-term effectiveness, the denigration of agonist maintenance and a few high-profile deaths that could probably have been avoided with better post-anaesthesia monitoring, made many academic addiction specialists both sceptical and angry.[56] That is unfortunate and also – for the many patients whose previous experiences of opiate withdrawal have been so distressing that they are reluctant to attempt it again – inhumane.[57] In experienced hands, humane ROD techniques have low morbidity and very low or absent mortality (see below) especially when compared with the morbidity and mortality of cosmetic surgery – a matter of vanity – or bariatric surgery, commonly used for another unhealthy addiction, that is, to food.[58] Further evidence of its safety comes from its use in two infants with severe congenital heart disease who had become therapeutically dependent on opiates and were unable to be withdrawn conventionally.[59] It might be thought that in the competitive and highly commercial medical atmosphere of the technology-loving United States, this approach would prove popular, but the anti-medical 'no pain, no gain' philosophy of most of the 12-step oriented clinics that still dominate US addiction treatment made them as opposed to simultaneous detoxification and NTX induction as they were (and often still are) to NTX treatment itself.

In Perth, where the longest-acting NTX implant was introduced about 20 years ago, over 10,000 patients have been rapidly detoxified and – in most cases – had an implant inserted during another non-anaesthetic rapid detoxification technique[60] with no deaths and only a small incidence of transient morbidity – mostly dehydration from persistent vomiting that needed some fluid replacement. The addition of octrectide to the list of anti-withdrawal medications has considerably reduced the incidence and severity of both vomiting and diarrhoea, and it is now routinely used as part of the pre-medication. The Perth technique uses very small but steadily increasing doses of i/v NLX to precipitate withdrawal in a controlled fashion. Midazolam provides both sedation and amnesia for the procedure, which may partly explain why Perth is unique in having had almost as many patients on NTX as on methadone or buprenorphine. Relatively light sedation is used because family members are present and can help to control the marked restlessness that is a feature of all rapid processes that do not use full anaesthesia. In combination with an excellent state-wide medical record linkage system, this programme has also provided academic researchers at the University of Western Australia with unparalleled opportunities to compare long-term mortality, medico-psychiatric morbidity and other outcomes in large numbers of patients treated with NTX or OAM. Their studies indicate that mortality is similar with both treatments, but the deaths that occur during methadone induction (from excessive methadone doses in the non- or barely tolerant or from inadequate methadone doses for which the patient compensates with excessive heroin that makes a lethal combination) are not a feature of NTX induction.[61] Depression and other psychiatric co-morbidity are common in addictions There is no evidence that NTX increases their incidence,[62] and, as with the OLITA study, the evidence suggests that consistent abstinence is associated with a steady decline in psychiatric symptoms without specific treatment and that antidepressant treatment does not accelerate the process, except perhaps in female patients to a non-significant extent. "HIV risk, psychiatric symptoms, and overall adjustment were markedly improved among all patients who remained on [DINTX] treatment and did not relapse, regardless of [antidepressant] assignment."[63]

Some NTX induction techniques can be described as accelerated or semi-rapid. Typically, all opiates are abruptly discontinued on admission, and the patient is generously medicated during 3–4 days of spontaneous withdrawal – preferably from a short-acting opiate or from buprenorphine which, with its partial antagonist properties, seems to facilitate the transition, although there are few comparative studies. NTX is given – usually after a NLX challenge – on day 3 or 4, by which time the resultant precipitated withdrawal is usually relatively mild, especially if NTX is initiated with very small but steadily escalating doses.[64] However, appropriate anti-emetic medication is important. The author knows of one patient, subsequently referred to him for NTX implantation, who was inadequately medicated during a 4–5 day detox and vomited so much after receiving his first dose of oral NTX that he acquired a gastric tear and required several units of blood for Mallory-Weiss syndrome.

FUTURE DEVELOPMENTS

NTX implants that can deliver effective blood levels for a year are already in development and will almost certainly improve outcomes that are already encouraging and both statistically and clinically significant. However, one of the most useful applications of DINTX may be in the management of pregnant opiate addicts, who are usually advised to begin or continue OAM and therefore deliver babies who nearly always need several days and sometimes weeks of care – sometimes relatively intensive – to recover from neo-natal withdrawal. Following the successful ROD and oral NTX induction of a patient in the second trimester, who subsequently had a full-term normal delivery of a healthy opiate-free child (who was a healthy 'normal' child 10 years later) the author collaborated in a publication with two other physicians who had treated pregnant women with oral or DINTX, usually after ROD procedures and with equally satisfactory obstetric outcomes.[65] In some cases, ROD was done without either patient or physician being aware of the pregnancy, but one of the authors – Pereira – so impressed his obstetric colleagues with the results that they referred further patients. Another of the authors – O'Neil – is an experienced and respected obstetrician-gynaecologist as well as an addiction physician and implant developer. In a large records-linked comparison of pregnant women treated with NTX, methadone or buprenorphine, NTX-treated patients did not greatly differ in the course of their pregnancies, but birth outcomes were superior, especially compared with methadone, and neonatal abstinence was, predictably, very uncommon.[66] Women treated with NTX also had higher fertility rates.

Since pregnant opiate addicts are quite often highly motivated to become opiate-free before delivery and since DINTX can facilitate both opiate-free deliveries and lasting post-partum abstinence, larger studies are surely indicated.

References

1. Martin WR, Sandquist V. A sustained release depot for narcotic antagonists. *Arch. Gen. Psychiat.* 1974;30(1):31–33.
2. Brahen L, Henderson R, Capone T. Naltrexone treatment in a jail work-release program. *J. Clin. Psychol.* 1984;45:49–52.
3. Krupitsky E, Nunes EV, Ling W, Illeperuma A, Gastfriend DR, Silverman BL. Injectable extended-release naltrexone for opioid dependence: A double-blind, placebo-controlled, multicentre randomised trial. *Lancet.* 2011;377(9776):1506–1513. doi: 10.1016/S0140-6736(11)60358-9
4. Krupitsky E, Zvartau E, Blokhina E, et al. Randomized trial of long-acting sustained-release naltrexone implant vs oral naltrexone or placebo for preventing relapse to opioid dependence. *Arch Gen Psychiatry.* 2012;69(9):973–981. doi: 10.1001/archgenpsychiatry.2012.1a.
5. Kelty E, Joyce D, Hulse G. A retrospective cohort study of mortality rates in patients with an opioid use disorder treated with implant naltrexone, oral methadone or sublingual buprenorphine. *Am J Drug Alcohol Abuse.* 2019;45(3):285–291. doi: 10.1080/00952990.2018.1545131.
6. Kunøe N, Lobmaier P, Ngo H, Hulse G. Injectable and implantable sustained release naltrexone in the treatment of opioid addiction. *Br J Clin Pharmacol.* 2014;77(2):264–271. doi: 10.1111/bcp.12011.
7. Dole VP, Nyswander M. A medical treatment for diacetylmorphine (heroin) addiction: A clinical trial with methadone hydrochloride. *JAMA.* 1965;193(8):646–650. doi: 10.1001/jama.1965.03090080008002.
8. Brewer C. Editorial (bilingual): Harm-reduction for unwanted pregnancies and unwanted addictions: An instructive analogy. *Adicciones,* 2008;20(1):5–13.
9. Brewer C. Fact, fiction, finance and effectiveness in alcoholism treatment. *Brit J Clin Pract.* 1987;41:39–46.
10. Kleber H. Personal communication.
11. Terg R, Coronel E, Sorda J, Munoz AE, Findor J. 2002. Efficacy and safety of oral naltrexone treatment for pruritus of cholestasis, a crossover, double blind, placebo controlled study. *J Hepatol,* 37(6):717–722.
12. Brewer C, Wong V-S. Naltrexone: A case report of lack of hepatotoxicity in acute viral hepatitis, with a review of the literature. *Addiction Biol.* 2004;9:81–87.
13. Wickler A. *Opioid dependence: Mechanisms and treatment.* Plenum Press. New York, 1980. *passim.*
14. Nunes EV, Bisaga A, Krupitsky E, et al. Opioid use and dropout from extended-release naltrexone in a controlled trial: Implications for mechanism. *Addiction.* 2020;115:239–246.
15. Kunøe N. Commentary on Nunes et al. Blocked opioid use in antagonist treatment-time for cognitive and user-centered perspectives. *Addiction.* 2020;115:247–248.
16. Ghosh A, Singh P. Extinction as the behavioral mechanism of naltrexone-extended release for opioid dependence: Could there be an alternate explanation? *Addiction.* 2020;115: doi: 10.1111/add.15105.
17. Chan KY. The Singapore naltrexone community-based project for heroin addicts compared with a drug-free community-based programme: The first cohort. *J Clin Forens Med.* 1996;3:87–92.
18. Chan KY. Singapore's probation-linked naltrexone programme. Paper presented at the 4th Stapleford international addiction conference, 1998, London, 9th Jan.
19. Cornish J, Metzger D, Woody G, et al. Naltrexone pharmacotherapy for opioid dependent federal probationers. *J Subst Abuse Tr.* 1997;14(6):529–534.
20. Azrin N, Sissons R, Meyer S, Godley M. Alcoholism treatment by disulfiram and community reinforcement therapy. *J Behav Ther Exp Psychiat.* 1982;13:105–112.
21. Azrin N. Disulfiram and behaviour therapy: A social-biochemical model of alcohol abuse and treatment. In: C. Brewer (Ed.), *Treatment options in addiction: Medical management of alcohol and opiate abuse.* Gaskell/Royal College of Psychiatrists. London, 1993.
22. Krampe H, Stawicki S, Wagner T, Bartels C, Aust C, Rüther E, Poser W, Ehrenreich H. Follow-up of 180 alcoholic patients for up to 7 years after outpatient treatment: Impact of alcohol deterrents on outcome. *Alc Clin Exp Res.* 2006;30(1):86–95.
23. Brewer C. Serum naltrexone and 6-beta-naltrexol levels from naltrexone implants can block very large amounts of heroin: A report on two cases. *Addiction Biol.* 2002;7:321–323.

24. Brewer C, Gastfriend DR. Rapid opioid detoxificiation. *JAMA*. 1998;279:172.
25. Nunes EV, Bisaga A, Krupitsky E, et al. Opioid use and dropout from extended-release naltrexone in a controlled trial: Implications for mechanism. *Addiction*. 2020;115:239–246.
26. De Sousa A, De Sousa A. A one-year pragmatic trial of naltrexone vs disulfiram in the treatment of alcohol dependence. *Alcohol*. 2004;39(6):528–531. doi:10.1093/alcalc/agh104
27. Johnsen J, Mørland G. Depot preparations of disulfiram: Experimental and clinical results. *Acta Psychiatrica Scandinavica*. 1992;86:27–30.
28. Skinner MD, Lahmek P, Pham H, et al. Disulfiram efficacy in the treatment of alcohol dependence: A meta analysis. *Plos One* 2014;9:e87366.
29. Newton-Howes G, Levack WM, McBride S, Gilmor M, Tester R. Non-physiological mechanisms influencing disulfiram treatment of alcohol use disorder: A grounded theory study. *Drug Alc Depend*. 2016;165:126–131.
30. Brewer C, Streel E. Ch.7 Components of effectiveness in disulfiram treatment and other interventions for alcoholism: Including placebo and non-specific effects. In: C. Brewer, E. Streel (Eds.), *Antabuse treatment for alcoholism: An evidence-based handbook for medical and non-medical clinicians*. Foreword by William R. Miller. CreateSpace IPP. North Charleston, SC, 2018.
31. Simpson SH, Eurich DT, Majumdar SR, Padwal RS, Tsuyuki RT, Varney J, Johnson JA. A meta-analysis of the association between adherence to drug therapy and mortality. *BMJ*. 2006 Jul 1;333(7557):15. Epub 2006 Jun 21.
32. Eklund, C. *Withdrawal from methadone maintenance treatment in Sweden*. Introduction, Uppsala University Press. Stockholm, Sweden, 1996.9–10.
33. de Jong C. Subcutaneous naltrexone implants: A one-year follow-up study. Paper presented at the 10th Stapleford international addiction conference, Athens, Feb 2011.
34. Brewer C. Hair analysis as a tool for monitoring and managing patients on methadone maintenance: A discussion. *Forensic Sci Int*. 1993 Dec;63(1–3):277–283. doi:10.1016/0379-0738(93)90281-e.
35. Brewer C, Streel E. Learning the language of abstinence in addiction treatment: Some similarities between relapse-prevention with disulfiram, naltrexone and other pharmacological antagonists and intensive "immersion" methods of foreign language teaching. *Subst Abuse*. 2003;24(3): 157–173.
36. Murphy S, Hoffman A. An empirical description of phases of maintenance following treatment for alcohol dependence. *J Subst Abuse*. 1993;5:131–143.
37. Newton-Howes G, Levack WM, McBride S, Gilmor M, Tester R. Non-physiological mechanisms influencing disulfiram treatment of alcohol use disorder: A grounded theory study. *Drug Alc Depend*. 2016;165:126–131.
38. Brewer C, Streel E. Current issues in the use of opioid antagonists: Naltrexone for opiate abuse: A re-educational tool as well as an effective drug. In: Reginald L. Dean III, Edward J. Bilsky, S. Stevens Negus III (Eds.), *Opioid Receptors and Antagonists: From Bench to Clinic*. Contemporary Neuroscience Series. Wiley. New York. 2009.
39. Foster J, Brewer C, Steele T. Naltrexone implants can completely prevent early (one month) relapse after opiate detoxification: A report on two cohorts totalling 101 patients with a note on blood levels of naltrexone. *Addiction Biol*. 2003;8:211–217.
40. Kunøe N, Lobmaier P, Vederhus JK, Hjerkinn B, Gossop M, Hegstad S, et al. Challenges to antagonist blockade during sustained-release naltrexone treatment. *Addiction*. 2010;105:1633–1639.
41. Nunes EV, Bisaga A, Krupitsky E, et al. Opioid use and dropout from extended-release naltrexone in a controlled trial: Implications for mechanism. *Addiction*. 2020;115:239–246.
42. Ghosh A, Singh P. Extinction as the behavioral mechanism of the naltrexone-extended release for opioid dependence: Could there be an alternative explanation? *Addiction*. 2020;115. doi: 10.1111/add.15105.
43. Kunøe N. Commentary on Nunes et al. Blocked opioid use in antagonist treatment: Time for cognitive and user-centered perspectives. *Addiction*. 2020;115:247–248.
44. Hulse GK, Tait RJ, Comer SD, et al. Reducing hospital presentations for opioid overdose in patients treated with sustained release naltrexone implants. *Drug Alc Depend*. 2005;79:351–357.
45. Krupitzky E, Burakov AMV, Tsoy M, Egorova V, Slavina T, Grinenko A, Zvartau E, Woody G. Overcoming opioid blockade from depot naltrexone (Prodetoxon®) *Addiction*. 2007 July;102(7):1164–1165.
46. Krupitsky EM, Masalov DV, Didenko TY, et al. Prevention of suicide by naltrexone in a recently detoxified heroin addict. *Eur Addict Res*. 2001;7(2):87–88. doi: 10.1159/000050722.
47. Koukidis E, Brewer C, Lagoudaki M. Changes in sexual interest and performance following opiate detoxification and oral naltrexone treatment: A prospective study. Paper presented at the 10th Stapleford international addiction conference, Athens, Greece, Feb 2011.

48. Strang J, McCambridge J, Best D, Beswick T, Bearn J, Rees S, Gossop M. Loss of tolerance and overdose mortality after inpatient opiate detoxification: Follow up study. *BMJ*. 2003;326:959–960.
49. Wood E, Albarqouni L, Tkachuk S, et al. Will this hospitalized patient develop severe alcohol withdrawal syndrome? The rational clinical examination systematic review. *JAMA*. 2018;320(8):825–833. doi: 10.1001/jama.2018.10574.
50. Blachly P, Casey D, Marcel L, et al. Rapid detoxification from heroin and methadone using naloxone: A model for study of the treatment of the opiate abstinence syndrome. In: E. Senay, V. Shorty, H. Alkesne (Eds.), *Devlopment in the field of drug abuse*. Schenkman Publishing Co. Cambridge, Mass. 1975.327–336.
51. Charney DS, Riordan CE, Kleber HD, et al. Clonidine and naltrexone: A safe, effective and rapid treatment of abrupt withdrawal from methadone therapy. *Arch Gen Psychiatry*. 1982;39:1327–1332.
52. Brewer C, Rezae H, Bailey C. Opiate withdrawal and naltrexone induction in 48–72 hours with minimal dropout using a modification of the clonidine-naltrexone technique. *British Journal of Psychiatry*. 1988;153:340–343.
53. Loimer N, Schmid R, Presslich O, Lenz K. Continuous naloxone administration suppresses opiate withdrawal symptoms in human opiate addicts during detoxification treatment. *J. Psychiatry Res*. 1988;23:81–86.
54. Brewer C. Taking the tears out of opiate withdrawal: High tech comes to the aid of heroin addicts. *Wellington Hospital News*. 1989 July.
55. Carreño JE, Bobes J, Brewer C, et al. 24-hour opiate detoxification and antagonist induction at home – the 'Asturian Method': A report on 1368 procedures. *Addict Biol*. 2002;7:243–250.
56. Brewer C, Williams J, Carreño JE, Bobes J. Unethical promotion of rapid opiate detoxification under anaesthesia (RODA). *Lancet*. 1998; 351:218.
57. Brewer C. Ultra-rapid, antagonist-precipitated opiate detoxification under general anaesthesia or sedation. (Invited review.) *Addiction Biol*. 1997;2:291–302.
58. Brewer C, de Jong CJ, Williams J. Rapid opiate detoxification and antagonist induction under general anaesthesia or intravenous sedation is humane, sometimes essential and should always be an option: Three illustrative case reports involving diabetes and epilepsy and a review of the literature. *J Psychopharmacol*. 2014 Jan;28(1):67–75.
59. Greenberg M. Ultra rapid opioid detoxification of two children with congenital heart disease. *J Addict Dis*. 2000;19:53–58.
60. Arnold-Reed D, Hulse GK. A comparison of rapid (opioid) detoxification with clonidine-assisted detoxification for heroin-dependent persons. *J Opioid Manag*. 2005 Mar–Apr;1(1):17–23. doi: 10.5055/jom.2005.0007.
61. Tait RJ, Ngo HT, Hulse GK. Mortality in heroin users 3 years after naltrexone implant or methadone maintenance treatment. *J Subst Abuse Treat*. 2008 Sep;35(2):116–124.
62. Ngo HT, Tait RJ, Arnold-Reed DE, Hulse GK. Mental health outcomes following naltrexone implant treatment for heroin-dependence. *Prog Neuropsychopharmacol Biol Psychiatry*. 2007;31(3):605–612. doi: 10.1016/j.pnpbp.2006.12.005.
63. Krupitsky EM, Zvartau EE, Masalov DV, et al. Naltrexone with or without fluoxetine for preventing relapse to heroin addiction in St. Petersburg, Russia. *J Subst Abuse Treat*. 2006;31(4):319–328. doi: 10.1016/j.jsat.2006.05.005.
64. Badaras R, Jovaisa T, Lapinskiene I, Ivaskevicius J. Dose escalation of naltrexone to reduce stress responses associated with opioid antagonist induction: A double-blind randomized trial. *J Addict Med*. 2020;14(3):253–260. doi: 10.1097/ADM.0000000000000560.
65. Hulse GK, O'Neill G, Pereira C, Brewer C. Obstetric and neonatal outcomes associated with maternal naltrexone exposure. *Aust N Z J Obstet Gynaecol*. 2001;41(4):424–428. doi: 10.1111/j.1479-828x.2001.tb01322.x.
66. Kelty E, Hulse G. A retrospective cohort study of obstetric outcomes in opioid-dependent women treated with implant naltrexone, oral methadone or sublingual buprenorphine, and non-dependent controls. *Drugs*. 2017;77(11):1199–1210. doi: 10.1007/s40265-017-0762-9.

29
Optimizing Patient Care – Suicide Prevention

Paul S. Links

Introduction	317
Assessment: Risk and Protective Factors (Adapted From Craven & Links, 2019)	318
Risk Assessment Is Not Suicide Prediction	318
Is Your Patient Suicidal?	319
Ask About Suicide	319
Special Situations	319
Investigate the Severity of the Suicidal Intent	319
Assess the Patient's Intent to Act	320
Self-Harm Versus Suicidality	320
Identify Factors That Increase Risk Substantially	320
Screening and Assessment Measures	321
Do Screening Questionnaires Help?	321
Using Questionnaires or Measures	322
Managing Patients at Risk (Adapted From Craven & Links, 2019; Sall et al., 2019; Weber et al., 2017)	322
Management of the Patient With a Suicide Plan and High Intent	323
Management of the Patient With Low Intent but With Serious Risk Factors	323
Management of the Patient With Suicidal Thoughts but No Plan	324
Transferring the High-Risk Patient for Emergency Psychiatric Consultation	324
If the Patient Is Co-Operative and Wants Help	325
If the Patient Is Not Co-Operative	325
Patients With a Chronic Risk for Suicide (Links et al., 2019)	325
Specific Strategies: Safety Planning; Removing Access to Means, Caring Contacts	326
Psychotherapy With Suicidal Patients	327
Psychotherapy Management of Patients With Suicide Risk	327
Conclusion	330

INTRODUCTION

The World Health Organization in 2012 estimated the global suicide rate to be 11.4 per 100,000, with the rate for men at 15.0 and women 8.0 per 100,000. Globally, 804,000 individuals died by suicide in 2012. However, the rates vary from country to country based on data from 172 countries with populations over 300,000; rates ranged from 0.4 to 44.2 per

100,000 (World Health Organization (WHO), 2014; p. 21). The highest suicide rates were found in low- and middle-income countries (LMICs) in South East Asia, accounting for 39% of global suicides, followed by high-income countries, with 25% of global deaths by suicide. Although estimates of the global suicide attempt rates were much more difficult to establish, the WHO report (2014) indicated that globally for each adult over 18 years of age who died by suicide, there were another more than 20 individuals who made one or more suicide attempts. The WHO report (2104) identified that a major strategy for the prevention of suicide is the use of evidence-based individual-level approaches to the assessment and management of persons with mental health disorders and/or who have attempted suicide.

Recently, new standards for assessing and managing mental health patients at risk for suicide have been widely adopted across the globe. In particular, the Zero Suicide approach aims to improve care for individuals at risk of suicide in healthcare systems and relies on a system-wide tactic to improve outcomes and close gaps rather than on the heroic efforts of individual health professionals (Hampton, 2010; Hogan, 2016; Suicide Prevention Resource Centre, 2015–2018). This quality improvement initiative has core components at three levels: a direct practice level that focuses on identifying the risk of suicidal behavior and necessitates treating the risk of suicide behavior as a distinct syndrome using best practice interventions; a process level related to quality and safety improvement to provide accessible, reliable and continuous care to patients and an organizational level that promotes a safety culture; and a system-wide commitment to the aspirational goal of zero suicides. (Mokkenstorm et al., 2018).

Although Zero Suicide has captured much attention and serves as a stimulus for this chapter, a recent systematic review of clinical practice guidelines in suicide prevention illustrates that many organizations and clinical specialties are working to inform emerging standards related to clinical practice, research and training in this area (Bernert et al., 2014). The current chapter will be informed by the evidence-based strategies coming from the Zero Suicide approach and will focus on the individual-level interventions that mental health clinicians can use in their community management of mental health patients. The chapter will begin by discussing the clinical assessment of suicide risk including a broad discussion of risk and protective factors; however, the reader must remember that these factors will vary from one community to the next. The role of screening and assessment measures of suicide risk will be introduced; however, no measure has sufficient strengthens to replace the necessary requirement for an assessment done by a clinician trained and experienced in suicide risk assessment and management. The chapter will highlight some specific interventions that should be under taken with patients at risk for suicide and introduce the approach to managing patients with a suicide plan and high intent, with low intent but with serious risk factors and with suicidal thoughts but no plan. The chapter will conclude with identifying important factors to imbed in the clinician-patient relationship and pinpointing that documentation and supervision are necessary to safeguard the clinician's welfare in managing patients at risk for suicide.

ASSESSMENT: RISK AND PROTECTIVE FACTORS (ADAPTED FROM CRAVEN & LINKS, 2019)

Risk Assessment Is Not Suicide Prediction

For the clinician to predict which individual will or will not attempt or die by suicide at any given point in time is impossible because suicide is a relatively rare event, and suicidal intent can change rapidly.

The clinician's job is to identify individuals at higher risk of suicide and take steps to lower and manage the patient's risk for suicide.

Is Your Patient Suicidal?

When seeing patients in the community, concern about suicide risk begins with one or more of the following:

- recognition that a patient is seriously distressed or mentally unwell.
- a clear or covert statement by the patient that he or she is considering suicide: "I'm not sure how long I can go on like this." "I'm just so tired of being down."
- communication from a family member or friend who is concerned about the patient: "He keeps talking about how we'd be better off without him."

Ask About Suicide

The clinician's responsibility is to investigate suicidal intent in the patient. The most direct, effective way to do this is to ask:

- "Have things gotten so bad that you've thought about hurting yourself or ending your life?"
- "Sometimes when people feel the way you do right now, they start to have thoughts about suicide. Has this ever happened to you?"

Why now? Identifying the most recent precipitants can help the clinician and patient target interventions to reduce risk. A calm, non-judgmental, concerned approach will tell the patient that you care and that you will be able to cope with his or her answer.

Note: Asking about suicidal intent does not cause the patient who is suicidal to more seriously consider this option. Talking openly about suicide typically can help relieve the patient's distress.

Special Situations

- After a romantic relationship has ended, ask the patient whether he or she has thoughts about harming/killing the former partner and/or children.
- In a female patient with postpartum depression and suicidality, ask about thoughts that the baby would be better off dead, intent to harm the child.

Investigate the Severity of the Suicidal Intent

If the patient endorses suicidal thoughts, the clinician's next task is to determine how serious the suicidal intent is.
  Ask the patient:

- "What kinds of thoughts have you been having?" (This is a high-yield question, so be sure to let the patient talk.)
- "How long have you been having these thoughts? When did they first start?"
- "How often are they happening? Daily? Weekly? All the time?"

Ask the patient to rate the severity of the suicidal thinking on a scale of 1 to 10, with 1 being very low intensity and 10 being extremely intense or severe.

Ask about a plan and access to means:

- "Do you have a plan for how you would kill yourself?"
- "Have you thought about any other methods?" (Patients may not reveal the most lethal method at first ask.)
- "Do you have any firearms or other weapons at home? Where are they?"

If the preferred method is overdose or hanging:

- "Have you bought or saved pills? Do you have poisons at home? Do you have a rope?"
- "Have you 'rehearsed' or 'gone through the motions' of killing yourself?"

Assess the Patient's Intent to Act

"In the next 24–48 hours, how likely is it that you will act on your suicidal plan?" (Ask the patient to rate the likelihood on a scale of 1 to 10, with 1 being very unlikely and 10 being certain.)

Consider whether the patient has a history of impulsivity (high-risk behaviors, overspending, fights, poorly thought-out decisions). If you don't know the patient well, ask:

- "Would you consider yourself an impulsive person?"
- "Have you recently felt out of control at times?"

Self-Harm Versus Suicidality

Not all patients who harm themselves by cutting, burning or other mutilating behaviors are actively suicidal. To differentiate self-harm from suicidal behavior, ask about the person's intentions. Was the cutting (burning, etc.) done to end the person's life, to gain relief from emotional distress or to overcome a feeling of numbness? Remember, patients who self-harm may have more than one intention for the behavior, and self-harm is a risk factor for future suicide attempts. Co-existence of both behaviors is common in borderline personality and other impulsive personality disorders.

Identify Factors That Increase Risk Substantially

Impaired Impulse Control

- Impulsivity or impaired reality testing
- Intoxication with alcohol or other drugs

Note: Do not permit the intoxicated suicidal patient to go home. Consider observing these patients until they are no longer intoxicated.

Hopelessness

- Ask the patient: "Are you feeling hopeless?" or "Can you see things getting better for you?"

Previous Attempted Suicide

- The more lethal the method used in previous attempts, the higher the risk.
- The risk increases with each attempt; the more recent the attempt, the higher the risk.
- People who have had multiple suicide attempts should be considered chronically at risk.
- People who were recently discharged from an inpatient psychiatric ward, particularly if suicide was attempted, are at higher risk.

Current Severe Psychiatric Disorder

- Major depression; mixed manic/depressive episodes
- Schizophrenia
- Alcohol abuse/dependence
- Borderline and antisocial personality disorders, especially in combination with major depression or active substance abuse

Other Factors Known to Increase Risk

- Family history of suicide or suicide attempts (there is likely a genetic as well as a family environment contribution)
- Alcohol/substance abuse
- Debilitating medical illness; chronic physical pain
- Recent loss (divorce, unemployment, death of someone close)

Assess Reasons for Living and Factors That May Be Protective

Ask the patient:

- "Things have been pretty rough. What keeps you going?"
- "You've been thinking about suicide, but you say you wouldn't follow through. What keeps you from harming yourself?"

Factors that may be associated with lower suicidal risk include:

- religious/moral beliefs that suicide is wrong
- married state
- children under 18 years of age living at home
- employment
- good social supports
- strong therapeutic relationship
- good problem-solving skills
- generally higher level of self-esteem

SCREENING AND ASSESSMENT MEASURES

Do Screening Questionnaires Help?

Self-administered screening tests are usually brief and easy to use, and they may help the clinician begin a difficult discussion or indicate further questioning. However, they often have a high percentage of false positives and a low positive predictive value when compared to the gold standard of the clinician interview or a more detailed clinician-administered assessment tool (Chan et al., 2016; LeFevre, 2014). Moreover, a single negative screen should not result in diminished clinical monitoring for suicidal ideation or intent. Ongoing assessment and a high index of suspicion are important in any patient with significant risk factors.

Using Questionnaires or Measures

New standards address the issues of using standard screening and assessment measures in the care of patients seen in emergency departments, mental health services and primary care. The Joint Commission in the United States called for the screening of all patients for suicidal ideation, using a brief, standardized, evidence-based screening tool (National Action Alliance for Suicide Prevention, 2018). The National Action Alliance for Suicide Prevention's "Recommended Standard Care for People with Suicide Risk" calls for primary care to screen all patients with mental illness and/or substance use disorders while recommending that emergency departments identify and assess all patients who have harmed themselves and those with mental illness and/or substance use disorders (National Action Alliance for Suicide Prevention, 2018). If the patient screens positive because of elevated risk, a more comprehensive assessment by a mental health professional using a standardized suicide risk assessment tool should follow.

The tools to utilize may vary by clinical settings; however, two examples of widely adopted and freely available tools are the Patient Health Questionnaire – 9 (PHQ-9) and the Columbia Suicide Severity Rating Scale (C-SSRS). The PHQ-9 is a screening tool used in primary care that asks about suicide and positive responses to the ninth item can identify patients having suicide rates 6 to 10 times higher in the subsequent year than patients with negative responses (Hogan, 2016). The C-SSRS has been adapted for use in a variety of settings and by various users, such as family, friends, first responders, researchers and healthcare providers and in many different countries. The scale can be used as a screening or assessment tool and is a reliable and validated measure that captures current and past suicide ideation, suicide attempts, preparatory behavior and non-suicidal self-injury (The Columbia Lighthouse Project, 2016). In addition, the necessary training to use the C-SSRS is available free of charge.

Reliable and valid measures help ensure clinicians cover the necessary content involved in assessing suicide risk. In addition, the scores from measure can improve the communication of suicide risk from one clinician to another during transitions in care. However, the gold standard assessment remains that done by a trained and experienced clinician.

MANAGING PATIENTS AT RISK (ADAPTED FROM CRAVEN & LINKS, 2019; SALL ET AL., 2019; WEBER ET AL., 2017)

All people who are suicidal are ambivalent, wanting to die and wanting to live. Keep in mind that suicidality is a fluid state and can change dramatically in the space of a few hours.

Management should focus on:

- Optimizing the safety of the person and removing access to means – take steps to have firearms, large amounts of medication and poisons removed from the home. If no reliable family member is available or willing to help with this, local police should be called to assist with removing guns. Document your actions to reduce the patient's access to means.
- Communicating concern, caring and support.
- Intervening wherever possible to decrease modifiable risk factors.
- Identifying and optimizing protective factors.

- Identifying coping strategies (e.g., distraction) and self-soothing behaviors (e.g., listening to music, going for a walk).
- Identifying people/resources the patient can turn to. Provide a phone number for local crisis service. Ask the patient's permission to involve family/friends in the safety plan.
- Providing immediate symptomatic relief for insomnia, agitation, anxiety.
- Treating identified psychiatric disorders.
- Offering hope of a positive treatment outcome.
- Identifying patients who require urgent/emergent consultation.
- Following up with an ongoing management plan.
- Documenting the management plan clearly.

Management of the Patient With a Suicide Plan and High Intent

If your patient has suicide ideation with a plan and tells you that he or she has a strong intent to follow through, or if the plan is highly lethal (e.g., firearm, poisons, hanging), the patient may require immediate transfer to a hospital emergency department. These patients will be unable to maintain safety independent of external support or help. Common risk factors may include a recent suicide attempt and/or ongoing preparatory suicidal actions.

These patients should be transferred immediately to the nearest emergency department, as these patients typically require psychiatric hospitalization. Until their transfer to a secure unit with limited access to lethal means, such persons may need to be directly observed.

Document your risk assessment and the steps you are taking to transfer these patients.

Management of the Patient With Low Intent but With Serious Risk Factors

If your patient denies a plan, or has low intent to follow through in the short term and has an ability to maintain safety independent of external support but has one or more serious risk factors, request an urgent psychiatric consultation (within 24 to 48 hours) and:

- Wherever possible (with the patient's agreement) get corroborative history from family, friends or co-workers to confirm your assessment of risk.
- Remove lethal weapons, poisons and medications from the home. Have a responsible family member or friend call you to report that this has been done. If no reliable family member is available or willing to help with this, local police should be called to assist with removing guns. Document your actions to reduce the patient's access to means.
- Ensure that the patient and his or her family know how to reach you/what to do if suicidal thoughts worsen. Make sure the family knows about crises services available 24/7.
- Provide symptomatic relief (e.g., small quantities of benzodiazepine for agitation or insomnia; prescribe a high enough dose to be effective). Mental health treatment may be required to address co-existing conditions.
- See the patient the next day to reassess and then frequently (as dictated by level of suicidal intent) until psychiatric consultation takes place or the patient's suicidal risk returns to baseline.
- Assess and support the patient's reasons for living.
- Evaluate the patient's ability to collaboratively develop a safety plan.
- Document your risk assessment, your safety plan, and your management plan clearly in the chart.

Management of the Patient With Suicidal Thoughts but No Plan

Patients who have suicidal thoughts but no plan, no current intent, no recent preparatory behaviors and *no serious risk factors* (e.g., previous attempt) can often be managed in the community. There should be collective (e.g., patient, care provider, family) high confidence in the ability of the patient to independently maintain safety. These patients will engage in appropriate safety planning and coping strategies during the during crisis period.

- Ask the patient for permission to talk to a family member, friend or co-worker to confirm your impressions and get additional history. If the patient is refusing permission to speak to others, then carefully reconsider your assessment of the patient's risk.
- Remove any lethal weapons, poisons or dangerous amounts of medication from the home. Have a responsible family member or friend call you to report that this has been done. If no reliable family member is available or willing to help with this, local police should be called to assist with removing guns. Document your actions to reduce the patient's access to means.
- Ensure that your patient and his or her family know how to reach you/what to do if suicidal thoughts worsen. Make sure the family knows about crises services available 24/7.
- If the patient lives alone, try to find a family member or friend who will stay with the person until treatment begins to have an effect.
- Provide symptomatic relief (e.g., small quantities of benzodiazepine for agitation or insomnia; prescribe a high enough dose for it to be effective).
- Start treatment for depression. Whenever possible, use selective serotonin reuptake inhibitors in preference to more lethal drugs such as tricyclic antidepressant medications. Educate your patient about depression and communicate hope and reassurance about a positive treatment outcome. Provide treatment for other mental health conditions that co-exist.
- Encourage the patient to reduce or eliminate the use of alcohol or other substances.
- Address relationship issues and other stressors – refer for counselling if you do not provide counselling yourself.
- See the patient at least weekly for the first month to monitor:
    - suicidality
    - compliance with treatment
    - side-effects of medication
    - response to treatment
- Assess and support the patient's reasons for living.
- Monitor and revise the patient's collaboratively developed safety plan.
- Document your risk assessment, your safety plan, and your management plan clearly in the chart.

Transferring the High-Risk Patient for Emergency Psychiatric Consultation

- Do not leave the patient alone.
- Place the patient in as safe an environment as is possible.
- Tell the patient you want him or her to be seen by a psychiatrist as soon as possible.
- Call for an urgent consultation.
- Give the emergency department physician or the on-call psychiatrist as much information as you can, including any history of psychiatric disorders, past suicide attempts, family history of suicide attempts, current stressors, current medical conditions and medications. Whenever possible send a brief note. For example:

- This 45-year-old male patient has a history of serious unipolar depression with one suicide attempt in the past. He is currently going through a difficult divorce, is depressed and expressing hopelessness, suicidal intent, with a plan to overdose on his antidepressants. He is medically well except for mild hypertension. His current medications are: hydrochlorothiazide 25 mg per day, and sertraline 150 mg per day.
- Place a call to a family member or friend of the patient.

If the Patient Is Co-Operative and Wants Help

If the patient is co-operative, he or she can be transferred to hospital as a voluntary patient with a responsible family member or friend. Let the emergency room know when the patient leaves your office and when they should expect the patient to arrive. Ask to be called if the patient does not arrive within a reasonable time. If the patient does not arrive, call the patient's home. If you cannot locate the patient, call police and tell them your concerns, and ask them to apprehend and take the patient to the nearest emergency room. Familiarize yourself with your jurisdiction's mental health legislation to be able to use its powers appropriately to help your patients.

If the Patient Is Not Co-Operative

If the patient refuses to go to the emergency room, tell the patient that you are very concerned and that you are obliged by law to ensure his or her safety. (Each community will have mental health legislation that deals with the clinicians' powers and responsibilities, and clinicians should be aware of these legal obligations.) Call police and request that they take the patient to the nearest emergency room. Be prepared to give a description of the patient if he or she leaves your office. Do not try to physically stop the patient.

Patients With a Chronic Risk for Suicide (Links et al., 2019)

The clinical assessment of patients with a chronic risk for suicide (e.g., patients with borderline personality disorder) is complicated and clinicians should ensure that they have supervision or collegial support when caring for these patients. Often these patients have made multiple suicide attempts and may have unstable or turbulent relationships and living situation. In patients with chronic risk, assessing the acute-on-chronic level of risk (i.e., the acute risk that occurs over and above the ongoing chronic risk) must be determined to decide the appropriate level of care.

Patients at chronic risk for suicide such as patients with borderline personality disorder (BPD) typically are at a chronically elevated risk of suicide much above that of the general population. This risk exists primarily because of a history of multiple previous attempts, although in some studies the patients' history of (non-suicidal) self-injurious behavior has also been shown to increase the risk for suicide (Linehan, 1993; Stanley et al., 2001). The patient's level of chronic risk can be estimated by taking a careful history of the previous suicidal behavior and focusing on the times when the patient may have demonstrated attempts with the greatest subjective intent, objective planning and medical lethality. By studying the patient's most serious suicide attempts, one can estimate the severity of the patient's ongoing chronic risk for suicide, particularly as the method of previous attempts tends to predict the seriousness of suicide vulnerability.

An acute-on-chronic risk will be present if the patient with chronic risk has comorbid major depression or if the patient is demonstrating high levels of hopelessness or depressive symptoms. In addition, patients with BPD are known to be at risk for suicide around times of hospitalization and discharge. The recently discharged hospitalized patient is potentially at an acute-on-chronic risk, and the assessment cannot be truncated because of the recent discharge. Proximal substance abuse can increase the suicide risk in a patient with BPD. The risk is acutely elevated in patients who have less immediate family support, those who have lost or perceive the loss of an important relationship or those who have suffered recent stressful events, including legal contacts (Yen et al., 2005). The acute level of risk should be evaluated and stratified as outlined previously (e.g., high acute risk versus low acute risk).

Using the acute-on-chronic model can be very effective for communicating in the health record the decisions regarding interventions. For example, if a patient is felt to be at a chronic but not acute-on-chronic risk for suicide, one can document and communicate that a short-term hospital admission will have little or no impact on a chronic risk that has been present for months and years. For these patients, evidence-based psychotherapy interventions as outlined subsequently are needed to build appropriate coping skills. However, an inpatient admission of a patient demonstrating an acute-on-chronic risk might well be indicated. In this circumstance, a short-term admission may allow the level of risk to return to chronic preadmission levels.

Specific Strategies: Safety Planning; Removing Access to Means, Caring Contacts

To manage patients at risk for suicide, according to the new standards clinicians should ensure that safety planning is carried out. A safety plan is a brief intervention collaboratively completed with the patient to develop a plan to recognize suicidal thoughts and to manage them safely. The plan includes five questions:

   a. What are your warning signs that you are going into a crisis?
   b. What coping strategies such as distraction or soothing techniques have you used successfully in the past?
   c. What social situations and/or people that can help distract you when you are in crisis?
   d. Who can you ask for help when you are in crisis (or note if a person is unhelpful when you are in crisis)?
   e. What professionals or agencies can you contact during a crisis?

(adapted from Stanley & Brown, 2012)

A crucial part of the safety plan is working with the patient and family to remove access to lethal means of suicide such as guns, poisons and large quantities of medication. The physician should work out the plan, ensure that the agreed-upon actions have been taken and document these actions in the health record.

The new standards call for providing "caring contacts" to patients with significant risk after hospital discharge or emergency department discharge, follow-up in primary care or mental health settings and when care is interrupted (e.g., missed appointments; transfers of care). "Caring contacts" encompass contacts via phone calls, texts and email as preferred by the patient and simply provide messages of support and encouragement (National Action Alliance for Suicide Prevention, 2018). The National Action Alliance for Suicide Prevention "Recommended Standard Care for People with Suicide Risk: Making Health Care Suicide Safe" provides specific guidelines for caring contacts by setting. For example, for emergency departments, one caring contact should be completed within 48 hours of the visit and a second caring contact within 7 days of visit. Similarly, following discharge from an inpatient psychiatric service the recommended standard of care calls for caring contacts within 48 hours of discharge and within 7 days of discharge.

PSYCHOTHERAPY WITH SUICIDAL PATIENTS

The Zero Suicide model also calls for adopting evidence-based interventions that directly address the patient's risk for suicide. These approaches require that staff be trained in evidenced-based psychotherapies that targets the individuals' risk of suicide (e.g., dialectical behavior therapy [DBT]; cognitive behavior therapy; Collaborative Assessment and Management of Suicidality; Attempted Suicide Short Intervention Program [see Mokkenstorm et al., 2018]). However, the National Action Alliance for Suicide Prevention has not included these treatment approaches as part of the "basic elements of suicide care" and at this time, they are considered additional "promising and desirable" elements (National Action Alliance for Suicide Prevention, 2018).

These various psychotherapies for patients at risk for recurrent suicide behavior have decreased the risk of future suicide attempts, lessened the medical risk from subsequent suicidal behavior and decreased the likelihood of emergency department visits for suicidal behavior. These findings have led experts to extract a limited number of psychotherapy principles that may be effective in reducing the risk of future suicide behavior in a variety of patients, and these elements are reviewed next (Schiavone & Links, 2013).

Psychotherapy Management of Patients With Suicide Risk

This chapter suggests techniques/therapeutic elements that community practitioners can incorporate in psychotherapy with patients who are at risk for suicide.

Construction of a Coherent Treatment Model

An effective treatment model for suicidal patients requires a coherent model that helps clinicians feel more confident in their conceptualization of the patient's suicidal risk. Despite many different views on the nature of suicidality, successful therapies are universally well structured and clearly focused (Bateman & Fonagy, 2000). Understanding the purpose of suicidal behavior (e.g., to regulate distressing emotions) helps the clinician to both understand the patient's difficulties and to avoid blaming the patient. Some strategies that have been suggested to maintain coherence to a model of understanding include supervision, training including access to a treatment manual and regular adherence checks (de Groot et al., 2008).

An Active Therapeutic Stance

In the context of suicidality, the active therapeutic stance encourages hope, models proactive problem solving, contains the patient's distress and behavioral disorganization and maintains the treatment focus on suicidal behavior (Livesley, 2007).

Two tools of the active therapist are a structured treatment frame and a strong therapeutic relationship (Bateman & Fonagy, 2000; Comtois & Linehan, 2006; Livesley, 2007; Weinburg et al., 2010). According to Gunderson, these two tasks represent stages of therapy that occur sequentially and are necessary precursors to the patient's becoming able to fully engage in treatment (Links et al., 2016). The first stage of therapy establishes the treatment frame or contract (Links et al., 2016). The contract establishes the structure of the therapy, including policies regarding therapist vacations, cancellations, termination of therapy, confidentiality, contact with the therapist between sessions, accepted and prohibited behaviors and frequency and duration of sessions. The contract also establishes the patient's goals and the roles of both patient and therapist in achieving these goals (Livesley, 2007; Weinburg et al.,

2010). Adherence to the treatment contract provides consistency and stability and models appropriate boundaries (Livesley, 2007; Weinburg et al., 2010).

The second task of the active therapist is to build "a powerful attachment relationship between therapist and patient" (Bateman & Fonagy, 2000, p. 141). Livesley considers the alliance a "generic intervention" which both addresses core pathology and underlies the treatment frame (Links et al., 2016; Livesley, 2007). The therapeutic relationship is strengthened through supportive interventions and deliberate attention to the "real" relationship as well as the transference relationship (Livesley, 2007; Weinburg et al., 2010). The repair of relationship ruptures and disruptive patterns within the therapeutic relationship can lead to a wider improvement in other interpersonal relationships (Links et al., 2016).

Through careful attention to the treatment frame, and to developing the therapeutic relationship, the active therapist is able to hold the patient in therapy and address core interpersonal deficits. The experience of an active therapist ultimately provides a corrective relational experience and motivates the patient to change and to reduce their use of suicidal behavior (Livesley, 2007).

Balance of Validation and Change

Validation is a component of building the therapeutic relationship and also an important technique in its own right (Links et al., 2016; Livesley, 2007; Weinburg et al., 2010). Validation is a patient-centered technique which "[affirms] existing thoughts, feelings or behaviors of the patient" (Weinburg et al., 2010). The use of validation alongside change oriented interventions balances acceptance of the patient as they are with demands for the patient to change; this helps the patient to tolerate change oriented interventions which may otherwise be perceived as invalidating and cause the patient to terminate treatment (Linehan, 1993).

Although Livesley considers validation useful at all times, it is particularly employed in the initial, or containment, phase of therapy, when the main goal is "settling crisis behavior, containing impulses and affects, and restoring behavioral control" (Livesley, 2007, p. 141). Validation is further indicated at times of crisis or dissociation or to soothe the patient when affect is too intense (Livesley, 2007). In this model, crisis behavior stems from a need for understanding, so validation can contain crisis behavior by meeting this need (Livesley, 2007). In *Cognitive Behavioral Treatment of Borderline Personality Disorder*, Linehan outlines several validation strategies used by DBT oriented therapists, and notes that certain strategies are "part of almost all therapy traditions" (1993, p. 223). For example, emotional validation identifies the patient's emotions and encourages their expression, reflects them with sympathy and non-judgment and acknowledges their validity within their context (Linehan, 1993). If the patient cannot identify their feelings, the therapist may offer a brief list of options (Linehan, 1993). The therapist conveys sympathy and acceptance and may encourage the patient to more fully express the emotion by identifying associated physical responses, action urges, cognitions and desires (Linehan, 1993). Linehan uses behavioral validation to directly address incidents of suicidal behavior while building the patient's tolerance for change (Linehan, 1993). The therapist validates the emotions that led up to the use of suicidal behavior and conveys that the behavior is understandable and makes sense but does not convey approval of the behavior itself (Linehan, 1993). The therapist conversely validates the patient's disappointment in the behavior and affirms the patient's worth and capacity for change (Linehan, 1993). The therapist thereby allows the patient to feel understood while still encouraging the patient to use other methods to tolerate their feelings (Linehan, 1993).

Validation in some form is employed by all therapies with suicidal patients to acknowledge and empathize with the patient's thoughts, feelings and behaviors and to build a therapeutic relationship. The use of validating interventions should be balanced with the use of change-oriented interventions in order to help the patient tolerate therapy while still promoting change.

Fostering a Sense of Self-Agency

Patients at risk for suicide often experience difficulties with self-agency, or the sense that that the environment is altered by and responsive to their actions and intentions (Knox, 2011). According to Knox, a sense of self-agency can be restored through a "co constructive relational process" between the patient and the therapist (Knox, 2011). The therapist models flexibility and responsiveness to the patient's concerns, so that the patient experiences self-agency without being rejected or ignored (Knox, 2011). The therapist specifically avoids interpretations that suggest that they have privileged knowledge of the patient's subconscious, which builds the patient's sense that they know their own mind best (Knox, 2011). If the therapist does offer an interpretation or opinion, the therapist uses qualifications like "I wonder if," and is willing to modify his or her opinion and admit to mistakes (Bateman & Fonagy, 2006). This attitude on the part of the therapist allows the patient to shape their environment and reflect on their experiences, thereby promoting self-agency (Bateman & Fonagy, 2006).

Improvement in Patient Ability to Connect Actions and Feelings

By giving the patient a model within which to understand their suicidality, the therapist engages with the healthier part of the patient's ego and encourages a more objective stance (Links et al., 2016). During the therapy, significant attention is devoted to psychoeducation around emotion processing (Links & Bergmans, 2016). Suicidality can be conceived as arising from an inability to name or describe the subjective experience of distressing emotions, and the intention is therefore to reduce suicidality by teaching patients to more objectively observe their emotional experience and to identify the feelings and needs prompting them to engage in suicidal behavior (Links & Bergmans, 2016). This begins with psychoeducation on the general role of emotions, their names and their natural lifecycle, with particular attention to the idea that emotions will pass naturally on their own whether or not suicidal behavior is used and to acceptance of feelings as they are (Links & Bergmans, 2016).

The therapist teaches the patient to observe themselves and their emotions as they occur by commenting on the patient's facial expressions and body language during the session and helping the patient to connect these cues their feelings in the moment (Links & Bergmans, 2016). This allows for the identification of the early warning signs that emotional intensity is increasing (Links & Bergmans, 2016). The patient is also encouraged to develop a method to scale their emotional intensity (e.g., based on the weather, where a storm represents a severe negative mood), and this scale allows them to monitor and communicate their distress (Links & Bergmans, 2016). When patients can more readily identify when their distress is rising and can observe their feelings rather than acting, they are more able to identify and use adaptive coping strategies (Links & Bergmans, 2016).

Similarly, in DBT, the therapist views suicidal behavior as a solution to a problem and attempts to clarify the problem with a careful chain analysis; a step by step description of the chain of events leading up to and following the suicidal behavior including feelings, behaviors, thoughts, imaginings and events in the environment (Linehan, 1993). The chain analysis helps the therapist and patient to identify the links between the patient's feelings and their eventual use of suicidality as a solution, with the goal of eventually identifying other ways in which the patient can respond to those feelings (Linehan, 1993).

When patients are more able to objectively observe their emotions and to identify the unmet needs that are prompting their responses, they are then able to link their emotions to actions such as suicidality and to come up with alternative responses.

Differentiation Between Lethal and Non-Lethal Suicide Intention

One important task with chronically suicidal individuals is to accurately gauge the intensity and potential lethality of suicidal ideation, since concerns about imminent death by suicide can cause the clinician significant anxiety and impair the therapy. It has been suggested, as outlined previously, that lethality assessment in this population should concentrate on the presence of an "acute on chronic" risk for suicide, as this population will likely have some level of chronic suicidal ideation. The assessment of acute on chronic risk focuses on identifying and targeting periods when environmental risk factors increase the risk of suicidal behavior beyond the patient's baseline.

Safety planning, as outlined previously, is typically a brief intervention for acutely suicidal patients which is collaborative, tailored to the individual patient and designed to both assess the immediate risk of suicide (acute on chronic risk) and to create a mutually agreed-upon plan for coping (Stanley & Brown, 2012). However, safety planning should be used in the context of long-term psychotherapy; the plan can be regularly evaluated and revised to ensure that it remains relevant (Stanley & Brown, 2012).

Therapist Access to Supervision

Supervision is a key component of psychotherapy for patients at risk for suicide, because this population tend to be unusually challenging to work with. Supervision can serve several functions: Livesley identifies therapist stress and countertransference as goals for supervision and adds that supervision helps to keep treatment coherent (Livesley, 2007). In the community, the clinician should adopt a "low threshold" for seeking consultation or supervision and carefully monitor and manage countertransference feelings which may interfere with treatment (Links et al., 2016). If a need for supervision is identified, the therapist should seek out a trusted colleague in whose presence they may reveal themselves, reflect on their experience of therapy and receive feedback (Links et al., 2016).

CONCLUSION

The prevention of suicide in patients receiving mental healthcare requires as a system-wide approach that provides accessible, reliable and continuous care and organizationally driven quality improvement. Individual clinicians should be informed to deliver evidence-based individual-level approaches to the assessment and management of persons with mental health disorders and/or who have attempted suicide. These approaches include using appropriate screening and assessment tools, developing collaborative safety plans, removing access to lethal means, providing caring contacts and delivering psychotherapeutic elements found to be effective for patients at risk for suicide. Adopting these new systematic approaches to care for patients at risk for suicide appears to hold great promise to keep patients under our care safe and well.

References

Bateman, A.W., & Fonagy, P. (2000). Effectiveness of psychotherapeutic treatment of personality disorder. *British Journal of Psychiatry, 177*(Aug.): 138–143.

Bateman, A.W., & Fonagy, P. (2006). Progress in the treatment of borderline personality disorder. *British Journal of Psychiatry, 188*(Jan.): 1–3.

Bernert, R.A., Hom, M.A., & Roberts, L.W. (2014). A review of multidisciplinary clinical practice guidelines in suicide prevention: Toward an emerging standard in suicide risk assessment and management, training and practice. *Academic Psychiatry*, 38(5): 585–592. doi: 10.1007/s40596-014-0180-1.

Chan, M.K., Bhatti, H., Meader, N., Stockton, S., & Kendall, T. (2016). Predicting suicide following self-harm: Systematic review of risk factors and risk scales. *British Journal of Psychiatry*, 209(4): 277–283.

The Columbia Lighthouse Project. (2016) *Columbia Suicide Severity Scale*. http://cssrs.columbia.edu

Comtois, K.A., & Linehan, M.M. (2006). Psychosocial treatments of suicidal behaviors: A practice friendly review. *Journal of Clinical Psychology*, 62(2): 161–170. doi:10.1002/jclp.20220

Craven, M., & Links, P.S. (2019). Assessment and management of suicide risk. In David S. Goldbloom & Jon Davine (Eds.) *Psychiatry in primary care: A concise Canadian pocket guide*, Second Edition (pp. 299–312). Centre for Addiction and Mental Health, Toronto.

de Groot, E.R., Verheul, R., & Trijsburg, R.W. (2008). An integrative perspective on psychotherapeutic treatments for borderline personality disorder. *Journal of Personality Disorders*, 22(4): 332–352. doi:10.1521/pedi.2008.22.4.332

Hampton, T. (2010). Depression care effort brings dramatic drop in large HMO population's suicide rate. *JAMA*, 303(19): 1903–1905.

Hogan, M.F. (2016). Better suicide screening and prevention are possible. *JAMA Psychiatry*, 73(11): 1111–1112. doi: 10.1001/jamapsychiatry.2016.2411

Knox, J. (2011). *Self-agency in psychotherapy*. New York: W.W. Norton.

LeFevre, M.L. (2014). Screening for suicide risk in adolescents, adults, and older adults in primary care: U.S. Preventive Services Task Force recommendation statement. *Annals of Internal Medicine*, 160(160): 719–726.

Linehan, M.M. (1993). *Cognitive-behavioral treatment of borderline personality disorder*. London: Guilford Press.

Links, P.S., & Bergmans, Y. (2016). Managing suicidal and other crises. In W.J. Livesley, G. Dimaggio, & J.F. Clarkin (Eds.) *Integrated treatment of personality disorder: A modular approach* (pp. 197–210). London: Guilford Press.

Links, P.S., Links, M., & Boursiquot, P. (2019). Evaluation et gestion du risque suicidaire aigu chez les patients avec un trouble de la personnalite borderline. In S. Kolly, P. Charbon, & U. Kramer (Eds.) *Trouble de la personnalite borderline. Pratiques therapeutiques*. (pp. 57–74). London: Elsevier Masson.

Links, P.S., Mercer, D., & Novick, J. (2016). Establishing a treatment framework and therapeutic alliance. In W.J. Livesley, G. Dimaggio, & J.F. Clarkin (Eds.) *Integrated treatment of personality disorder: A modular approach* (pp. 101–119). London: Guilford Press.

Livesley, W. (2007). An integrated approach to the treatment of personality disorder. *Journal of Mental Health*, 16(1): 131.

Mokkenstorm, J.K., Kerkhof, J.F.M., Smit, J.H., & Beekman, A.T.F. (2018). Is it rational to pursue Zero Suicides among patients in health care? *Suicide Life Threaten Behavior*, 48(6): 745–754.

National Action Alliance for Suicide Prevention. (2018). *Transforming health system initiative work group 2018: Recommended standard of care for people with suicide risk: Making health care suicide safe*. Washington, DC: Education Development Center, Inc. www.actionallianceforsuicideprevention.org

Sall, J., Brenner, L., Milliken Bell, A.M., & Colston, M.J. (2019). Assessment and management of patients at risk for suicide: Synopsis of the 2019 U.S. department of veterans affairs and U.S. department of defense clinical practice guidelines. *Annals of Internal Medicine*, 171(5): 343–353. doi:10.7326/M19-0687

Schiavone, F.L., Links, P.S. (2013). Common elements for the psychotherapeutic management of patients with Self Injurious Behavior. *Child Abuse and Neglect*, 37(2–3): 133–138 doi: 10.1016/j.chiabu.2012.09.012

Stanley, B., & Brown, G.K. (2012). Safety planning intervention: A brief intervention to mitigate suicide risk. *Cognitive Behavior Practice*, 19(2):256–265. doi: 10.1016/j.cbpra.2011.01.001

Stanley, B., Gameroff, M.J., Michalsen, V., & Mann, J.J. (2001). Are suicide attempters who self-mutilate a unique population? *American Journal of Psychiatry*, 158(3): 427–432.

Suicide Prevention Resource Centre. (2015–2018). *Zero Suicide Toolkit. Education Development Center Inc. 2015–2018* [cited July 31, 2018]. https://zerosuicide.sprc.org/toolkit

Weber, A.N., Michail, M., Thompson, A., & Fiedorowicz, J.G. (2017). Psychiatric emergencies: Assessing and managing suicidal ideation. *Medical Clinics of North America*, 101(3): 553–571.

World Health Organization. (2014). *Preventing suicide: A global imperative 2014* [cited March 23, 2020]. ISBN: 978 92 4 156477 9. www.who.int/mental_health/suicide-prevention/world_report_2014/en/

Yen, S., Pagano, M.E., Shea, M. T., Grilo, C.M., & Zanarini, M.C. (2005). Recent life events preceding suicide attempts in a personality disorder sample: Findings from the collaborative longitudinal personality disorders study. *Journal of Consulting and Clinical Psychology, 73*(1), 99–105.

30
Optimising Patient Care in Psychiatry – Focus on Consultation Liaison Psychiatry

Parijat Roy and Avinash De Sousa

Historical Background	333
Psychiatric Consultation in the General Hospital	334
Optimising the Consultation	335
Speaking Directly With the Referring Doctor	335
Reviewing Current and Past Records	335
Reviewing Patient Medications	335
Gathering Collateral Data	336
Interviewing the Patient	336
Examining the Patient	336
Formulation of Diagnosis and Therapeutic Strategies	337
Writing a Note	338
Speaking Directly With the Referring Clinician	338
Periodic Follow-Ups	338
Role of Other Providers in Optimising the Consultation	338
Consultation in the Outpatient Setting	339
Practice Guidelines	339
Benefits of Consultation Liaison Psychiatry	339
Conclusion	339

Consultation liaison (C-L) is the study, practice and teaching of the relation between medical and psychiatric disorders. The C-L psychiatrist serves as a bridge between psychiatry and other specialities. In the ward, C-L psychiatrists play a plethora of roles; skilful interviewer, able psychiatrist and psychotherapist and a teacher. This specialised field goes by various names; medical-surgical psychiatry, psychological medicine, psychiatry care of the complex medically ill and psychosomatic medicine.

HISTORICAL BACKGROUND

C-L psychiatry has a rich history. It started with the Rockefeller Foundation's funding of C-L units in various hospitals in the United States in the year 1935. The National Institute of Mental Health (NIMH), in 1975, started giving training grants for C-L psychiatry. In 2001, the Academy of Psychosomatic Medicine applied for recognition of the branch as a subspeciality of psychiatry, which was approved in 2003. In 2018, the American Board of Psychiatry and Neurology officially renamed the subspeciality as consultation-liaison psychiatry. Various organisations are working globally in this field, the prominent among them are listed below:

Academy of Consultation Liaison Psychiatry
American Psychosomatic Society
American Neuropsychiatric Association
European Association for Psychosomatic Medicine
International Organization for Consultation-Liaison Psychiatry
World Psychiatric Association-Section of General Hospital Psychiatry
International College of Psychosomatic Medicine

PSYCHIATRIC CONSULTATION IN THE GENERAL HOSPITAL

Psychiatrists working in medical settings are charged with providing consultation to medical and surgical patients. Constraints of the modern hospital with respect to comfort, quiet and privacy make it different from the treatment of patients in a psychiatric clinic. It is worth mentioning that the consultant's bedside manner is important in compensating for this. Common categories of differential diagnoses which a C-L psychiatrist encounters are as follows

- Psychiatric presentations of medical conditions
- Psychiatric complications of medical conditions/treatments
- Psychological reactions to medical conditions or treatments
- Medical presentations of psychiatric conditions
- Medical complications of psychiatric conditions/treatments
- Comorbid medical and psychiatric conditions

Common C-L problems encountered are:

- Deliberate self harm (DSH): DSH rates are higher in patients with medical illness. Male gender, substance use, poor social support and chronic pain increase the risk further. If suicide risk is present, then the patient should be transferred to a psychiatric unit.
- Depression: Depression with or without suicidal intent is commonly encountered in the medical and surgical ward. A careful assessment of the drug interaction must be made before prescribing an antidepressant.
- Agitation: Agitation is often encountered in withdrawal states or dementia. Hallucinations and paranoid ideations to which the patient may be responding in an agitated manner must always be ruled out, as should toxic reactions to medications that cause agitation. Low-dose antipsychotics are of great help in managing agitation and physical restraint should be the last resort.
- Sleep-wake disorders: Pain is the commonest cause of insomnia in the hospitalised patient. Early morning awakening is seen in depression and anxiety causes difficulty in initiating sleep. Early substance withdrawal as a cause should also be considered. Based on the aetiology appropriate agents are prescribed.
- Confusion: Delirium is the most common cause of confusion in a hospitalised patient. The aetiology can be metabolic, infectious, toxic, neurological or substance among a myriad of others. Low-dose antipsychotics are particularly useful in controlling the agitation, along with non-pharmacological interventions. The mainstay, however, remains the correction of the aetiology.

- Non-compliance: Refusal to take medications or give consent to a procedure is often encountered in the hospital setting. Careful exploration of the doctor-patient relationship along with education and reassurance often solves the problem. Cognitive disorders are an important cause of impaired judgement and hence carefully assessed for.
- No organic basis for symptoms: Various psychiatric conditions must be considered when no medical or surgical basis for the presenting symptoms can be determined, even on repeated investigations, important among which are somatisation disorder, conversion disorder, factitious disorder and malingering.
- Specialised situations: Intensive care units (ICUs), haemodialysis units, burn units, oncology wards and transplantation wards are some of the specialised situations wherein a C-L psychiatrist plays a major role before, during and after the procedure.

OPTIMISING THE CONSULTATION

A procedural approach to psychiatric consultation goes a long way in optimising patient care. A consultation should incorporate the following components in a linear fashion:

- Speaking directly with the referring doctor
- Reviewing current and past records
- Reviewing patient's medications
- Gathering collateral data
- Interviewing the patient
- Examining the patient
- Formulation of diagnosis and therapeutic strategies
- Writing a note
- Speaking directly with the referring clinician
- Periodic follow-ups

Speaking Directly With the Referring Doctor

Due to the vague and often imprecise nature of psychiatric referrals, speaking directly with the referring physician assumes a great deal of importance. The referrals sometimes signify that the treating physician recognises that a problem exists; the problem maybe an untreated psychiatric disorder or countertransferential feelings that the treating physician might develop towards the patient. This brief interaction provides a window to the psychiatrist to understand how the consultation may be useful to the physician and the patient.

Reviewing Current and Past Records

Reviewing the records provides a general orientation to the case. Many details which may have been overlooked previously come into focus. For example, nurses often note salient behavioural data like level of awareness, agitation, orientation; occupational therapists estimate functional abilities crucial to the diagnosis of cognitive disorders. These notes thus provide unique clues for the better understanding of the case and complement independent history taking and examination.

Reviewing Patient Medications

Reviewing the patient's medications is an extremely valuable practice. Special attention must be given to medications with psychoactive effects; anticholinergics; and those that produce withdrawal symptoms, like benzodiazepines, opiates antidepressants. Medication administration records should also be reviewed, as the patient may not always receive prescribed medications.

Gathering Collateral Data

History from the hospitalised patient can often be unreliable especially if the patient is drowsy, delirious or comatose. Data from collateral sources like family members and friends become critical in these circumstances. However the source of the data should be objective, adequate and reliable, as family members often tend to be overinvolved or in denial or have a personal agenda. Confidentiality must be valued, and ideally the patient's consent must be taken first, which may not be possible practically. Ultimately it is upon the psychiatrist's clinical acumen to weigh each bit of information according to the reliability of its source.

Interviewing the Patient

Interviewing is critical for an independent assessment. The interview process must be adapted to the consultation setting. An engaging, spontaneous stance is essential to establish rapport. A brief introduction, explaining the purpose of the visit, and enquiry into physical health are the stepping stones. Neither a rigid biological approach nor an exclusively psychoanalytical inquiry should be adopted. Patient's beliefs about his/her illness should be elicited so that emotional responses and behaviours can be placed in perspective. Open-ended interviews should be used whenever possible.

Examining the Patient

Mental status examination (MSE) is central to the psychiatric consultation, even in a hospital setting. It should be taken in a systematic fashion and consist of:

1. Level of consciousness: alert, drowsy, somnolent, stuporous, comatose, fluctuating
2. Appearance and behaviour: grooming, hygiene, cooperation, eye contact, psychomotor activity, abnormal movements
3. Attention: active attention and passive attention
4. Orientation and memory: orientation to time/place/person; immediate, recent and remote memory
5. Language: rate, volume, fluency, prosody of speech; comprehension and naming; abnormalities like aphasia, dysarthria, alexia, echolalia, clanging
6. Constructional ability: clock drawing, intersecting pentagons to assess for neglect, executive function and parietal function
7. Mood: subjective sustained emotion
8. Affect: observed emotion, range, intensity, stability, lability, appropriateness
9. Thought: form, content, stream, possession
10. Perception: auditory, visual, olfactory, gustatory, tactile hallucinations
11. Judgement: social, personal and test judgement
12. Insight into one's illness

Physical Examination

The importance of physical examination should never be discounted, especially in a hospital setting. The C-L psychiatrist should at least review the physical examinations performed by the treating physician. Examination of the central nervous system (CNS) functions relevant to the differential diagnosis is often critical. Even in a sedated or comatose patient, simple manoeuvres may potentially yield significant findings. Some common findings on physical examination and their significance are given in the following:

1. General appearance healthier than expected: somatic symptom disorder
2. Fever: NMS
3. Pulse/BP abnormality: withdrawal
4. Body habitus: eating disorders, PCOS, Cushing's syndrome
5. Diaphoresis: NMS, withdrawal
6. Piloerection: opioid withdrawal
7. Dry skin: anticholinergic toxicity
8. Characteristic stigmata: cirrhosis, syphilis, self-mutilation
9. Bruises: physical abuse
10. Mydriasis: opiate withdrawal
11. Miosis: opiate intoxication
12. Kayser-Fleischer ring: Wilson's disease
13. Tremors: delirium, lithium toxicity, parkinsonism
14. Primitive reflexes: frontal lobe dysfunction
15. Ophthalmoplegia: Wernicke's encephalopathy, dystonia
16. Papilledema: raised ICT
17. Abnormal movements: Parkinson's disease, Huntington's disease, EPS
18. Abnormal gait: normal pressure hydrocephalus
19. Loss of position and vibratory sense: vitamin B12 deficiency

Formulation of Diagnosis and Therapeutic Strategies

Before arriving at a diagnosis, the C-L psychiatrist reviews the tests already done and considers what additional tests are required. Common tests routinely ordered in psychiatric consultation are as follows:

1. Complete blood count
2. Serum electrolyte
3. Blood glucose levels
4. Liver function tests
5. Renal function tests
6. TSH levels
7. Vitamin B12 levels
8. Toxicology, serum/urine
9. Serology for syphilis
10. HIV tests
11. Urinalysis
12. Electrocardiogram

These tests assume more importance in cases like delirium and dementia to ascertain the aetiology.

Apart from the previous investigations, the C-L psychiatrist must also be familiar with neuroimaging. It often aids in the differential diagnosis of neuropsychiatric conditions. Magnetic resonance imaging (MRI) is preferred over computerised tomography (CT) owing to its higher resolution. CT is preferred in cases of suspected intracranial haemorrhages and in situations where MRI is contraindicated. New-onset psychosis, new-onset dementia, delirium of unknown cause and acute mental status change with an abnormal neurological examination are some of the conditions that warrant neuroimaging. The C-L psychiatrist should also read the radiologist's report, as even small abnormalities have diagnostic and therapeutic implications.

Electroencephalogram (EEG) is often indicated in patients with suspected complex partial seizure or pseudoseizure often assisted by video recording. An EEG maybe helpful in documenting the presence of generalised slowing in a delirious patient, whom the primary treatment team insists on transferring to the psychiatric unit because of a mistaken belief that the symptoms of delirium represent schizophrenia, although it cannot ascertain the aetiology behind delirium.

Neuropsychological testing, although not feasible at times, may be helpful in diagnosis, prognosis and treatment planning.

Writing a Note

The consultation note should be clear and concise and focus on specific diagnostic and therapeutic recommendations. A full psychosocial formulation has little place in C-L psychiatry. Criticism of the primary care team should be avoided. Flexibility in the mode of management is also preferred.

An ideal note should begin with a summary of the patient's medical and psychiatric history, reason for admission and referral. Next comes a brief summary of the current medical illness. Relevant physical and neurological findings, laboratory investigations and neuroimaging should also be summarised. The C-L psychiatrist should then list the differential diagnoses in order of decreasing likelihood, making clear which is the working diagnosis. Finally, the consultant should make recommendations in order of decreasing importance. For medication recommendations, a brief notation of the side effects and their management is useful. Finally, a statement mentioning that the consultant will provide follow-up will reassure the consulting team.

Speaking Directly With the Referring Clinician

Personal contact is crucial especially when diagnostic or therapeutic suggestions are time sensitive. Some information, owing to its sensitive nature, is better conveyed verbally than fully documented in the notes.

Periodic Follow-Ups

A large number of consultations require several encounters and cannot be completed in a single visit. New issues commonly arise during the course of the consultative process, requiring periodic follow-ups. All follow-up visits should be documented in the notes. Finally, if a patient is stabilised or the consultant's recommendations are not followed, it is appropriate to sign off a case.

ROLE OF OTHER PROVIDERS IN OPTIMISING THE CONSULTATION

It is to be noted that teamwork rather than individual work plays a crucial role in optimising consultation and patient care. Psychologists play an important role in performing neuropsychological assessments and providing psychotherapeutic and behavioural interventions. The psychiatric clinical nurse provides services to the nursing staff that parallel those the psychiatrist provides to the medical team. They are particularly helpful in conducting nursing behavioural treatment plans that include behavioural contracts with patients. Social workers facilitate transfers and concessions and set up aftercare.

CONSULTATION IN THE OUTPATIENT SETTING

An even greater impact can be achieved by working collaboratively with the primary care physicians in the outpatient setting. It is well known that more people with mental disorders present to general physicians than to psychiatrists, the reason being incorrect identification of symptoms by the patient, attached stigma, lack of mental healthcare training for primary care providers, and restrictions in insurance coverage for mental healthcare services, among others. Although adequate screening, use of practice guidelines, provider training and referral to specialists are important in improving mental healthcare in general setting, these alone are inadequate. The development of collaborative care models, which refers to the coming together of mental healthcare providers with primary care physicians to deliver specialised care within the outpatient primary care setting, represents a solution to this problem. The first piece in collaborative care is care management undertaken by a trained nurse, social worker or psychologist and helps identify patients in need, educates them, provides follow-up, monitors progress and alters the treatment course as needed. The next piece is consultation and appropriate sharing of information among the primary care provider, the care manager and the consulting psychiatrist.

PRACTICE GUIDELINES

Several countries have developed psychosomatic medicine practice guidelines that detail professional standards for consultation in non-psychiatric settings, delineating integrated clinical approaches, effective methods and methods to improve adherence to recommendations made by the consulting psychiatrist.

BENEFITS OF CONSULTATION LIAISON PSYCHIATRY

The link between comorbid psychopathology and increased length of hospital stay and thus increased in patient costs is well established. Apart from cost reduction, patients also benefit from the reductions in mental suffering and improvements in psychological well-being that result from more appropriate treatment.

CONCLUSION

The C-L psychiatrist is an expert in the diagnosis and treatment of psychopathology in the medically ill. Consultation offers a unique ability to offer a panoramic view of the patient, the illness and the relationship between the two and hence is essential in providing comprehensive care in the medical setting.

Bibliography

- Alpay M, Park L: Laboratory tests and diagnostic procedures, in *Massachusetts General Hospital Psychiatry Update and Board Preparation*, 2nd Edition. Edited by Stern TA, Herman JB. New York, McGraw-Hill, 2004, pp 251–265.
- Bronheim HE, Fulop G, Kunkel EJ, et al., The Academy of Psychosomatic Medicine: The Academy of Psychosomatic Medicine practice guidelines for psychiatric consultation in the general medical setting. *Psychosomatics* 39(4):S8–S30, 1998 9691717.

- Carter G, Page A, Large M, et al: Royal Australian and New Zealand College of Psychiatrists clinical practice guideline for the management of deliberate self-harm. *Aust N Z J Psychiatry* 50(10):939–1000, 2016 27650687.
- Dougherty DD, Rauch SL: Neuroimaging in psychiatry, in *Massachusetts General Hospital Psychiatry Update and Board Preparation*, 2nd Edition. Edited by Stern TA, Herman JB. New York, McGraw-Hill, 2004, pp 227–232.
- Eshel N, Marcovitz DE, Stern TA: Psychiatric consultations in less-than-private places: Challenges and unexpected benefits of hospital roommates. *Psychosomatics* 57(1):97–101, 2016 26671624.
- Folstein MF, Folstein SE, McHugh PR: "Mini-mental state": A practical method for grading the cognitive state of patients for the clinician. *J Psychiatry Res* 12(3):189–198, 1975 1202204.
- Gitlin DF, Levenson JL, Lyketsos CG: Psychosomatic medicine: A new psychiatric subspecialty. *Acad Psychiatry* 28(1):4–11, 2004 15140802.
- Goldberg DP, Blackwell B: Psychiatric illness in general practice: A detailed study using a new method of case identification. *BMJ* 1(5707):439–443, 1970 5420206.
- Hackett TP, Cassem NH, Stern TA, et al: Beginnings: Psychosomatic medicine and consultation psychiatry in the general hospital, in *Massachusetts General Hospital Handbook of General Hospital Psychiatry*, 6th Edition. Edited by Stern TA, Fricchione GL, Cassem NH, et al. Philadelphia, PA, Saunders/Elsevier, 2010, pp 1–6.
- Hodges B, Inch C, Silver I: Improving the psychiatric knowledge, skills, and attitudes of primary care physicians, 1950–2000: A review. *Am J Psychiatry* 158(10):1579–1586, 2001 11578983.
- Katon WJ, Schoenbaum M, Fan MY, et al: Cost-effectiveness of improving primary care treatment of late-life depression. *Arch Gen Psychiatry* 62(12):1313–1320, 2005 16330719.
- Leentjens AFG, Boenink AD, Sno HN, et al., Netherlands Psychiatric Association: The guideline "consultation psychiatry" of the Netherlands Psychiatric Association. *J Psychosom Res* 66(6):531–535, 2009 19446712.
- Perry S, Viederman M: Adaptation of residents to consultation-liaison psychiatry, I: working with the physically ill. *Gen Hosp Psychiatry* 3(2):141–147, 1981 7250694.
- Royal Colleges of Physicians and Psychiatrists: *The Psychological Care of Medical Patients: Recognition of Need and Service Provision: A Joint Working Party Report*. London, Royal College of General Practitioners, 1995.
- Simon GE: Evidence review: Efficacy and effectiveness of antidepressant treatment in primary care. *Gen Hosp Psychiatry* 24(4):213–224, 2002 12100832.
- Spitzer RL, Kroenke K, Williams JB: Validation and utility of a self-report version of PRIME-MD: The PHQ primary care study: Primary care evaluation of mental disorders: Patient health questionnaire. *JAMA* 282(18):1737–1744, 1999 10568646.
- Spitzer RL, Kroenke K, Williams JB, et al: A brief measure for assessing generalized anxiety disorder: The GAD-7. *Arch Intern Med* 166(10):1092–1097, 2006 16717171.
- Stern TA, Herman JB, Slavin PL (eds): *Massachusetts General Hospital Guide to Primary Care Psychiatry*, 2nd Edition. New York, McGraw-Hill, 2004.
- Unützer J, Katon W, Callahan CM, et al., IMPACT Investigators: Improving mood-promoting access to collaborative treatment: Collaborative care management of late-life depression in the primary care setting: A randomized controlled trial. *JAMA* 288(22):2836–2845, 2002 12472325.
- Unützer J, Schoenbaum M, Druss BG, et al: Transforming mental health care at the interface with general medicine: Report for the presidents commission. *Psychiatr Serv* 57(1):37–47, 2006 16399961.
- Worth JL, Stern TA: Benefits of an outpatient Psychiatric TeleConsultation Unit (PTCU): Results of a one-year pilot. *Prim Care Companion J Clin Psychiatry* 5(2):80–84, 2003 15156235.

31
Differential Awareness of Some Psychiatric Presentations

Tarek Okasha

Introduction	343
Self-Neglect	343
Organic Causes	*343*
Psychotic Disorders	*344*
Mood Disorders	*344*
Neurotic Disorders	*344*
Personality Disorders	*344*
Other Causes	*344*
Agitation	344
Organic Causes	*344*
Substance Abuse	*344*
Psychotic Disorders	*345*
Mood Disorders	*345*
Neurotic Disorders	*345*
Personality Disorders	*345*
Other Causes	*345*
Bizarre Behaviour	345
Organic Causes	*345*
Substance Abuse	*345*
Psychotic Disorders	*345*
Mood Disorders	*346*
Neurotic Disorders	*346*
Personality Disorders	*346*
Catatonia	346
Organic Causes	*346*
Substance Abuse	*346*
Psychotic Disorders	*347*
Mood Disorders	*347*
Neurotic Disorders	*347*
Personality Disorders	*347*

DOI: 10.4324/9780429030260-34

- Excitement — 347
    - *Organic Causes* — *347*
    - *Substance Abuse* — *347*
    - *Psychotic Disorders* — *347*
    - *Mood Disorders* — *348*
    - *Neurotic Disorders* — *348*
    - *Personality Disorders* — *348*
    - *Other Causes* — *348*
- Psychomotor Retardation — 348
    - *Organic Causes* — *348*
    - *Substance Abuse* — *348*
    - *Psychotic Disorders* — *349*
    - *Mood Disorders* — *349*
    - *Neurotic Disorders* — *349*
    - *Personality Disorders* — *349*
    - *Other Causes* — *349*
- Aggression — 349
    - *Organic Causes* — *349*
    - *Substance Abuse* — *350*
    - *Psychotic Disorders* — *350*
    - *Mood Disorders* — *350*
    - *Neurotic Disorders* — *350*
    - *Personality Disorders* — *350*
    - *Other Causes* — *350*
- Hallucinations — 350
    - *Organic Causes* — *350*
    - *Substance Abuse* — *350*
    - *Psychotic Disorders* — *351*
    - *Mood Disorders* — *351*
    - *Neurotic Disorders* — *351*
    - *Personality Disorders* — *351*
    - *Other Causes* — *351*
- Attempted Suicide — 351
    - *Organic Causes* — *351*
    - *Substance Abuse* — *351*
    - *Psychotic Disorders* — *352*
    - *Mood Disorders* — *352*
    - *Neurotic Disorders* — *352*
    - *Personality Disorders* — *352*
    - *Other Causes* — *352*
- Unexplained Somatic Symptoms — 352
    - *Organic Causes* — *352*
    - *Substance Abuse* — *352*
    - *Psychotic Disorders* — *352*
    - *Mood Disorders* — *353*
    - *Neurotic Disorders* — *353*
    - *Personality Disorders* — *353*
    - *Other Causes* — *353*
- Conclusion — 353

INTRODUCTION

Differential awareness is similar to differential diagnosis; however, here we try to emphasise the awareness of the non-psychiatrist of the different disorders that can cause or lead to the presentation of this particular symptom or sign not only to reach a diagnosis but also to eliminate important aetiologies. Differential diagnosis is developing a list of the possible conditions that might produce a patient's symptoms and/or signs and is an important part of clinical reasoning. It ensures that doctors consider all possibilities before they make a diagnosis of a patient's illness.

The process of DSM-5 differential diagnosis can be broken down into six basic steps: 1) ruling out malingering and factitious disorder, 2) ruling out a substance aetiology, 3) ruling out an etiological medical condition, 4) determining the specific primary disorder(s), 5) differentiating adjustment disorder from the residual other specified and unspecified conditions and 6) establishing the boundary with no mental disorder (DSM5, 2013).

In developing countries, both psychiatrists and non-psychiatrists have to be good physicians and neurologists in order to practice and understand different psychiatric presentations, as these presentations in both outpatient clinics can emergency rooms can be caused by many organic disorders in the brain or systemic disorders. Therefore, the order of differential awareness will be slightly different than that in the DSM5: 1) ruling out organic disorders and medical conditions, 2) ruling out substance abuse, 3) ruling out psychotic disorders, 4) ruling out mood disorders, 5) ruling out neurotic disorders, 6) ruling out personality disorders and 7) ruling out malingering and establishing the boundary with no mental disorder. (Okasha & Okasha, 2018).

SELF-NEGLECT

Self-neglect is a behavioural condition in which an individual neglects to attend to their basic needs, such as personal hygiene, appropriate clothing, feeding or tending appropriately to any medical conditions they have.

More generally, any lack of self-care in terms of personal health, hygiene and living conditions can be referred to as self-neglect (Lamkin et al., 2017).

Examples of self-neglect include not eating or drinking enough food and water, homelessness or living in a home or space that is very unclean or unsafe and not bathing or taking care of personal hygiene.

Self-neglect can either be intentional (by choice) or non-intentional (secondary). Intentional self-neglect occurs when a person makes a conscious choice to engage in self-neglect. Non-intentional self-neglect occurs as a result of health-related conditions that contribute to the risk of developing self-neglect, as in the case of some psychiatric disorders.

Upon being confronted by a patient with self-neglect, we should methodologically go through the different psychological causes that can lead to self-neglect (Day et al., 2016; Kutame, 2007; Day, 2013; Okasha & Okasha, 2018).

Organic Causes

These include many disorders, such as frontal lobe tumours; dementia, mainly Alzheimer's dementia, frontal dementia and front temporal dementia; disorders that affect cognition and behaviour; or chronic non-controlled medical disorders leading to delirium. One of the commonest causes of self-neglect secondary to substance abuse is alcoholism, especially in the elderly. Other causes include long-term heroin abuse with social and financial deterioration.

Psychotic Disorders

One of the commonest psychotic disorders with self-neglect is schizophrenia, which can be seen in chronic patients and patients with marked residual and negative symptoms, as well as in patients with marked paranoid ideations, mainly delusions of reference and persecution.

Mood Disorders

Self-neglect can be seen in patients with depression, mainly in patients with melancholic features and severe retardation living alone without any family or social support.

Neurotic Disorders

Self-neglect can be a feature in neurotic disorders, mainly in obsessive compulsive disorder (OCD), mainly seen in patients with obsessions related to cleanliness and fear of germ transmission who have a compulsion to excessively wash, and instead of excessive washing, they avoid contact with anyone and anything, including water.

Personality Disorders

These are not commonly accompanied by self-neglect.

Other Causes

These include poverty, homelessness, nutritional deficiency, social isolation and social dependency.

AGITATION

Agitation is a serious, disruptive and pathological complication of many chronic psychological disorders. Agitation is defined as excessive motor activity associated with a feeling of inner tension. It should be differentiated from irritability, which is defined as a deficit in filtering environmental stimuli combined with a faulty inhibitory capacity, leading to impulsive and exaggerated reactions to common situations.

Upon being confronted by a patient with agitation, we should methodologically go through the different psychological causes that can lead to agitation (Karttunen et al., 2011; Scott Zeller et al., 2017; Zeller & Citrome, 2016; Benazzi et al., 2004; Correll et al., 2017; Okasha & Okasha, 2018).

Organic Causes

They include delirium, dementia, brain tumours, stroke, brain haemorrhage, CNS infection, hypothyroidism, hypoglycaemia and hyperglycaemia (diabetic ketoacidosis).

Substance Abuse

Commonly seen in alcohol intoxication or alcohol withdrawal. It is also seen in stimulant intoxication with substances like cocaine and amphetamine.

Psychotic Disorders

Can be seen in patients suffering from schizophrenia, which can be secondary to the delusions or hallucinations.

Mood Disorders

Agitation can occur in depression and is referred to as agitated depression. The patient can be irritable as well. It can also occur in bipolar disorder during a depressive or manic episode. Agitation can also be a presentation in some women suffering from premenstrual dysphoric disorder.

Neurotic Disorders

Obsessive-compulsive disorder can present with agitation, especially if the obsessions are accompanied by a high level of anxiety. Some patients with extreme generalised anxiety disorder can also suffer from agitation.

Personality Disorders

When patients are frustrated or confronted by legal, social or family norms and/or restrictions like in borderline and antisocial personality disorders.

Other Causes

They include work stress, peer pressure, being burnt out from work and premenstrual syndrome (PMS).

BIZARRE BEHAVIOUR

Behaviour that is self-contradictory or inconsistent. It may include childlike silliness, purposeless behaviour, unpredictable agitation or extreme emotional reaction (e.g., laughing after a catastrophe). A typical example is dressing in clothing inappropriate for the weather (e.g., wearing several layers on a warm summer day).

Upon being confronted by a patient with bizarre behaviour, we should methodologically go through the different psychological causes that can lead to bizarre behaviour (Okasha & Okasha, 2018).

Organic Causes

These include dementia, frontal lobe tumours, frontal lobe epilepsy.

Substance Abuse

Usually occurs in drug intoxication and alcohol intoxication.

Psychotic Disorders

In patients with schizophrenia, bizarre behaviour is common, and the behaviour is mainly related to the delusions and auditory hallucinations.

Mood Disorders

It is not common in mood disorder unless there are severe psychotic symptoms; even in mania, disinhibited behaviour is more common than bizarre.

Neurotic Disorders

Bizarre behaviour can be seen in some cases of dissociative disorders, in the form of fugue, for example.

Personality Disorders

Bizarre behaviour is not common but might appear in some extreme behavioural changes in antisocial personality disorder.

CATATONIA

Catatonia is a neuropsychiatric condition that affects both behaviour and motor function and results in unresponsiveness in someone who otherwise appears to be awake. Catatonia is sometimes referred to as catatonic syndrome, because there is not just one identifying sign or symptom associated with this condition or symptoms that appear separately from one another but rather a collection of several symptoms that appear together at the same time. These specific signs and symptoms do not vary, regardless of the underlying reason for the condition. According to the DSM5 (2013), catatonia can present as: 1) stupor (oblivious inability to move or respond to stimuli), 2) catalepsy (rigid body posture), 3) mutism (little to no verbal communication), 4) waxy flexibility (body remains in whatever position it is placed by another), 5) negativism (lack of verbal response), 6) posturing (holding a posture or position that goes against gravity), 7) mannerisms (extreme or odd movements and mannerisms), 8) stereotypy (frequent repetitive movements for no reason), 9) agitation (for no reason) or grimacing (distorted facial expressions), 10) echolalia (repeating others' words) and 11) echopraxia (repeating others' movements).

Upon being confronted by a patient with catatonia, we should methodologically go through the different psychological causes that can lead to catatonia (Moskowitz, 2004; Ungvari et al., 2010; Grover et al., 2015; Okasha & Okasha, 2018).

Organic Causes

They include encephalitis, neurodegenerative disorders, brain tumours and folate deficiency. It can also occur in some cases of dementia, mainly frontal dementia.

Substance Abuse

It can be secondary to some neuroleptics and in its severe form is known as neuroleptic malignant syndrome accompanied by fever, rigidity, clouding of consciousness and autonomic instability. It can also be seen in cases of increased serotonin, known as serotonin syndrome, accompanied by myoclonic jerks, fever and clouding of consciousness. In a mild form, it can be a side effect of neuroleptics as a severe presentation of neuroleptic-induced extra-pyramidal side effects.

Psychotic Disorders

This can be seen in patients with schizophrenia and is termed catatonic schizophrenia. The term catatonic schizophrenia is used as long as the catatonic symptoms are present, and the diagnosis is revised once it has improved.

Mood Disorders

Depression can present with catatonic symptoms and is an indication of the severity of depression, which needs immediate attention as it could lead to death. Also, in mania, catatonic symptoms can occur alternating with periods of clear manic symptoms; this is also known as manic stupor.

Neurotic Disorders

Catatonia can occur in neurotic disorders and can be seen as motor symptom in conversion disorder.

Personality Disorders

Can be present in patients with cluster B personality disorders known to be emotionally erratic and dramatic, like histrionic personality disorder and borderline personality disorder.

EXCITEMENT

Excitement is a response to stimuli, often used specifically to denote excessive responsiveness to stimuli, particularly of an emotional nature, and often leading to impulsive activity. Psychomotor excitement is a form of psychomotor acceleration.

Upon being confronted by a patient with excitement, we should methodologically go through the different psychological causes that can lead to excitement (Ewen Cameron, 2006; Mavrogiorgou, 2011; Okasha & Okasha, 2018).

Organic Causes

They include delirium, and this is referred to as excited delirium; it can also occur in any form of dementia when delirium is a comorbidity. Other physical disorders include hypothyroidism, myocardial infarction and hypoglycaemia.

Substance Abuse

Mainly occurs with alcohol intoxication and withdrawal; also, missed use of benzodiazepines can lead to excitement, especially during withdrawal and sometimes as a paradoxical side effect of the drug.

Psychotic Disorders

Occurs in patients suffering from schizophrenia as a behavioural change in response to the delusions of hallucinations.

Mood Disorders

Excitement can occur in depressed patients, mainly in the form of depression known as agitated depression. It can similarly occur in both patients with hypomania and mania.

Neurotic Disorders

Excitement can be a presentation in some patients with generalised anxiety disorder and panic disorder, mainly during the phase of the attack.

Personality Disorders

Patients with cluster B personality disorders are more prone to excitement (hysterical, borderline, narcissistic and antisocial).

Other Causes

May include frustration or heightened physiological arousal during watching and playing competitive sports.

PSYCHOMOTOR RETARDATION

Psychomotor retardation involves a slowing down of thought and a reduction of physical movements in an individual. Psychomotor retardation can cause a visible slowing of physical and emotional reactions, including speech and affect. This can include unaccountable difficulty in carrying out what are usually considered "automatic" or "usual" self-care tasks for healthy people, such as taking a shower, dressing, self-grooming, cooking, brushing one's teeth and exercising or physical difficulty performing activities which normally would require little thought or effort such as walking up a flight of stairs, getting out of bed, preparing meals and clearing dishes from the table, household chores or returning phone calls. Tasks requiring mobility suddenly (or gradually) may inexplicably seem to be "impossible." Activities such as shopping, getting groceries, caring for the daily needs of one's children and meeting the demands of employment or school are commonly affected. Activities usually requiring little mental effort can become challenging, such as balancing one's cheque book, making a shopping list or making decisions.

Upon being confronted by a patient with psychomotor retardation, we should methodologically go through the different psychological causes that can lead to psychomotor retardation (Allgulander et al., 2003; Buyukdura et al., 2011; Bennabi et al., 2013; Okasha & Okasha, 2018).

Organic Causes

Can occur in patients suffering from Parkinson's disease and other forms of neurodegenerative disorders, such as Huntington's disease. Other physical disorders include hypothyroidism and chronic uncontrolled physical illnesses.

Substance Abuse

Usually seen in doses of sedatives, but can also be seen in benzodiazepine abuse.

Psychotic Disorders

Patients suffering from schizophrenia can present with psychomotor retardation as a behavioural disturbance.

Mood Disorders

It is a common presentation in severe depression and is sometimes referred to as retarded depression. Psychomotor retardation is a central feature of depression that can have clinical and therapeutic implications. This includes both motor and cognitive impairments, affecting speech, motility and ideation. These symptoms may severely impact patient's psychosocial functioning and are closely linked with severity of depression.

Neurotic Disorders

May be present in extreme forms of anxiety when the patient reaches the exhaustion period and in patients with obsessive-compulsive disorder, especially with checking, and repetitive rituals can manifest with psychomotor retardation.

Personality Disorders

Commonly not seen but can be a symptom of presentation in histrionic personality disorder.

Other Causes

Psychomotor retardation can be present in eating disorders like anorexia nervosa in late stages and in undernourished individuals.

AGGRESSION

Is a behaviour that is intended to harm another individual who does not wish to be harmed. Since it involves the perception of intent, what looks like aggression from one point of view may not look that way from another, and the same harmful behaviour may or may not be considered aggressive depending on its intent. Intentional harm is, however, perceived as worse than unintentional harm, even when the harms are identical.

Aggression needs to be differentiated from the term "violence" to refer to aggression that has extreme physical harm, such as injury or death, as its goal. Thus, violence is a subset of aggression. All violent acts are aggressive, but only acts that are intended to cause extreme physical damage, such as murder, assault, rape and robbery, are violent. Slapping someone really hard across the face might be violent, but calling people names would only be aggressive.

Upon being confronted by a patient with aggression, we should methodologically go through the different psychological causes that can lead to aggression (Baron & Richardson, 1994; Ames & Fiske, 2013; Okasha & Okasha).

Organic Causes

These include dementia; brain tumours, mainly in the amygdala and frontal lobe; some cases of stroke; meningitis; hormonal changes, especially involving testosterone; and genetic disorders involving the Y chromosome.

Substance Abuse

Seen with patients suffering from alcoholism and drug abuse, especially benzodiazepine abuse and opiates.

Psychotic Disorders

Present in some patients suffering from schizophrenia, and it is usually a behavioural response to delusions and hallucinations.

Mood Disorders

Can be seen in an episode of mania, especially when the patient is restricted from his/her activities. Aggression can be seen in some forms of depression but is not a common presentation.

Neurotic Disorders

Particularly see in patients with post-traumatic stress disorder (PTSD) when suffering from flashbacks or waking up during a dream. It can also be secondary to substance abuse, which is a common comorbidity of PTSD.

Personality Disorders

Can be present in patients with cluster B personality disorders known to be emotionally erratic and dramatic, like borderline personality disorder and antisocial personality disorder.

Other Causes

Secondary to frustration or in response to aggression and violence like bullying, domestic abuse and so on.

HALLUCINATIONS

Hallucination is perception without a stimulus. It can affect any of the five senses; hence, there are auditory, visual, olfactory, gustatory and tactile hallucinations.

Upon being confronted by a patient with hallucinations, we should methodologically go through the different psychological causes that can lead to hallucinations (Honig et al., 1998; Ffytche, 2008; Okasha & Okasha, 2018).

Organic Causes

Usually present more with visual hallucinations, whether well or ill formed, which are usually scary to the patient. Sometimes patients may present with auditory and tactile hallucinations. They can also occur in cases of delirium, dementia and brain tumours (temporal lobe and occipital lobe tumours).

Substance Abuse

Visual hallucinations mainly occur with hallucinogens like LSD, ecstasy and magic mushrooms, as well as in alcoholism and sometimes with stimulants like cocaine and amphetamine. Proper drug screening should be done in younger patients with sudden onset of hallucinations.

Psychotic Disorders

Hallucinations occur in most psychotic disorders but mainly in schizophrenia, where hallucinations are usually auditory hallucinations characterised by beings ordering, insulting or offering running commentary, also known as a third voice. In schizophrenia, hallucinations can also be olfactory, gustatory or tactile.

Mood Disorders

Auditory hallucinations can mainly occur in both mania and psychotic depression and are usually coloured by the patient's mood. The hallucinations in depression are depressive in nature, with shame, sin and guilt as a content, while those in mania are more joyful and grandiose.

Neurotic Disorders

Usually do not present with hallucinations, but if they do, they are usually fragmented and non-vivid and occur in conversion and dissociative disorders.

Personality Disorders

Personality disorders usually do not present with hallucinations unless substance abuse is a comorbidity.

Other Causes

People with sensory impairments many present with hallucinations; for example, patients with loss of vision many present with hallucinations in syndrome called Charles Bonnet syndrome.

ATTEMPTED SUICIDE

Suicide, taking your own life, is a tragic reaction to stressful life situations and all the more tragic because suicide can be prevented. Following attempted suicide, high intention to kill oneself is a significant risk factor for both death from all causes and suicide.

Upon being confronted by a patient with attempted suicide, we should methodologically go through the different psychological causes that can lead to attempted suicide (Suominen et al., 2004; Okasha & Okasha 2018).

Organic Causes

Can be seen in patients with chronic pain not responding to medication and neurodegenerative disorders with intact mental abilities and impaired motor activities.

Substance Abuse

Alcohol and drug abuse may be a cause, especially if the patient is suffering from comorbid depression.

Psychotic Disorders

Attempted suicide can occur in schizophrenia in response to auditory hallucinations and sometimes secondary to akathesia, which is a movement disorder that makes it hard for the patient to stay still. It causes an urge to move that the patient cannot control. Patients might need to fidget all the time, walk in place or cross and uncross their legs. Usually, akathesia is a side effect of antipsychotic medication.

Mood Disorders

Nearly 15% of patients with depression will commit suicide, and double that number will attempt suicide. This usually occurs in patients with severe and psychotic depression. Also, patients suffering from bipolar disorder have a 19% chance of suicide and nearly 50% chance of attempted suicide.

Neurotic Disorders

Patients with panic disorder have a 19% chance of suicide, especially if accompanied by agoraphobia. Similarly, patients with PTSD may attempt suicide especially if depression or substance abuse is a comorbidity.

Personality Disorders

Attempted suicide is one of the features of borderline personality disorder and is usually impulsive in nature rather than planned, like in depression.

Other Causes

Less commonly, eating disorders, extreme social and financial problems and strong history of physical or sexual abuse.

UNEXPLAINED SOMATIC SYMPTOMS

Patients presenting with multiple somatic complaints which are not related to any known anatomical or physiological distribution, are patients have been to see several doctors and undergone several investigations without any specific findings.

Upon being confronted by a patient with unexplained somatic symptoms, we should methodologically go through the different psychological causes that can lead to unexplained somatic symptoms (Okasha & Okasha, 1999, 2018, 2019a, 2019b).

Organic Causes

They need to be excluded by proper history taking, clinical examination and investigations if needed.

Substance Abuse

Can occur especially during withdrawal of opiates.

Psychotic Disorders

In schizophrenia, can be secondary to delusions of control (thought insertion, thought withdrawal) or in delusions of persecution when the patient believes that there is a device planted in the body causing the symptoms.

Mood Disorders

In some patients with depression, somatic presentation is a way of expressing depression, especially in communities where psychological and emotional complaints are considered weakness or lack of faith.

Neurotic Disorders

The physical symptoms can be part of the autonomic hyperactivity seen in generalised anxiety disorder (palpitations, chest tightness, nausea, vomiting, frequency of micturition, etc.); panic, especially during a panic attack and anticipatory anxiety phases; conversion, which includes motor, sensory and visceral somatic presentations; somatisation, where patients complain of multiple somatic complaints affecting multiple systems in the body; and hypochondriasis, where the patients attributes the physical symptoms present to a serious disorder.

Personality Disorders

Uncommon except in the anxious and fearful (cluster C) group (avoidant, obsessive, dependent and passive aggressive personality disorders).

Other Causes

Include mainly malingering.

CONCLUSION

Differential awareness is an important clinical skill for both psychiatrists and non-psychiatrists working in developing countries, especially when the burden falls on doctors to be both a general practitioner and a specialist at the same time. The aim of this chapter was to improve the clinical skills of both the psychiatrist and non-psychiatrist working in the emergency room and outpatient clinics in order to help in better diagnosis, leading to better management and, more importantly, a better quality of life for our patients.

References

Allgulander, C., Bandelow, B., Hollander, E., Montgomery, S. A., Nutt, D. J., Okasha, A., Pollack, M. H., Stein, D. J., et al. (Aug 2003). WCA recommendations for the long-term treatment of generalized anxiety disorder. *CNS Spectr.* 8(8 Suppl 1), 53–61. doi:10.1017/S1092852900006945

Ames, D. L., & Fiske, S. T. (2013). Intentional harms are worse, even when they're not. *Psychological Science*, 24(9), 1755–1762.

Baron, R. A., & Richardson, D. R. (1994). *Perspectives in social psychology: Human aggression* (2nd ed.). New York, NY: Plenum Press.

Benazzi, F., Koukopoulos, A., & Akiskal, H. (2004). Toward a validation of a new definition of agitated depression as a bipolar mixed state (mixed depression). *European Psychiatry*, 19(2), 85–90. doi:10.1016/j.eurpsy.2003.09.008

Bennabi, D., Vandel, P., Papaxanthis, C., Pozzo, T., & Haffen, E. (2013). Psychomotor retardation in depression: A systematic review of diagnostic, pathophysiologic, and therapeutic implications. *BioMed Research International*, Article ID 158746, 18 pages. https://doi.org/10.1155/2013/158746

Buyukdura, J. S., McClintock, S. M., & Croarkin, P. E. (2011). Psychomotor retardation in depression: Biological underpinnings, measurement, and treatment. *Prog Neuropsychopharmacol Biol Psychiatry*, 35(2), 395–409. doi:10.1016/j.pnpbp.2010.10.019

Correll, C. U., Yu, X., Xiang, Y., Kane, J. M., & Masand, P. (May 2017). Biological treatment of acute agitation or aggression with schizophrenia or bipolar disorder in the inpatient setting. *Annals of Clinical Psychiatry: Official Journal of the American Academy of Clinical Psychiatrists*, 29(2), 92–107.

Day, M. R., Leahy-Warren, P., & McCarthy, G. (2013). Perceptions and views of self-neglect: A client-centered perspective. *Journal of Elder Abuse & Neglect*, 25(1), 76–94. DOI: 10.1080/08946566.2012.712864

Day, M. R., Leahy-Warren, P., & McCarthy, G. (2016). Self-neglect: Ethical considerations. *Annual Review of Nursing Research*, 34(1), 89–107.

Dominic, H. (2008). The hodology of hallucinations. *Cortex*, 44(8), 1067–1083. ISSN 0010-9452. https://doi.org/10.1016/j.cortex.2008.04.005.

DSM5 (Diagnostic and Statistical Manual 5th Revision). (2013). *American psychiatric association*. New York, NY: American Psychiatric Publishing.

Ewen Cameron. (2006). Some relationships between excitement, depression and anxiety. *American Journal of Psychiatry*. Published Online: 1 Apr. https://doi.org/10.1176/ajp.102.3.385

Grover, Sandeep, Chakrabarti, Subho, Ghormode, Deepak, Agarwal, Munish, Sharma, Akhilesh, & Avasthi, Ajit. (2015). Catatonia in inpatients with psychiatric disorders: A comparison of schizophrenia and mood disorders. *Psychiatry Research*, 229(3), 919–925. ISSN 0165-1781. https://doi.org/10.1016/j.psychres.2015.07.020

Honig, Adriaan, Romme, Marius, Ensink, Bernardine, Escher, Sandra, Pennings, Monique, & Devries, Marten. (October 1998). Auditory hallucinations: A comparison between patients and nonpatients. *The Journal of Nervous & Mental Disease*, 186(10), 646–651.

Karttunen, K., Karppi, P., Hiltunen, A., et al. (2011). Neuropsychiatric symptoms and quality of life in patients with very mild and mild Alzheimer's disease. *Int J Geriatr Psychiatry*, 26, 473–482.

Kutame, M. M. (2007). Understanding self-neglect from the older person's perspective (Doctoral dissertation, The Ohio State University, Columbus, OH).

Lamkin, J., Nguyen, P. T., Coverdale, J. H., & Gordon, M. R. (Sep 2017). Towards a definition of "self-neglect" in psychiatric patients: Descriptions of a case series. *Psychiatr Q.* 88(3), 553–560. doi: 10.1007/s11126-016-9467-6. PMID: 27682463.

Mavrogiorgou, P., Brüne, M., & Juckel, G. (2011). The management of psychiatric emergencies. *Deutsches Arzteblatt International*, 108(13), 222–230. https://doi.org/10.3238/arztebl.2011.0222

Moskowitz, A. K. (2004). "Scared stiff": Catatonia as an evolutionary-based fear response. *Psychological Review*, 111(4), 984–1002. https://doi.org/10.1037/0033-295X.111.4.984

Okasha, A., & Okasha, T. (1999). Somatoform disorders – An Arab perspective. In *Somatoform disorders: A worldwide perspective*. Y. Ono, A. Janca, M. Asai, & N. Sartorius (eds.). Berlin: Springer. pp. 38–46.

Okasha, A., & Okasha, T. (eds.). (2018). *Contemporary psychiatry*. 18th edition. Cairo, Egypt: Anglo Egyptian Bookshop (In Arabic).

Okasha, T. (2019a). Major trends of psychosomatic medicine in North Africa and Middle East. Chapter 8. In *Global psychosomatic medicine and consultation-liaison psychiatry*. Hoyle Leigh (ed.). Switzerland AG: Springer Nature. pp. 147–161.

Okasha, T. (2019b). Psychosomatic medicine in Egypt and North Africa: Development, research, education and practice. Chapter 21. In *Global psychosomatic medicine and consultation-liaison psychiatry*. Hoyle Leigh (ed.). Switzerland AG: Springer Nature. pp. 451–470.

Suominen, K., Isometsä, E., Ostamo, A., et al. (2004). Level of suicidal intent predicts overall mortality and suicide after attempted suicide: A 12-year follow-up study. *BMC Psychiatry*, 4, 11. https://doi.org/10.1186/1471-244X-4-11

Ungvari, Gabor S., Caroff, Stanley N., & Gerevich, Jozsef. (March 2010). The catatonia conundrum: Evidence of psychomotor phenomena as a symptom dimension in psychotic disorders. *Schizophrenia Bulletin*, 36(2), 231–238. https://doi.org/10.1093/schbul/sbp105

Zeller, S. L., & Citrome, L. (2016). Managing agitation associated with schizophrenia and bipolar disorder in the emergency setting. *The Western Journal of Emergency Medicine*, 17(2), 165–172. https://doi.org/10.5811/westjem.2015.12.28763

Zeller, S. L., Nordstrom, Kimberly D., & Wilson, Micheal P. (eds.). (2017). *The diagnosis and management of agitation*. Cambridge: Cambridge University Press.

Section 4
Innovations in the Model of Care

32
Optimising Patient Care in Psychiatry Using Cognitive Behaviour Therapy

Pragya Lodha

Introduction	357
A-B-C of Cognitive Behaviour Therapy	358
What Entails a CBT Session?	359
CBT for Psychoeducation	360
CBT Approach to Psychiatric Illnesses	361
CBT and Psychiatric Disorders	361
Mood Disorders	362
Anxiety and Related Disorders	362
Eating Disorders	362
Somatoform Disorders	362
Schizophrenia and Psychosis	362
Substance Use Disorders	363
Sexual Disorders	363
Personality Disorders	363
Suicidality and Non-Suicidal Self Injury	363
Utility of CBT in Community Mental Health Approach	363
CBT and Crisis Intervention	364
Cognitive Behavioural Group Therapy	365
Plurality and Effectiveness of CBT	366
CBT: The Third Wave	367
CBT With Children and Adolescents	367
Criticism of CBT	367
Conclusion	368

INTRODUCTION

Optimal patient care in psychiatry has often adopted the bio-psycho-social model of health to explain the effectiveness of combination treatment entailing psychopharmacology and psychotherapy. cognitive behaviour therapy, better known as CBT, is a psychotherapeutic school proposed by Aaron T. Beck in the 1960s. Beck, a psychiatrist, dissatisfied with the totality of psychoanalysis for the treatment of depression, was convinced that people with depression experienced negative thoughts. Thus, his development of CBT was oriented in the management of negative thoughts in patients with depression. To date, CBT has grown as a psychological treatment that is used with a wide range of psychiatric illnesses, like mood disorders (depression, dysthymia and bipolar disorder), anxiety disorders (generalised disorder, social anxiety disorder, panic attack and phobias), personality disorders, somatoform disorders, obsessive compulsive disorder, eating disorders and substance use disorders, as well other general stress, chronic pain, mental health problems such as relationship and marital discord, exam anxiety and adjustment-related problems. It has also shown success with psychotic disorders like schizophrenia (most effective in the prodromal phase and first episode) as well. The strongest support exists for CBT for anxiety disorders, somatoform disorders, bulimia, anger control problems and general stress. Cognitive behaviour therapy was established as one of the most dominant therapy over behaviour therapy and psychoanalysis by 1976 (Gaudiano 2008) and continues to remain popular.

Cognitive behaviour therapy largely comes under the umbrella of cognitive therapy. Cognitive therapy (CT) perceives psychological problems as stemming from commonplace processes such as faulty thinking, making incorrect inferences on the basis of inadequate or incorrect information and failing to distinguish between fantasy and reality. Cognitive therapy and the cognitive behavioural approaches are quite diverse, but they do share these attributes: (1) a collaborative relationship between client and therapist, (2) the assumption that psychological problems are mainly a function of disturbances in cognitive processes, (3) a focus on changing cognitions to produce desired changes in affect and behaviour, (4) a present-centred and time-limited focus, (5) an emphasis on the client's responsibility for assuming an active role in the therapy process and (6) making use of a variety of cognitive and behavioural strategies to bring about change (Corey, 2001).

Generally, CBT falls under CT with a premise that the way situations are perceived influences the way one feels emotionally. Thus, it is not a situation that directly affects how people feel emotionally but their thoughts in that situation. When in distress, people often have an inaccurate perception, and their thoughts may be unrealistic. Cognitive behaviour therapy helps people identify the distressing thoughts and evaluate how realistic the thoughts are/can be. Then, people learn to change their distorted thinking. When they think more realistically, they feel better. The consistent emphasis of CBT is also on solving problems and initiating behavioural changes as part of better coping mechanisms.

CBT is rooted in the present functioning with adequate attention to patient's history. CBT therapists emphasise what is going on in the person's current life rather than what has led up to their difficulties. There is an intake of information about patient's history that is necessary, but the primary focus of CBT-based treatment is to focus on present problems and on moving forward in time to develop more effective ways of coping with stressors in life.

A-B-C OF COGNITIVE BEHAVIOUR THERAPY

Though a general expectation of CBT being a cognitive therapy would focus on thought processes, the practice of CBT goes beyond cognition to address behavioural and affective aspects as well. Effective CBT addresses the intellect of thoughts and thought processes, experience of emotions and dysfunctional(/maladaptive) behaviours. The process of CBT is divided into several steps, with an insistence on distinct therapeutic mechanisms (establishing a therapeutic relationship, practicing collaborative empiricism and managing the maladaptive cognitions and behaviours).

Cognitive behaviour therapy, in essence, also draws from the foundations of REBT (rational emotive behaviour therapy) proposed by Albert Ellis (1950s). REBT is a precursor to CBT. Albert Ellis's infamous ABC model also extends to explain the CBT modality. A typical CBT model is graphically understood by the triad relationship of A-B-C, where A represents

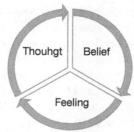

Figure 32.1 Core principles of cognitive behavioral therapy.

the 'antecedent or activating event', B represents the 'belief' and C is the 'consequence'. This explains to patients that it is the irrational belief (IB) that leads to the consequences (negative). Simply put, CBT explains the inter-relationship between thoughts, feelings and behaviours. CBT helps to build a set of skills that enables an individual to be aware of thoughts and emotions; identify how situations, thoughts and behaviours influence emotions; and improve feelings by changing dysfunctional thoughts and behaviours.

CBT is based on several core principles, including (APA 2020):

1. Psychological problems are based, in part, on faulty or unhelpful ways of thinking.
2. Psychological problems are based, in part, on learned patterns of unhelpful behaviour.
3. People suffering from psychological problems can learn better ways of coping with them, thereby relieving their symptoms and becoming more effective in their lives.

CBT treatment usually involves one making efforts in order to change thinking patterns/thought processes. These strategies might include:

- Learning to recognise one's distortions in thinking that are creating problems and then to re-evaluate them in light of reality.
- Gaining a better understanding of the behaviour and motivation of others.
- Using problem-solving skills to cope with difficult situations.
- Learning to develop a greater sense of confidence is one's own abilities.

CBT treatment also involves efforts to bring about change in behavioural patterns, and some of these strategies might include:

- Facing one's fears instead of avoiding them.
- Using role-playing to prepare for potentially problematic interactions with others.
- Learning to calm one's mind and relax one's body.

WHAT ENTAILS A CBT SESSION?

Case formulation for cognitive behaviour therapy, like any other therapeutic modality, acts as a backbone for each therapy session and provides a sense for the course of treatment. The goal of the initial sessions is to psycho-educate the patient about the problem and elicit a close relationship between cognition and emotion. This helps for some insight creation that leads the way to better reception of concepts in therapy. Therapist and patient engage in "collaborative empiricism" to identify, evaluate, modify and replace distorted thinking with more accurate and adaptive cognitions.

CBT as a psychotherapeutic modality is quite structured (as opposed to person-centred therapy or psychoanalysis). A conventional therapy session begins with establishing an agenda that lists the current problems that the patient may be experiencing, followed by cognitive restructuring of maladaptive cognitions (negative automatic thoughts, cognitive distortions, assumptions and unhealthy schema). At the end, the session is summarised. Most often, homework assignments are designed to help the patient in applying the specific skills and concepts learned from the session to his/her real-life problems. Exercises in the session, as well as "homework" exercises outside of sessions, help to develop coping skills, whereby patients can learn to change their own thinking, problematic emotions and behaviour.

In each therapy session, cognitive behaviour therapists help patients specify the problems they have encountered during the week or that they expect to encounter in the current week. They then identify the ideas and behaviours that have interfered with patients' ability to solve problems themselves. Therapists get patients to actively engage in deciding where to start working. Mutually, they develop an "action plan" or homework for patients to do during the week in order to implement solutions to problems or to make changes in their thinking and actions. This process is to get patients actively involved in their own treatment; they begin to recognise that the way to get better is to make small changes in how they think and what they do every day. When treatment ends, patients are able to use the skills and tools they have learned in therapy in their day-to-day lives. This is the principle of self-determination that is built during therapy sessions in order to help people realise that they are capable of solving their own problems.

Over the course of therapy, the session contents progress from superficial automatic thoughts to deeper beliefs and schemas. Training in cognitive restructuring skills is offered through didactic or Socratic means. In the didactic approach, the therapist explains the concept of cognitive distortion and discusses the types of distortions which is followed by application to real world examples. In the Socratic approach, the idea of guided discovery is emphasised through the usage of a series of questions to help the patients evaluate the validity and utility of their cognitions (Beck et al. 1979; Hofmann and Reinecke 2010; Tarrier 2006).

CBT FOR PSYCHOEDUCATION

As discussed, this section is to highlight how cognitive behaviour therapy plays a very important role in building awareness about the illness for the patient. However, in nearly all therapeutic sessions, therapists ground a basic psychoeducation about the illnesses/problems that

Examples of Various Techniques Used in CBT	
Cognitive reconstruction	Psychoeducation
Self-monitoring (e.g. Thought Record)	Cognitive continuum
Descending Arrow Technique	Acceptance
Socratic Questioning Techniques	Behavioral Activation
Advantages and disadvantages	Relapse Prevention
Rational-emotional role-play	Mindfulness
Relaxation	Self-disclosure
Acting "as If"	Core Belief worksheet
Behavioral experiments	Extreme contrasts
Homework	Developing metaphors
Exposure	Historical tests
Skills development	Restructuring early memories
Reconstructing personal history	Coping cards
Balcony method	Problem-solving
Response Prevention	Pie Chart

Figure 32.2 Various components of cognitive behaviour therapy.

patients come in with, which is done to equip patients about the nature and source of their problems for better understanding. However, what is unique about CBT is that the modality in itself is psycho-educative in nature. The core principles and strategies deployed in CBT are tools that also fulfil the required component of psychoeducation, helping the patient become aware.

In several disorders, such as bipolar disorder, schizophrenia and sexual disorders, explaining to the patient why and how the course of disorder takes place can be complex. When CBT is utilised as a mode of treatment, this is explained in the therapy framework, for example, with the help of explaining faulty cognitions, cognitive distortions and unhealthy processing of emotions leading to unhelpful behaviours – people can learn what to correct in order to experience healthier emotions and fruitful behaviours. A lot of times, patients may not be engaged in a psychoeducation session separately and for several reasons – they may not have the bandwidth to understand because of a lack of education or poverty of insight, and sometimes they may not be ready enough to be able to take that information, as denial acts as protection initially (it is only once there is a comfortable rapport that patients gain the courage to confront their real problems as is). CBT as a therapy is credited for its unembellished framework, which makes it quite accessible for people across ages and beyond formal education.

CBT APPROACH TO PSYCHIATRIC ILLNESSES

The CBT approach to understanding psychopathology poses that psychopathological states are a result of faulty information processing. Distorted and dysfunctional cognitions produce negative affective states and maladaptive behaviours that underlie the presentation of pathological symptomatology. Each disorder can be explained with the characterisation by different but predictable patterns of information processing distortions. There is a plethora of techniques designed to modify dysfunctional beliefs and faulty information processing that are characteristic to every disorder. These techniques fall under four broad areas that involve identifying distorted thinking, modifying beliefs, relating to others in different ways and changing behaviours. CBT identifies the cognitive formulations (the beliefs and behavioural strategies that characterise a specific disorder) for disorders in order to cater to the specific deficits and needs in every patient. There is a two-fold goal in the treatment course; one is to reduce symptomatology, and the second, larger goal is to obtain functional restoration. This goal is met by engaging in an active, goal-oriented and problem-solving approach by the therapist and patient mutually. As discussed, the core premise of work with CBT is to work on the distorted (unhealthy) thought processes and combine them with behavioural strategies as and when required, in order to achieve healthy emotional processing and day-to-day functioning.

CBT AND PSYCHIATRIC DISORDERS

Having discussed the nature of CBT, the therapy can be understood to have two broad aspects:

1. One in which cognitive restructuring is the core element of the treatment.
2. The other in which though cognitive restructuring remains an important component, but at least two other components also have a prominent place. These components could be behavioural modification, social skills training, relaxation or coping skills.

Mood Disorders

Meta-analyses conducted to study the effect of CBT on depression (dysthymia and depression) have found that in comparison to controls who did not receive treatment or were waitlisted for treatment, CBT has been found to be effective. However, when compared to other psychological treatment, the results were mixed. Some studies showed the efficacy of modalities like interpersonal and psychodynamic therapy over CBT, whereas contrary results were found in other studies. Research has also indicated the aided effect of CBT when given in conjunction with pharmacotherapy. With therapy and medication, there have been mixed results regarding the efficacy of CBT post treatment and after a follow-up period.

For bipolar disorder, CBT does not promise efficacy as a stand-alone treatment and must be given in addition to medication. Therapy usually addresses the depressive moods in bipolar disorder; this is likely understood since the genesis of several therapies has stemmed from that that of unipolar depression; clinically, we also don't see patients presenting or finding the need for therapy during their uplifted moods.

Anxiety and Related Disorders

Cognitive behaviour therapy is the first line of treatment for this class of disorders and has shown positive effects on the treatment of primary (restlessness, palpitations) and secondary symptoms (sleep dysfunction) of anxiety. CBT delivered through the internet medium and self-guided help has also shown to be effective for anxiety disorder. For social anxiety disorder, generalised anxiety disorder, specific phobia, panic attacks and agoraphobia, the CBT technique was found to be highly effective as a standalone treatment as well as with relaxation treatments.

Eating Disorders

Not all eating disorders have been found to improve with CBT. Bulimia nervosa has been found to have some improvement with CBT; however, behaviour therapy was found more effective than CBT. However, in remission, response rates for bulimia nervosa benefitted most from CBT interventions as compared to several other psychotherapies.

Somatoform Disorders

Hypochondriasis and body dysmorphic disorders are the most-studied somatoform conditions with regard to CBT, and results have shown CBT to be fairly effective therapeutic treatment modality that outperformed other psychological treatments as well as pharmacotherapy treatment.

Schizophrenia and Psychosis

CBT has been found to have a marked effect on positive symptoms of schizophrenia (hallucinations/delusions), though the effect on negative symptoms has been debatable. CBT has been found to be efficacious with pharmacotherapy. CBT has been found to have a positive effect on acute conditions versus more chronic schizophrenia. Better efficacy has been reported in the treatment of secondary outcomes (that were indirect targets of treatment), such as general functioning, mood and social anxiety.

Substance Use Disorders

Caffeine and nicotine dependence have been reported to have reduced in patients when CBT was administered in adjunct with other non-pharmacological treatments. CBT was also found effective as monotherapy treatment. However, CBT was found less effective than brief interventions as compared to pharmacological treatment.

Sexual Disorders

The use of CBT has been found to be effective in male and female sexual dysfunctions. Frequently, sexual dysfunctions (and some disorders) are rooted in various factors such as the anxiety to perform well (performance anxiety); lack of communication between the partners; lack of communication regarding the act of sex, especially when there are discrepant sexual behaviours; interpersonal problems; suspicion of infidelity; and unrealistic expectations about the act of intercourse. CBT therapists teach these clients relaxation and refocusing tools to heighten awareness of their sensations, to focus on pleasure and to reduce anxiety and the demand to perform.

Personality Disorders

In comparison to the use of long-term therapies like psychodynamic therapy, CBT was found to be less effective for treatment of personality disorders such as antisocial personality disorder and borderline personality disorder. Interesting to note is that self-reports indicate CBT to be more effective than long-term therapies.

Suicidality and Non-Suicidal Self Injury

Cognitive behaviour therapy has been found to be effective when used as intervention for suicidal thoughts and suicidal behaviours. This was likely because CBT targets these two aspects of suicidality. Presently, there is less evidence from clinical trials to suggest that CBT focusing on mental illnesses also reduces suicidal cognitions and behaviours. Effective reduction in suicidal ideation has been reported with the administration of CBT practices. Though dialectical behaviour therapy has a higher rate of success in dealing with and managing suicidality, CBT is the next-best approach to psychotherapy. DBT is also a version of CBT.

Non-suicidal self-injury (NSSI) or deliberate self-harm (DSH) are conditions usually seen with psychiatric illnesses such as personality disorder, depression, eating disorders and bipolar disorder. CBT has been shown to be the most promising treatment for NSSI. Manually assisted cognitive behaviour therapy (MACT) is a form of CBT used as a treatment developed for DSH.

UTILITY OF CBT IN COMMUNITY MENTAL HEALTH APPROACH

Cognitive behaviour therapy was initially used in private clinic settings, making it a treatment measure more for the higher socio-economic classes. However, with adaptations, CBT was also translated into community mental health practice for the benefit of a lot more people.

Cognitive behaviour therapy, being time-bound, usually entails 12–20 sessions in therapy. The straightforward and simple-to-understand core principles of CBT give it great appeal in applications in a community mental health approach. A variant of CBT that makes it especially useful in a community mental health approach is brief CBT. In brief CBT, the concentration is on specific treatments for a limited number of the patient's problems. The sessions usually range from four to eight sessions in the brief version of therapy. Treatment is required to be specific because of the limited number of sessions and because the patient is required to be diligent in using extra reading materials and homework to assist in their therapeutic growth. In brief CBT, the sessions are directed towards managing specific problems at hand that are seen at a community level and largely entail psychoeducation, awareness, focus on cognitive distortions and absorbing behavioural techniques for quicker results. Brief CBT can be used for the management of adjustment-related stress, adjustment anxiety, depressive thinking, anxiety and depression related to chronic/acute medical conditions, pain management, coping with a (new) diagnosis (medical/psychiatric) and enhancing adjustment. It also includes lifestyles changes, diet, exercise and medication compliance. Brief CBT works well as the basic coping ability is in place. However, there are also certain contraindications for the use of brief CBT, such as for personality disorders, severe comorbid conditions, trauma, PTSD and other severe mental illnesses. Sometimes, training in CBT can also be applied for crisis situations such as suicidal ideation and non-suicidal self-injury; however, the efficacy and use are questionable (this discussed in the following section).

CBT can very easily be taught to community mental health workers and positively impacts the treatment burden and overall treatment gap. Since a larger proportion of the population suffering from mental illnesses also benefit from community mental health services, CBT equips community mental health workers to provide comprehensive services to these patients. With therapy coming along with pharmacological treatment given to patients, patients have better chances for recovery. CBT being used by community mental health workers also increases the chances for better rehabilitation of patients with mental illnesses.

CBT AND CRISIS INTERVENTION

As discussed, the cognitive-behavioural approach involves an individual first focusing on the individual's automatic thoughts and schemata. This deals with the individual's belief systems, assumptions about oneself, the world, their experiences, the future in general and their usual perceptions. This initial therapeutic work is thus intrapersonal/intrapsychic in nature. The second focus of the therapy is interpersonal and deals with the manner in which the individual relates to others. The third focus of the therapy is external, where the person learns and applies healthier behaviours for better productive coping. This generally involves learning new behaviours/responses, trying the new behaviours, evaluating the result of the new behaviours and developing and using available resources. The use of CBT in crisis situations such as that of suicidal ideation, suicide attempts and non-suicidal self-injury is questionable, though there are certain attributes of cognitive therapy make it a good fit for crisis intervention work. Following are eight aspects of CBT that make it a viable tool in crisis situations:

1. Activity model: this allows the patient to be an active member in the process of therapy, also helping them to feel a sense of control for driving change in themselves.
2. Directiveness: allows the therapist to take an active role of guiding and directing the therapy session, giving a sense of resourcefulness to the patient.
3. Structured session: the practice of establishing discrete goals and evaluating how progress is taking place helps the therapist and patient to understand how therapy is going ahead and if any re-focus is required.
4. Short-term nature: people prefer time-bound therapy for faster results, cost effectiveness and a framework for establishing agenda for maximum success.

5. Collaboration: it is the backbone of CBT sessions, where the therapist and patient work together on deciding on the goals and course of therapy.
6. Dynamic model: a dynamic cognitive approach to therapy promotes rapid self-disclosure of individual cognitions in order to increase understanding through enhanced knowledge and an understanding of thoughts, beliefs and attitudes.
7. Psychoeducational model: this allows CBT therapy sessions to garner awareness and understanding about the nature of mental illnesses, understanding what triggers are and how can they be best prevented. CBT is a skill-building and coping model of therapy.
8. Social/interpersonal model: CBT well integrates the interpersonal relationships that the patient has with family members, friends and peers, along with the intrapsychic function of therapy.

Clinically, what must be adhered to when it comes to crisis situations is that CBT may address the initial disorganisation, upset and emotional instability, and the end goal is to reduce the potential of a radical outcome.

Natural disasters are another kind of an emergency/crisis situation. CBT plays a role of intervention in post-disaster situations where there is a need to relieve people of the (stressful and traumatic) effects of the calamity. It is often referred to as CBT-post disaster (CBT-PD). CBT addresses several post-disaster stress reactions that encompass a wide range of affective, cognitive and behavioural reactions: depression, post-traumatic stress disorder, stress vulnerability, panic attacks and routine dysfunction. CBT-PD is usually a ten-session therapy substructure which works with a primary focus on identifying, challenging and replacing disaster-related maladaptive beliefs. CBT-PD has three components: psychoeducation, management of anxiety and cognitive restructuring.

Nevertheless, not all situations can be managed by CBT alone and may demand a long-term intervention. Thus, most CBT plays an intermediate role between crisis counselling and long-term psychotherapy in order to provide immediate (brief) relief and coping. The efficacious use of CBT as crisis intervention depends on the situation in context, severity and the need for urgent help. Situations such as those involving domestic violence, sexual abuse and suicidal ideations may benefit from immediate supportive counselling and CBT but maybe not long-term care.

COGNITIVE BEHAVIOURAL GROUP THERAPY

Cognitive-behavioural group therapy (CBGT) is a group approach under the CBT spectrum of therapies that deploys behavioural, cognitive, relational and group procedures to enhance the coping skills of the participants. CBGT focuses on working on the interpersonal and intrapersonal problems of patients. In CBGT, the group provides a rich source of ideas in brainstorming, suggestions for alternative strategies and models for role-playing in order to help people cope with their challenges. Another advantage is that patients get reinforcement from each other, which is far more powerful than reinforcement by a therapist. Patients get a chance to learn from each other's lived experiences and also find motivation in others' coping (personal experience). Starting in the 1970s, group CBT has shown huge support efficacy. CBGT can be used with children, adolescents, adults and the elderly. Considerable efficacy for CBGT has been shown for depression, anxiety, panic disorder, eating disorder, chronic pain and general stress.

Group therapy is found to be one of the most effective non-pharmacological interventions with children and adolescents. CBGT for younger populations involves sessions that cover psychoeducation, parent training, organisation and planning, problem-solving, social skill training and emotional regulation. CBGT has been found to be most effective with children who suffer from anxiety disorders. However, successful outcomes have also been seen for anxiety, depression, post-traumatic stress disorder, behaviour problems and substance abuse; the group settings allows for learning to take place and new relationships to form, and thus internal reinforcements allow for better impact.

Cognitive-behavioural therapy can help children to reframe how they identify, interpret and evaluate their emotional and behavioural reactions to negative experiences. The group experience may enrich this learning given that children and adolescents go through a transitioning time and seek to identify and belong where they feel understood.

PLURALITY AND EFFECTIVENESS OF CBT

Cognitive behaviour therapy continues to remain as a popular choice of therapy not just with clinicians but equally with patients as well. Some reasons for its popularity are its common-sense approach and clear and simple principles, along with its extensive use in self-help books that makes it an understandable approach to the receiver. Another crucial factor that makes CBT favourable among an empirically driven clinical approach is its short-term nature of treatment. Colloquially understood, in a time where no one has the time and patience to wait, CBT seems to come around with faster results. The *Washington Post* once proclaimed that, for better or worse, cognitive therapy is fast becoming what people mean when they say they are "getting therapy."

CBT is one of the few psychotherapies that has been scientifically tested across hundreds of clinical trials to show efficacious outcomes with several disorders. Along with empirical grounding, the several aforementioned aspects make CBT a better choice of therapy among the patient group as well as among practitioners. CBT can be very easily blended with other modalities in an eclectic practice of psychotherapy as well, which adds to its efficacy. Not only does CBT use a variety of cognitive and behavioural techniques, but it also borrows from many psychotherapeutic modalities, including dialectical behaviour therapy, acceptance and commitment therapy, gestalt therapy, compassion-focused therapy, mindfulness, solution-focused therapy, motivational interviewing, positive psychology, interpersonal psychotherapy and psychodynamic psychotherapy.

Empirically, CBT has also shown success with varied age groups, right from children to adolescents, adults and the geriatric population (Hofmann et al. 2012).

Another aspect that makes CBT a favoured choice of therapy is the nature of the psycho-educative model it has, which makes it fit the bill with almost all disorders. Even if CBT may not be the long-term monotherapy of choice, it plays a role in the initial phases of the treatment and may be used as and when needed during the psychotherapeutic treatment phase. As mentioned, CBT makes the explanation of understanding the aetiology of illness simple by bringing the explanation to the atomic level of thoughts, feelings and behaviours. The elements of altering unhealthy thoughts and incorporating healthier behaviours, even if they aren't rooted in insight, serve as helpful to bring about the first layer of change and relief for the patient.

Some other factors that make CBT a favourable therapeutic modality are:

1. As discussed, it can be used as a supportive measure in crisis situations.
2. Given the nature of the therapy, it is suitable to be deployed in online/virtual mediums.
3. It can easily be made available for mass readership, as in self-help books and manuals.
4. CBT can be easily be used for group therapy as well.
5. The common-sensical approach appeals to more people.
6. It can be successfully used with patients with average and lower-than-average intellectual capacity as well.

CBT: THE THIRD WAVE

Though the tenets of CBT are fairly straightforward, there are several other treatment modalities that are categorised under the spectrum of CBT. These treatment modalities are specific, as they are targeted towards specific symptom clusters or psychiatric disorders (empirically proved to be evidence based). Some of the many among the family of interventions are problem-solving therapy, dialectical behaviour therapy, meta-cognitive therapy, rational-emotive behaviour therapy, cognitive processing therapy, positive CBT, mindfulness-based cognitive therapy, cognitive-behavioural analysis system of psychotherapy and schema-focused therapy. These interventions are also referred to as the third wave of CBT that arose in 2003–2004 (Hayes 2004), where the identification is more with a contextual concept focused more on the person's relationship to the thoughts and emotions than just the content of it. The third wave of CBT emphasises issues such as mindfulness, emotions, acceptance, the relationship, values, goals and meta-cognition. Comprehensively, therapies that fall under cognitive and cognitive behaviour therapy are nearly 22 in total and can be categorised under three broad areas: cognitive restructuring, coping skills training and problem-solving skills training. All CBTs share common features of a comprehensive cognitive and behavioural assessment of thoughts, emotions and behaviours using a functional analysis, a therapeutic model for psychopathology based on cognitive theory, recognition of thought patterns and subsequently strategies to modify them using behavioural and cognitive strategies.

CBT WITH CHILDREN AND ADOLESCENTS

CBT is an evidence-based treatment modality used successfully with the younger population as well. CBT has been used for the management of several psychiatric conditions seen in the younger population, including anxiety, mood disorders such as bipolar disorder, depression, eating disorders, disruptive and oppositional behaviours, self-injurious behaviours, anger and aggressive behaviours, along with major psychiatric disorders such as schizophrenia and substance use disorders. However, research claims that CBT is best effective for anxiety disorders and obsessive-compulsive disorder; the results for depression and NSSI were scarce and limited. A mixed result was obtained for efficacy of CBT in disruptive classroom behaviour, aggressive behaviours and antisocial behaviours.

However, CBT was primarily developed for adults with a core need for adults to become aware, identify and understand distortions and then learn healthier thought processes. Taking the cognitive theories into consideration, some changes need to be made to suit the cognitive level and demands of a younger clientele. The developmental age of the adolescent is important to consider before applying CBT with them, as that would determine if the adolescent is receptive to the therapeutic treatment. Is it important to note that there is no cut-off for the developmental age of the child, as it may vary from child to child irrespective of their chronological ages. For effective results, CBT is preferably used after the child has reached adolescence. Since behavioural strategies and therapies work better with the younger age group, CBT for adolescents incorporates several behavioural strategies. Contrary to adults, adolescents may not always develop insight with talk therapy about social cognitions and attachment styles (which play a very important role in development), and thus therapy sessions are a lot more activity- and exercise-oriented to imbibe CBT principles (personal experience).

CRITICISM OF CBT

Despite the proven efficacy and the popularity that CBT has garnered, it is apparent that it has received its share of criticism as well. First, though CBT has shown empirical evidence for its efficacy, there haven't been clear indications of the causality of which of the tenets of

CBT principles really led to the change – most often behavioural change has been found to show improvement in patients with no demonstration in change of cognitive distortions (Jacobson et al. 1996). It is quickly labelled as mechanistic and superficial, as the therapy doesn't endorse the patient as a "whole." Second, the theoretical aspects of CBT have often not found orientation in cognitive psychology and neuroscience; thus, it is understood that the empirical nature of theoretical therapy is amiss. Third, when it comes to the treatment of depression and anxiety, CBT often fails to differentiate between cognitive symptoms and cognitive distortions and thus may actually backfire as a treatment modality in the absence of psychopharmacological support or if used as a monotherapy treatment.

Linguistic and pragmatic criticism has also revolved around the synonymous and interchangeable use of terms like negative self-concepts, irrational beliefs about the self, dysfunctional self-concept and biased cognitions about the self. Psychodynamic therapists argue that CBT falls short of addressing the deeper-rooted causes of troubles, and unless the underlying causes are left unaddressed, problems are likely to re-occur. There is a hustle around the short-term effectiveness of CBT that makes it more popular with altering automatic thoughts in depression and anxiety (best results with milder and moderate forms). The psychodynamic take is that depression and anxiety protect us from the vulnerable feelings associated with the true source of our distress, and CBT helps with altering these automatic thoughts on the surface to bring back functionality, which is helpful in the short term but fails to prolong impact in the long run (Kendall & Southam-Gerow 1996). Research has supported less-promising results for the long-term efficacy of CBT. Likewise, several psychodynamic therapists and trauma therapists laud the effectiveness of CBT but find it ineffective for long-term well-being and have also identified the need to blend CBT with psychotherapeutic modalities that have long-lasting effects like psychodynamic and integrative forms of therapy (Knekt et al. 2008).

In an intriguing aspect of comparative research, Johnsen and Friborg analysed 70 studies between the years 1977 and 2014 and found that CBT is roughly half as effective in treating depression as it used to be. There are two theories to support this; one is a positive correlation between the popularity of therapy and increase in incompetent therapists – as therapy grows more popular, the proportion of incompetent practitioners increases in number. Second is the placebo effect. As CBT rapidly grew to be known as a measure of treatment for depression and anxiety, people claimed it was a miraculous cure. However, what is suspect about it is that not many people today really report similar miraculous efficacy. The demands and expectations of people (patients) are far more realistic, and thus the lowered effectiveness of CBT is no longer a revelation. To understand the meaning of placebo when it comes to talk therapy, one must reflect the discrepancy between the belief and the therapy that may have caused the positive outcome. Beliefs are an integral part of our psychological system and existence – if one can believe, the chances it will happen increase.

Last, therapists also claim that CBT is not the best for all types of patients; there are patients who prefer working on an insight level, patients who are already aware of their distortions and unhealthy patterns and rather want to understand the source of them, patients with a higher intellect quotient and patients who are sensitive to affectional states – these are the patients who may not do the best with CBT as a therapeutic modality.

CONCLUSION

Cognitive behaviour therapy is here to stay, and progressive research in modifying the therapeutic school will aid to the benefit of its utility and efficacy with patients. Though insight-oriented and integrative therapies have an edge over CBT, cognitive behavioural techniques have their share of success as well. One must crucially see that before the efficacy of any psychotherapeutic modality is considered, it is indispensable to note the quality of therapist-patient rapport/alliance. This is crucial to the success of any therapeutic relationship. What also needs consideration when it comes to a better choice of therapy is for the clinician to be able to gauge whether CBT is to be used alone or as an admixture with other schools. The patient's personality factors also play a decisive role. What research needs to bridge is the rigorous use of CBT in diverse yet specific aspects (behavioural and cognitive) of psychopathological states in order to provide for continuous efficacy. Thus, there needs to be hand-in hand research on understanding psychopathological states/symptoms as well as the treatment modalities addressing them. Emphatically, the needs of the evolving patient has to be the core niche for surmounting changes and modifications that CBT should incorporate.

Bibliography

1. American Psychological Association. (2020). What is cognitive behavioural therapy? *APA Div. 12, Society of Clinical Psychology.* www.apa.org/ptsd-guideline/patients-and-families/cognitive-behavioral
2. Beck, A. T. (Ed.). (1979). *Cognitive therapy of depression.* London: Guilford press.
3. Beck, A. T. (2010). *Cognitive-behavioral strategies in crisis intervention.* London: Guilford Press.
4. Bond, F. W., & Dryden, W. (Eds.). (2005). *Handbook of brief cognitive behaviour therapy.* New York: John Wiley & Sons.
5. Butler, A. C., Chapman, J. E., Forman, E. M., & Beck, A. T. (2006). The empirical status of cognitive-behavioral therapy: A review of meta-analyses. *Clinical Psychology Review, 26*(1), 17–31.
6. Carpenter, J. K., Andrews, L. A., Witcraft, S. M., Powers, M. B., Smits, J., & Hofmann, S. G. (2018). Cognitive behavioral therapy for anxiety and related disorders: A meta-analysis of randomized placebo-controlled trials. *Depression and Anxiety, 35*(6), 502–514. https://doi.org/10.1002/da.22728
7. Clark, G. I., & Egan, S. J. (2015). The Socratic method in cognitive behavioural therapy: A narrative review. *Cognitive Therapy and Research, 39*(6), 863–879.
8. Corey, G. (2001). *Case approach to counselling and therapy.* London, UK: Sage Publications.
9. David, D., Cristea, I., & Hofmann, S. G. (2018). Why cognitive behavioral therapy is the current gold standard of psychotherapy. *Frontiers in Psychiatry, 9,* 4.
10. Dobson, K. S., & Jackman-Cram, S. U. S. A. N. (1996). Common change processes in cognitive-behavioral therapies for depression. *Advances in Cognitive-Behavioral Therapy, 63*–82.
11. Gautam, M., Tripathi, A., Deshmukh, D., & Gaur, M. (2020). Cognitive behavioral therapy for depression. *Indian Journal of Psychiatry, 62*(Suppl 2), S223–S229. https://doi.org/10.4103/psychiatry.IndianJPsychiatry_772_19
12. Hamblen, J. L., Norris, F. H., Symon, K. A., & Bow, T. E. (2017). Cognitive behavioral therapy for postdisaster distress: A promising transdiagnostic approach to treating disaster survivors. *Psychological Trauma: Theory, Research, Practice, and Policy, 9*(S1), 130.
13. Halder, S., & Mahato, A. K. (2019). Cognitive behavior therapy for children and adolescents: Challenges and gaps in practice. *Indian Journal of Psychological Medicine, 41*(3), 279–283. https://doi.org/10.4103/IJPSYM.IJPSYM_470_18
14. Hayes, S. C., & Hofmann, S. G. (2017). The third wave of cognitive behavioral therapy and the rise of process-based care. *World Psychiatry, 16*(3), 245.
15. Hofmann, S. G., Asnaani, A., Vonk, I. J., Sawyer, A. T., & Fang, A. (2012). The efficacy of cognitive behavioral therapy: A review of meta-analyses. *Cognitive Therapy and Research, 36*(5), 427–440. https://doi.org/10.1007/s10608-012-9476-1
16. Johnsen, T. J., & Friborg, O. (2015). The effects of cognitive behavioral therapy as an anti-depressive treatment is falling: A meta-analysis. *Psychological Bulletin, 141*(4), 747.
17. Kabat-Zinn, J. (2013). *Full catastrophe living, revised edition: How to cope with stress, pain and illness using mindfulness meditation.* London: Hachette.
18. Kendall, P. C. (1994). Treating anxiety disorders in children: Results of a randomized clinical trial. *Journal of Consulting and Clinical Psychology, 62*(1), 100.
19. Knekt, P., Lindfors, O., Sares-Jäske, L., Virtala, E., & Härkänen, T. (2013). Randomized trial on the effectiveness of long-and short-term psychotherapy on psychiatric symptoms and working ability during a 5-year follow-up. *Nordic Journal of Psychiatry, 67*(1), 59–68.

20. Lodha, P., & Sousa, A. D. (2020). Cognitive behavioural therapy and its role in the outcome and recovery from schizophrenia. In *Schizophrenia treatment outcomes* (pp. 299–312). Cham: Springer.
21. Schaub, A., Hippius, H., Möller, H. J., & Falkai, P. (2016). Psychoeducational and cognitive behavioral treatment programs: Implementation and evaluation from 1995 to 2015 in Kraepelin's former hospital. *Schizophrenia Bulletin, 42* (Suppl 1), S81–S89. https://doi.org/10.1093/schbul/sbw057
22. Stirman, S. W., Gutiérrez-Colina, A., Toder, K., Esposito, G., Barg, F., Castro, F., Beck, A. T., & Crits-Christoph, P. (2013). Clinicians' perspectives on cognitive therapy in community mental health settings: Implications for training and implementation. *Administration and Policy in Mental Health, 40*(4), 274–285. https://doi.org/10.1007/s10488-012-0418-8
23. van der Gaag, M. (2014). The efficacy of CBT for severe mental illness and the challenge of dissemination in routine care. *World Psychiatry: Official Journal of the World Psychiatric Association (WPA), 13*(3), 257–258. https://doi.org/10.1002/wps.20162
24. Veltro, F., Falloon, I., Vendittelli, N., Oricchio, I., Scinto, A., Gigantesco, A., & Morosini, P. (2006). Effectiveness of cognitive-behavioural group therapy for inpatients. *Clinical Practice and Epidemiology in Mental Health, 2*(1), 1–6.

33
Optimising Patient Care in Psychiatry With Policy and Practice of ECT in Malaysia

Chee Kok Yoon

Introduction	371
ECT and Neuropsychiatry in Kuala Lumpur Hospital	372
Nationwide ECT Survey 2020	373
ECT and COVID-19 in Malaysia	374
Future Directions	374

INTRODUCTION

There has not been much research done in Malaysia concerning electroconvulsive therapy (ECT) in the past. The first survey of ECT service in Malaysia was reported by Chanpattana et al. in 2010[1] as part of the ECT therapy practice survey in Asia. His paper included only 11 hospitals from Malaysia, and 1 out of the 11 hospitals did not have ECT service. Medical officers performed ECT, and no institution had any formal teaching program for the procedure. Three hospitals did not use anaesthesia during ECT, and most of the respondents did not know the type of ECT machine used. fewer than half of the hospitals in the survey carried out electroencephalogram (EEG) monitoring. There was another smaller study on ECT performed at a university hospital in Kuala Lumpur. Lai et al.[2] studied 31 patients who underwent ECT over three weeks in October 1982 and found the main indications were an inadequate response to pharmacotherapy, depression with suicidal ideation, and aggressive behaviour. Among the most common side effects reported were memory impairment and headache.

Before 2001, mental healthcare in Malaysia was governed by three laws: the Mental Health Disorders Ordinance 1952 for peninsular Malaysia, Mental Health Ordinance 1961 for Sarawak and Lunatic Ordinance 1951 for Sabah. None of these laws had any provision for ECT treatment. When the Malaysian parliament passed the Mental Health Act 2001 (MHA 2001), it was a significant turning point for Malaysia's mental healthcare. In this act and the subsequent Mental Health Regulation 2010 (MHR 2010), ECT is classified as a surgical procedure. Therefore, how an ECT session is performed must be the same as how a surgical procedure is carried out. In MHA 2001, ECT is mentioned explicitly in Part IV. This section contains the law required for the procedure for ECT, operation theatre or treatment suite, oxygen supplies in the treatment and recovery room or area, equipment and supplies in the treatment room, ECT device, maintenance, and logbook. When the Ministry of Health Malaysia's Psychiatric and Mental Health Service Operational Policy was published in November 2011,

ECT was included only in the appendix instead of as a stand-alone psychiatric service. In the appendix, the ECT procedure is minimally elaborated on in term of its indication, frequency, investigations needed and consent-related issues. Nevertheless, there are still wide variations in how ECT is prescribed and performed across the country. There was no standardised format in prescribing ECT to patients, managing an individual ECT session, recovery assessment, and ECT training in general.

ECT AND NEUROPSYCHIATRY IN KUALA LUMPUR HOSPITAL

In the past, ECT service is considered only one of the treatment procedures for a patient with a severe mental disorder. It is included as part of the general psychiatric service, and no specific psychiatrist has been assigned to coordinate the service. When I established the neuropsychiatry service in Kuala Lumpur Hospital (KLH) in 2012, ECT service was included to coordinate the procedure more optimally.

The first step in standardising and optimising the ECT procedure in KLH was by organising training for the mental health staff in the Department of Psychiatry and Mental Health, KLH. The Neuropsychiatry Unit KLH organised the first ECT training course in 2013; among the topics were the indications, adverse events, electrophysiology, dosing of ECT, ECT and the law in Malaysia, concomitant medications during ECT, special populations and ECT, and the proper way to prescribe and implement ECT. It also contained a practical session on troubleshooting when a problem arises with the ECT machine. Since then, the ECT workshop has been organised annually. The workshop's participation has grown from KLH to all hospitals in Malaysia with ECT and other Asian countries.

The second step in standardising the ECT procedure in KLH was the publication of the Hospital Kuala Lumpur Handbook on Electroconvulsive Therapy in 2014. This handbook was a joint effort from me, Salina Abdul Aziz, and Kenny Ong Kheng Yee. The aim of producing this handbook for KLH was to provide a document with the clearly defined ECT practise method, including the indication, placement of electrodes, dose management using titration method, and so on. The director-general of health, Datuk Sri Dr Nor Hisham Abdullah, officiated this handbook in 2014 during the 9th Kuala Lumpur Mental Health Conference.

The third step was to revamp the ECT prescription and individual treatment forms and the standard operating procedure (SOP) for ECT in KLH. The new ECT prescription and individual treatment form were officially used in 2017 and subsequently modified several times. The first objective of the new prescription and individual treatment forms is a privileged medical officer or specialist must be accountable for whether the ECT is needed, the placement of electrodes, and so on. The second objective is which time-out is introduced to ensure the right patient and the correct procedure prescribed. The ECT procedure must also have an accountable ECT coordinator and practitioner. In 2020, the Neuropsychiatric Unit (NEURON) made a new change to the individual treatment form, the EEG quality rating scale based on the duration of recruitment, the EEG's amplitude, termination of EEG recording, duration of seizure, and post-suppression index score (PSI) or adequacy score. This change aims to improve reliability on evaluation of EEG quality. Monthly ECT review meetings with the ECT coordinators and medical officers have been carried out to ensure the practice of ECT is audited and following the proposed SOP.

The fourth step is the establishment of the Neuropsychiatry Centre for Neuromodulation Therapies (SYNAPSE) unit in KLH. SYNAPSE is part of the Neuropsychiatry & Neuromodulation Unit of the Department of Psychiatry and Mental Health, KLH. Currently, SYNAPSE is headed by Dr Kenny Ong Kheng Yee, a consultant neuropsychiatrist, and assisted by Mr

Bunyamin Taufik, the ECT coordinator head. SYNAPSE is responsible for producing the National Guideline for ECT, which will be completed by September 2021.

The fifth step is preparing the Ministry of Health Malaysia National ECT Guideline, which began in February 2021 and aims to complete by September 2021. The guideline is chaired by Kenny Ong Kheng Yee, a neuropsychiatrist and the current head of the ECT committee in KLH, and consists of other psychiatrists and anaesthetists. This guideline will be an improved version of the 2014 Hospital Kuala Lumpur Handbook on ECT, and a significant portion of the guideline will include anaesthesia in ECT.

NATIONWIDE ECT SURVEY 2020

The first Nationwide ECT Survey was a voluntary effort by all Ministry of Health (MOH) Hospitals with psychiatric service. It was completed in March 2020. The survey aimed to determine the current ECT service in the country. A questionnaire was created using SurveyMonkey, and a link to the survey was sent to either the head of the department of the psychiatric service or the ECT coordinator. Among the questions asked were the type of psychiatric facility, place where ECT is performed, kind of ECT machine, the procedure itself (including dose management and anaesthesia related), and so on.

There were 53 MOH hospitals with psychiatric service that participated in the survey (49 general hospitals and 4 mental institutions). Thirty-six (67.9%) of these centres provide ECT service, and 69.4% of those centres with ECT service performed the procedure in an operation theatre consistent with the recommendation by MHA 2001 and MHR 2010 that ECT be a surgical procedure. The META SpECTrum 5000 (M & Q) was the most common machine used (69.4%), followed by Thymatron (33.3%). Bitemporal placement was the most common electrode placement (91.2%), and only a small percentage of centres preferred a right unilateral electrode placement as their first choice. Most of the respondents chose 1.0 ms as their preferred pulse width (71.4%).

Concerning anaesthesia, all centres performed ECT with anaesthesia. The most common anaesthetic agent used is propofol (97.3%). Succinylcholine is the most common muscle relaxant used (97.1%). All ECT had pre-oxygenation before anaesthetic induction. Pre-ECT anaesthetic evaluation is almost entirely done by a medical officer or specialist from anaesthetic unit. Before ECT was commenced, the medical officer in charge performed blood tests (97.3%) and an electrocardiogram (83.8%).

In terms of ECT dose management, a privileged medical officer performed the ECT. 88.9% of the dosing was based on the titration method, and only 11.1% was based on the patient's age. Seizure duration, EEG quality, and clinical response were the three main criteria whether the dose of ECT should be increased throughout the procedure. The majority (94.4%) of the ECT monitoring was done using EEG.

The three primary clinical diagnoses that required a prescription of ECT were bipolar I disorder in manic phase, schizophrenia, and major depressive disorder with psychotic features. High suicidal risk was the main indication for ECT, followed by severe aggression and pharmacotherapy failure. Many centres also prescribe ECT to elderly more than 65 years old (78.1%), adolescents (75.0%), and pregnant women (65.6%). None of the centres in the survey has prescribed ECT to children under the age of 12 years.

Three ECT sessions per week were the most common practice in Malaysia (91.7%), but several centres practised two sessions per week. Two sessions per week was due to the availability of an anaesthesiology service. On average, 6–9 sessions of ECT were administered in an acute course of ECT (77.8%). An acute course of ECT was terminated after the targeted symptoms were resolved (75.0%). However, several centres still focused on a certain number of ECT sessions that must be completed regardless of the symptoms' resolution.

Augmentation of ECT with ketamine, hyperventilation, and remifentanil was highly infrequent. Concerning concomitant medications during ECT, most centres would withhold anticonvulsants (86.1%), benzodiazepines (86.1%), and lithium (75.0%).

All centres would review the patients prescribed for ECT at least once per week, and 72.2% of the centres surveyed reviewed these patients after every ECT session. Formal rating scales to assess the clinical states of patients receiving ECT were uncommon; almost 80% of the centres' surveys did not use any objective assessment. On the other hand, the cognitive side effects of ECT were assessed at least in one-fourth of the centres surveyed; the Montreal Cognitive Assessment Tool and Mini-Mental State Examination were the two most common cognitive screening tools used. The three most common side effects of ECT reported were headache, cognitive side effects, and muscle pain.

More than 97% of the centres surveyed prescribed continuation and maintenance ECT. Continuation and maintenance ECT is extremely common in Malaysia. Schizophrenia, bipolar I disorder, and major depressive disorder were the three primary diagnoses prescribed with maintenance ECT. Most of the centres (66.7%) used a flexible protocol in determining the frequency of ECT, and most of them (83.3%) did not have a specific timeline to terminate the course of maintenance ECT.

Privileging mental health professionals to perform ECT is very important in Malaysia. Almost 90% of the centres have a formal process to privilege medical officers and specialists to prescribe and perform ECT treatment independently without supervision. Such privileging is commonly determined by either a credentialed psychiatrist or a privileged medical officer who has completed evaluation using a logbook.

ECT AND COVID-19 IN MALAYSIA

During the unfortunate period of the COVID-19 pandemic in Malaysia, ECT in KLH remains functioning but with modification to its procedure to provide safety measures to the medical staff and patients. SYNAPSE KLH developed the guideline on the management of ECT during the COVID-19 pandemic. The latest version was published and distributed nationwide on 3 January 2021.

In the SOP for ECT during the COVID-19 period, all patients must complete a self-declaration form before the informed consent for ECT. Only a minimal number of essential healthcare workers assigned for ECT are allowed in the ECT suite or operation theatre. Students and visitors are not permitted in the vicinity during the ECT procedure. All essential healthcare workers involved in the ECT are needed to don appropriate personal protective equipment, which are a three-ply surgical mask, face shield, disposable sleeveless apron, and gloves. There shall be physical distancing of at least 1 meter. The ECT suite or operation theatre is required to have disinfection before and after ECT procedures for the day.

All patients going for ECT are required to screen for the COVID-19 virus with RTK-PCR 72 hours before ECT and must be tested negative for the virus. All acute and maintenance ECT COVID-19 testing is done via the RTK-PCR method. The RTK-Ag test is only performed for urgent cases.

FUTURE DIRECTIONS

There is still much to be done to ensure optimal ECT treatment in Malaysia. In 2013 we focused on training mental health professionals on properly prescribing and performing ECT, which is something we will need to do annually. We have standardised the evaluation and prescription of ECT to patients and individual ECT treatment sessions. We are moving forward to establish the National Guideline on ECT Management, which hopefully will complete by September 2021. After the completion of the guideline, SYNAPSE will carry out nationwide training on ECT management. SYNAPSE will also focus on research in the coming years. Currently, SYNAPSE is studying fNRI patterns on patients undergoing acute ECT and doing another study on maintenance ECT.

References

1. Chanpattana W, Kramer BA, Kunigiri G, Gangadhar BN, Kitphati R, Andrade C. A Survey of the Practice of Electroconvulsive Therapy in Asia. *J ECT*. 2010;26(1):5–10. doi:10.1097/YCT.0b013e3181a74368.
2. Pin AL, Tho OS, Hun YB, Koh L. The Use of Electroconvulsive Therapy in the University Hospital, Kuala Lumpur: A Study of 31 Patients. *Med J Malaysia*. 1983;38(2):145–149. doi:10.1016/j.yebeh.2006.06.013.

34
Rehabilitation and Case Management Using Cognitive Remediation Therapy

Akshata Mulmule and Aniket Bansod

Introduction	376
Rehabilitation and Recovery	377
Principles of Recovery-Oriented Practice	378
Types of Rehabilitation	378
Recovery-Oriented Rehabilitation Workforce	378
Factors That Aid Clinicians in Rehabilitation Setup Includes	379
Service Provision Influenced by Worker Behavior	379
Assessment	379
Partnership	379
Supporting Self-Management Skills	380
Motivational Interviewing	380
Strength-Based Interventions	380
Therapeutic Use of Environment	380
Workforce and Professional Development	380
Supervision and Reflective Practice	381
Meeting Everyone's Needs	381
Safety and Quality of Service Delivery	381
Challenges	382
Measuring Personal Recovery (Shanks et al., 2013)	382
Conclusion	382

INTRODUCTION

Across the world, mental health is being transformed in terms of structure and services, with an emphasis on a recovery-oriented approach (SA Health, 2012). National and state policies are being updated to match this, which is further emphasized by the growth of the non-governmental organisations (NGO) sector as a key service provider in mental health. This has resulted in increasing access to rehabilitation services.

The aim is to enable support of a person's unique and personal journey towards creating a fulfilling, hopeful and contributing life despite the limitations posed by the experience of mental illness. It is vital that the person get access to right type of support at the right time. Not every person needs access to rehabilitation services, and the need is not limited to a specific phase of recovery but is driven by a person's motivation for change. However, it should be considered proactively for the mental health clients. A hopeful, inspiring and stable environment without any unrealistic expectations promotes recovery from the experience of mental illness (Heras et al., 2003). Access to rehabilitation has been linked to positive individual and cost-benefit outcomes. The literature supports more than 50% reduction in cost of care secondary to a decrease in hospitalization (Branch, 2008).

Thorough assessment forms an innate aspect of rehabilitation framework and is a team effort involving all service providers, clients and their families. Every mental health client needs a comprehensive assessment with a focus on a strengths-based approach, including their recovery goals and rehabilitation needs (Department of Health, 2010a).

Motivation building and goal setting work as tools for recovery-based approach, including the mental healthcare plan, which places the client and carers at the center of their recovery. Goal setting is a key evidence-based coping strategy that is incorporated into recovery-oriented rehabilitation practice, and when based on a person's values, desires and skills, it can assist with motivation.

It is highly recommended that mental health clinicians have knowledge of a rehabilitation approach and skills to assist individual recovery. With standardized care models and established guidelines, an equally crucial role is played by skilled clinicians in this change implementation.

REHABILITATION AND RECOVERY

The World Health Organization (WHO; 2010) defines 'rehabilitation' as:

> A process aimed at enabling (people who experience disabilities) to reach and maintain their optimal physical, (spiritual, occupational) sensory, intellectual, psychological and social functional levels. Rehabilitation provides (people who experience disabilities) with the tools they need to attain independence and self-determination.

Rehabilitation is experienced on a spectrum. It encompasses processes, skills and strategies aimed at supporting individuals to develop the required skills that assist them to learn or build on their existing skills necessary to participate in all domains of life. Clinicians are expected to assimilate the principles of rehabilitation in regular interactions with clients. It enables them to assist individuals in gaining independence and striving for recovery. A positive therapeutic alliance forms an important part of rehabilitation intervention. However, it is not imperative that rehabilitation always lead to positive gains. It is a journey with obstacles in the form of setbacks, and overcoming them leads to progress. It should be offered and accessible to clients repeatedly during the management phase. Historically, mental health rehabilitation services have been limited. However, national and international reforms tend to guide this approach with an increase in the number of services.

It is essential to understand the alliance between recovery and rehabilitation if the service aims to adopt and integrate this prototype shift. Recovery underpins the development and delivery of rehabilitation services with a personalized approach. Clinicians must embrace the approach of 'potential for recovery'. However, it's not an intervention, and professionals cannot 'do' recovery 'to' people; there is no fixed timeline, and each individual journey is unique (SA Health, 2012). Recovery is the potential and actualization of person's individual journey.

There is no straightforward definition of recovery, as it's a personal experience. 'Recovery' is a concept that is values based and focuses on the inherent value and capacity of every individual to engage in a personalized journey of growth in living a meaningful life. The term 'recovery', as informed by people who have a lived experience, implies a process whereby a person constantly utilizes their ability to influence things that stand in the way of living a good life.

Patricia E Deegan describes the personal experience of recovery as:

> not an equivalent thing as being cured. Recovery may be a process not an endpoint or a destination. Recovery is an attitude, a way of approaching the day and facing the challenges. Being in recovery means recognising limitations so as to ascertain the limitless possibilities. Recovery means being in control . . . to recover, psychiatrically disabled persons must be willing to try and try again.
>
> (H, 2010)

She has pointed out the difference between the two concepts: Rehabilitation refers to the services and technologies that are made available to people who experience disabilities so they may learn to adapt to their world. Recovery refers to the lived or real-life experiences of persons as they accept and overcome the challenge of the incapacity (Deegan, 1988).

PRINCIPLES OF RECOVERY-ORIENTED PRACTICE

Principles of recovery-oriented mental health practice are outlined by the National Standards for Mental Health Services 2010. The objective is to ensure service delivery that supports recovery of the mental health clients (Branch, 2020).

The following are the recovery principles:

1. Uniqueness of the individual: Belief in empowering individual to be at the center of care. Recovery is proposed to be a combination of exposure to opportunities, to be able to lead a meaningful, satisfying and purposeful life as a valued community member.
2. Real choices: Supports the individual to recognize and build on their strengths, take responsibility, creatively explore and empower them to make meaningful choices.
3. Attitudes and rights: Instills hope and encourages them to maintain social, recreational, occupational and vocational activities. To promote and protect individual's legal, citizenship and human rights.
4. Dignity and respect: Respect and a sensitive approach to the individual's values, beliefs and culture. Confronting discrimination and stigma within the service or the community and advocating for the clients.
5. Partnership and communication: Facilitating partnership and understanding that every individual is self-expert in their care.
6. Evaluating recovery: It ensures that the mental health system addresses some of the key outcomes which indicate recovery such as housing, employment, education and social and family relationships as well as health and wellbeing measures.

TYPES OF REHABILITATION

Though there are multiples types of rehabilitation facilities available, they do not work independently and most often overlap or are approached in various combinations based on the individual needs. Out of a long list of rehabilitation services, frequently accessed ones include psychosocial rehabilitation, vocational and educational rehabilitation, drug and alcohol rehabilitation, physical rehabilitation and clinical rehabilitation (SA Health, 2012).

RECOVERY-ORIENTED REHABILITATION WORKFORCE

Mental health clinicians need to understand and practice the principles of recovery-oriented rehabilitation. A recovery orientation in mental health is an approach in which multidisciplinary teams and NGOs strive to provide services which focus on the potential and capacity of individuals to recover from mental illness. They provide supportive environments and meaningful opportunities to explore possibilities and meet basic needs (SA Health, 2012).

As simply expressed by Anthony and Farkas, 'Recovery is what people with disabilities do. Treatment, case management, rehabilitation and other services are what helpers do to facilitate recovery' (2012). Assistance with recovery should be fundamental to the role of professionals. In relation to service delivery, a recovery approach requires clinicians to be passionately involved in flexible partnership with clients and their families, to strengthen and reinforce their recovery and personal empowerment (Warner, 2009).

Mental health clinicians in rehabilitation settings who aspire to develop a recovery orientation need to embrace a recovery approach by visualizing the inherent individual possibilities with their clients and endeavor to offer appropriate supports and opportunities for their development. The emphasis is on every individual as a complete person, and the focus is on their entire wellbeing rather than solely becoming symptom free. In their recovery journey, clinicians need to 'walk alongside' the clients. This could be achieved by building a strong therapeutic relationship and understanding the individual's values, interests and motivation and creating safe and supportive environment to boost exploration and ability to master new skills (SA Health, 2012).

FACTORS THAT AID CLINICIANS IN REHABILITATION SETUP INCLUDES

Service Provision Influenced by Worker Behavior

It has been proposed in the literature that factors that impact individual experience and prognosis include the clinician's approach, including the therapeutic relationship and implementation of recovery-oriented rehabilitation interventions. Words account for just 7–10% of how we perceive meaning in face-to-face communication; 35% of interpretation is associated with voice tone and 55% with body language (Eggert, 1997)

For the efficiency of rehabilitation practices, it is important to ensure that the core recovery principles are embedded in rehabilitation practices during every interaction with the clients and the carers. The therapeutic relationship forms an important component of success in rehabilitation process which can be achieved by being respectful, empathetic and an active listener (Anthony, 2012).

Assessment

Per the Personal Recovery Framework analysis, there is a difference in the person diagnosed with mental illness and the specific mental illness and the subsequent importance of a focus on the individual and not on the illness. As a part of the recovery journey, it is crucial for the person experiencing mental illness to integrate that experience into their overall identity. It cannot be imposed upon the person, so part of the assessment includes involving the person to assist them in establishing their own explanation. The clinical formulation and diagnosis should be shared but with a degree of flexibility in the way it is used in the assessment process. It should not be taken as an answer but as a resource to the client for better understanding of the phenomenon. Assessment can be a means to validate personal meaning, amplify strengths, foster personal responsibility, support a positive identity and instill hope.

Partnership

The process of developing a clinician-client relationship is as vital as the outcome of the partnership. The basis of the partnership is that the clients and their carers are expert in client's life. The purpose is to empower clients, create enabling opportunities for recovery and promote safety. Essential aspects of effective partnerships include shared values, vision and purpose, focus on relationships, working together, accountability, community and information sharing (SA Health, 2012).

Peers are people with personal experience of mental illness and can notably influence the recovery journey of others (Clay et al., 2005; Network, 2005; S, 2005). It is considered a creative approach towards recovery-oriented practices. They can inspire clients to express themselves, talk about their experience with recovery and be part of peer-run programs.

Supporting Self-Management Skills

This can be achieved by the development of client confidence (a self-belief that the person can impact their own life), empowerment and supporting identity during crisis and motivation. It involves managing self-medication; positive risk-taking relates to behaviors which involve the person taking on challenges leading to personal growth and development.

Motivational Interviewing

It is a person-centered approach directed towards collaboration and autonomy and supporting behavioral changes with the aim of resolution of ambivalence by exploration (S. M, 2009).

Motivational interviewing presumes equity in the client-clinician relationship and prioritizes the client's rights to define issues and choose solutions. Thus, it is, in a sense, a counselling style emphasizing collaboration instead of confrontation, evocation instead of education and autonomy over the authoritarian style, as opposed to a set of techniques (Barrowclough et al., 2001).

Strength-Based Interventions

It enables workers to reflect upon the internal capacities, strengths and potential to flourish of the people they are working with. On most occasions, clients work on their situation. Thus, as a clinician, it is expected that one will tap into that capacity and demonstrate it and find and build on the possibilities (Cohen, 1999).

Strength-based practice builds on individual success and has a strong theoretical foundation. One of the key principles of rehabilitation is focusing on strengths. There is strong evidence informing outcomes associated with strength-based approaches. Extensive evidence over nearly 30 years has shown that people with serious mental illness, down the line, learn to live with it and recover. However, it involves encouraging clients to understand their life purpose, to foster positive self-image, assist in spiritual and cultural experiences and witness self-growth.

Therapeutic Use of Environment

There is a dynamic interaction between an individual and their environment: change in one aspect affects the other and vice versa (Townsend, 2002). The environment can work as an enabler or opposer of an individual aiming to be involved in a meaningful activity important to them.

Workforce and Professional Development

There is an equal responsibility of the individual and the organization to access recovery orientation and maintain individual competence. Organizations must ensure that the infrastructure and resources are in place so that the workforce has the opportunity to continue to progress and deliver the finest practicable services. Systemic and clinical pathways are important for the applicability of training in practice. However, it also involves dedication to recovery-oriented practices and to seek support in supervision sessions, team discussions and implementing management planning. Workforce professional standards can also be promoted by using tools such as the National Practice Standards for the Mental Health Workforce 2013 (Department of Health, 2013). These are standards that apply to professionals and should be used in conjunction with the National Standards for Mental Health Services 2010. The practice standards should be met by mental health professionals within 2 years of commencing work in a mental health service (Department of Health, 2010b).

Supervision and Reflective Practice

It is speculated that standards of recovery-oriented rehabilitation services are strengthened by regular access to supervision and consultation. It's a fundamental right of every clinician (Townsend, 2002). Supervision is consistently reported to be an effective strategy in improving recovery-oriented practice. It is an important strategy to promote quality control, maintain and facilitate the supervisee's competence and capabilities and help supervisees to work more effectively with reducing burnout. It has also been associated with an increase in workers' self-awareness and resilience, evidence-based practice skills, promotion of standardized performance across the organization, increased job satisfaction and self-confidence and improved worker retention, and supervision enables the pursuit of a lifelong learning process (Kilminster & Jolly, 2000; B. M, 1997; Milne, 2007; Thomsen et al., 1999). Supervision therefore has an important role to play in ensuring that recovery-oriented rehabilitation practice is integrated into all aspects of every individual worker's practice.

Meeting Everyone's Needs

Specific consideration must be given to best meet the distinct needs of diverse populations. Regular effective interactions between service as a whole and clients and their carers must be ensured involving various modalities. It is true that no one service can meet every individual need; however, it is always imperative that mental health services be culturally embracing and sensitive towards communities such as 'culturally and linguistically diverse' (CALD) communities (Australia, 2001).

Mental health issues should be managed in the broader aspect with innovative means of supporting individual recovery and healing along with families and communities. For Aboriginal Australians, mental health constitutes 15.5% of the total disease burden (D. o. Health, 2010).

Safety and Quality of Service Delivery

All services are expected to perform to specific set standards. Best practice is steady service improvement based on feedback from clients, carers and other partners. Consumer-centered practice is characterized by collaborative and partnership approaches to practice that encourage and respect a person's autonomy, control and choice and support their right to enact these choices (Hammell, 2001; Law et al., 1995).

A safe, respectful relationship between the client and the clinician is vital in nurturing a safe environment in which both parties can exchange feedback, discuss recovery goals and possibilities and assist the person's self-efficacy and self-determination (S. Health, 2012).

CHALLENGES

All services are expected to work per the set standards, and services are measured against these. Continuous service improvement is considered a best practice. Feedback from clients and their significant others assist in improving services. Quality and safety are everyone's responsibility and need to be integrated into everyday practices.

MEASURING PERSONAL RECOVERY (SHANKS ET AL., 2013)

The CHIME (connectedness, hope and optimism, identity, meaning and purpose and empowerment) framework for personal recovery is one example which was developed through a systematic review and narrative synthesis of recovery. It helps to evaluate measures of recovery rather than other aspects of good practice in mental health services. There are more than 30 recovery measures available. Here are some of the most studied and most relevant per the CHIME framework.

1. Illness Management and Recovery (IMR) Scale
2. Recovery Assessment Scale (RAS), most widely used
3. Recovery Process Inventory (RPI)
4. Stages of Recovery Instrument (STORI)
5. Psychosis Recovery Inventory (PRI)
6. Questionnaire About the Process of Recovery (QPR)

CONCLUSION

There is still a long way to go in terms of developing a recovery-oriented approach in mental health systems. Foundational transformation forms the basis of evolving towards a recovery vision. The intellectual challenge emerges from outside the dominant scientific paradigm that is understanding recovery from peers, shifting attention from robust clinical preoccupations such as risk assessment, symptom profile, hospitalization and so on, with the patient's perspective becoming central to assessment.

A recovery approach involves the experience of mental illness as a part of the person; the presence of valued social roles improves the symptoms, with reductions in hospitalization, their contribution towards sharing and working towards goals, strength-focused assessment and partnership in achieving goals with motivation and crisis management.

The implications for both service users and staff of embarking on a recovery journey are profound. It most obviously has the potential to empower clients but also to liberate mental health staff from unrealistic expectations. Thus, a focus on recovery is in the interests of all. However, ongoing research is required to ensure best practices around recovery-oriented rehabilitation remain up to date.

References

Anthony, W. F., MD. (2012). *The essential guide to psychiatric rehabilitation practice*. Melbourne, Australia: Center for Psychiatric Rehabilitation.

Australia, G. o. W. (2001). *A trans culturally-oriented mental health service for Western Australia*. Western Australia.

Barrowclough, C., Haddock, G., Tarrier, N., Lewis, S. W., Moring, J., O'Brien, R., . . . McGovern, J. (2001). Randomized controlled trial of motivational interviewing, cognitive behavior therapy, and family intervention for patients with comorbid schizophrenia and substance use disorders. *Am J Psychiatry*, *158*(10), 1706–1713. doi:10.1176/appi.ajp.158.10.1706

Branch, M. H. (2008). NSW Community mental health strategy 2007 2012 from prevention and early intervention to recovery. Retrieved from www.health.nsw.gov.au/mentalhealth/resources/Pages/mental-health-strategy.aspx

Branch, M. H. (2020). Principles of recovery oriented mental health practice. Retrieved from www.health.nsw.gov.au/mentalhealth/psychosocial/principles/Pages/recovery.aspx

Cohen, B.-Z. (1999). Intervention and supervision in strengths-based social work practice. *Fam Soc, 80*(5), 460–466. doi:10.1606/1044-3894.1475

Deegan, P. E. J. P. r. j. (1988). Recovery: The lived experience of rehabilitation. *Psychosoc Rehab J, 11*(4), 11.

Department of Health, S. A. (2010a). Adult community mental health services, model of care, prepared by the mental health unit, department of health, adelaide, South Australia. Retrieved from www.sahealth.sa.gov.au/wps/wcm/connect/public+content/sa+health+internet/services/mental+health+and+drug+and+alcohol+services/mental+health+services/mental+health+services

Department of Health, S. A. (2010b). National standards for mental health services 2010. Retrieved from www1.health.gov.au/internet/main/publishing.nsf/Content/mental-pubs-n-servst10

Department of Health, S.A. (2013). National practice standards for the mental health workforce. Retrieved from www1.health.gov.au/internet/main/publishing.nsf/Content/mental-pubs-n-wkstd13

Eggert, M. (1997). *Assertiveness pocketbook*. Hampshire, UK: Management Pocketbooks.

H, G: (2010). *Unpacking practices that support personal efforts of 'recovery'*. Australia: Enlightened Consultants Pty Ltd.

Hammell, K. W. (2001). Using qualitative research to inform the client-centred evidence-based practice of occupational therapy. *Brit J Occup Ther, 64*(5), 228–234. doi:10.1177/030802260106400504

Health, D. o. (2010). *Aboriginal health care plan 2010–2016*. Adelaide: Department of Health.

Health, S. (2012). The framework for recovery-oriented rehabilitation in mental health care. Retrieved from www.sahealth.sa.gov.au/wps/wcm/connect/public+content/sa+health+internet/clinical+resources/clinical+resources

Heras, C. G. d. l., Llerena, V., Kielhofner, G., University of, I., & Model of Human Occupation, C. (2003). *A user's manual for remotivation process: Progressive intervention for individuals with servere volitional challenges: (version 1.0)*. Chicago: University of Illinois: Model of Human Occupation Clearinghouse. Dept. of Occupational Therapy.

Kilminster, S. M., & Jolly, B. C. (2000). Effective supervision in clinical practice settings: A literature review. *Med Educ, 34*(10), 827–840. doi:10.1046/j.1365-2923.2000.00758.x

Law, M., Baptiste, S., & Mills, J. (1995). Client-centred practice: What does it mean and does it make a difference? *Can J Occup Ther, 62*(5), 250–257. doi:10.1177/000841749506200504

M, B. (1997). *Relational learning: A strategy for providing supervision for child and family support workers, Cross borders*. Paper presented at the Australian College for Child and Family Protection Practitioners, Melbourne, Melbourne.

M, S. (2009). 100 ways to support recovery: A guide for mental health professionals. *Rethinking Recovery Series*. Retrieved from www.rethink.org/advice-and-information/living-with-mental-illness/treatment-and-support/100-ways-to-support-recovery/

Milne, D. (2007). An empirical definition of clinical supervision. *Br J Clin Psychol, 46*(Pt 4), 437–447. doi:10.1348/014466507x197415

Network, S. R. (2005). *The role and potential development of peer support services*. Glasgow, Scotland: Scottish Recovery Network.

Organisation, W. H. (2010). Health topics, rehabilitation. Retrieved from www.who.int/topics/rehabilitation/en

S, M. (2005). *Intentional peer support: An alternative approach*. New York: Plainfield.

Shanks, V., Williams, J., Leamy, M., Bird, V. J., Le Boutillier, C., & Slade, M. (2013). Measures of personal recovery: A systematic review. *Psychiatr Serv, 64*(10), 974–980. doi:10.1176/appi.ps.005012012

Thomsen, S., Soares, J., Nolan, P., Dallender, J., & Arnetz, B. (1999). Feelings of professional fulfilment and exhaustion in mental health personnel: The importance of organisational and individual factors. *Psychotherapy and Psychosomatics, 68*(3), 157–164. doi:10.1159/000012325

Townsend, E., & Bognetti, Giovanni. (2002). *Enabling occupation: An occupational therapy perspective*. Ottawa: Canadian Association of Occupational Therapists.

Warner, R. (2009). Recovery from schizophrenia and the recovery model. *Curr Opin Psychiatry, 22*(4), 374–380. doi:10.1097/YCO.0b013e32832c920b

35
Optimizing Patient Care With Effective Psychotherapeutic Interventions

Tanya Malik and Urveesha Nirjar

Interpersonal Psychotherapy	385
Group IPT	386
Group IPT for Depression	387
Cognitive Processing Therapy	387
CPT for Victims of Sexual Assault	389
Dialectical Behavior Therapy	389
DBT for BPD	391
Rational Emotive Behavior Therapy	391
REBT for Depression	392
Conclusion and Future Directions	392

The current need is communal engagement. Far too much time has passed with a focus on independent, individual development. The community lifts the individual higher than before – it is the community to which we return. Communal being or engagement is predicated on simple facets of health, inclusivity and education. The stakeholders of any community have the greatest responsibility, as well as the highest power, to encourage worthwhile change for their citizens.

When we think about mental health, we are typically limited to a one-on-one interaction. We envision physicians and therapists counseling in isolation. While the focus has been on the negative impact environmental factors have on the mental health of individuals, often overlooked is the overall health of the community. This book aims to fill these gaps, and this chapter shall serve as the bedrock of communal interventions that have been implemented. It is important we look around the world to see what has been done, so we know what to do for our communities.

The most common psychotherapies that are evidence based are cognitive behavioral therapy (CBT), interpersonal psychotherapy (IPT), and cognitive processing therapy (CPT). Other evidence-based therapies also include dialectical behavior therapy (DBT), and rational emotive behavior therapy (REBT). Therapeutic inclination such as psychodynamic and psychanalytic therapies, which are focused on the interpretation of emotional and mental processes as compared to behavioral outcomes, have been a point of contention in the greater psychology community. The arguments range from efficacy to generalizability, the strength of randomized controlled trials (RCTs), limitations on types of mental illness, and the lengthy time taken.

As CBT has been addressed in other chapters, we take this opportunity to offer details on alternative forms of therapies, discuss the strength and limitations of interventions already taken place, and finally make note of key determinants that need to be kept in mind when contemplating community care.

INTERPERSONAL PSYCHOTHERAPY

Interpersonal psychotherapy is an empirically supported, diagnosis-targeted, time-limited treatment. Compared to the other well-known therapeutic treatments available, IPT is a relatively young psychotherapy that was originally developed to treat depression. Over time substantial evidence has emerged supporting the clinical effectiveness of IPT in treating depression and a variety of other problems. This has further led to the development of various adaptations of IPT for groups; subpopulations of patients with mood disorders; postpartum depression; and mental disorders such as anxiety, bulimia nervosa, and borderline personality disorder, to name a few. The treatment alliance formed between the patient and the therapist is considered the base of the foundation of IPT. The therapist engages with the patient emphatically, helps the patient to feel understood, arouses effect, presents a clear rationale and treatment ritual, and yields successful experiences.

IPT is structured and time limited, so there are only about 6–20 sessions, ideally weekly and 45–60 minutes in length. Essentially, the treatments are divided into three phases – the initial phase, the middle phase, and termination.

Phase 1 or the initial phase usually consists of the first one to three sessions. This phase includes diagnostic evaluation and psychiatric history and sets the framework for the treatment. There are three main tasks – dealing with depression, linking the depression to interpersonal problems, and identifying the primary problems areas and providing psychoeducation on IPT. Giving hope regarding the treatment and assigning the patient the temporary "sick role" is an important aspect of IPT. Another important facet is conducting an interpersonal inventory, that is, gathering information about the important people, alive or dead, in the person's life and mobilizing support resources.

The second or middle phase incorporates sessions 4–13. During these sessions interpersonal changes and symptom improvement occur as the therapist explores the problem area/s further and strategies are implemented. These sessions start with a check of the patient's symptoms and mood ratings. Scales such as the Patient Health Questionnaire-9 (PHQ-9) and Hopkins Depression Symptom Checklist are commonly used. These are conducted at the beginning of every session, and progress is also discussed.

Linking the mood to interpersonal events is an important strategy which provides a way to demystify depression by showing that being depressed is a two-way street – it is affected by relationships but also affects relationships. Communication analysis is another strategy commonly employed by the therapist to analyze communications from the previous weeks. The main goal is to help the patient have a better understanding of verbal and non-verbal communication and the impacts of these communications on the patient as well as the impact of others' communication on the patient. The therapist also encourages the patient's ability to change these interactions and therefore change feelings associated with the relationships.

The strategy of decision analysis is actively utilized in the middle phase. First, an interpersonal situation that is causing distress is selected. Possible ways of managing the issues are discussed while evaluating the pros and cons of each option. The patient further chooses an option or a combination and tries it by rehearsing the interaction with the therapist in the form of a "role play". Role playing gives the patient a safe place to practice a new interpersonal skill and receive feedback prior to applying it outside of therapy. Termination is also actively brought up during sessions leading to it in order to re-establish the time-limited nature of the psychotherapy and preparing the patient.

The last phase of treatment, or termination, occurs in sessions 14–16. It is explicitly discussed throughout treatment, and the patient's feelings about termination are also explored. The patient's progress such as changes in symptoms and in the interpersonal problem area are extensively reviewed. Symptoms of relapse are discussed, as well as the possibility of continuation of treatment depending on the progress made.

Based on its foundations, IPT has two principles, also known as the IPT Model of Depression. These two basic principles explain the patient's depression and situation (Bleiberg & Markowitz, 2014). First, depression is a medical illness, and the therapist explains depression as a common illness with a discrete and predictable set of symptoms that are treatable. Through this, the symptoms seem less overwhelming and more manageable, and the patient is excused, as the blame is taken away from him/her. The second principle is that the patient's depression or their mood and life situation are related. Building on the interpersonal theories of, as well as John Bolwby's attachment theory (psychosocial theories of depression, the patient's mood and disturbing life events can either trigger or follow from the onset of depression. The purpose of IPT is to solve an interpersonal crisis (grief or complicated bereavement, a role dispute, a role transition, or interpersonal deficits) so that the person can improve their life situation and simultaneously relieve depressive symptoms.

The four key interpersonal problems have specific strategies that will aid the therapist:

- Grief addresses a patient's complicated bereavement following the death of a significant other, family member, or any other individual in the person's life. It can either be in the past or in the present. Through IPT the therapist engages with patient by facilitating the mourning process of the patient. The ultimate goal is achieved by encouraging catharsis and helping the patient compensate for the loss by forming new relationships and new activities.
- Role transitions are associated with depression when a person has difficulty coping with life change, including the beginning or ending of a relationship, a geographic move, starting or losing a job, becoming a parent, or even being diagnosed with a medical illness. Using IPT the therapist helps mourn the loss of the old role and finally adjust to the new role and gain a sense of mastery. Role disputes include conflicts with a significant other, friend, parent, spouse, employer, or close friend. This relationship and the nature of the dispute are explored, and the therapist guides the patient in exploring the options to resolve it.
- Interpersonal deficits are the focus when the other three problem areas are not present and the patient is or has been struggling in terms of interpersonal functioning. These depressed patients have few social supports and a history of inadequate or unsustaining interpersonal relationships. The strategies would include relating the depressive symptoms to isolation, assisting the patient in finding opportunities to break social isolation, and using extensive role play and feedback in preparing and reviewing the new social communication of the patient.

GROUP IPT

Group IPT is also possible and has been extensively adapted and researched for various populations. The format is similar to the individual treatment, with the exception of pre-group individual meetings and the number of total sessions. Pre-group individual meetings are set up to both find appropriate patients for the intervention and for the IPT group facilitator or clinician to assess the needs of the group as a whole. In most adapted group versions of IPT, there are a total of eight sessions. The initial phase is one session, the middle is sessions two to seven, and the last session is termination. Sessions can either be conducted weekly or biweekly if necessary. The first initial group session is 60–90 minutes, and the ongoing sessions last 45–60 minutes.

Group IPT has been found to be a particularly ideal intervention for collectivistic or community-centered cultures. In many collectivistic cultures around the globe, people tend to see themselves as part of a family and community before they see themselves as individuals, and IPT-G has appeared to be a more relevant approach in such cases (Verdeli et al., 2003). The group format also allows patients to feel that they are not alone, that they are not the only ones struggling with depression. An environment of collective support, where patients also provide feedback to other patients as the clinician facilitates the session, can prove beneficial.

GROUP IPT FOR DEPRESSION

Because of the structured and manual nature of this therapeutic intervention, it can be easily adapted as community-based intervention. Especially in areas where there exists a dearth of mental health practitioners, for example, developing countries like India or Africa, trained clinicians and practitioners can further train and supervise lay workers to deliver IPT.

Verdeli and colleagues successfully adapted group interpersonal psychotherapy for depression in rural southwest Uganda in a randomized controlled trial. A number of studies conducted in Uganda indicated substantial levels of depressive symptoms in the community (Orley & Wing, 1979; Wilk & Bolton, 2002; Bolton et al., 2002; Judd et al., 1997). In a total of 15 villages, 107 depressed men and women in single-gender groups of 5–8 patients each received IPT over a period of 16 weeks. The treatment was sanctioned by the local leaders' council and approved by the traditional healers. Besides delivering the treatment, the researchers also assessed the efficacy and acceptability of the treatment as perceived by the patients and their community. They found that IPT-GU (Group IPT in Uganda) was accepted in the community with a high attendance rate. The drop-out rate was 7.8% versus 18% in the control group. No conflicts were reported in the acceptability of the treatment amongst the patients, group leaders, or relatives. The trial also showed that group leaders were successfully trained in administering the treatment, and the principles and strategies of the intervention were easily graspable. The termination assessment also indicated a strong effect for IPT-GU in reducing depressive symptoms and impairment.

COGNITIVE PROCESSING THERAPY

Cognitive processing therapy was initially developed to treat the symptoms of PTSD of female rape victims. This type of therapy encourages clients to feel overwhelming emotions that are usually avoided or suppressed after a sexual trauma. CPT has three components: education on PTSD symptoms, exposure, and cognitive therapy. Exposure includes writing and reading vivid accounts of the incident, while cognitive therapy includes identifying the relationship of thoughts and emotions; challenging maladaptive beliefs; and developing the areas of safety, trust, power, esteem, and intimacy (Resick & Schnicke, 1992). Individual CPT sessions typically consist of 12 one-hour weekly sessions as based on CPT treatment manual.

The first session will be the introduction and education phase – where recommendations for attendance and homework completion will be made. There is an emphasis on rapport building during this session. Homework will include writing about the meaning of the assault to identify stuck points.

In the second session, the meaning of the event will be broken down. The therapist will describe how interpretations of events can affect emotions. A (activating event) – B (belief) – C (consequence) worksheets will be given as homework.

The third session serves to identify thoughts and feelings, to understand generalized anxieties and trigger points. Homework for this week will be to write a detailed account of the incident.

Session four is remembering the assault in order to recover memories and experience emotions. Avoidance and recovery options will be discussed. Homework for this week will be a repeat – write the whole incident once again.

Session five is an analysis of feelings and the identification of stuck points. By now it is expected that the intensity of emotions would have reduced. A Challenging Questions Sheet will be given following this session, where the client is asked to write out two stuck points and respond to the set of questions in the sheet.

The sixth session is based on challenging questions and focuses of the self-blame that may accompany the participants. Homework for this week includes identifying faulty thinking patterns.

The seventh session will address these patterns by addressing how they may have affected the client's reaction to the assault. The Challenging Beliefs worksheet will be completed in session. The homework will be to analyze and confront one of the stuck points.

Session eight will bring up safety issues and help the client confront faulty cognitions. The homework from the previous week will be continued to be analyzed.

Session nine will address trust issues that the client may have, including distrust. A Power Issues worksheet will be given as homework to confront these beliefs.

Session ten will be an overview of power and control issues to alleviate any feelings of incompetence that may have arisen from the assault. An Identifying Assumptions (acceptance, competence, control).

The eleventh session will deal with esteem issues and will have the therapist reinforcing the client's efforts to enhance their self-esteem. Theories of intimacy will be introduced and discussed. The homework for this week will be to write one page on what it means to the client that they were sexually assaulted.

The twelfth and final session will be a scope into discovering the meaning of the event. Self-intimacy and self-comforting issues will be dealt with. The client will be encouraged to write an essay on how their views have changed as a result of the work done in therapy.

Group CPT is also possible, typically consisting of groups of five to six individuals receiving 90-minute sessions once a week, with two therapists present. A longer time is allowed for group therapy due to the number of participants. One therapist facilitates the conversation, and the other observes reactions, providing feedback as necessary and bringing it into the discussion. At the first session, education on symptoms will be presented and a homework assignment will be given on writing about how the participant's event occurred and what it meant for them. At the second session, clients in the group will be taught how to separate feelings from thoughts and see how self-statements and emotions are connected. A-B-C worksheets will be given as homework. In the following two sessions, each participant will write a detailed, sensory-oriented account of their sexual assault, with all thoughts and emotions included. They will be fully allowed to feel their emotions in the group environment. The fifth session will focus on becoming aware of maladaptive beliefs about their sexual assault, to better understand self-blame and find acceptance of the event. The sixth session will focus on identifying negative thinking patterns. The seventh session will focus on the five areas of belief: safety, trust, power, esteem, and intimacy, and how each could be disrupted by the sexual assault. One area of belief will be focused on for weeks 7–11, with homework given and discussed, and group members helping one another on areas they feet difficulty confronting. At session 11, the participants will write again about the meaning of the traumatic event. The final and twelfth session concludes with beliefs about intimacy and the participants' hopes and goals for the future (Resick & Schnicke, 1992).

CPT FOR VICTIMS OF SEXUAL ASSAULT

A study in Australia conducted in 2016 by Reginald Nixon and his team examined the effectiveness of CPT when compared with regular treatment options for survivors of recent sexual assault with a diagnosis of acute stress disorder (ASD). For their study, they delivered CPT by community clinicians at a sexual assault center. Their participants underwent an initial assessment, as well as at 3 months, 6 months, and 12 months following treatment in order to check for reduction in post traumatic stress disorder (PTSD) and depression symptoms. The researchers discovered that both CPT and the usual form of therapy had merit; however, there were some indications that CPT led to better outcomes due to a reduction in PTSD symptoms 12 months after follow-up. This study, which involved 158 participants, demonstrates the effectiveness of an evidence-based, trauma-focused therapy like CPT when delivered as an early intervention in a routine mental health setting (Nixon et al., 2016).

Another study in the midwest of the United States was conducted amongst 121 victims of rape to discuss the efficacy of CPT combined with prolonged exposure (PE) techniques in treatment for PTSD and depression (Resick et al., 2002). CPT was selected as its initial focus is on assimilated–distorted beliefs such as denial and self-blame. A second step of shifting focus to overgeneralized beliefs about the self and the trauma are taken into consideration. By having participants challenge their beliefs through Socratic questioning and the utilization of daily worksheets, the prevalence of balanced self-statements increases. The incorporation of PE encourages participants to write detailed accounts of their trauma, aimed at experiencing their emotions and identifying areas of blind assumptions and conflicting beliefs. Researchers concluded that the presence of CPT provided improved scores on guilt subscales, and CPT combined with PE is highly efficacious even 9 months posttreatment.

Cognitive processing therapy in the treatment of PTSD has gained rousing acclaim with the success of empirical studies that provide evidence of its efficacy. The advantage of this form of therapy is its ability to be combined with other therapies also typically used for the treatment of traumatic experiences. Other studies utilizing CPT has discovered minor differences in successful outcomes when compared on the basis of sex; there has also been a marked difference in rates of depression when CPT has been provided via video conferencing to rural areas (Galovski et al., 2013; Hassija & Gray, 2011).

DIALECTICAL BEHAVIOR THERAPY

Dialectical behavior therapy was developed in the late 1980s by Marsha Linehan and her colleagues (Linehan, 1993) for individuals diagnosed with borderline personality disorder (BPD) with chronic parasuicidal problems. It is a structured, time-limited, emotion-focused treatment and an extension of CBT. It is currently the only empirically supported treatment for BPD. Linehan found that CBT alone did not work as well as expected in patients with BPD and suicide and parasuicidal behaviors, as they perceived CBT as non-validating, as it revolved around the idea that they had a problem that needed to be fixed. Their focus on changing cognitions and behaviors in patients made them feel criticized and misunderstood and eventually led to dropping out. By adding techniques to CBT researchers were able to develop DBT, a psychotherapy that would meet the unique needs of this population.

Individuals diagnosed with BPD have been universally recognized as a patient population which is difficult to treat effectively because of the range of multi-problematic symptoms shown and the tendencies to engage in suicidal or self-harm behavior. Based on cognitive-behavioral principles, several critical and unique elements were woven into the treatment by Linehan to convey acceptance of the patient and aid in the patient's acceptance of herself, her emotions, thoughts, and the world (Chapman, 2006). Since DBT is conceptualized as a disorder of emotion dysregulation, one of the primary goals of DBT is to improve the quality of life by helping patients to regulate their emotions. This is achieved through a blend of three theoretical positions – dialectical philosophy, behavioral science, and Zen practice. Dialectical philosophy or dialectics became the guiding principle of the treatment. Dialectics means holding two conflicting ideas at the same time, and within DBT, it refers to the integration of acceptance and change, which are both necessary for improvement (Linehan, 1993). The position of behavioral science, that is, the principles of behavior change adapted from CBT are countered by the acceptance of the client, and Zen practices include principles of mindfulness.

DBT was developed as a comprehensive program comprising individual therapy, group therapy or skills training, telephone consultation, and a therapist consultation team, instead of just a single mode of treatment (Linehan, 1993). These individual components work together to teach behavioral skills that target common symptoms of BPD, including an unstable sense of self, fear of abandonment, chaotic relationships, impulsivity, and self-injurious behaviors (May et al., 2016). This was done by Linehan as a means of providing the best possible treatment to individuals with BPD and as it was also found to be daunting when done by a single practitioner in isolation (Chapman, 2006). However, it can also be modified to accommodate any treatment setting (Linehan, 1993).

The standard DBT treatment program consists of weekly 60-minute individual therapy sessions, a weekly group skills training session lasting 90–150 minutes, and a therapist consultation team meeting approximately 60–120 minutes long.

DBT specifically focuses on providing therapeutic skills in four key areas – emotional regulation, distress tolerance, interpersonal effectiveness, and mindfulness.

- Emotional regulation: Individuals with DBT are known to have issues regulating their emotions. This area covers strategies to manage and change intense emotions that are causing problems in the patient's life.
- Distress tolerance: Rather than escaping from negative emotion, the goal is to increase the tolerance towards negative emotions.
- Interpersonal effectiveness: Individuals with BPD usually have issues with interpersonal relationships. They have trouble maintaining relationships and are usually referred as "chaotic." This area consists of techniques that allow a person to communicate with others in a way that is assertive, maintains self-respect, and strengthens relationships.
- Mindfulness: A skill that is crucial to DBT is helping patients stay and focus in the present rather than focusing on the past or future concerns that might cause them distress. This area focuses on improving the patient's ability to accept and be able to attend to the current moment.

Linehan listed five functions of treatment unique to DBT which are critical to any adaptation of DBT:

1. Enhancing capabilities: Individuals with DBT require many skills building resources to effectively regulate emotions, navigate interpersonal situations, tolerate distress, and achieve mindfulness. This function is completed using didactics, homework assignments, active practice, and weekly skills group sessions.

2. Generalizing capabilities: This function is critical in order to make sure that the skills being learned during sessions are effectively being used in patients' daily lives. This is achieved by providing homework assignments to practice skills learned.
3. Improving motivation and reducing dysfunctional behaviors: Accomplished through individual therapy, the therapist's goal uses various strategies such as a self-monitoring diary card maintained by the patient where he or she tracks their treatment targets such as emotional misery and self-harm. The therapist then encourages the patient to explore reasons for their maladaptive behaviors and the consequences that might be reinforcing and maintaining these behaviors. Actively encouraging the patient to commit to behavior change and build on skills of problem solving fall under this function as well.
4. Enhancing and maintaining therapist capabilities and motivation: As mentioned before, treating BPD patients is difficult, and sometimes the motivations and skills of the therapist and/or treatment providers can be effected. This is why effective treatment includes multiple resources for support, validation, training and skill-building, feedback, and encouragement to therapists. Linehan's component of team consultation meetings helps serve this function.
5. Structuring the environment: This function focuses around structuring the patient's environment in a way that the effective behavior is reinforced. This also involves guiding patients to modify their environment, for example, avoiding social circles that promote drug use or any other maladaptive behavior.

DBT FOR BPD

DBT has the most empirical support for parasuicidal women with borderline personality disorder but has also been proven successful for patients with binge-eating disorder, patients with BPD and substance use disorders (SUDs), and post-traumatic stress disorder, as well as depressed elderly patients through various randomized control trials. DBT has been shown to improve outcomes for individuals with emotion regulation difficulties in adolescence through adulthood (Groves et al., 2012).

Soler and colleagues conducted a 3-month randomized controlled clinical trial comparing DBT Skills Training (DBT-ST) to standard group therapy in individuals with BPD. They conducted 13 weekly group psychotherapy sessions of 120 minutes of either standard group therapy or DBT-skills training. Results showed that DBT-ST was associated with a dropout rate of 34.5% compared to 63.4% with standard group therapy. The 13-week DBT-ST proved more useful in improving depression, anxiety, irritability, anger, and affect instability. The group concluded that its straightforward implementations, cost effectiveness, and greater clinical improvements make it an ideal intervention for individuals with BPD.

RATIONAL EMOTIVE BEHAVIOR THERAPY

Rational emotive behavior therapy was developed by the American psychotherapist Albert Ellis in 1956. He embraced the idea "people are disturbed not by events, but by the views which they take of them," as expressed by the philosopher Epictetus, in order to help adopt a more rational way of thinking. He believed that people contribute to their own problems by maintaining rigid, extreme beliefs. By using REBT, clients learn tools to identify and dispute irrational beliefs. It is an attempt to bypass the "absolutes" in our thinking like "should" and the like. It takes a directive and educational approach by assuming that our thoughts, feelings, and behaviors influence one another. He believed that the emotions that create distress arise from our beliefs, evaluations, interpretations, and reactions to life situations

The ABC framework of REBT are tools to understand the interplay of thoughts, feelings, and behaviors.

A Activating/Aggravating Event.
   What you were doing (objectively) that led to some unpleasant experience.
B Beliefs.
   Thinking/cognitions surrounding the activating event. Thoughts about the event that seem to come up automatically/habitually.
C Consequences.
   What's happening (behavioral/emotional/sensations that arise). Your emotional experience as a result of the event and any behavioral actions.
D Disputes.
   New/more rational beliefs after examining the events. The reframing/new beliefs after an examination of the helpful/unhelpful aspects of your automatic thought.
E New Effect.
   Potential new emotional experiences/behavioral consequences after a consideration of disputes.
F New Feeling.

The key therapeutic technique involved in REBT are cognitive restructuring, which is the disputing of irrational beliefs, identifying unhelpful self-talk, and substituting with more adaptive self-talk. Cognitive homework, for example, the completion of "thought records," is also widely used. As the final goal of REBT is to attain unconditional self-acceptance, bibliotherapy, humor, role play, and shame-attacking exercises are also utilized. Another cognitive and behavioral intervention that is a part of this form of therapy is rational emotive imagery which serves as a form of exposure technique by the vivid imagination of a worst-case scenario.

As systematic desensitization is also involved, the further applications of REBT include the utilization of its educational approach that lends itself to group interventions. Group members can help each other learn and implement new skills and keep each other accountable.

REBT FOR DEPRESSION

Rational-emotive behavior therapy has had considerable success in the treatment of depressive disorders. In a randomized clinical trial in Romania, researchers compared REBT (14 weeks) with pharmacotherapy (14 weeks; fluoxetine) in 170 patients and discovered that while immediately at posttest there were no differences in depression levels, at the 6-month follow-up, there was a significantly larger effect of REBT on scales for depression (David et al., 2008).

This study examined the effects of the cognitive restructuring intervention program of REBT on irrational thoughts/behaviors arising from adverse childhood stress in Nigeria. Twenty-six participants who were identified as victims of adverse childhood stress went through 12 weeks of full intervention and 2 weeks of follow-up meetings. Through this intervention program, irrational thoughts/behaviors were significantly reduced in the treatment group when compared to the control group. Significant improvement was also observed at the end of the intervention of the treatment group (Eseadi et al., 2016).

CONCLUSION AND FUTURE DIRECTIONS

Community-based psychotherapy is a growing field, marked by the needs of the population. Research has shown us that it is certainly possible and a remarkable feat when lay workers can be efficiently trained to reduce the burden on psychologists and psychiatrists. Training lay workers in psychoeducation and therapeutic practices provides an interesting opportunity and shines light onto the true state of mental health needs in rural areas around the world.

Telecommunication when utilized by psychologists is also an interesting area by which to reduce the mental health gap within our societies. The truth is that when high rates of stigmatized practice surrounding therapy are present, we need to call on community stakeholders and leaders to serve as the channel for communication.

The therapies we have discussed in this chapter have their independent merits. Cognitive processing therapy, for example, when coupled with prolonged exposure, has seen great success in reducing rates of depression following sexual assault. Rational emotive behavior therapy is beneficial in the pursuit of overall mental health. Interpersonal therapy is well structured, follows the path of CBT, and is remarkably efficient in a group setting. Dialectical behavioral therapy is important when considering patients with BPD and suicidal ideation. Altogether this chapter has served as an overview for possible therapies in an outpatient setting.

Barriers for efficacious therapy are most profoundly the high rates of stigma and discrimination against this form of care. Individuals in many parts of the world, despite the growing conversation around mental health, actively refrain from seeking out and engaging in therapy, increasing the treatment gap that already exists in the field of mental health. This serves as a roadblock for patients to access mental health resources, thereby further impairing their functioning.

Concerning the relationship between psychotherapy and the community, we would like to end this chapter with a few suggestions regarding areas of improvement, directed at communal and individual well-being. A major aspect of research that limits our understanding of different societies is the absence of culturally adaptable measures. By encouraging researchers and physicians to take part in these efforts, we will obtain a closer view of the needs of the population. In order for these interventions to be adapted and accepted, communities need to be provided with more psychoeducation to decrease the stigma associated with mental illnesses. Some ways that this can be achieved are through an increased collaboration between researchers and community stakeholders within developing countries, as well as increased investment and participation by governments in community mental health interventions.

Finally, this chapter was designed to separately review theoretical and empirical dimensions of psychotherapies and the fledgling research on the relationship between them. Both phenomena are critical in human behavior and interaction. Further research is warranted, and it may well result in an enhanced ability to contribute to the well-being of individuals and groups.

Bibliography

Bolton, P., Neugebauer, R., & Ndogoni, L. (2002). Prevalence of depression in rural Rwanda based on symptom and functional criteria. *The Journal of Nervous and Mental Disease*, 190(9), 631–637.

Chapman, A. L. (2006). Dialectical behavior therapy: Current indications and unique elements. *Psychiatry (Edgmont)*, 3(9), 62.

David, D., Szentagotai, A., Lupu, V., & Cosman, D. (2008). Rational emotive behavior therapy, cognitive therapy, and medication in the treatment of major depressive disorder: A randomized clinical trial, posttreatment outcomes, and six-month follow-up. *Journal of Clinical Psychology*, 64(6), 728–746.

Ellis, A. (1995). Rational emotive behavior therapy. *Current Psychotherapies*, 5, 162–196.

Ellis, A., & Dryden, W. (2007). *The Practice of Rational Emotive Behavior Therapy*. UK: Springer Publishing Company.

Ellis, A., & MacLaren, C. (1998). *Rational Emotive Behavior Therapy: A Therapist's Guide*. London, UK: Impact Publishers.

Eseadi, C., Anyanwu, J. I., Ogbuabor, S. E., & Ikechukwu-Ilomuanya, A. B. (2016). Effects of cognitive restructuring intervention program of rational-emotive behavior therapy on adverse childhood stress in Nigeria. *Journal of Rational-Emotive & Cognitive-Behavior Therapy*, 34(1), 51–72.

Frank, J. D. (1971). Therapeutic factors in psychotherapy. *American Journal of Psychotherapy*, 25(3), 350–361.

Galovski, T. E., Blain, L. M., Chappuis, C., & Fletcher, T. (2013). Sex differences in recovery from PTSD in male and female interpersonal assault survivors. *Behaviour Research and Therapy*, 51(6), 247–255.

Groves, S., Backer, H. S., van den Bosch, W., & Miller, A. (2012). Dialectical behaviour therapy with adolescents. *Child and Adolescent Mental Health*, 17(2), 65–75.

Hassija, C., & Gray, M. J. (2011). The effectiveness and feasibility of videoconferencing technology to provide evidence-based treatment to rural domestic violence and sexual assault populations. *Telemedicine and E-Health*, 17(4), 309–315.

Herschell, A. D., Lindhiem, O. J., Kogan, J. N., Celedonia, K. L., & Stein, B. D. (2014). Evaluation of an implementation initiative for embedding dialectical behavior therapy in community settings. *Evaluation and Program Planning*, 43, 55–63.

Judd, L. L., Akiskal, H. S., & Paulus, M. P. (1997). The role and clinical significance of subsyndromal depressive symptoms (SSD) in unipolar major depressive disorder. *Journal of Affective Disorders*, 45(1–2), 5–18.

Linehan, M. M. (1993). *Skills training Manual for Treating Borderline Personality Disorder*. UK: Guilford Press.

Linehan, M. M. (2018). *Cognitive-Behavioral Treatment of Borderline Personality Disorder*. UK: Guilford Publications.

Markowitz, J. C., & Weissman, M. M. (2004). Interpersonal psychotherapy: Principles and applications. *World Psychiatry*, 3(3), 136.

May, J. M., Richardi, T. M., & Barth, K. S. (2016). Dialectical behavior therapy as treatment for borderline personality disorder. *Mental Health Clinician*, 6(2), 62–67.

Nixon, R. D., Best, T., Wilksch, S. R., Angelakis, S., Beatty, L. J., & Weber, N. (2016). Cognitive processing therapy for the treatment of acute stress disorder following sexual assault: A randomised effectiveness study. *Behaviour Change*, 33(4), 232–250.

Orley, J., & Wing, J. K. (1979). Psychiatric disorders in two African villages. *Archives of General Psychiatry*, 36(5), 513–520.

Resick, P. A., Nishith, P., Weaver, T. L., Astin, M. C., & Feuer, C. A. (2002). A comparison of cognitive-processing therapy with prolonged exposure and a waiting condition for the treatment of chronic posttraumatic stress disorder in female rape victims. *Journal of Consulting and Clinical Psychology*, 70(4), 867.

Resick, P. A., & Schnicke, M. (1992). Cognitive processing therapy for sexual assault victims. *Journal of Consulting and Clinical Psychology*, 60(5), 748.

Swales, Heidi, Heard, L, Mark, J. G., & Williams, M. (2000). Linehan's dialectical behaviour therapy (DBT) for borderline personality disorder: Overview and adaptation. *Journal of Mental Health*, 9(1), 7–23.

Verdeli, H., Clougherty, K., Bolton, P., Speelman, L., Lincoln, Bass, J., Neugebauer, R., & Weissman, M. M. (2003). Adapting group interpersonal psychotherapy for a developing country: Experience in rural Uganda. *World Psychiatry*, 2(2), 114–120. London: Oxford University Press.

Weissman, M. M., Markowitz, J. C., & Klerman, G. (2008). *Comprehensive Guide to Interpersonal Psychotherapy*. London, UK: Basic Books.

Wilk, C. M., & Bolton, P. (2002). Local perceptions of the mental health effects of the Uganda acquired immunodeficiency syndrome epidemic. *The Journal of Nervous and Mental Disease*, 190(6), 394–397.

36
Telepsychiatry as a Means to Optimizing Psychiatric Care

Mary V. Seeman

Advantages of Videotherapy	396
Difficulties	397
Outcomes	398
Effectiveness	398
The Pandemic	399
Variety of Uses of Telepsychiatry	399
Psychiatric Epidemiology	*399*
Clinical Assessment	*399*
Psychotherapy	*400*
Training and Supervision of Trainees	*400*
Psychoeducation and Self-Help	*400*
Legal Issues	*401*
Uses in Research	*401*
Conclusion	401

Telepsychiatry is a method of providing mental healthcare to patients in the community without the service user and care provider needing to meet face to face. Because a substantial number of psychiatric patients prefer to remain socially isolated, treatment at a safe remove from human contact is, in most cases, very welcome. This is not a new concept. Over a hundred years ago, the psychoanalytic couch already put "physical/social distance" between patient and doctor. Freud, the founder of psychoanalysis, probably instituted this practice more for his own needs than for those of his patients; reportedly, he did not like to be stared at all day. He wrote: "They (the patients) ask to be allowed to go through the treatment in some other position, for the most part because they are anxious not to be deprived of a view of the doctor. Permission is regularly refused" (Freud, 1958, p. 139). Later generations of mental health professionals, practising their profession in small offices with little spare space for couches, began to sit *with*, rather than *away from*, their patients. Nonetheless, psychoanalytic opinion, for the most part, continues to endorse the value of the Freudian couch, on which the patient relaxes and stares at a blank ceiling while confiding in a disembodied voice positioned behind and out of sight. According to Jacobson (1995), not seeing the therapist decreases the influence of his or her facial expressions and, thus, encourages patients' engagement with their own inner thoughts, fantasies, feelings, and bodily sensations (Jacobson,

DOI: 10.4324/9780429030260-40

1995). At the same time, it has been noted, this traditional positioning stops the psychiatrist from directly witnessing the emotional impact on the patient of therapeutic interventions intended to deepen emotional insight.

The advent of the COVID-19 pandemic, which shut down face-to-face medical and paramedical contacts and imposed telephone, online, or video therapy on patients and therapists, has brought into sharp focus both the advantages and the disadvantages of therapy at a distance. The year 2020 will be seen in history as the year of birth of a widespread use of telepsychiatry.

In Ontario, Canada, where I practise, on March 16, 2020, the provincial COVID-19 lockdown had already begun. The provincial ministry of health and long-term care announced that physicians would temporarily be reimbursed for care that was other than face-to-face, formerly disallowed by the Ontario health insurance plan. The ministry provided an online platform designed to improve access to virtual care, hoping in this way to relieve pressure on hospitals during the pandemic. The platform included a health services directory, access to e-consults and to confidential therapy and support over the internet. Most psychiatrists tried it, but they encountered frequent glitches and crashes on a system that was not prepared for the overwhelmingly high demand that resulted from the corona crisis. Many ended up using the service for the initial meeting with new patients and then reverting to the telephone, which most found easier to use and more reliable. Some also used video communication systems such as Skype and Zoom, but worried about confidentiality. Because therapeutic conversations are considered exquisitely personal and private, guarantees of confidentiality are perceived as essential (Aref-Adib et al., 2018; Freundlich et al., 2017; Lattie et al., 2020).

ADVANTAGES OF VIDEOTHERAPY

Both patients and therapists have commented on unquestionable advantages of videotherapy over office-based therapy. For instance, videos allow virtual entry into patients' homes. Case managers and social workers had always had entry into their clients' homes, a practice that, reportedly, was not always safe (Lyter and Abbot, 2007). By contrast, virtual entry is danger free but still permits glimpses of a patient's habitual surroundings and way of life, something never before accessible to psychologists and psychiatrists. From the patient's viewpoint, doing therapy from home has many practical advantages; it saves time, trouble, and cost of travel to and from appointments. It obviates babysitting arrangements. One early study in rural Canada found that patients could save $210 per consultation by communicating with their psychiatrists from a distance (Simpson et al., 2001). Younger generations, familiar with the technology, invariably prefer telepsychiatry to face-to-face encounters (Chan et al., 2015). Even older patients with little past technology experience have been eager to try something new and have shown surprising ability to adapt relatively quickly (Christensen et al., 2020). Motivation is important and, practical issues apart, for shy or distrusting, nervous or antisocial persons, confiding across a digital barrier, may prove less intimidating than being in the same room with a stranger.

Although there is a constant danger of unencrypted internet communications falling into the wrong hands, paradoxically, therapy from home has considerable confidentiality advantages. My patients used to be afraid of entering the psychiatric centre where I worked, afraid to be seen entering, afraid to meet a neighbour on the elevator and be forced to explain their presence in a psychiatric institution. Virtual therapy protects people from such awkward encounters. It also facilitates treatment of agoraphobia, or severe obsessive disorder, or the marked reclusiveness that accompanies severe forms of anxiety, depression, and psychosis. Individuals with these conditions are often stopped, by the nature of their symptoms, from seeking traditional help.

There are certain privacy advantages for care providers as well. Once again, they can, like Freud, choose to be invisible to patients, an invisibility that can be put to practical use. Freud was able to review notes of past visits and take new notes of his patients' free associations as he sat, unobserved, behind the couch. With telepsychiatry, mental health staff can also review the patient's file while the patient speaks and they can type up the current session as it unfolds, an extra efficiency, although it could be argued that it takes their mind away from what the patient is saying. Whether it does or not, the practice may offend patients if they see it (Gutheil and Hilliard, 2001). Many persons perceive note taking as showing a lack of interest, but research into this topic indicates that the patient-doctor relationship is, on the whole, not harmed by seeing a doctor take notes. For instance, a systematic review of the impact of electronic medical records (EMRs) found that, while physicians typing during medical visits often interrupted conversation and directed the gaze away from the patient, it did not change patient satisfaction with the session, nor was ease of interpersonal communication affected (Alkureishi et al., 2016).

Telepsychiatry is of theoretical benefit when dealing with a suicidal or potentially aggressive patient who requires involuntary psychiatric admission. In the office, it is very difficult to make civil commitment and hospitalization arrangements with the patient in front of you ready to run or attack. At a distance, this process should be able to proceed much more smoothly and safely.

A convenience for both patient and therapist is that therapy can take place in essentially any physical location, which offers flexibility to both parties. If necessary, one can continue seeing patients even when on vacation. Patients have potential access to their therapist even they are sick, or hospitalized, or imprisoned.

DIFFICULTIES

Difficulties have been noted when using both video and telephone therapy. A very talkative or emotional patient is difficult to interrupt or redirect, and instances of patient and therapist talking over each other occur with some frequency. The sound and visual quality of audio or video can be a significant problem. According to Cowan et al. (2019), sound quality on telephone or other device affects the doctor-patient encounter more than video quality.

Poor visual or audio transmission limits mutual connection and understanding and impairs a diagnostician's ability to detect potentially critical features such as vocal tics, tremors, subtle facial expressions, or eye gaze deviances. In a 2007 survey, only about one-third of medical respondents felt they could conduct a proper physical examination remotely (Barton et al., 2007). Technology has vastly improved since then, however.

Kate Murphy (2020) wrote an article in the New York Times entitled "Why Zoom Is Terrible." She enumerated all the reasons the helping professions should be wary of using Zoom (a free-of-charge videoconferencing application). The opinion of the experts she interviewed was that human beings were exquisitely sensitive to the meaning of small muscle contractions observed on each other's faces. When these clues to emotion appear asynchronous with the speaker's voice, or when they are blurred or distorted by the camera or the transmission, it makes it impossible to read the other person's intent. From the health provider's perspective, it is hard, via video, to look people in the eye when delivering hard truths. Because the two parties are not in the same space, they may be preoccupied with something more immediately present, their minds not fully on the task of therapy. Ms. Murphy recommends the ordinary telephone, because this is a technology most people find familiar and easy to use. Her belief is that a total lack of facial cues is better than the transmission of faulty ones. She suggest that the absence of all visual input on the phone might even heighten people's sensitivity to shifts of tone, momentary hesitations, and the meanings inherent in the changes of rhythm in a person's breathing.

OUTCOMES

Whatever its current failings, the more technology is used, the more technical issues will gradually resolve. In the Canadian province of Ontario, telepsychiatry consultations have been practised for decades to serve patients in the remote north of the province when travel in winter is difficult. A study in 2007 compared the outcomes of 495 randomized psychiatric consultations – telepsychiatry versus face-to-face visits. At completion, patients in the two groups (roughly 250 in each) expressed similar levels of satisfaction with the service they received. Most measured outcomes were the same except that telepsychiatry incurred less cost per patient (O'Reilly et al., 2007). A review of internet-based versus face-to-face cognitive therapy conducted in 2014 also found similar results (Andersson et al., 2014) although, at the time, very few therapists were offering the service by remote (Chan et al., 2014).

EFFECTIVENESS

Many pre-COVID effectiveness studies and reviews have been published over the last decade (Hilty et al., 2013; Parish et al., 2017; Rees and Maclaine, 2015), but the evidence base for telepsychiatry is still considered relatively sparse (Cowan et al., 2019). While a concern has been expressed about the ability of therapists to form an alliance with the patients virtually, most studies have found that only clinicians are concerned with the alliance being impaired; patients are, for the most part, satisfied with the quality of the telehealth alliance (Lopez et al., 2019).

Internet-delivered CBT has been shown to be as effective as face-to-face CBT for anxiety (Axelsson et al., 2020), post traumatic SD (Turgoose et al., 2018) and for depression (Kerst et al., 2019). In a 2016 review that included over 150 studies, Bashshur et al. had already concluded,

> Effective approaches to the long-term management of mental illness include monitoring, surveillance, mental health promotion, mental illness prevention, and biopsychosocial treatment programs. The empirical evidence ... demonstrates the capability of [telepsychiatry] to perform these functions more efficiently and as well as or more effectively than in-person care.

Costs of teletherapy are significantly lower (Axelsson et al., 2020). Several studies have supported its cost-effectiveness, such as equal effect at lower cost (Cowan et al., 2019; Yilmaz et al., 2019)

According to research by Chakrabarti (2015), online psychotherapy can be as efficient, effective, and efficacious as traditional therapy (if not more so).) This research shows it to be more accessible and flexible. Therapeutic conversations are easier to record and document and can be revisited at any time by both parties. Sessions can continue when the client is experiencing emergency situations which usually preclude access to therapy. These include postpartum crises, acute bereavement, serious illness, or imprisonment, situations when individuals are in most need. Moreover, online therapy is good for the environment. In Canada in 2019 (prior to the pandemic), it had been estimated that virtual healthcare reduced travel-related carbon (CO_2) emissions by 120,000 metric tonnes (Centre, 2020).

THE PANDEMIC

Disasters have, in the past, brought telepsychiatry to centre stage (Augusterfer et al., 2015), but the corona virus 2019 pandemic has been a game changer in this respect. It has been said that the future will view virtual therapy in terms of pre- and post–COVID-19 (Shore et al., 2020) because, due to fear, bereavement, isolation, loss of income, and despair about the future, the number and severity of psychiatric problems grew as never before (Zarghami, 2020), with support and counselling in high demand. Teletherapy was, and is at the time of writing, the only form of therapy available where I live. It became widely available in the United States because of the temporary governmental waiving of numerous telehealth regulations on March 17, 2020 (Torous et al., 2020). Regulatory barriers were loosened to allow for therapy across state lines (Freeman, 2020). Because of the pandemic, similar provisions for access to and reimbursement of telehealth services were made across the world. The mobile phone (Torous and Keshavan, 2020), especially the smart phone (Bauer et al., 2020), and, to a lesser extent, video technology, became a valued lifeline for people isolated in their homes or in hospitals (Zhou et al., 2020).

VARIETY OF USES OF TELEPSYCHIATRY

Frank et al. (2020) suggest in their recent review that telepsychiatry is feasible and useful in many settings, such as emergency departments in hospitals, correctional facilities, geriatric nursing homes, children's schools, addiction rehabilitation programs, assertive community treatment teams, and in essentially all psychiatric conditions, including the treatment of people for whom offices visits were previously inaccessible, namely disabled children, geriatric patients, and members of distant rural and indigenous communities.

The following sections briefly describe some of the potential uses of telepsychiatry:

Psychiatric Epidemiology

Online surveys are an excellent way to determine rates of mental illness in different geographic regions and to categorize respondents by age and sex and variables such as socioeconomic class, ethnicity, education, and potential etiological factors. Survey results can be used not only for statistical purposes but also for decision-making about public health messaging or determinations of new sites of psychology/psychiatric clinics or training centres for mental health personnel. Surveys conducted online have been used to probe opinions about mental health stigma (Seeman, 2015; Seeman et al., 2016), about accessibility and quality of available mental health services (Liu et al., 2020), about risks of suicidality (Seeman et al., 2017), or other questions of concern to epidemiologists.

Clinical Assessment

Video mental health consults to hard-to-reach populations have long been provided by personnel of academic centres. In this way, far-away specialists have been able to establish a working diagnosis and recommend appropriate treatment strategies to local practitioners. Since the COVID pandemic, this model has been adapted to video assessment for the general public, including referral for appropriate tests as necessary, and recommendations for treatment given directly to patients, with prescriptions, when necessary, forwarded to pharmacies (Zhou et al., 2020).

Psychotherapy

There is now strong evidence for the efficacy of online cognitive-behavioural therapy, but other forms of virtual therapies have not been sufficiently evaluated. Patients have reported, however, that working with a therapist online is less inhibiting than face-to-face therapy and that it enables comparatively greater disclosure and interaction (Cook and Doyle, 2002; Drum and Littleton, 2014). Concerns about a negative influence on therapeutic alliance have been expressed, but only, as stated earlier, by therapists (Lopez et al., 2019). The technical aspects of virtual therapy are more familiar to young people than to older generations (Kauer et al., 2014) but, for all age groups, access is reportedly easier currently than access to traditional therapy (McDonald et al., 2020).

The main concerns have been with privacy, confidentiality, and data security. Questions have also surfaced about the lack of appropriate training for staff moving into this area for the first time. Additional concerns expressed in the literature are a) therapists missing non-verbal cues in virtual therapy and b) therapists unable to respond to emergencies (Stoll et al., 2020; Van Wynsberghe and Gastmans, 2009).

There are also reported problems with respect to reimbursement, insurance coverage for patients, and malpractice coverage for practitioners (Shore et al., 2020) and currently unresolved technical problems such as the use of different electronic health record systems by different healthcare organizations (Frank et al., 2020).

Ease of tele-treatment of mental illnesses may well differ depending on the nature of the problems being treated. Psychosis treatment, for instance, is multifaceted and usually requires the involvement of families, the monitoring of pharmacotherapy for effectiveness and side-effects, and extra care with respect to suicide threat, plus interventions such as psychoeducation, cognitive remediation, exercise programs, smoking cessation programs, and vocational rehabilitation (Kumar et al., 2018; Lal et al., 2020; Naslund et al., 2015; Niendam et al., 2018; Torniainen-Holm et al., 2016). These can all be delivered virtually but patient-centred co-ordination is critical and may be difficult to achieve.

Training and Supervision of Trainees

Case supervision of trainees can also be done virtually. It takes many years of practice and mentoring feedback for practitioners to become effective therapists (Watkings, 2020). Supervisory sessions teach case formulation and model ways of thinking about oneself in relation to the patient. The relationship with the supervisor is often mirrored in trainees' dealings with their own patients. One advantage of video sessions of supervision is that they can be saved and referred to later.

The availability of online training modules in various aspects of mental health have proven usefulness in promoting knowledge in students of all mental health disciplines (Covell et al., 2014; Dixon and Patel, 2020). Online teaching can involve patients to a greater degree than standard teaching. Patients writing about their symptoms, evaluating their treatments, and documenting their side effects is effective in pressing governments and health systems to provide improved services (Whitley et al., 2020).

Psychoeducation and Self-Help

Telepsychiatry is not restricted to one-to-one encounters. It can consist of forums and blogs in which practitioners offer psychoeducational services to a wide audience and recommendations on what to do or not do to keep mentally healthy. This has been a common practice during COVID-19. In China, a mental health service digital platform has provided around-the-clock psychological support during the COVID-19 outbreak (Liu et al., 2020).

There has been widespread dissemination in China since the beginning of the pandemic of advice about diet and exercise, when to reach out for medical help, and what health-enhancing applications to purchase, among other examples of health promotion (Zhou, 2020). The communication of public health messages to vast populations is increasingly feasible over the internet (Seeman et al., 2016).

Legal Issues

Case law is lacking in the area of telepsychiatry, which, at present, creates a barrier to widespread use because of concerns about liability, the possibility of litigation, and the skyrocketing costs of malpractice insurance. Practitioners are usually required to be licensed in their own geographic district as well as in that in which their patient is located, constituting a formidable barrier to treatment across jurisdictions. Some regions offer special telemedicine licenses that allow clinicians to practice across jurisdictional borders. The dispensing of medications or instituting civil commitment procedures may, however, not be feasible outside one's own jurisdiction. Each region has its own regulations and legal procedures, creating difficulties for all concerned parties, especially since laws periodically change (Cowan et al., 2019).

Uses in Research

Virtual and mobile device-based methodologies are particularly suited to research. Digital technologies can quickly collect vast amounts of data. It is possible, for instance, to conduct real-time measurement of variables in patients' own environments and to monitor symptom fluctuations in response to everyday events (Park et al., 2020).

Besides the ease of conducting random, anonymous, privacy-compliant surveys about a variety of topics of interest to psychiatry, as mentioned earlier, it is now even possible to do imaging research remotely. Mobile EEG devices and mobile MRI scanners that use a forehead band or a bonnet worn over the head are now available (Park et al., 2020).

CONCLUSION

Telepsychiatry guidelines are currently available but will undoubtedly change with time and may substantially differ for different mental health disciplines (Am Telemed, 2019; Lin et al., 2020; Von Hafften, 2020).

Freud and his couched patients may not have seen each other's faces during therapy, but they, at least, shared the same environment, were exposed to the same extraneous noises, the same smells, the same room temperature and humidity. At the end of the session, they were able to shake hands and look each other directly in the eye. Therapy at a distance does not provide these subtle extras. Are they necessary to effective therapy? Will therapy become less effective with the advent of widespread telepsychiatry? Only time will tell.

References

Alkureishi MA, Lee WW, Lyons M, Press VG, Imam S, Nkansah-Amankra A, et al. Impact of electronic medical record use on the patient-doctor relationship and communication: A systematic review. *J Gen Intern Med.* 2016;31:548–560. doi: 10.1007/s11606-015-3582-1
American Telemedicine Association. 2019. www.americantelemed.org/. Accessed: July 9, 2020.

Andersson G, Cuijpers P, Carlbring P, Riper H, Hedman E. Guided internet-based vs. face-to-face cognitive behavior therapy for psychiatric and somatic disorders: A systematic review and meta-analysis. *World Psychiatry*. 2014;13:288–295.

Aref-Adib G, McCloud T, Ross J, et al. Factors affecting implementation of digital health interventions for people with psychosis or bipolar disorder, and their family and friends: A systematic review. *Lancet Psychiatry*. 2018;6:257–266. doi: 10.1016/S2215-0366(18)30302-X

Augusterfer EF, Mollica RF, Lavelle J. A review of telemental health in international and post-disaster settings. *Int Rev Psychiatry*. 2015;27:540–546. doi: 10.3109/09540261.2015.1082985

Axelsson E, Andersson E, Ljótsson B, et al. Effect of internet vs face-to-face cognitive behavior therapy for health anxiety: A randomized noninferiority clinical trial. *JAMA Psychiatry*. 2020. doi: 10.1001/jamapsychiatry.2020.0940

Barton PL, Brega AG, Devore PA, et al. Specialist physicians' knowledge and beliefs about telemedicine: A comparison of users and nonusers of the technology. *Telemed J E Health*. 2007;13:487–499.

Bauer M, Glenn T, Geddes J, et al. Smartphones in mental health: A critical review of background issues, current status and future concerns. *Int J Bipolar Disord*. 2020;5:2. doi: 10.1186/s40345–019–0164-x

Centre for Sustainable Health Systems. June 10, 2020. www.sustainablehealthsystems.ca/events/webinar-how-the-rise-of-virtual-care-is-contributing-to-sustainable-health-care Accessed: July 9, 2020.

Chakrabarti S. Usefulness of telepsychiatry: A critical evaluation of video-conferencing-based approaches. *World J Psychiatry*. 2015;5:286–304. doi: 10.5498/wjp.v5.i3.286

Chan SR, Parish M, Yellowlees P. Telepsychiatry today. *Curr Psychiatry Rep*. 2015;17:89. doi: 10.1007/s11920-015-0630-9

Chan SR, Torous J, Hinton L, Yellowlees P. Mobile tele-mental health: Increasing applications and a move to hybrid models of care. *Healthcare*. 2014;2:220–233; doi: 10.3390/healthcare2020220

Christensen LF, Moller AM, Hansen JP, et al. Patients' and providers' experiences with video consultations used in the treatment of older patients with unipolar depression: A systematic review. *J Psychiatr Ment Health Nurs*. 2020;27:258–271. doi: 10.1111/jpm.12574

Cook JE, Doyle C. Working alliance in online therapy as compared to face-to-face therapy: Preliminary results. *Cyberpsychol Behav*. 2002;5:95–105.

Covell N, Margolies P, Myers R, et al. State mental health policy: Scaling up evidence-based behavioral health care practices in New York state. *Psychiat Serv*. 2014;65:713–715.

Cowan KE, McKean AJ, Gentry MT, Hilty DM. Barriers to use of telepsychiatry: Clinicians as gatekeepers. *Mayo Clin Proc*. 2019;94:2510–2523. doi: 10.1016/j.mayocp.2019.04.018

Dixon LB, Patel SR. The application of implementation science to community mental health. *World Psychiatry*. 2020;19:173–174.

Drum KB, Littleton HL. Therapeutic boundaries in telepsychology: Unique issues and best practice recommendations. *Prof Psychol Res Pract*. 2014;45:309–15. doi: 10.1037/a0036127

Frank B, Peterson T, Gupta S, Peterson T. Telepsychiatry: What you need to know. *Current Psychiatry*. 2020;19:16–23.

Freeman MP. COVID-19 from a psychiatry perspective: Meeting the challenges. *J Clin Psychiatry*. 2020;81(2): doi: 10.4088/JCP.20ed13358

Freud S. *On beginning the treatment*. Standard Edition, 12:121–144. London: Hogarth Press, 1958, p. 139.

Freundlich RE, Freundlich KL, Drolet BC. Pagers, smartphones, and HIPAA: Finding the best solution for electronic communication of protected health information. *J Med Syst*. 2017;42:9. doi: 10.1007/s10916-017-0870-9

Gutheil TG, Hilliard JT. "Don't write me down": Legal, clinical, and risk-management aspects of patients' requests that therapists not keep notes or records. *Am J Psychotherapy*. 2001;55:157–165. doi: 10.1176/appi.psychotherapy.2001.55.2.157

Harris B, Birnbaum R. Ethical and legal implications on the use of technology in counselling. *Clin Soc Work J*. 2015;43:133–141.

Hilty DM, Ferrer DC, Parish MB, et al. The effectiveness of telemental health: A 2013 review. *Telemed J E Health*. 2013;19:444–454.

Jacobson JG. The analytic couch: Facilitator or sine qua non? *Psychoanalytic Inquiry*. 1995;15:304–313. doi: 10.1080/07351699509534038

Kauer SD, Mangan C, Sanci L. Do online mental health services improve helpseeking for young people? A systematic review. *J Med Internet Res*. 2014;16:e66.

Kerst A, Zielasek J, Gaebel W. Smartphone applications for depression: A systematic literature review and a survey of health care professionals' attitudes towards their use in clinical practice. *Eur Arch Psychiatry Clin Neurosci*. 2019;1–14.

Kumar D, Tully LM, Iosif AM, et al. A mobile health platform for clinical monitoring in early psychosis: Implementation in community-based outpatient early psychosis care. *JMIR Ment Health*. 2018;5:e15.

Lal S, Abdel-Baki A, Sujanani S, et al. Perspectives of young adults on receiving telepsychiatry services in an urban early intervention program for first-episode psychosis: A cross-sectional, descriptive survey study. *Front Psychiatry*. 2020;11:117.

Lattie EG, Nicholas J, Knapp AA, et al. Opportunities for and tensions surrounding the use of technology-enabled mental health services in community mental health care. *Adm Policy Ment Health*. 2020;47:138–149. doi: 10.1007/s10488-019-00979-2

Lin LA, Fernandez AC, Bonar EE. Telehealth for substance-using populations in the age of coronavirus disease 2019: Recommendations to enhance adoption. *JAMA Psychiatry*. 2020. doi: 10.1001/jamapsychiatry.2020.1698

Liu S, Yang L, Zhang C, Xiang YT, Liu Z, Hu S, et al. Online mental health services in China during the COVID-19 outbreak. *Lancet Psychiatry*. 2020;7:E17–E18.

Lopez A, Schwenk S, Schneck CD, et al. Technology-based mental health treatment and the impact on the therapeutic alliance. *Curr Psychiatry Rep*. 2019;21:76. doi: 10.1007/s11920-019-1055-7

Lyter SC, Abbott AA. Home visits in a violent world. *Clin Supervisor*. 2007;26:17–33. doi: 10.1300/J001v26n01_03

McDonald A, Eccles JA, Fallahkhair S, Critchley HD. Online psychotherapy: Trailblazing digital healthcare. *B J Psych Bull*. 2020;44:60–66. doi: 10.1192/bjb.2019.66

Murphy K. Why zoom is terrible. *New York Times*. 2020. www.nytimes.com/2020/04/29/sunday-review/zoom-video-conference.html Accessed: July 9, 2020.

Naslund JA, Marsch LA, McHugo GJ, Bartels SJ. Emerging mHealth and eHealth interventions for serious mental illness: A review of the literature. *J Ment Health*. 2015;24:321–332. doi: 10.3109/09638237.2015.1019054

Niendam TA, Tully LM, Iosif A-M, et al. Enhancing early psychosis treatment using smartphone technology: A longitudinal feasibility and validity study. *J Psychiat Res*. 2018;96:239–246.

O'Reilly R, Bishop J, Maddox K, Hutchinson L, Fisman M, Takhar J. Is telepsychiatry equivalent to face-to-face (individual or group) psychiatry? Results from a randomized controlled equivalence trial. *Psychiatr Serv*. 2007;58:836–843. doi: 10.1176/ps.2007.58.6.836

Parish MB, Fazio S, Chan S, Yellowlees PM. Managing psychiatrist-patient relationships in the digital age: A summary review of the impact of technology-enabled care on clinical processes and rapport. *Curr Psychiatry Rep*. 2017;19:90.

Park HS, Moitra E, Gaudiano BA. Lessons learned when using mobile ecological momentary assessment in patients with psychotic-spectrum disorders following a psychiatric hospitalization. *SAGE Res Meth Cases: Med Health*. 2020. doi: 10.4135/9781529722758

Rees CS, Maclaine EJAP. A systematic review of videoconference-delivered psychological treatment for anxiety disorders. *Aust Psychol*. 2015;50:259–264.

Seeman N. Use data to challenge mental-health stigma. *Nature*. 2015;528:309. doi: 10.1038/528309a

Seeman N, Reilly DK, Fogler S. Suicide risk factors in US college students: Perceptions differ in men and women. *Suicidol Online*. 2017;8:20–26.

Seeman N, Tang S, Brown AD, Ing A. World survey of mental illness stigma. *J Affect Disord*. 2016;190:115–121. doi: 10.1016/j.jad.2015.10.011

Shore JH, Schneck CD, Mishkind MC. Telepsychiatry and the coronavirus disease 2019 pandemic: Current and future outcomes of the rapid virtualization of psychiatric care. *JAMA Psychiatry*. 2020. doi: 10.1001/jamapsychiatry.2020.1643

Simpson J, Doze S, Urness D. Telepsychiatry as a routine service: The perspective of the patient. *J Telemed Telecare*. 2001;3:155–160. doi: 10.1258/1357633011936318

Stoll J, Muller JA, Trachsel M. Ethical issues in online psychotherapy: A narrative review. *Front Psychiatry*. 2020. doi: 10.3389/fpsyt.2019.00993

Torniainen-Holm M, Pankakoski M, Lehto T, et al. The effectiveness of email-based exercises in promoting psychological wellbeing and healthy lifestyle: A two-year follow-up study. *BMC Psychology*. 2016;4:21.

Torous J, Keshavan M. COVID-19, mobile health and serious mental illness. *Schizophr Res*. 2020. doi: 10.1016/j.schres.2020.04.013

Touros J, Myrick KJ, Rauseo-Ricupero N, Firth J. Digital mental health and COVID-19: Using technology today to accelerate the curve on access and quality tomorrow. *JMIR Ment Health*. 2020;7:e18848. doi: 10.2196/18848

Turgoose D, Ashwick R, Murphy D. Systematic review of lessons learned from delivering tele-therapy to veterans with post-traumatic stress disorder. *J Telemed Telecare*. 2018;24:575–585.

Van Wynsberghe A, Gastmans C. Telepsychiatry and the meaning of in-person contact: A preliminary ethical appraisal. *Med Health Care Philos.* 2009;12:469–476. doi: 10.1007/s11019-009–9214-y

Von Hafften A. Telepsychiatry practice guidelines. American Psychiatric Association. 2020. www.psychiatry.org/psychiatrists/practice/telepsychiatry/toolkit/practice-guidelines. Accessed: July 9, 2020.

Watkings CE, Jr. Psychotherapy supervision: An ever-evolving signature pedagogy. *World Psychiatry.* 2020;19:244–245. doi: 10.1002/wps.20747

Whitley R, Sitter KC, Adamson G, et al. Can participatory video reduce mental illness stigma? Results from a Canadian action-research study of feasibility and impact. *BMC Psychiatry.* 2020;20:16. doi: 10.1186/s12888-020-2429-4

Yilmaz SK, Horn BP, Fore C, et al. An economic cost analysis of an expanding, multi-state behavioural telehealth intervention. *J Telemed Telecare.* 2019;25:353–364.

Zarghami M. Psychiatric aspects of coronavirus (2019-nCoV) infection. *Iran J Psychiatry Behav Sci.* 2020;14:e102957. doi: 10.5812/jpbs.102957

Zhou X. Psychological crisis interventions in Sichuan province during the 2019 novel coronavirus outbreak. *Psychiatry Res.* 2020;286:112895. doi: 10.1016/j.psychres.2020.112895

Zhou X, Snoswell CL, Harding LE, et al. The role of telehealth in reducing the mental health burden from COVID-19. *Telemed J E Health.* 2020;26:377–379. doi: 10.1089/tmj.2020.0068

37
Smartphone Technology to Optimize Psychiatric Care in the Community

Boniface Harerimana and Cheryl Forchuk

Introduction	405
Enhanced Access to Psychiatric Care	406
Improvements in Clients' Engagement and Satisfaction With Treatment	406
Optimized Community Psychiatric Care Outcomes	407
Examples of the Implementation of Smartphone-Based Psychiatric Care Interventions	408
The Healthcare Provider's Side of the CHR Interface	411
CHR Interface From the Patient's Side	411
Conclusion	411

INTRODUCTION

The use of smartphone technologies for delivery of healthcare has seen a substantial expansion over the last few decades (Aguilera & Muñoz, 2011; Franklin et al., 2003; Leong et al., 2006; Miloh et al., 2009). Smartphone technologies that are used in healthcare include phone apps and web-based automated access to database networks (Luxton et al., 2011). Several healthcare disciplines implement smartphone technology interventions to achieve different health benefits. For example, short text messages are used to send reminders for appointments (Leong et al., 2006) and taking medications (Miloh et al., 2009), as well as to collect health information (Franklin et al., 2003) and monitor symptoms and behaviors during the post-discharge period (Bauer et al., 2003). Given the health benefits established by smart technology-based interventions across several health disciplines, the delivery of community psychiatric care using smartphones is rapidly expanding (Carras et al., 2014; Radovic et al., 2016) and has strengthened prospects of improving clients' access to care from their communities (Bauer et al., 2003; Goodwin et al., 2016; Niendam et al., 2018; Torous et al., 2014). Smartphone technology interventions make psychiatric care services more accessible and readily available to people in their community (Lappalainen et al., 2013; Morris et al., 2010; Reid et al., 2013). Also, smartphone-delivered interventions have demonstrated effectiveness in reducing mental illness symptoms (Enock et al., 2014; Moëll et al., 2015) and detecting related changes earlier (Ben-Zeev et al., 2015; Garcia Ceja et al., 2015; Osmani, 2015) as a result of enhanced client engagement with treatment (Ben-Zeev et al., 2018). However, the provision of psychiatric care through smartphone technologies has practical issues that require attention. This chapter evaluates how the implementation of smartphone interventions optimizes community psychiatric care by enhancing access to care, improving clients' engagement and satisfaction with treatment, and improving community psychiatric care outcomes. The chapter also discusses real-life practical considerations through examples of the implementation of smartphone-based psychiatric care interventions that have been conducted in London, Ontario, Canada.

ENHANCED ACCESS TO PSYCHIATRIC CARE

Smartphone-based psychiatric care holds the potential for improving clients' confidentiality and providing pragmatic solutions to travel distance burdens, disclosure issues, and mental health stigma. Psychiatric care delivered with smartphone technologies has enhanced the prospect of reaching people who would otherwise not receive treatment for mental illness (Price et al., 2014). Smartphone technology has helped to negate barriers to psychiatric treatment, such as burden related to travel distance (Marcus et al., 1997; Rost et al., 1998; Syed et al., 2013) and limited access to services in remote areas (Thomas et al., 2009), as well as mental health stigma (Happell et al., 2018; Henderson & Gronholm, 2018; Nyblade et al., 2019) and difficulties with self-disclosure (Mohr et al., 2006). For example, confidentiality and accessibility may be enhanced by the fact that smartphones are not geographically tied and are somewhat flexible and privately owned by individuals. As such, some smartphones have devices that enable users to carry out measurement and dynamic management of their mental health check-ups in real time without limitations of time and place (Oyama-Higa et al., 2016).

Additionally, clients with an urgent need for help can get support through mental health apps that are readily downloadable and easy to utilize on smartphones (Wilson et al., 2011). Research has indicated that smartphone technologies can improve access to psychiatric care from the community by providing clients with web-based self-help support materials that are delivered in familiar and comfortable conditions (Martinez & Williams, 2010). Moreover, the use of smartphone technology can mitigate issues related to conventional in-person healthcare delivery, such as rescheduled and missed appointments, along with delayed healthcare and medication (Syed et al., 2013). Subsequently, smartphone-based psychiatric care can contribute to the prevention of unmet healthcare needs and cumulative or worsened healthcare outcomes, such as sleep, mobility, conservation (Wang et al., 2016), and level of stress changes (Chang et al., 2011).

IMPROVEMENTS IN CLIENTS' ENGAGEMENT AND SATISFACTION WITH TREATMENT

Smartphone-based interventions optimize psychiatric care through enhanced client engagement and satisfaction with treatment. Currently, smartphones have several apps that allow clients to complete preloaded monitoring tools and therapy-related assignments while enabling healthcare providers to follow up on client implications and rating scores (Matthews et al., 2008; Rizvi et al., 2011; Rizvi et al., 2016). As such, smartphone technologies facilitate the immediate transmission of completed tools to care providers depending on the scores, and care providers may initiate virtual visits that allow real-time assessment and treatment outcomes (Matthews et al., 2008; Rothbaum et al., 2006; Shore et al., 2020). Research on client engagement and satisfaction with smartphone-based psychiatric care has indicated that clients who receive smartphone-based psychiatric care for severe mental illness, such as schizophrenia, schizoid-affective disorder, major depression, and bipolar disorder, are more likely to start treatment, remain fully engaged, and have a high level of satisfaction (Ben-Zeev et al., 2018). These positive experiences with smartphone-based interventions were supported in a review by Hind and Sibbald (2014). The review results indicated that clients who received smartphone-based psychiatric interventions not only had positive perceptions and experiences but also exhibited an enhanced willingness to use applications to impact their mental wellbeing (Hind & Sibbald, 2014).

OPTIMIZED COMMUNITY PSYCHIATRIC CARE OUTCOMES

Community psychiatric care delivery has significantly benefited from the use of smartphone technologies. Substantial research has shown that the use of smartphones for the delivery of community psychiatric care services reduces the severity of symptoms, psychological distress (Enock et al., 2014; Firth, Torous, Nicholas, Carney, Rosenbaum et al., 2017; Ivanova et al., 2016; Moëll et al., 2015), and delays in hospital readmissions and improves self-esteem and perceived recovery (Petros & Solomon, 2015). These clinical benefits were supported by two recent meta-analyses of randomized trials of smartphone based care (Firth, Torous, Nicholas, Carney, Pratap et al., 2017; Firth, Torous, Nicholas, Carney, Rosenbaum et al., 2017). A meta-analysis of randomized trials that tested 22 different smartphone apps demonstrated that not only were depression symptoms significantly reduced among clients in the intervention group, but the apps also showed the potential for enhanced self-management of depression (Firth, Torous, Nicholas, Carney, Pratap et al., 2017). Similarly, another meta-analysis found significant improvements in the treatment outcomes of anxiety disorders among community-dwelling clients who participated in randomized trials of smartphone interventions (Firth, Torous, Nicholas, Carney, Rosenbaum et al., 2017). Clinical benefits pertaining to the use of smartphone technologies for the delivery of psychiatric care may be associated with enhanced subjective social support and therapeutic relationships between care providers and clients (Aguilera & Berridge, 2014; Aguilera & Muñoz, 2011), as well as improved monitoring and early detection of changes (Aguilera et al., 2015; Chang et al., 2011; Wang et al., 2016).

A handful of evidence supports that the use of smartphone technologies for community psychiatric care delivery enhances clients' positive experiences and engagement with treatment interventions (Aguilera & Berridge, 2014; Aguilera & Muñoz, 2011; Hind & Sibbald, 2014), which in turn promotes compliance with treatment plans and improves treatment outcomes (Agyapong et al., 2012). For example, clients with comorbid unipolar depression and alcohol use disorders had reduced depression symptoms and enhanced alcohol cumulative abstinence scores when they were allocated to a 3-month intervention that involved providing twice-daily positive feedback support with text messaging (Agyapong et al., 2012). Another investigation of text-messaging intervention by Aguilera and Berridge (2014) revealed that client participants with a diagnosis of depression felt socially supported and exhibited enhanced introspection and awareness of mood state. Likewise, an adjunctive intervention to psychotherapy that consisted of 2-month text messaging increased the sense of closeness to a social group and therapists among clients with depression (Aguilera & Muñoz, 2011). In sum, the use of smartphone interventions for delivery of community psychiatric care can lead to clients' positive perceptions and experiences of participating in the process of treatment as well as the willingness to use the apps to impact their mental health (Hind & Sibbald, 2014).

The use of smartphone technologies also improves community psychiatric care by facilitating early detection of adverse changes and enabling the delivery of necessary support in a timely manner. This was exemplified by a community psychiatric care intervention that used automatic text messages designed for PHQ9 tool administration (Aguilera et al., 2015). The study results indicated that not only did the intervention facilitate timely clinical assessment of mood changes but also alleviated practical limitations, such as long length and higher literacy required for the assessment (Aguilera et al., 2015). In addition, smartphone technologies enable care providers to identify relapse signatures by intercepting changes in sleep, mobility, speech, and other self-reported mental health indicators earlier (Chang et al., 2011; Wang et al., 2016). More specifically, some smartphone apps provide avenues for accurate monitoring and analysis of clients' emotion changes and mental distress from their own homes (Chang et al., 2011). A review of studies that tested smartphone apps for delivery of psychiatric care showed that these apps have the ability to provide accurate and detailed symptom monitoring and to facilitate the implementation of psychotherapy interventions that are appropriate to the client needs (Hind & Sibbald, 2014).

Although clinical benefits of the use of smartphone technologies for community psychiatric care are indisputable, they are critical aspects for consideration for their effective implementation. Smartphone technology-based interventions supplement the effect of usual psychiatric care by primarily increasing client engagement and compliance with treatment plans (Bauer et al., 2018; Forchuk, Reiss et al., 2016; Henson et al., 2019; Mackie et al., 2017). Second, clinical benefits linked to the use of smartphone technologies for community psychiatric care are very much tied to improved therapeutic relationships through their potential for enhancing communication and sharing information with care providers outside the usual healthcare settings (Bauer et al., 2018; Forchuk, Reiss et al., 2016; Mackie et al., 2017; Richards & Simpson, 2015). The extent to which the use of smartphone technologies impacts the effectiveness of community psychiatric care depends on several factors, including client attributes and learning capacity and feedback systems, along with particular clinical, peer, and technical support (Henson et al., 2019).

EXAMPLES OF THE IMPLEMENTATION OF SMARTPHONE-BASED PSYCHIATRIC CARE INTERVENTIONS

Between 2010 and 2017, the mental health research group at the Lawson Health Research Institute (LHRI) hospital-based research arm set up a 7-year strategic plan to implement smart technologies for community healthcare delivery. The present chapter discusses three examples of smartphone projects that stemmed from the LHRI strategic plan.

Initially, we discuss the Mental Health Engagement Network (MHEN) intervention conducted to support persons with psychiatric illness dwelling in the community (Forchuk et al., 2014; Forchuk et al., 2013; C Forchuk et al., 2015). Individual beneficiaries of the MHEN intervention were enabled to access, maintain, and share their personal health information, including medications, medical history, allergies, and their mental healthcare professionals' contact information (Cheryl Forchuk et al., 2015; Forchuk et al., 2014; Forchuk et al., 2013; C Forchuk et al., 2015). Individual beneficiaries accessed health maintenance applications enabling mood monitoring, health journal entries, and sending reminders to support daily living (Cheryl Forchuk et al., 2015; Forchuk et al., 2013). In addition, the MHEN intervention included applications that provided person beneficiaries with functionalities for clients in tracking physiological measures, such as blood pressure, blood glucose, and weight. The MHEN intervention also included functionalities for informing care providers of their clients' health information and enabling them to contact clients through a secure messaging system.

The MHEN intervention took place between 2011 and 2014 in London, Ontario, Canada, and the surrounding areas. In total, 400 persons with a major mood or psychotic disorder received a smartphone with a separate account each. Participating care providers were also given a tablet and space account. Results of the MHEN intervention showed that intervention supplemented community psychiatric care by enhancing communication between individual beneficiaries and their care providers (Cheryl Forchuk et al., 2015; Forchuk et al.,

2013). The intervention results also supported that the use of smartphone technologies enhanced access to mental healthcare and reduced the financial burden of mental illness on the healthcare system by decreasing the use of more costly services, including outpatient visits, psychiatric admissions to hospital, and visits to emergency and crisis services (Cheryl Forchuk et al., 2015; Forchuk et al., 2014; Forchuk et al., 2013; C Forchuk et al., 2015).

The second example consists of a research project that implemented smartphone technology, Telemedicine and Patient-Reported Outcome Measurement (TELEPROM-Y), among the youth aged 14–25 with symptoms of depression or anxiety. TELEPROM-Y had the capacity to facilitate synchronous and asynchronous communication between care providers and the youth through the Collaborative Healthcare (CHRR) Platform and virtual visits (Forchuk et al., 2020). The project evaluation indicated that care providers and youth participants rated the use of the smartphone as a device and the apps highly. Both participating groups noted that a particular strength of the intervention was the enhanced ability to communicate more efficiently, an aspect that may improve access to care and support the therapeutic relationships (Forchuk et al., 2020). Data from focus groups also emphasized that the youth participants had a positive experience and were satisfied with receiving care from the comfort of their environment using the CHR app. Such findings indicate that the use of smartphone technologies has the potential for optimizing community psychiatric care delivery by minimizing missed appointments or concerns going unchecked, thereby enabling early intervention and prevention. In this regard, perspectives of care providers highlighted that the CHR facilitated closer monitoring of clients for early intervention and prevention. This was mainly associated with the fact that clinical assessment questionnaires were completed in real time by smartphone apps, and the care providers could be alerted to any potential mental healthcare crises that may have otherwise been unreported or unacknowledged.

The last example is a pilot study that used a mixed-methods design for evaluating smartphone technology, Telemedicine and Patient-Reported Outcome Measurement for Geriatric population (TELEPROM-G), among community-dwelling seniors with depressive symptoms (Forchuk, Cassidy et al., 2016). The study recruited participants from older adult outpatient services of two hospitals in Ontario, Canada. The sample included eight care providers and 30 individual patients who met the study criteria. Recruitment entailed enrolling care providers, who then referred client participants from their caseloads. The inclusion criteria for clients were being an outpatient on the caseload of community mental health services affiliated with one of the two participating hospitals, being aged 65 years or older, having depressive symptoms, not having significant cognitive deficits (as determined by a Mini-Mental State Examination [MMSE] (Tombaugh & McIntyre, 1992) score of 19 or less), and scoring over 5 on the Geriatric Depression Scale (GDS) (Yesavage, 1988). Care providers were included in the study if they were employed in a community mental health team that provided service to adults ages 65 and older who had depressive symptoms.

Client participants received a Wi-Fi–enabled computer tablet device that allowed in-cloud storage of anonymized information with encrypted and password-protected access. Twenty enrolled patient-participants already had in-home Wi-Fi. In cases where participants did not have access to Wi-Fi in the home, the cost of the Wi-Fi service was provided for the duration of the study. Participants were trained to use the tablet device and a web-based CHR platform. The CHR in this study recorded personal health information and ratings from self-administered questionnaires. It also used digital prompts and reminders to support care planning and enabled secure HCP-patient communication by video. See the CHR interface, which is presented in Figures 37.1 and 37.2.

Qualitative data were gathered during four focus groups, of which two took place 2 months after the intervention had started. Clients and care providers participated in separate groups, and both focused on the barriers and facilitators of adopting TELEPROM-G and on

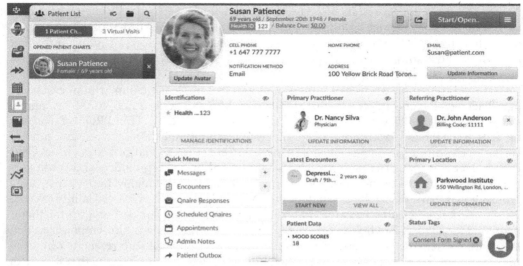

Figure 37.1 The healthcare provider's side of the CHR interface.

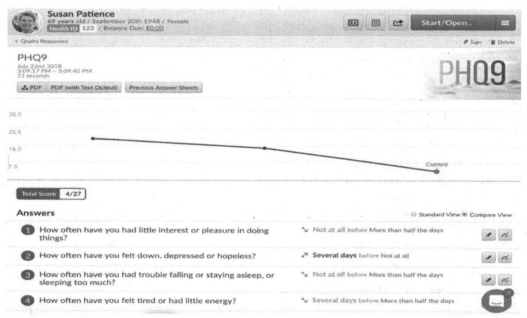

Figure 37.2 CHR interface from the patient's side.

perceptions of the program. Discussions in each group were audio-recorded, and the recordings were subsequently transcribed verbatim.

Findings showed that the use of smart technologies for delivery of psychiatric care to seniors is feasible, as exemplified by the fact that the study achieved full enrolment of 30 clients and retained 26 until the end of the 1-year intervention period. All clients were over 65 years of age, with an average age of 72.83 (SD = 4.84), and 12 (40%) were male. Findings also showed that client participants had a varied level of education. That is, 3 (10%) had grade (primary) school, 14 (46.7%) had high (secondary) school, and 13 (43.3%) had post-secondary (university) education. Sixteen were living alone, and the remainder lived with family members.

Twenty participants were diagnosed with two or more psychiatric conditions, of which anxiety disorders ($n = 17$; 56.7%) and mood disorders ($n = 27$; 90%) were the most prevalent. Twenty-seven had concurrent physical and psychiatric conditions, which included arthritis ($n = 10$; 33.3%), hypertension ($n = 10$; 33.3), and anxiety disorders ($n = 17$; 56.7%). All clients were taking prescribed medications for mental health issues, and 15 (50%) had been admitted to a psychiatric hospital at some point in their lives.

The Healthcare Provider's Side of the CHR Interface

Qualitative findings highlighted that using the CHR platform was beneficial in the sense that it was associated with enhanced communication, greater convenience, and user-friendliness. As for experienced difficulties of using the CHR platform, client participants underlined technical device-related issues and concerns with privacy and confidentiality. During focus groups, participants made several suggestions for improvements, such as tailoring features and functionalities to the clients and making modifications to address concerns about confidentiality.

CHR Interface From the Patient's Side

The quantitative of the study evaluated potential modifications to the current TELEPROM-G through clients' perceptions of smart technologies. Clients' perception of TELEPROM-G device and CHR platform was generally positive. For example, on a scale of 1 to 7, clients rated the simplicity and helpfulness of device as 3.20 and 4.92, respectively. Scores were highly positive among clients with prior experience of internet use, higher education, young age, and living with a relative. Concerning the impact of the intervention on client participants health outcomes, the quantitative data analysis found no statistically significant effect on the client' measures, such as community integration, depression, and quality of life, along with social, health, and justice service utilization. Nonetheless, subjective medication adverse effects were significantly lower between two-time points of data collection.

CONCLUSION

The present chapter discusses the potential of implementing smartphone-based intervention for optimizing community psychiatric care. Both reviewed literature and real-life examples drawn from the LHRI smart technology strategic plan underscored that the use of smartphones improves access to and optimizes the delivery of community psychiatric care by negating travel distance burdens, disclosure issues, mental health stigma, and other negative experience with mental health services. Smartphone-based interventions, such as TELEPROM-Y and TELEPROM-G, have the potential for providing timely assistance to individuals with mental illness through enhanced access to resources and support, as well as further prospects for communication with care providers. Moreover, the use of smartphones may represent a more convenient approach to mental healthcare as opposed to in-person appointments or printed resources, such as brochures and information sheets, that can be easily lost or damaged. The use of smartphone technologies may also allow care providers to see and communicate with more individuals in one day. While the use of smartphone-based interventions improves interactions between care providers' clients, several aspects should be considered for enhancing their effectiveness. Such aspects include client attributes and learning capacity, previous experience with technologies, and feedback systems, along with particular clinical, peer, and technical support.

References

Aguilera, A., & Berridge, C. (2014). Qualitative feedback from a text messaging intervention for depression: Benefits, drawbacks, and cultural differences. *JMIR mHealth and uHealth*, *2*(4), e46.

Aguilera, A., & Muñoz, R. F. (2011). Text messaging as an adjunct to CBT in low-income populations: A usability and feasibility pilot study. *Professional Psychology: Research and Practice*, *42*(6), 472.

Aguilera, A., Schueller, S. M., & Leykin, Y. (2015). Daily mood ratings via text message as a proxy for clinic based depression assessment. *Journal of Affective Disorders*, *175*, 471–474.

Agyapong, V. I., Ahern, S., McLoughlin, D. M., & Farren, C. K. (2012). Supportive text messaging for depression and comorbid alcohol use disorder: Single-blind randomized trial. *Journal of Affective Disorders*, *141*(2–3), 168–176.

Bauer, A. M., Iles-Shih, M., Ghomi, R. H., Rue, T., Grover, T., Kincler, N., Miller, M., & Katon, W. J. (2018). Acceptability of mHealth augmentation of Collaborative Care: A mixed methods pilot study. *General Hospital Psychiatry*, *51*, 22–29.

Bauer, S., Percevic, R., Okon, E., Meermann, R. U., & Kordy, H. (2003). Use of text messaging in the aftercare of patients with bulimia nervosa. *European Eating Disorders Review: The Professional Journal of the Eating Disorders Association*, *11*(3), 279–290.

Ben-Zeev, D., Brian, R. M., Jonathan, G., Razzano, L., Pashka, N., Carpenter-Song, E., Drake, R. E., & Scherer, E. A. (2018). Mobile health (mHealth) versus clinic-based group intervention for people with serious mental illness: A randomized controlled trial. *Psychiatric Services*, *69*(9), 978–985.

Ben-Zeev, D., Scherer, E. A., Wang, R., Xie, H., & Campbell, A. T. (2015). Next-generation psychiatric assessment: Using smartphone sensors to monitor behavior and mental health. *Psychiatric Rehabilitation Journal*, *38*(3), 218.

Carras, M. C., Mojtabai, R., Furr-Holden, C. D., Eaton, W., & Cullen, B. A. (2014). Use of mobile phones, computers and internet among clients of an inner-city community psychiatric clinic. *Journal of Psychiatric Practice*, *20*(2), 94.

Chang, K.-h., Fisher, D., & Canny, J. (2011). Ammon: A speech analysis library for analyzing affect, stress, and mental health on mobile phones. *Proceedings of PhoneSense*, 2011.

Enock, P. M., Hofmann, S. G., & McNally, R. J. (2014). Attention bias modification training via smartphone to reduce social anxiety: A randomized, controlled multi-session experiment. *Cognitive Therapy and Research*, *38*(2), 200–216.

Firth, J., Torous, J., Nicholas, J., Carney, R., Pratap, A., Rosenbaum, S., & Sarris, J. (2017). The efficacy of smartphone-based mental health interventions for depressive symptoms: A meta-analysis of randomized controlled trials. *World Psychiatry*, *16*(3), 287–298.

Firth, J., Torous, J., Nicholas, J., Carney, R., Rosenbaum, S., & Sarris, J. (2017). Can smartphone mental health interventions reduce symptoms of anxiety? A meta-analysis of randomized controlled trials. *Journal of Affective Disorders*, *218*, 15–22.

Forchuk, C., Cassidy, K.-L., Burhan, A. M., Booth, R., Vasudev, A., Hoch, J. S., Lewis, M., Isaranuwatchai, W., Lizotte, D., & Rudnick, A. (2016). TELEPROM-G: A study evaluating access and care delivery of telehealth services among community-based seniors. 2016 Future Technologies Conference (FTC), New York.

Forchuk, C., Donelle, L., Ethridge, P., & Warner, L. (2015). Client perceptions of the mental health engagement network: A secondary analysis of an intervention using smartphones and desktop devices for individuals experiencing mood or psychotic disorders in Canada. *JMIR Mental Health*, *2*(1), e1.

Forchuk, C., Fisman, S., Reiss, J. P., Collins, K., Eichstedt, J., Rudnick, A., Isaranuwatchai, W., Hoch, J. S., Wang, X., & Lizotte, D. (2020). Improving access and mental health for youth through virtual models of care. International Conference on Smart Homes and Health Telematics, New York.

Forchuk, C., Reiss, J., Eichstedt, J., Singh, D., Collins, K., Rudnick, A., Walsh, J., Ethridge, P., Kutcher, S., & Fisman, S. (2016). The youth-mental health engagement network: An exploratory pilot study of a smartphone and computer-based personal health record for youth experiencing depressive symptoms. *International Journal of Mental Health*, *45*(3), 205–222.

Forchuk, C., Rudnick, A., Hoch, J. S., Donelle, L., Campbell, R., Osaka, W., Edwards, B., Osuch, E., Norman, R., & Vingilis, E. (2014). Mental health engagement network: Innovating community-based mental healthcare. *Journal of General Practice*, *2*(1).

Forchuk, C., Rudnick, A., Hoch, J. S., Godin, M., Donelle, L., Rasmussen, D., Campbell, R., Osoka, W., Edwards, B., & Osuch, E. (2013). Mental health engagement network (MHEN). *International Journal on Advances in Life Sciences*, *5*(1–2), 1–10.

Forchuk, C., Rudnick, A., Reiss, J., Hoch, J., Donelle, L., Corring, D., Godin, M., Osaka, W., Campbell, R., & Capretz, M. (2015). Mental health engagement network: An analysis of outcomes following a mobile and web-based intervention. *J Technol Soc, 11*(2), 1–10.

Franklin, V., Waller, A., Pagliari, C., & Greene, S. (2003). "Sweet Talk": Text messaging support for intensive insulin therapy for young people with diabetes. *Diabetes Technology & Therapeutics, 5*(6), 991–996.

Garcia Ceja, E., Osmani, V., & Mayora Ibarra, O. A. (2015). Automatic stress detection in working environments from smartphones\textquoteright accelerometer data: A first step. *IEEE Journal of Biomedical and Health Informatics, 20*(4), 1053–1060.

Goodwin, J., Cummins, J., Behan, L., & O'Brien, S. M. (2016). Development of a mental health smartphone app: Perspectives of mental health service users. *Journal of Mental Health, 25*(5), 434–440.

Happell, B., Platania-Phung, C., Bocking, J., Scholz, B., Horgan, A., Manning, F., Doody, R., Hals, E., Granerud, A., & Lahti, M. (2018). Nursing students' attitudes towards people diagnosed with mental illness and mental health nursing: An international project from Europe and Australia. *Issues in Mental Health Nursing, 39*(10), 829–839.

Henderson, C., & Gronholm, P. C. (2018). Mental health related stigma as a 'wicked problem': The need to address stigma and consider the consequences. *International Journal of Environmental Research and Public Health, 15*(6), 1158.

Henson, P., Wisniewski, H., Hollis, C., Keshavan, M., & Torous, J. (2019). Digital mental health apps and the therapeutic alliance: Initial review. *BJPsych Open, 5*(1).

Hind, J., & Sibbald, S. L. (2014). Smartphone applications for mental health: A rapid review. *Western Undergraduate Research Journal: Health and Natural Sciences, 5*(1).

Ivanova, E., Lindner, P., Ly, K. H., Dahlin, M., Vernmark, K., Andersson, G., & Carlbring, P. (2016). Guided and unguided acceptance and commitment therapy for social anxiety disorder and/or panic disorder provided via the Internet and a smartphone application: A randomized controlled trial. *Journal of Anxiety Disorders, 44*, 27–35.

Lappalainen, P., Kaipainen, K., Lappalainen, R., Hoffrén, H., Myllymäki, T., Kinnunen, M.-L., Mattila, E., Happonen, A. P., Rusko, H., & Korhonen, I. (2013). Feasibility of a personal health technology-based psychological intervention for men with stress and mood problems: Randomized controlled pilot trial. *JMIR Research Protocols, 2*(1), e1.

Leong, K. C., Chen, W. S., Leong, K. W., Mastura, I., Mimi, O., Sheikh, M. A., Zailinawati, A. H., Ng, C. J., Phua, K. L., & Teng, C. L. (2006). The use of text messaging to improve attendance in primary care: A randomized controlled trial. *Family Practice, 23*(6), 699–705.

Luxton, D. D., McCann, R. A., Bush, N. E., Mishkind, M. C., & Reger, G. M. (2011). mHealth for mental health: Integrating smartphone technology in behavioral healthcare. *Professional Psychology: Research and Practice, 42*(6), 505.

Mackie, C., Dunn, N., MacLean, S., Testa, V., Heisel, M., & Hatcher, S. (2017). A qualitative study of a blended therapy using problem solving therapy with a customized smartphone app in men who present to hospital with intentional self-harm. *Evidence-Based Mental Health, 20*(4), 118–122.

Marcus, S. C., Fortney, J. C., Olfson, M., & Ryan, N. D. (1997). Travel distance to outpatient treatment for depression. *Psychiatric Services (Washington, DC), 48*(8), 1005–1006.

Martinez, R., & Williams, C. (2010). Matching clients to CBT self-help resources. *Oxford Guide to Low Intensity CBT Interventions*, 113–120.

Matthews, M., Doherty, G., Coyle, D., & Sharry, J. (2008). Designing mobile applications to support mental health interventions. In *Handbook of research on user interface design and evaluation for mobile technology* (pp. 635–656). USA: IGI Global.

Miloh, T., Annunziato, R., Arnon, R., Warshaw, J., Parkar, S., Suchy, F. J., Iyer, K., & Kerkar, N. (2009). Improved adherence and outcomes for pediatric liver transplant recipients by using text messaging. *Pediatrics, 124*(5), e844–e850.

Moëll, B., Kollberg, L., Nasri, B., Lindefors, N., & Kaldo, V. (2015). Living SMART: A randomized controlled trial of a guided online course teaching adults with ADHD or sub-clinical ADHD to use smartphones to structure their everyday life. *Internet Interventions, 2*(1), 24–31.

Mohr, D. C., Hart, S. L., Howard, I., Julian, L., Vella, L., Catledge, C., & Feldman, M. D. (2006). Barriers to psychotherapy among depressed and nondepressed primary care patients. *Annals of Behavioral Medicine, 32*(3), 254–258.

Morris, M. E., Kathawala, Q., Leen, T. K., Gorenstein, E. E., Guilak, F., DeLeeuw, W., & Labhard, M. (2010). Mobile therapy: Case study evaluations of a cell phone application for emotional self-awareness. *Journal of Medical Internet Research, 12*(2), e10.

Niendam, T. A., Tully, L. M., Iosif, A.-M., Kumar, D., Nye, K. E., Denton, J. C., Zakskorn, L. N., Fedechko, T. L., & Pierce, K. M. (2018). Enhancing early psychosis treatment using smartphone technology: A longitudinal feasibility and validity study. *Journal of Psychiatric Research, 96*, 239–246.

Nyblade, L., Stockton, M. A., Giger, K., Bond, V., Ekstrand, M. L., Mc Lean, R., Mitchell, E. M., La Ron, E. N., Sapag, J. C., & Siraprapasiri, T. (2019). Stigma in health facilities: Why it matters and how we can change it. *BMC Medicine, 17*(1), 25.

Osmani, V. (2015). Smartphones in mental health: Detecting depressive and manic episodes. *IEEE Pervasive Computing, 14*(3), 10–13.

Oyama-Higa, M., Wang, W., Kaizu, S., Futaba, T., & Suzuki, T. (2016). Smartphone-based device for checking mental status in real time. BIOSIGNALS.

Petros, R., & Solomon, P. (2015). Reviewing illness self-management programs: A selection guide for consumers, practitioners, and administrators. *Psychiatric Services, 66*(11), 1180–1193.

Price, M., Yuen, E. K., Goetter, E. M., Herbert, J. D., Forman, E. M., Acierno, R., & Ruggiero, K. J. (2014). mHealth: A mechanism to deliver more accessible, more effective mental health care. *Clinical Psychology & Psychotherapy, 21*(5), 427–436.

Radovic, A., Vona, P. L., Santostefano, A. M., Ciaravino, S., Miller, E., & Stein, B. D. (2016). Smartphone applications for mental health. *Cyberpsychology, Behavior, and Social Networking, 19*(7), 465–470.

Reid, S. C., Kauer, S. D., Hearps, S. J., Crooke, A. H., Khor, A. S., Sanci, L. A., & Patton, G. C. (2013). A mobile phone application for the assessment and management of youth mental health problems in primary care: Health service outcomes from a randomized controlled trial of mobiletype. *BMC Family Practice, 14*(1), 84.

Richards, P., & Simpson, S. (2015). Beyond the therapeutic hour: An exploratory pilot study of using technology to enhance alliance and engagement within face-to-face psychotherapy. *British Journal of Guidance & Counselling, 43*(1), 57–93.

Rizvi, S. L., Dimeff, L. A., Skutch, J., Carroll, D., & Linehan, M. M. (2011). A pilot study of the DBT coach: An interactive mobile phone application for individuals with borderline personality disorder and substance use disorder. *Behavior Therapy, 42*(4), 589–600.

Rizvi, S. L., Hughes, C. D., & Thomas, M. C. (2016). The DBT coach mobile application as an adjunct to treatment for suicidal and self-injuring individuals with borderline personality disorder: A preliminary evaluation and challenges to client utilization. *Psychological Services, 13*(4), 380.

Rost, K., Zhang, M., Fortney, J., Smith, J., & Smith, Jr, G. R. (1998). Rural-urban differences in depression treatment and suicidality. *Medical Care*, 1098–1107.

Rothbaum, B. O., Anderson, P., Zimand, E., Hodges, L., Lang, D., & Wilson, J. (2006). Virtual reality exposure therapy and standard (in vivo) exposure therapy in the treatment of fear of flying. *Behavior Therapy, 37*(1), 80–90.

Shore, J. H., Schneck, C. D., Mishkind, M., Caudill, R., & Thomas, M. (2020). Advancing treatment of depression and other mood disorders through innovative models of telepsychiatry. *Focus, 18*(2), 169–174.

Syed, S. T., Gerber, B. S., & Sharp, L. K. (2013). Traveling towards disease: Transportation barriers to health care access. *Journal of Community Health, 38*(5), 976–993.

Thomas, K. C., Ellis, A. R., Konrad, T. R., Holzer, C. E., & Morrissey, J. P. (2009). County-level estimates of mental health professional shortage in the United States. *Psychiatric Services, 60*(10), 1323–1328.

Tombaugh, T. N., & McIntyre, N. J. (1992). The mini-mental state examination: A comprehensive review. *Journal of the American Geriatrics Society, 40*(9), 922–935.

Torous, J., Chan, S. R., Tan, S. Y.-M., Behrens, J., Mathew, I., Conrad, E. J., Hinton, L., Yellowlees, P., & Keshavan, M. (2014). Patient smartphone ownership and interest in mobile apps to monitor symptoms of mental health conditions: A survey in four geographically distinct psychiatric clinics. *JMIR Mental Health, 1*(1), e5.

Wang, R., Aung, M. S., Abdullah, S., Brian, R., Campbell, A. T., Choudhury, T., Hauser, M., Kane, J., Merrill, M., & Scherer, E. A. (2016). CrossCheck: Toward passive sensing and detection of mental health changes in people with schizophrenia. Proceedings of the 2016 ACM International Joint Conference on Pervasive and Ubiquitous Computing.

Wilson, C. J., Rickwood, D. J., Bushnell, J. A., Caputi, P., & Thomas, S. J. (2011). The effects of need for autonomy and preference for seeking help from informal sources on emerging adults' intentions to access mental health services for common mental disorders and suicidal thoughts. *Advances in Mental Health, 10*(1), 29–38.

Yesavage, J. A. (1988). Geriatric depression scale. *Psychopharmacol Bull, 24*(4), 709–711.

38
Optimizing School Mental Health Services

Avinash De Sousa

Introduction	415
The Role of the School Counselor	415
Challenge 1: Move Away From Just the Special Children	416
Challenge 2: Making Your Presence Felt	416
Challenge 3: Building Partnerships With Teachers	416
Challenge 4: Using Age-Appropriate Interventions	417
Challenge 5: Reaching Out to All Age Groups	417
Challenge 6: Need to Incorporate School Counseling in Teacher and Psychologist Training and Education	418
Challenge 7: Maintaining Commitment Despite Poor Gains	418
Future Strategies	418

INTRODUCTION

Schools have always been the second family of our children. They have been conducive to the mental and emotional development of our children, avenues for them to learn cultural norms and the path towards skill acquisition. A child spends on an average 6–8 hours a day in his or her school. If we are in any way concerned about the mental health of children or counseling with children, then there is no doubt that schools are the place to be. Today more and more consultants are providing interventions in schools. A school is an area that in fact needs the skills of all mental health disciplines. Mini clinics have become more frequent on school campuses, and 'school intervention' as a broader term has now replaced school counseling [1].

School-based interventions are essential, as studies worldwide have reported that 3–10% of school-going children have some psychopathology [2]. The heartening fact remains that 75% of the studies on school interventions have reported positive outcomes of interventions [3]. This chapter looks at the status of school counseling today, the multiple roles a school counselor has to play and the various challenges they face.

THE ROLE OF THE SCHOOL COUNSELOR

The most important function of the school counselor is to recognize the diverse needs of everyone in the school. It is important to realize that just like other human beings, different people in schools have different priorities. The teachers aim at good teaching and classroom behavior control, and the parents want their children to do well and get the best from the school. It is important that parents realize that school counseling does not undo bad parenting and is not a substitute for good parenting. It helps in repairing a certain amount of damage that is done. Their job does not end once the counselor starts working. Many principals, on the other hand, aim to protect the name and integrity of the school at all costs while aiming for a 100% result in scores for the school. The counselor has to handle all of this [4]. The school counselor has to provide direct consultation to students without losing out on classes (a distant dream), help teachers in classroom behavior interventions and advise the principal on various policy matters that may benefit the school. The counselor must share the anxiety of the parents and the teachers and help in building alliances between the students, parents and staff. They must cultivate respect for everyone and help in constructing effective alliances that will help in future collaboration. Their role is to view the child holistically from a biopsychosocial point of view and help others to see the child in different lights at times. They have to assume various roles of a teacher, guide and friend in order to get the maximum from and empower the staff [5,6].

CHALLENGE 1: MOVE AWAY FROM JUST THE SPECIAL CHILDREN

It is noted that only one-third of children in all schools receive effective mental health consultations from counselors. With schools in countries like ours, where there is no funding for child mental health either from the government or private agencies, the counselor has to learn to be cost effective and to maximize the limited resources in the schools. The first daunting task is to not just focus on the special children. Very often it is felt that the role of the school counselor is to help the child with special needs, and the other children can manage themselves. The special child is already in the limelight and often is getting help from and outside the school. These often are just 1–3% of the normal school population. The school counselor in a mainstream school must move away from just helping special children, their parents and the problems of inclusive education and must focus on the remaining non-disabled children who also need help [7]. Very often the school authorities keep referring these children time and again to the counselor with the same problems, and the children who may need help for study problems, time management and exam stress are often left out.

CHALLENGE 2: MAKING YOUR PRESENCE FELT

It is important that school authorities be made aware of what the roles and responsibilities of the counselors are. They must be told why counselors are there and what their abilities are. From time to time, presentations have to be made to the staff about various mental health problems, academic issues and problems like developmental disabilities or learning disabilities that are seen in schools and the role of the counselor in alleviating them [8]. It is important to remember that in schools, we are dealing with diverse stakeholder groups, and hence each group must realize that the counselor is the neutral authority and has the best interests of the child at heart. It is important to note that school-based interventions have greater acceptance and often are an early intervention. The parents often view the counselor as part of the school authority and respect what he/she says. It is important to exploit this viewpoint to the maximum to enhance the effectiveness of the intervention [9,10].

CHALLENGE 3: BUILDING PARTNERSHIPS WITH TEACHERS

It is very important for the counselor to build good relationships with the teachers. This enables the counselor to be their most effective in their interventions and also involve them in the therapeutic process. Often with children, involving a teacher who is dear to them enhances the intervention, and the child may even open up more easily [11].

Teachers can be educated easily and even made to rectify their errors if the counselor has a good working relationship with them. The expectations from the intervention must be clarified with a particular teacher and time frame needed to achieve results must be specified. Teachers often feel that with one referral to the counselor, there will be a rapid resolution of the child's problems, which is not always the case. Teachers must also be made aware of the various referrals that have to be made to the counselor. Very often in schools, the counselor is viewed as an adjunct disciplinarian, and children the teacher cannot handle in school are often referred to the counselor when all their problems are in fact a part of normal adolescence and different facets of child development [12].

Building relationships with teachers also helps in effective classroom interventions that should be carried out. This is all the more important in secondary schools, where unlike primary schools, where the same teacher is present most of the day, teachers change every half-hour, so a uniformity of classroom handling is needed. Teachers must be sensitized to the child's needs, and the importance of confidentiality in many cases must be stated. Teachers often have a habit of talking about children to other teachers, and slowly the word of particular child's problems may spread in the school. A child who loses trust in the confidentiality in the counselor will never be receptive to any intervention thereafter [13,14]. It is important that the counselor take building partnerships further in playing a pivotal role in partnerships between parents and teachers, thus completing the school triangle.

CHALLENGE 4: USING AGE-APPROPRIATE INTERVENTIONS

It is important that the counselor make the school authorities aware regarding the appropriate age of referral. It is important that the teachers be taught not to jump prematurely and label children and to judge the severity of the problem and thereby choose appropriate referrals [15]. It is also important that premature psychological testing and intelligence assessments not be encouraged by the counselor, reports of which may at times prove detrimental to the further progress of the child. The awareness of appropriate age-associated interventions and psychological tests as well as their proper use is essential for the counselor. Sometimes behavior interventions are tried prematurely in children with hyperactivity, which at times may a part of the normal developmental process, and are not effective [16]. With the aim of judging age-appropriate interventions, it is essential that the counselor have an in-depth knowledge of normal child development and also be adept at differentiating between what is normal and what is not [17].

CHALLENGE 5: REACHING OUT TO ALL AGE GROUPS

It is important that the counselor reach out to various age groups in the school. It is important to realize that psychopathology and the need for counselors may often exist in areas where we feel them least. The kindergarten (KG) is an area of the school where counselors rarely venture, but it is important to note that problems needing attention may be lurking here. Successful early child development is a must for further development. The isolated, banal and beleaguered atmosphere of the KG class may be an area where the child develops separation anxiety that may at times be difficult to tackle. The kindergarten child has to deal with daily separations and reunions with his parents, and parents need to be trained to handle their children [18].

It is important that teenagers in a school be handled in a proper manner. Often, many schools are large and impersonal to teenagers. The counselor must be sensitive to the developmental needs of adolescents and must exhort school authorities to realize the same [19]. Teenagers often develop a detachment from their parents in their search for independence. Appropriate student-parent conferences organized by the counselor may play a pivotal role in promoting respect and healthy relationships between parents and teenagers [20]. Teenagers also need to be watched, and early detection and interventions in problems for them are a must. Problems like violence and substance abuse are common among teenagers, and these issues need to be addressed regularly in schools [21,22]. Educating the teenager on issues like sexuality and substance abuse as well as handling relationships maturely in the form of regular lectures and workshops is a must on the part of the counselor [23]. Very often teenagers find solace in the counselor when they feel no one understands them. It is important that the counselor be equipped to handle teenage infatuations and feelings that may arise from the teenager during the counseling process and during their interactions with the counselor [24]. It is also important that the counselor be well equipped to handle transitions seen as a result of children from different schools and cities who may develop psychological symptoms adjusting to a new environment.

CHALLENGE 6: NEED TO INCORPORATE SCHOOL COUNSELING IN TEACHER AND PSYCHOLOGIST TRAINING AND EDUCATION

There is a growing need for training in school counseling both at the college and post-degree level for both psychologists and teachers. Exposure to school mental health and child psychiatry will be helpful to both psychologists and teachers in their later contacts with students. In the past, it was often difficult to find counselors who were trained in school mental health. It is necessary for the psychologist and psychiatrist to be familiar with school settings, classroom format, potential and terminology to be able to present relevant and clinical views of children and adolescents in schools [25].

Psychologists undergoing training in the university as well as psychiatrists in training must be posted in schools to enhance their skills in dealing with children. It is important to remember that the school is not just an area that encompasses child psychiatry, but often the counselor deals with adults (parents) who may have psychopathology, as well as grandparents, which in turn leads to exposure to a wide variety of people across all ages, sexes, races and religions. The school counselor also sometimes has the opportunity to participate in special projects that may be carried out in the school. Thus schools are a fertile ground for a myriad of experiences that may be challenging, frustrating and rewarding at the same time [26].

CHALLENGE 7: MAINTAINING COMMITMENT DESPITE POOR GAINS

Finally, though we all do not always work for money, it is important that we earn enough to be happy and earn what we think is a fair sum for our efforts. One major deterrent in the stability of school counselors in various schools is the poor pay scale for both full- and part-time counselors, as well as the reluctance of schools to spend more than a certain amount on counseling services while a lot is spent on sports, extracurricular activities and academic pursuits. Counselors in India earn far less than those abroad, leading to many seeking greener pastures from time to time as well as many going overseas for better prospects. This has lead to a paucity of school counselors and instability in school counseling and mental health services. It is high time our school authorities gave school counselors their dues.

FUTURE STRATEGIES

The world is progressing, and we are progressing at the same pace. Yet today in certain sectors, visits to counselors, psychologists and psychiatrists are viewed as stigmatizing. There is a need to make people accept the basis and rationale of school interventions today. A child benefits from intervention by people who understand him or her and the environment he or she is in along with the stressors he or she faces. Parents and certain elders in the family feel that visits to the school counselor may mean that their child is singled out and labeled as having a psychological problem. Sometimes a good counselor may be undermined by an external opinion sought by parents that may suit their minds and then be imposed on the school. It is essential that the school and its teachers have full faith in their counselors and the interventions that they suggest. People have to realize that interventions take time and waiting is definitely rewarding.

There is a need for expert clinicians and experts from various fields to come out of their glass houses and move into schools if we are to achieve the objective of positive school mental health for all. These clinicians have to realize that moving into schools does not degrade or undermine them but rather enhances their own skills and makes them accessible to a wider audience. Their suggestions and expertise will go a long way in building a committed team of school mental health experts working hand in hand with counselors.

Child psychiatry and psychology have taken a back seat here in India. We hear every day of suicides in children, children having exam stress and the aftermath of bad parenting in our dailies and newspapers. This must serve as a wake-up call to all those in the field of child mental health to work towards the betterment of all our children. Practicing child psychology, child psychiatry and school counseling in India is a grave challenge, but once the challenge is taken up, it must be met!

References

1. Pearson G, Jennings J, Norcoss J. A program of comprehensive school based mental health services in a large urban school district: The Dallas model. *Adolescent Psychiatry* 1999; 23: 209–231.
2. Bostic JQ, Rauch PK. The 3 Rs of school consultation. *Journal of the American Academy of Child & Adolescent Psychiatry* 1999; 38: 339.
3. Sheridan SM, Welch M, Orme SF. Is consultation effective: A review of research. *Remedial & Special Education* 1996; 17: 341–344.
4. Erchul WP, Martens BK. *School Consultation: Conceptual and Empirical Bases of Practice*. 1997, New York; Plenum Press.
5. Kampwirth TJ. *Collaborative Consultation in Schools*. 1999, Upper Saddle River; Prentice Hall.
6. Marks M, Edwards S. *Entry Strategies for School Consultation*. 1995, New York; Guilford Press.
7. Comer JP. *Waiting for a Miracle: Why Schools Can't Solve Our Problems and How We Can*. 1997; New York: Dutton Books.
8. Evans SW. Mental health services in schools: Utilization, effectiveness and consent. *Clinical Psychology Review* 1999; 19: 165–179.
9. Lonigan CJ, Elbert JC, Johnson SB. Empirically supported psychosocial interventions for children: An overview. *Journal of Clinical Child Psychology* 1998; 27: 138–145.
10. Flaherty LT, Weist MD. School based mental health services: The Baltimore models. *Journal of Psychology in Schools* 1999; 36: 379–389.
11. Weist MD, Schlitt JJ. Alliances in school based health care. *Journal of School Health* 1998; 68: 401–403.
12. Sedlak MW. The uneasy alliance of mental health services and schools: A historical perspective. *American Journal of Orthopsychiatry* 1997; 67: 374–384.
13. Waxman R, Weist MD, Benson D. Toward collaboration in the growing education: Mental health interface. *Clinical Psychology Review* 1999; 19: 239–253.
14. Adelman HS. Restructuring education support services and integrating community resources: Beyond the full service school model. *School Psychology Review* 1996; 25: 431–445.
15. Berlin IN. Mental health consultation in schools: Who can do it and why. *Community Mental Health Journal* 1965; 1: 19–22.
16. Adelman HS, Taylor L. Mental health in schools and systems restructuring. *Clinical Psychology Review* 1999; 19: 137–163.
17. Berkovitz IH, Sinclair E. Teaching child psychiatrists about interventions in the school systems. *Journal of Psychiatric Education* 1984; 8: 240–245.

18. Furman E. Play and work in early childhood. In *Child Analysis: Clinical, Theoretical and Applied Perspectives* Vol. 1. 1990, UK: Taylor and Francis; Pp. 60–76.
19. Brener ND, Collins JL. Co-occurrence of health risk behaviors among adolescents in the United States. *Journal of Adolescent Health* 1998; 22: 209–213.
20. Mattison RE. School consultation: A review of research on issues unique to the school environment. *Journal of the American Academy of Child and Adolescent Psychiatry* 2000; 39: 1–12.
21. Milstein SG, Irwin CE. Accident related behavior in adolescents: A bio-psychosocial perspective. *Alcohol, Drugs and Driving* 1987; 4: 21–29.
22. Newcomer S, Baldwin W. Demographics of adolescent sexual behavior, contraception and pregnancies. *Journal of School Health* 1992; 62: 265–270.
23. Symons CW, Cinelli B, James TC. Bridging student health risks and academic achievement through comprehensive school health programs. *Journal of School Health* 1997; 67: 220–227.
24. Sofalvi AJ, Birch DA. Working with education reporters to advocate for comprehensive school health education. *Journal of School Health* 1997; 67: 185–186.
25. Adelsheim S. Addressing barriers to development and learning: School, family and agency partnerships in New Mexico. *Counseling and Human Development* 2000; 32: 1–12.
26. Berkovitz IH. The benefits of clinician consultation in schools of education. *Child & Adolescent Psychiatric Clinics of North America* 2001; 10(1): 199–204.

39
Optimising Patient Care in Psychiatry – Focus on Forensic Psychiatry

Jason Quinn, Ajay Prakash, Jared Scott and Arun Prakash

Introduction	421
The "Insanity Defense"	422
The Forensic System	422
Assessing Risk for Violence	423
Unstructured vs. Structured Risk Assessment	423
Actuarial vs. Structured Professional Judgment Instruments	423
Unique Considerations in Forensic Rehabilitation	425
Personality Disorder and Psychopathy	425
Substance Use Disorders in the Forensic Context	425
Problematic Sexual Behaviours	427
Forensic Outreach: Providing Care for Patients in the Community	429
Models of Community Care: ACT and FACT Teams	430
Forensic Outreach Service Delivery	430
The Compulsory Nature of Forensic Mental Healthcare	431
A System of Transitions	431

INTRODUCTION

Forensic psychiatry is a broad field, encompassing the assessment and treatment of individuals with mental illness who come into contact with the law. Forensic psychiatrists can assist the justice system in both civil and criminal matters. They work in different contexts, including in correctional institutions, hospitals, and the community. They often function as assessors and provide expert opinion evidence in courts of law. They also serve a more treatment-oriented rehabilitative role, functioning within multidisciplinary teams, providing care for mentally ill offenders.

This chapter reviews some of the considerations unique to the care of forensic patients, especially those living in the community setting. We will consider *forensic patients* individuals who have committed criminal offences but have been diverted from the traditional punishment-oriented sentences (such as jail time) to a supervised mental healthcare system (the *forensic system*). Community-dwelling forensic patients receive care and supervision from multidisciplinary teams (*outreach teams*), working towards the ultimate goal of community reintegration.

Forensic patients are generally individuals with severe and persistent mental illness. They are typically diagnosed with psychotic and/or major mood disorders and often have comorbid personality, substance use, and/or paraphilic disorders. During their crimes, their behaviour was likely seriously influenced by psychopathology. Prior to their entry into the forensic system, they were often heavy users of mental healthcare services (defined as those who have had a minimum of two hospitalizations in one year[1]). We will briefly review the history of the "Insanity Defense," the general structure of forensic systems in the English-speaking world, and issues inherent to forensic mental healthcare, including violence risk assessment. We will also review a few unique clinical considerations in the forensic context, including issues related to psychopathy/personality disorder, substance use disorders, and problematic sexual behaviours. Finally, we will review the structure and function of forensic outreach teams.

The "Insanity Defense"

Throughout history, societies around the world debated the ethics of guilt and punishment as it pertained to obviously mentally ill offenders. Although many early cultures recognized some version of the "insanity defense," (which can be even found in the Code of Hammurabi, dating to around 1772 BCE[2]), the treatment of mentally ill offenders was variable in pre-Norman times, influenced by local customs and culture.

In 1843 in England, Daniel McNaughton shot Edward Drummond, secretary to the prime minister, who died 5 days later. During his trial, he was found to have been acting under the influence of persecutory delusions relating to the prime minister's political party. His defence successfully argued that his "insanity" deprived him of responsibility for his actions, and he was ultimately acquitted. The resultant public controversy led to the development of the McNaughton Rules in the House of Lords, variations of which have since guided legal decisions relating to criminal responsibility throughout much of the English-speaking world.

The McNaughton Rules state that

> to establish a defense on the ground of insanity, it must be clearly proved that, at the time of the committing of the act, the party accused was labouring under such a defect of reason, from disease of the mind, as not to know the nature and quality of the act he was doing; or, if he did know it, that he did not know he was doing what was wrong.[3]

The Forensic System

Individuals who pass the test laid out in the McNaughton Rules are found not criminally responsible on account of mental disorder (NCRMD) in Canada (or not guilty by reason of insanity, NGRI, elsewhere). Further legislation and judicial interpretation of the legal test has led to variable precedents in different jurisdictions. Professionals asked to evaluate accused for the suitability of an NCRMD defence should thus be aware of the specifics of legislation and case law in their jurisdictions.

Although accused who are found NCRMD do not continue along the traditional crime-and-punishment pathway, they are not acquitted altogether. NCRMD-accused are generally diverted into the forensic system, where their level of liberty and community access is decided on by mental health review boards (quasi-judicial tribunals). In many Western forensic systems, review boards hold regular hearings to help them craft dispositions, based on evidence presented by forensic professionals (who are often treating clinicians, presenting unique ethical and therapeutic challenges). Dispositions (similar to judicial orders) are documents that detail the restrictions on patients' liberties and other conditions required to maintain their liberty (such as living in hospital or at a specific address, limits on geographic travel, providing random urine samples for drug screening, and so on.) Ideally, the intensity of the restrictions and conditions are matched to the risk a given patient has for violence, as opposed to the seriousness of their crime. Although it may be theoretically practical, this principal has occasionally proven controversial for both the public and the patients themselves, as it runs contrary to popular intuitions about justice and victim's rights[4] ("do the crime, do the time.") This is especially the case during high-profile cases which are popularized in the media (foreshadowed in McNaughton).

In Canada, once a given patient's risk is so low that a "significant threat" to the safety of the public can no longer be proven (on balance of probabilities), they are granted an "absolute discharge." Their forensic journey, and restrictions, are over. The period of time between entry into the forensic system to leaving it can thus be few or many years, depending on a given patient's risk profile.

ASSESSING RISK FOR VIOLENCE

Evaluating risk for violence is a core competency of forensic mental health practitioners. Violence risk assessment informs numerous decisions clinicians are called to make, including determining the level of risk patients pose to the community and what management strategies could mitigate specific risk factors. In addition to informing clinical decision-making, risk assessment ultimately guides review boards in making decisions about the appropriate levels of liberty to afford patients managed within forensic systems. It is thus important to have an understanding of the processes and tools used clinically to assess risk for violence. We will also review unique considerations within forensic mental healthcare, including psychopathy and sexual violence.

Unstructured vs. Structured Risk Assessment

Clinical strategies for assessing violence risk can be broadly divided into two categories: unstructured or structured.[5] Prior to the development of modern risk assessment instruments, clinicians had no choice but to use unstructured clinical judgment. Such judgment relies on a clinician's subjective impression as to whether an individual is likely to behave violently, based on professional experience and intuition.[6,7] All mental health clinicians are familiar with unstructured risk assessment: general psychiatrists, for example, conduct suicide and violence risk assessments as part of routine practice.

Clinicians typically form their impressions of violence risk based on their knowledge of the patient's history, collateral information from caregivers and other clinicians, psychiatric interviewing, and mental status examination. Known antecedents to violence in a given patient, such as medication nonadherence, emergent psychiatric symptoms, substance use, and stressors are risk factors often considered. However, unstructured risk assessments are compromised by the subjective element and poor inter-rater reliability between clinicians; in some cases, forensic psychiatrists' unstructured opinions on violence risk prediction are inconsistent and no better than that of non-professionals.[6]

In recent decades, a number of formalized, validated risk assessment tools have been developed. Such tools guide clinicians to consider risk factors with empirical support. Structured risk assessment strategies significantly outperform unstructured approaches in predicting violent recidivism.[8] Consequently, the use of such tools is typically preferred in the at-times high stakes context of forensic mental healthcare.

Actuarial vs. Structured Professional Judgment Instruments

Structured risk assessment tools differ in the questions they answer (for example, predicting general violence or sexual violence specifically), the populations they apply to, and their underlying approach. Actuarial tools, such as the Violence Risk Appraisal Guide (VRAG),[9] provide probabilistic estimates of recidivism risk over a set period of time. Such tools typically use demographic and recidivism data from one or more reference samples. A patient is then scored using the actuarial tool (there are 12 items on the VRAG, which are variably weighted) and then "matched" to a pre-existing set of patients with the same risk factor profile. The tool then generates a numerical estimate of risk over a period of time (such as over the next 10 or 15 years.) It is important to ensure the given actuarial tool is appropriate and validated for the relevant patient population – for example, the VRAG (and many other actuarial tools) is not validated for female patients, as there were no female offenders in the original reference sample. Although actuarial tools, as a group, perform reasonably well at predicting violent recidivism,[8] they do not provide information on when a given patient is at a relatively higher or lower risk for violence, or what interventions may be helpful in mitigating that risk. They focus purely on historical, or static, variables, such as the presence of childhood behavioural problems, psychiatric diagnoses, and the presence of past criminal convictions.

In contrast, structured professional judgment (SPJ) tools incorporate both historical/static and dynamic, or changeable, variables. A widely used SPJ tool used in violence risk prediction is the HCR-20 (currently in its third iteration).[10] The HCR-20 incorporates 10 historical risk factors (such as a history of violence), 5 clinical risk factors (such as recent problems with insight or symptoms of major mental disorder), and 5 risk management items (such as the likelihood an individual will experience significant stress over the coming supervision period, or the likelihood they will have difficulties with housing or supervision/treatment responsiveness.) After considering the risk factors outlined in the HCR-20 manual, the clinician makes an informed opinion on whether the level of risk for the upcoming supervision period is low, moderate, or high (in contrast with actuarial tools, which provide a more specific percentile estimate of recidivism). Aside from the HCR-20, there are many SPJ tools available to address specific types of violence or populations, such as youth violence, spousal violence, or sexual violence.

Recently, there has been a push to consider patient strengths when assessing risk for violence. The Structured Assessment of Protective Factors for Violence Risk (SAPROF) is an example of a strength based SPJ tool, which can complement the more traditional deficit-focused considerations in tools such as the HCR-20.[11] The SAPROF considers internal factors (such as intelligence, copping, and self-control), motivational factors (such as work, goals, and motivation for treatment), and external factors (such as a social network or intimate relationships) which serve to mitigate risk. There is some evidence that the use of strength-based instruments by forensic teams improves feelings of hope and can assist teams in refocusing their interventions.[12]

There has been an at-times heated debate about the relative utility of actuarial or SPJ tools.[13] SPJ tools may be more helpful in managing risk in forensic outpatients, as they provide information around how risk can be mitigated, and when risk may be relatively higher or lower. For example, when a patient loses their housing, experiences increased stress, and has a relapse of symptoms, appropriate strategies can be implemented to address those clinical and risk management variables.

Formalized training is often recommended or required when using specific risk assessment instruments. Such training is typically done by accredited in-person or online workshops. Although risk assessment instruments are traditionally administered by forensic psychologists or psychiatrists, certain tools, such as the HCR-20, may benefit from the input of other allied healthcare staff, such as forensic social workers or occupational therapists.[10] It is typically necessary to conduct a comprehensive file review and interview patients and caregivers to generate an accurate risk assessment. Regardless of the tool being used, clinicians should be aware of their limitations, as they are likely to be examined on the same in court or review board hearings.

UNIQUE CONSIDERATIONS IN FORENSIC REHABILITATION

Personality Disorder and Psychopathy

All mental health clinicians will be familiar with the diagnosis and treatment modalities recommended for personality disorders, as defined in the DSM-5 or ICD, which will not be covered in this chapter. Forensic patients often have comorbid personality disorders, which can increase their risk for violence and complicate their care. Psychopathy, a personality construct of particular relevance to forensic mental healthcare, can be conceived of as a form of personality disorder. Although it is not a DSM-5 or ICD diagnosis, psychopathy shares feature with the cluster B personality disorders, including antisocial personality disorder and narcissistic personality disorder.[14] Psychopathic individuals tend to have affective deficits (for example, the prototypical psychopath is interpersonally superficial, has shallow affective experiences, lacks empathy, and lacks remorse), are interpersonally exploitative, and live impulsive, parasitic lifestyles.[15,16] Psychopathy is highly correlated to criminal behaviour, including violence, although not all psychopathic individuals are violent.[17] It is thus often more clinically useful to forensic clinicians than the traditional personality disorder diagnoses, especially when assessing violence risk.

A comprehensive review of psychopathy as a construct is beyond the scope of this chapter; but interested readers should be aware that a wide body of research exists on the subject in the published literature. As it pertains to risk assessment, an individual's level of psychopathy can be measured using the Psychopathy Checklist-Revised[16] (PCL-R), a validated psychological assessment instrument developed by the Canadian psychologist Robert Hare. Specialized training is required to administer the PCL-R, which is widely used in forensic risk assessment. As with most other risk assessment instruments, scoring individuals on the PCL-R typically involves patient and family/caregiver interviews, and reviewing collateral and historical information. The PCL-R manual describes the specific meaning of 20 items (glibness/superficial charm, poor behavioural controls, lack of empathy, juvenile delinquency, criminal versatility, etc.); individuals are then given a total psychopathy score out of 40. Although a PCL-R score alone does not provide a probabilistic risk estimate, it is highly relevant in other risk assessment instruments, such as the VRAG or the HCR-20, and is heavily weighted in risk evaluation.[13]

Substance Use Disorders in the Forensic Context

Individuals with severe mental illnesses, who make up the bulk of the forensic patient population, are frequently diagnosed with comorbid substance use disorders.[18,19] The negative outcomes related to substance misuse in this clinical population include risk of re-emergent psychosis, rehospitalization, homelessness, and incarceration.[20] Substance use is also a major risk factor for violence, especially when related to personality disorders and/or major mental illness,[21] making its management particularly relevant in the forensic context.

Forensic outreach teams should incorporate evidence-based substance use treatment modalities as part of their comprehensive care plans. The provision of support, assertive outreach, motivational interventions, and functional skill development all play a role in identifying and mitigating the risks related to substance abuse.[22] Assertive outreach, which may involve providing care in patient residences, helps to prevent relapses or treatment dropout.[18,22,23] Integrating mental health and substance abuse interventions under one clinical team allows interventions to be delivered in a coordinated fashion.[22]

Monitoring Substance Use

Monitoring patients for substance use in the community setting relies on a combination of self-report and drug testing. Accurate self-reporting relies on a trusting relationship between patients and clinicians, and may provide an economical and convenient means of monitoring for substance use when appropriate.[24]

Forensic clinicians strive to remain recovery-focused in managing substance use disorders, rather than appear punitive, which is at times challenging in the supervisory context of the forensic system. Admitting to drug use may have negative consequences for forensic patients, such as involuntary rehospitalization or a slower progression to freedom. Naturally, patients facing such a situation are incentivized to underreport or deny active substance use.[25,26] As such, objective drug testing is usually part of forensic risk management.

Random urine drug screening reduces illicit drug use.[27] Random drug testing should be completed as clinically relevant to a given patient, with those at a higher risk of relapse being screened more often than those who have progressed further in their recovery.[28] Urine drug tests are useful tools for assessing and monitoring substance use as they provide objective evidence indicating if a patient has consumed drugs or alcohol and may support or negate a patient's self-report.[28] Urine drug testing allows for a relatively non-invasive means of detecting if a patient has consumed illicit substances and typically has a detection window of several days, depending on the substance.[29] The appropriate use of urine drug testing can strengthen the therapeutic relationship and promote healthy behaviours and patient recovery.[28]

There are several different kinds of urine drug tests; clinicians should be aware of the strengths and limitations of available test methods in their areas. Rapid drug screening is often based on immunoassays, using antibodies to detect the presence of drug metabolites. Such tests are typically sensitive and cost-effective and provide a rapid turnaround time, allowing teams to make timely patient care and risk management decisions.[29,30] Unfortunately, immunoassay-based tests have significant false-positive and false-negative rates due to cross-reactivity and sensitivity inherent in the tests.[28,30,31] Test results should thus be considered provisional and paired with clinical judgement, patient history, collateral information related to changes in mental status/patient presentation; consideration should be given to confirmatory testing when appropriate.[32,33] The decision as to whether hospital readmission is required or not is still based on an overall risk assessment, as individuals actively using substances may still be manageable in the community. However, if a patient had a relapse of psychotic and/or affective symptoms, and began to pose a greater risk to public safety, hospital readmission may be indicated, regardless of the specific aetiology.

Gas chromatography-mass spectrometry (GC-MS) is regarded as the gold standard in confirmatory testing for drug analysis.[31,34] GC-MS is highly sensitive and specific and is able to identify both specific substances and the quantities likely consumed.[28,31,35] GC-MS testing is more expensive than immunoassay testing and requires specialized machinery. It also has a longer turnaround time (up to 1 week) and so should be used in conjunction with rapid drug screening and ordered when needed.[28]

Forensic outreach teams need to be mindful that urine drug testing is susceptible to patient tampering, especially if patients provide samples without direct observation.[24] There are many ways that patients can tamper with test samples which impair the accuracy of detection and may mask the presence of substances in the urine.[36] Additional testing of the specimen to determine if tampering has occurred may be prudent if there is an apparent dissonance between a change in presentation and a negative drug test result. Additional testing may include creatinine, specific gravity, pH, and oxidants (nitrites), which can help to determine if the specimen has been diluted, substituted, adulterated, or is otherwise invalid.[33] Further, designer drugs (such as synthetic cannabinoids) are increasing in prevalence and present some challenge in testing due to continual changes in synthetic compounds.[32]

While drug testing is useful in identifying substance use, effective management of substance use disorders requires integration of clinical/therapeutic skills and supports into the care model. Forming shared goals around that care can be difficult, as many patients with comorbid major mental illness and substance use disorders have little readiness or engagement with abstinence-oriented treatment, and relapse in that context is a common occurrence.[22,37,38]

Keeping a Therapeutic Focus Within a Compulsory Abstinence-Based System

Abstinence-based substance use disorder programs have some drawbacks. Programs often label relapse a failure, rather than part of the recovery process, and can both negatively impact the therapeutic relationship and result in attempts to conceal substance use.[39] Harm reduction models represent relatively new and effective approaches to assisting in substance use recovery.[40] Such models generally tolerate ongoing substance use, instead focusing on reducing the harms associated with the same, while gradually moving patients forward in their insight and motivation to change. However, due to the legal restrictions outlined by review board dispositions, harm reduction models of care are often not practical or possible for forensic patients (if substance use is a violence risk factor in a given patient, review boards in Canada generally prohibit substance use altogether).

While harm reduction may not be practical in the forensic context, many principals are still useful. Effective substance use interventions should incorporate counselling that promotes cognitive and behavioural skill development (to manage cravings and reduce the frequency of use), motivational interventions (to help patients perceive develop insight and motivation to change, and recognize the relationship between their substance use and other mental health problems), social skill and relationship development to increase engagement with prosocial activities, and a focus on developing and employing strategies of relapse prevention to maintain recovery.[22,41]

Forensic outreach team members share responsibility for substance abuse service delivery. They seek to provide appropriate treatments and modify traditional interventions to fit the forensic context as necessary.[18,22] Throughout their interventions, they provide psychoeducation, support goal-setting, and seek to foster insight and instil hope into individuals with comorbid substance use disorders.[22,41]

Problematic Sexual Behaviours

Individuals with major mental illness and comorbid sexual behaviour problems often enter the forensic system following episodes of sexual violence. Consequently, understanding how to formulate sexually violent behaviours, assess risk for re-offence, and implement management strategies is an important component of forensic mental healthcare.

The factors driving sexually violent behaviours can be diverse.[42] For example, sexual behaviours may occur in the context of mood problems, disorganized psychotic symptoms, or poor social skills, amongst others. Individuals who would not otherwise be sexually violent may act with impaired judgment under the influence of a substance use disorder. Empathy deficits (related to psychopathy, for example) may lead to all manner of antisocial behaviours, including sexual violence. A comprehensive sexological assessment is thus recommended to assist in understanding a given patient's pathway to sexual violence and implement appropriate interventions.

Table 39.1 Paraphilic disorders described in DSM-5.

- Voyeuristic disorder: sexual arousal is associated with observing an unsuspecting person who is naked, in the process of disrobing, or engaging in sexual activity.
- Exhibitionistic disorder: arousal from exposing genitals to an unsuspecting person.
- Frotteuristic disorder: arousal from touching or rubbing against a nonconsenting person.
- Sexual masochism disorder: arousal from experiencing humiliation, bondage, or suffering.
- Sexual sadism disorder: arousal from inflicting humiliation, bondage or suffering on another.
- Paedophilic disorder: sexual arousal from children and/or pre-pubescent adolescents
- Fetishistic disorder: sexual arousal from specific non-living objects or having a highly specific focus on non-genital body parts.
- Transvestic disorder: sexual arousal from cross-dressing.

When a patient has a history of problematic sexual behaviours, special consideration is given to the possible diagnosis of a paraphilic disorder (although not all individuals with sexual violence history have paraphilias).

Paraphilias are defined in DSM-5 as any intense and persistent sexual interest other than sexual interest in genital stimulation or preparatory fondling with phenotypically normal, physically mature, consenting human partners.[43] Hundreds of unique paraphilic interests have been described.[44] The DSM-5 outlines eight specific paraphilic disorders, wherein sexual arousal is associated with specific fantasies or behaviours, as outlined in Table 39.1.

The designation of paraphilias as a mental disorder can be controversial, with many objecting to pathologizing sexual practices, however unusual, between consenting adults. However, individuals experiencing distress from their sexual fantasies/behaviours continue to be referred to mental health services.[45] The DSM-5 distinguishes between simply having a paraphilia (essentially, an atypical sexual preference) and having a *paraphilic disorder*. To be considered a disorder, a paraphilia must be causing distress or impairment to the individual, or the satisfaction of the sexual behaviour has to entail personal harm (or risk of harm) to others.[43]

The Sexological Assessment

Formal sexological evaluation often occurs in the context of specialized sexual behaviour clinics. A sexual behaviours assessment includes the demographic and clinical issues typically reviewed during a general psychiatric consultation, including taking a detailed demographic, psychiatric, and substance use history. However, additional consideration is given to sexual history. Clinicians pay special attention to early childhood experiences with sexuality and family beliefs, as well as pubertal developmental history. The number and nature of past sexual partners is considered, including the use of sex trade workers or telephone sex lines. Masturbatory practices and genera of pornography viewed also provides clues to guide a sexological formulation. As individuals in the forensic context are typically referred for sexological evaluation following problematic sexual behaviours, risk issues have to be considered, including access to children, capacity for empathy, and typical stress-coping mechanisms.[46] Patients with sex offence histories often have insight deficits and deploy typical cognitive distortions, such as minimization or denial of their violence, to facilitate their behaviour.[42] As patients are often understandably not forthcoming with information, interviewing partners, caregivers, and reviewing legal histories is also relevant.

Beyond the psychiatric interview and collateral information review, phallometric testing can be helpful both diagnostically and in assessing risk for violence.[47] Different techniques have been used, but all phallometric testing methods involve measuring changes in penile tumescence in response to visual or auditory sexual stimuli. For example, images of individuals of different age groups and genders are often shown to clarify the possible presence of a paedophilic disorder, or audiotapes of consenting and non-consenting sexual encounters may reveal a coercive sexual preference (such as in sexual sadism disorder). A positive result on a phallometric testing is associated with an increased risk for future violence.[48] However, such test should be considered in the context of a comprehensive sexual violence risk assessment, which includes the use of relevant actuarial and SPJ tools.

Treatment of Problematic Sexual Behaviours

Prior to treating patients with sexual offence histories, clinicians have to consider ethical issues,[49] including how the at-times coercive nature of the legal system impacts informed consent[46] and the serious risks of many sex-drive reducing medications.

The formulation generated by a comprehensive sexological assessment ultimately guides treatment interventions. Recall that there are many pathways to sexual violence, and not all of them include an underlying paraphilic disorder. For example, if substance use, psychosis, or mood issues underlie historical problematic behaviours, those variables should be individually addressed.

Both psychotherapy and pharmacotherapy play a role in managing problematic sexual behaviours; combining modalities likely leads to better outcomes.[8,50] Psychotherapy can be individual or group based and often involves insight-oriented, cognitive-behavioural, and supportive modalities. Such therapies generally attempt to address underlying cognitive distortions which facilitate offending behaviour (such as beliefs that children can consent to sex or are not harmed by abuse). Therapists also assist patients in recognizing dangerous situations and preventing relapse.[51]

Pharmacotherapeutic treatments are often used to reduce sex drive and are thought to decrease the risk of recidivism, although evidence of their effectiveness in that regard is limited.[52] The World Federation of Societies of Biological Psychiatry Guidelines provide an algorithm for when and which sex drive reducing medications are indicated.[46] Generally, more mild cases of problematic sexual behaviours (such as distressing fantasies alone) are treated with psychotherapy, plus or minus serotonin-reuptake inhibitors (SSRIs), which reduce sex drive as a side effect. As the seriousness and frequency of sexual offending behaviour increases, GnRH agonists (such as leuprolide acetate), and antiandrogen medications (such as cyproterone acetate) become indicated. Such hormonal medications come with a host of serious endocrine and metabolic risks and thus require careful monitoring.

Of course, aside from simply providing psychotherapy and medication to patients within the forensic system, an overarching supervisory and rehabilitative framework is required. If and when such patients are permitted to live in the community, supervision and treatment is typically delivered by forensic outreach teams.

FORENSIC OUTREACH: PROVIDING CARE FOR PATIENTS IN THE COMMUNITY

Forensic patients often begin their journey as hospital inpatients, but ideally, as their symptoms and risk profile improve, they are transitioned into the community, where their care continues, provided by outpatient clinicians. Community outreach mental health teams have a unique set of challenges. Their goal is not only to support the functional recovery of their patients (harnessing the perspectives and interventions from multiple disciplines) but also to manage their risk for violence and thus protect public safety. They have to monitor and address risk factors (such as medication non-adherence or substance use) and rely on legal tools for support when risk is elevated, especially if a patient's insight and internal motivation are underdeveloped. Outreach teams also have to provide care that is variably intensive, in order to meet the needs of patients at various stages of recovery.

Models of Community Care: ACT and FACT Teams

Assertive community treatment (ACT) teams involve multidisciplinary teams (psychiatrists, mental health nurses, allied healthcare staff, and case managers), which assist with a range of services (including clinical care and housing) with a high ratio of staff to patients, relative to traditional outpatient mental healthcare.[53,54,55,56] The ACT model is an effective means of providing care to high-needs community-dwelling patients who are otherwise not easily engaged.[53,57] Patients served with a community-focused ACT model are generally more engaged and satisfied with their care than with traditional outpatient programs.[54,58,59,60]

Forensic assertive community treatment (FACT), a relatively new model, differs from ACT in that it targets individuals with legal histories.[61,62,63] The multidisciplinary staff on FACT teams have specialized legal knowledge and coordinate with the justice system. They also have expertise in violence risk assessment and management. Within a forensic system, FACT teams are supported by legal structures to enforce at-times compulsory engagement in care.[61,64] Like traditional ACT teams, FACT teams reduce re-hospitalizations, treatment adherence, and quality of life, but they also reduce arrest frequency and time spent in jail.[1,65,66]

FACT teams generally comprise 11–12 clinicians who provide varying levels of service to up to 200 patients living in the community.[67] Practically, staff endeavour to support patients with whatever their recovery goals may be, and may provide care in home, school, work, or other settings as required. Each clinician on the FACT team contributes a discipline-specific skillset: the guiding philosophy is one of holistic rehabilitation and recovery. Team members typically include nurses (who assist with medication administration, psychoeducation, and assessment), occupational therapists (who formally assess functional and implement strategies to assist with living skills, education, and employment), social workers (who focus on psychosocial functioning and may provide specialized supports with substance use, for example), therapeutic recreation specialists (who support community participation and leisure activities), and psychiatrists.[68]

Forensic Outreach Service Delivery

All team members share in providing direct patient care, which may include traditional therapeutic modalities such as medication and evidence-based psychotherapies. Concurrently, they assess and manage violence risk factors, including active psychotic symptoms, substance use, and personality disorder.[61,69,70] As patients progress in their recovery, the emphasis shifts from purely pharmacological interventions to linking individuals with stable housing, meaningful structured activity (including, but not limited to, employment), social support networks, and positive stress-management mechanisms, which all reduce the risk for violence.[10]

The intensity of support forensic outreach teams deliver exists on a continuum. Some patients may require daily, assertive care, including mental status assessments, medication delivery/monitoring, and random urine drug screening. Members of the team thus have to be "on call" 24 hours a day.[73] Other patients may only need a less "hands-on" approach, such as occasional assistance with their goals, and are supervised only as required by their review board dispositions (for example, they may be required to "report to" their team four times per month, akin to a probation officer). Forensic teams thus match specific patient strengths and risk factors to specific interventions, stepping forward and backward as appropriate to manage risk and support recovery. Such flexibility enhances continuity of care and reduces disengagement.[67]

Forensic clinicians are responsible for discussing risk issues with their patients. As insight develops, they assist patients in recognizing of early warning signs of psychological decompensation and developing (and reviewing) safety plans.[71] Ideally, as patients require less and less active service provision during the process of their recoveries, their professional supports transition from intensive forensic outreach (such as FACT teams) to community mental health partners, in preparation for eventual discharge from the forensic system.

The Compulsory Nature of Forensic Mental Healthcare

Tenure in a forensic system can create a complicated narrative for both patients and providers. An ethical tension exists when care providers, in a traditional clinician-patient treatment role, also serve as risk assessors. From the patient perspective, although they are managed within a healthcare paradigm, their liberties are still significantly curtailed by review boards. Ultimately, however, incorporating legal authority through the compulsory nature of forensic mental healthcare prevents unnecessary incarceration and allows patients to live in the community. It also helps ensure treatment adherence (and thus reduces risk) when internal motivation or insight are lacking.[63] In general, judicial orders that compel patients with significant mental health challenges to participate in community treatment reduce time spent in hospital and paradoxically increase personal freedoms.[72]

Forensic healthcare providers should be mindful not to use the legal leverage inherent in judicial orders or review board dispositions as a form of punishment. Using the legal tools afforded within the forensic system should be used only when carefully considered risk assessment indicates they are required to prevent violence.[61] For example, if a patient in the community, previously doing well in their recovery, becomes nonadherent with their medication, relapses into substance use, withdraws from their volunteering placement, and develops psychotic symptoms, returning them to hospital against their will may be necessary to both manage risk to the community and re-engage them in their recovery. Such actions should be guided by the principle of using the least restrictive intervention necessary to manage risk. The combination of assertive outreach and legal leverage represents a critical balance in creating and maintaining a mental healthcare rehabilitation program that also addresses and mitigates risk.[63]

A System of Transitions

Transition is a major theme in forensic mental healthcare, for both patients and providers. Ideally, acutely unwell hospital inpatients transition into the community, community patients transition to less restrictive legal orders as their risk for violence decreases, and successful patients in the community transition to non-forensic professional supports in preparation for discharge from the forensic system.

It is important to be mindful of the at-times stressful nature of transition into the community and ultimately to freedom. Although patients may be moving forward, they face new challenges that could result in psychological decompensation during this vulnerable period. The process of transitioning to community care typically begins while a given patient is still a hospital inpatient. Forensic inpatients gradually develop community contacts and structure while still living in hospital: for example, patients may gain employment or begin attending school programs. When they transition and become forensic outpatients, they can thus continue to their pre-existing routines. "Testing the waters" in the community, while still living in hospital, allows for a more informed risk assessment and discharge plan.

When it becomes foreseeable that a forensic inpatient will likely be living in the community before long, the forensic outreach team begins to develop a therapeutic alliance, even prior to their move. They coordinate with the inpatient team and transfer important clinical information while establishing community-based goals to guide their rehabilitation after discharge.[73]

Once living in the community, the forensic outreach team begins to focus on transitioning care to other community services. To that end, the team prioritizes rehabilitative work related to community living and participation skills, which are necessary for enhanced independence or transition to less intensive levels of care.[53] Transferring patients back to local, traditional mental health services ideally occurs in a graduated way, following a period of stability under the care of the forensic team in the community. Given the wide range of communities (both urban and rural) overseen by forensic outreach teams, this may also involve the team advocating for and supporting the development of appropriate local services if none exist.

Over time, as patients progress in their recovery, review boards typically reduce the restrictiveness of legal orders, in concert with risk assessment. The increased level of patient liberty ultimately enables them to connect with local community services.[69,74,75] Outreach teams coordinate with local non-forensic care providers, sharing information about successful care strategies. Local providers begin to establish therapeutic relationships while the legal authority of the forensic system still remains in place. Such a gradual process mitigates the risk of losing clinical gains (and ultimately liberties) realized while patients were in the forensic system while still moving towards greater independence.[54,76,77,78]

References

1. Cuddeback, G. S., Morrissey, J. P., & Cusack, K. J. (2008). How many forensic assertive community treatment teams do we need?. *Psychiatric Services*, 59(2), 205–208.
2. Harper, R. F. (Ed.). (1999). *The Code of Hammurabi, King of Babylon: About 2250 BC: Autographed Text, Transliteration, Translation, Glossary Index of Subjects, Lists of Proper Names, Signs, Numuerals . . .* UK: The Lawbook Exchange, Ltd.
3. Schneider, R. D. (2013). History of mens rea and the evolution of the concept of criminal responsibility. In H. Bloom & R. D. Schneider (Eds.), *Law and Mental Disorder: A Comprehensive and Practical Approach* (pp. 249–261). Toronto, ON: Irwin Law.
4. Quinn, J., & Simpson, A. I. (2013). How can forensic systems improve justice for victims of offenders found not criminally responsible? *Journal of the American Academy of Psychiatry and the Law*.
5. Singh, J. P., Grann, M., & Fazel, S. (2011). A comparative study of violence risk assessment tools: A systematic review and metaregression analysis of 68 studies involving 25,980 participants. *Clinical Psychology Review*, 31(3), 499–513.
6. Quinsey, V. L., & Ambtman, R. (1979). Variables affecting psychiatrists' and teachers' assessments of the dangerousness of mentally ill offenders. *Journal of Consulting and Clinical Psychology*, 47(2), 353.
7. Bonta, J. (1996). Risk-needs assessment and treatment. In A. T. Harland (Ed.), *Choosing Correctional Options That Work: Defining the Demand and Evaluating the Supply* (pp. 18–32). Thousand Oaks, CA: Sage.
8. Hanson, R. K., & Morton-Bourgon, K. E. (2009). The accuracy of recidivism risk assessments for sexual offenders: A meta-analysis of 118 prediction studies. *Psychological Assessment*, 21(1), 1.
9. Harris, G. T., Rice, M. E., & Quinsey, V. L. (1993). Violent recidivism of mentally disordered offenders: The development of a statistical prediction instrument. *Criminal Justice and Behavior*, 20, 315–335.
10. Douglas, K. S., Hart, S. D., Webster, C. D., & Belfrage, H. (2013). *HCR20V3: Assessing Risk for Violence: User Guide*. Burnaby, Canada: Mental Health, Law, and Policy Institute, Simon Fraser University.

11. Robbé, M., de Vogel, V., & Stam, J. (2019). Protective factors for violence risk: The value for clinical practice. *Psych*, 3(12), 1259–1263.
12. Domjancic, T., Wilkie, T., Darani, S., Williams, B., Maheru, B., & Jamal, Z. (2019). Clinicians' perceptions of the implementation of the Structured Assessment of Protective Factors for Violence Risk (SAPROF) on an inpatient forensic unit. *International Journal of Risk and Recovery*, 2(2), 18–27.
13. Bloom, H., Webster, C., Hucker, S., & De Freitas, K. (2005). The Canadian contribution to violence risk assessment: History and implications for current psychiatric practice. *The Canadian Journal of Psychiatry*, 50(1), 3–11.
14. Wulach, J. S. (1988). The criminal personality as a DSM-III-R antisocial, narcissistic, borderline, and histrionic personality disorder. *International Journal of Offender Therapy and Comparative Criminology*, 32(3), 185–199.
15. Cleckley, H. M. (1951). The mask of sanity. *Postgraduate Medicine*, 9(3), 193–197.
16. Hare, R. D. (2003). *The Hare Psychopathy Checklist: Revised* (2nd ed.). Toronto, ON: Multi-Health Systems.
17. Lilienfeld, S. O., & Arkowitz, H. (2007). What "psychopath" means. *Scientific American Mind*, 18(6), 80–81.
18. Essock, S. M., Mueser, K. T., Drake, R. E., et al. (2006). Comparison of ACT and standard case management for delivering integrated treatment for co-occurring disorders. *Psychiatric Services*, 57(2), 185–196. doi: 10.1176/appi.ps.57.2.185
19. Rossman, S. B., Willison, J. B., Mallik-Kane, K., Kim, K., Debus-Sherrill, P., & Downey, P. M. (2012). *Criminal Justice Interventions for Offenders with Mental Illness: Evaluation of Mental Health Courts in Bronx and Brooklyn, New York*. Washington, DC: US Department of Justice, National Institute of Justice.
20. Essock, S. M., Mueser, K. T., Drake, R. E., et al. (2006). Comparison of ACT and standard case management for delivering integrated treatment for co-occurring disorders. *Psychiatric Services*, 57(2), 185–196. doi: 10.1176/appi.ps.57.2.185
21. Van Dorn, R., Volavka, J., & Johnson, N. (2012). Mental disorder and violence: Is there a relationship beyond substance use? *Social Psychiatry and Psychiatric Epidemiology*, 47, 487–503. doi: 10.1007/s00127-011-0356-x
22. Drake, R. E., Essock, S. M., Shaner, A., Carey, K. B., Minkoff, K., Kola, L., Lynde, D., Osher, F. C., Clark, R. E., & Rickards, L. (2001). Implementing dual diagnosis services for clients with severe mental illness. *Psychiatric Services (Washington, D.C.)*, 52(4), 469–476. doi: 10.1176/appi.ps.52.4.469
23. Beach, C., Dykema, L.-R., Appelbaum, P. S., Deng, L., Leckman-Westin, E., Manuel, J. I., & Finnerty, M. T. (2013). Forensic and nonforensic clients in assertive community treatment: A longitudinal study. *Psychiatric Services*, 64(5), 437–444. doi: 10.1176/appi.ps.201200170
24. Kilpatrick, B., Howlett, M., Sedgwick, P., & Ghodse, A. H. (2000). Drug use, self report and urinalysis. *Drug and Alcohol Dependence*, 58(1–2), 111–116. doi: 10.1016/s0376-8716(99)00066-6
25. Jackson, C. T., Covell, N. H., Frisman, L. K., & Essock, S. M. (2005). Validity of self-reported drug use among people with co-occurring mental health and substance use disorders. *Journal of Dual Diagnosis*, 1, 49–63. doi: 10.1300/J374v01n01_05
26. Connors, G. J., & Volk, R. J. (2003). Self: Report screening for alcohol problems among adults. In J. P. Allen & V. B. Wilson (Eds.), *Assessing Alcohol Problems: A Guide for Clinicians and Researchers* (2nd ed.). New York: U.S. Department of Health and Human Services.
27. Manchikanti, L., Manchukonda, R., Pampati, V., Damron, K. S., Brandon, D. E., Cash, K. A., & McManus, C. D. (2006). Does random urine drug testing reduce illicit drug use in chronic pain patients receiving opioids? *Pain Physician*, 9(2), 123–129.
28. Li, X., Moore, S., & Olson, C. (2019). Urine drug tests: How to make the most of them: Effective use of UDTs requires carefully interpreting the results, and modifying treatment accordingly. *Current Psychiatry*, 18(8), 10–20.
29. Thomas, S. N., & Knezevic, C. E. (2019). Urine drug screens: Caveats for interpreting results. *Contemporary Pediatrics*, 36(6).
30. Taylor, E. H., Oertli, E. H., Wolfgang, J. W., & Mueller, E. (1999). Accuracy of five on-site immunoassay drugs-of-abuse testing devices. *Journal of Analytical Toxicology*, 23(2), 119–124. doi.org/10.1093/jat/23.2.119
31. Moeller, K. E., Lee, K. C., & Kissack, J. C. (2008). Urine drug screening: Practical guide for clinicians. *Mayo Clinic Proceedings*, 83(1), 66–76. doi.org/10.4065/83.1.66
32. Moeller, K. E., Kissack, J. C., Atayee, R. S., & Lee, K. C. (2017). Clinical interpretation of urine drug tests: What clinicians need to know about urine drug screens. *Mayo Clinic Proceedings*, 92(5), 774–796. doi.org/10.1016/j.mayocp.2016.12.007

33. Smith, M. P., & Bluth, M. H. (2016). Forensic toxicology: An introduction. *Clinics in Laboratory Medicine*, 36(4), 753–759. doi.org/10.1016/j.cll.2016.07.002
34. Harper, L., Powell, J., & Pijl, E. (2017). An overview of forensic drug testing methods and their suitability for harm reduction point-of-care services. *Harm Reduction Journal*, 14. doi: 10.1186/s12954-017-0179-5
35. Jannetto, P. J., & Fitzgerald, R. L. (2016). Effective use of mass spectrometry in the clinical laboratory. *Clinical Chemistry*, 62(1), 92–98. doi.org/10.1373/clinchem.2015.248146
36. Jaffee, W. B., Trucco, E., Levy, S., & Weiss, R. D. (2007). Is this urine really negative? A systematic review of tampering methods in urine drug screening and testing. *Journal of Substance Abuse Treatment*, 33(1), 33–42. doi.org/10.1016/j.jsat.2006.11.008
37. Ziedonis, D. M., & Trudeau, K. (1997). Motivation to quit using substances among individuals with schizophrenia: Implications for a motivation-based treatment model. *Schizophrenia Bulletin*, 23(2), 229–238. doi.org/10.1093/schbul/23.2.229
38. Hubbard, R. L., Craddock, S. G., & Anderson, J. (2003). Overview of 5-year followup outcomes in the drug abuse treatment outcome studies (DATOS). *Journal of Substance Abuse Treatment*, 25(3), 125–134. doi: 10.1016/s0740-5472(03)00130-2
39. Mancini, M. A., Linhorst, D. M., Broderick, F., & Bayliff, S. (2008). Challenges to implementing the harm reduction approach. *Journal of Social Work Practice in the Addictions*, 8(3), 380–408. doi: 10.1080/15332560802224576
40. Henwood, B. F., Padgett, D. K., & Tiderington, E. (2014). Provider views of harm reduction versus abstinence policies within homeless services for dually diagnosed adults. *Journal of Behavioral Health Services and Research*, 41(1), 80–89. doi:10.1007/s11414-013-9318
41. Greenfield, S. F., Weiss, R. D., & Tohen, M. (1995). Substance abuse and the chronically mentally ill: A description of dual diagnosis treatment services in a psychiatric hospital. *Community Mental Health Journal*, 31(3), 265–277. doi.org/10.1007/BF02188753
42. Barbaree, H., Greenberg, D., & Fugere, R. (2013). Overview of sex offenders and the paraphilias. In H. Bloom & R. D. Schneider (Eds.), *Law and Mental Disorder: A Comprehensive and Practical Approach* (pp. 765–782). Toronto, ON: Irwin Law.
43. American Psychiatric Association. (2013). *Diagnostic and Statistical Manual of Mental Disorders* (5th ed.). Arlington, VA: American Psychiatric Press.
44. Fedoroff, J. P., & Marshall, W. L. (2010). *Paraphilias*. New York: APA.
45. Thibaut, et al. (2010). The world federation of societies of biological psychiatry, guidelines for the biological treatment of paraphilias. *The World Journal of Biological Psychiatry*, 11(1), 604–655. BJ Psych, 20(3).
46. Freund, K., & Blanchard, R. (1989). Phallometric diagnosis of pedophilia. *Journal of Consulting and Clinical psychology*, 57(1), 100.
47. Quinsey, V. L., Harris, G. T., Rice, M. E., & Cormier, C. A. (2006). *Violent Offenders: Appraising and Managing Risk*. New York: American Psychological Association.
48. Yakeley, J., & Wood, H. (2014). Paraphilias and paraphilic disorders: Diagnosis, assessment and management. *Advances in Psychiatric Treatment*, 20(3), 202–213.
49. Belgian Advisory Committee on Bioethics. (2006). *Opinion no. 39 of December 18th 2006 on Hormonal Treatment of Sex Offenders*. Brussels, Belgium: Belgium Advisory Committee on Bioethics. Retrieved from www.health.belgium.be/en/opinion-no-39-hormonal-treatment-sex-offenders.
50. McConaghy, N. (1998). Paedophilia: A review of the evidence. *Australian & New Zealand Journal of Psychiatry*, 32(2), 252–265.
51. Hall, Ryan, & Hall, Richard. (2007). A profile of pedophilia: Definition, characteristics of offenders, recidivism, treatment outcomes, and forensic issues. Mayo Clinic proceedings, Mayo Clinic. 82.
52. Khan, O., Ferriter, M., Huband, N., Powney, M. J., Dennis, J. A., & Duggan, C. (2015). Pharmacological interventions for those who have sexually offended or are at risk of offending. *Cochrane Database of Systematic Reviews*, (2).
53. Heard, C. P., Scott, J., Tetzlaff, A., et al. (2019). Transitional housing in forensic mental health: Considering consumer lived experience. *Health Justice*, 7, 8. doi: 10.1186/s40352-019-0091-z
54. Finnerty, M. T., Manuel, J. I., Tochterman, A. Z., et al. (2015). Clinicians' perceptions of challenges and strategies of transition from assertive community treatment to less intensive services. *Community Mental Health Journal*, 51, 85–95. doi: 10.1007/s10597-014-9706-y
55. Allness, D. J., & Knoedler, W. H. (1998). *The PACT Model of Community-Based Treatment for Persons with Severe and Persistent Mental Illness: A Manual for PACT Start-Up*. Arlington: NAMI.
56. Anthony, W. A., Cohen, M. R., & Farkas, M. D. (1990). *Psychiatric Rehabilitation*. Boston: Boston University, Center for Psychiatric Rehabilitation.

57. Salyers, M. P., & Tsemberis, S. (2007). ACT and recovery: Integrating evidence based practice and recovery orientation on assertive community treatment teams. *Community Mental Health Journal*, 43(6), 619–641. doi: 10.1007/s10597-007-9088-5
58. Stein, L. I., & Santos, A. B. (1998). *Assertive Community Treatment of Persons with Severe Mental Illness*. New York: Norton.
59. Rosen, A., Killaspy, H., & Harvey, C. (2013). Specialisation and marginalisation: How the assertive community treatment debate affects individuals with complex mental health needs. *The Psychiatrist*, 37(11), 345–348. doi: 10.1192/pb.bp.113.044537
60. Edwards, T., Macpherson, R., Commander, M., Meaden, A., & Kalidindi, S. (2016). Services for people with complex psychosis: Towards a new understanding. *BJPsych Bulletin*, 40(3), 156–161. doi: 10.1192/pb.bp.114.050278
61. Lamberti, J. S., Weisman, R. L., Cerulli, C., Williams, G. C., Jacobowitz, D. B., Mueser, K. T., Marks, P. D., Strawderman, R. L., Harrington, D., Lamberti, T. A., & Caine, E. D. (2017). A randomized controlled trial of the Rochester forensic assertive community treatment model. *Psychiatric Services*, 68, 1016–1024. doi: 10.1176/appi.ps.201600329
62. Jennings, J. L. (2009). Does assertive community treatment work with forensic populations? *Review and Recommendations*.
63. Lamberti, J. S., Weisman, R., & Faden, D. I. (2004). Forensic assertive community treatment: Preventing incarceration of adults with severe mental illness. *Psychiatric Services (Washington, D. C.)*, 55(11), 1285–1293.
64. Lamberti J. S. (2007). Understanding and preventing criminal recidivism among adults with psychotic disorders. *Psychiatric Services*, 58, 773–781.
65. Nugter, M. A., Engelsbel, F., Bähler, M., et al. (2016). Outcomes of FLEXIBLE assertive community treatment (FACT) implementation: A prospective real life study. *Community Mental Health Journal*, 52, 898–907. doi: 10.1007/s10597-015-9831-2
66. Firn, M., Hindhaugh, K., Hubbeling, D., Davies, G., Jones, B., & White, S. J. (2012). A dismantling study of assertive outreach services: Comparing activity and outcomes following replacement with the FACT model. *Social Psychiatry and Psychiatric Epidemiology*, 48, 997–1003.
67. Van Veldhuizen, J. R., & Bahler, M. (2015). *Manual flexible assertive community treatment (FACT)*. doi: 10.13140/RG.2.1.3925.1683
68. Bitter, N., Roeg, D., van Nieuwenhuizen, C., et al. (2016). Identifying profiles of service users in housing services and exploring their quality of life and care needs. *BMC Psychiatry*, 16, 419. doi: 10.1186/s12888-016-1122-0
69. Kent, A., & Burns, T. (2005). Assertive community treatment in UK practice: Revisiting . . . Setting up an assertive community treatment team. *Advances in Psychiatric Treatment*, 11(6), 388–397. doi: 10.1192/apt.11.6.388
70. Weisman, R., Lamberti, J., & Price, N. (2004). Integrating criminal justice, community healthcare, and support services for adults with severe mental disorders. *Psychiatric Quarterly*, 75, 71–85. doi: 10.1023/B:PSAQ.0000007562.37428.52
71. Van Veldhuizen, J. R. (2007). FACT: A Dutch version of ACT. *Community Mental Health Journal*, 43, 421–433. doi: 10.1007/s10597-007-9089-4
72. Frank, D., Perry, J. C., Kean, D., et al. (2005). Effects of compulsory treatment orders on time to hospital readmission. *Psychiatric Services*, 56(7), 867–869. doi: 10.1176/appi.ps.56.7.867
73. Beach, C., Dykema, L.-R., Appelbaum, P. S., Deng, L., Leckman-Westin, E., Manuel, J. I., & Finnerty, M. T. (2013). Forensic and nonforensic clients in assertive community treatment: A longitudinal study. *Psychiatric Services*, 64(5), 437–444. doi: 10.1176/appi.ps.201200170
74. Kent, A., & Burns, T. (2005). Assertive community treatment in UK practice: Revisiting . . . Setting up an assertive community treatment team. *Advances in Psychiatric Treatment*, 11(6), 388–397. doi: 10.1192/apt.11.6.388
75. Edwards, T., Macpherson, R., Commander, M., Meaden, A., & Kalidindi, S. (2016). Services for people with complex psychosis: Towards a new understanding. *BJPsych Bulletin*, 40(3), 156–161. doi: 10.1192/pb.bp.114.050278
76. Rosenheck, R. A., & Dennis, D. (2001). Time-limited assertive community treatment for homeless persons with severe mental illness. *Archives of General Psychiatry*, 58, 1073–1080.
77. Rosenheck, R. A., Neale, M. S., & Mohamed, S. (2010). Transition to low intensity case management in a VA assertive community treatment model program. *Psychiatric Rehabilitation Journal*, 33(4), 288–296.
78. Hackman, A., & Stowell, K. (2009). Transitioning clients from assertive community treatment to traditional mental health services. *Community Mental Health Journal*, 45, 1–5.

40
Optimising Patient Care in the Community Using Psychopharmacology

Shorouq Motwani and Sagar Karia

Caregivers	437
Social Health Care Workers	438
Nurses	439
Pharmacists	440

Whenever the term 'psychosis' or 'psychiatric disorder' is said out loud, it usually has a negative connotation. The general trend is to avoid and shame psychiatric patients and their families. This aspect of psychiatric disorders contributes significantly to the delay in receiving diagnosis and treatment for psychiatric patients. Most commonly, such patients are given all of sorts of alternate treatment modalities except bringing them to appropriate psychiatric care by a qualified psychiatrist. The reasons for such a significant delay in appropriate management are also multiple.

Based on age-old traditions, the general community even today believes that any deviance from normal behaviour has either a spiritual component and can be relieved through specific rituals and customs or that the psychiatric patient is malingering or well under the control of his or her symptoms and can control his/her behaviour independently. The second major reason for the low success rate of remission in psychiatric disorders is stigma. Stigma as a term is often used synonymously with psychiatric or mental disorders, which simply means that not just the psychiatric patient but their family often are excluded from integrating into community activities. Such families are also shamed as being the reason for the patient's odd behaviour and are given the role of the accused in such scenarios. Thus, stigma serves as major impediment in delivering mental healthcare services.

Unfortunately, it is not just the general community but even medical professionals who are highly trained individuals in the subject of medical specialties and other healthcare professionals who stigmatise psychiatric patients. This contributes to the lack of knowledge and awareness about psychiatric disorders and mental health problems. Moreover, due to the relatively recent growth of the importance of psychiatric disorders and their treatment, the number of psychiatrists and other mental healthcare professionals remains severely low and thus creates a dire need for more mental health professionals. These issues cumulatively make psychiatric disorders one of the major causes of global disease burden. The treatment gap in developing countries has been 76–85%, according to WHO. According NMHS, it is 83% in India for psychiatric disorders and 86% for alcohol use disorders, indicating that mental morbidity above the age of 18 years is 10.6%, with a lifetime prevalence of 13.7%. This means that 150 million Indians need active psychiatric intervention. Mental and addictive disorders affected more than 1 billion people globally in 2016. Seven percent of the total global burden of disease as measured in disability adjusted life years and 19% of all years lived with disability are due to psychiatric disorders. Depression was the leading cause of disability in the world, and suicide was the tenth leading cause of death in 2015. Major depressive disorder (MDD) is the fourth cause of disability around the world and is estimated to become the second leading cause of disability by 2020, signifying the desperate need to optimise psychiatric patient care.

However, there is a ray of sunshine in this abysmal darkness: effective treatment of psychiatric disorders in the form of pharmacotherapy and psychotherapy provides much-needed relief for patients of various psychiatric disorders and thus gives proof that such treatments work and catalyse the process of getting patients adequate and appropriate care. Examples of such treatment include cognitive behavioural therapy, exposure therapy, dialectical behaviour therapy, and so on, in addition to various psychotropic medications. In order to provide such extensive services to patients, a multidisciplinary team provides the optimum support where not just psychiatrists but mental healthcare professionals coming into contact with patients at various points of treatment contribute to the care of the patient in sometimes ambiguous and at other times direct manners. Efforts to improve the outcomes of psychiatric patients have often involved incorporating the skills of a variety of healthcare professionals into collaborative care models. A multidisciplinary team providing psychiatric care often includes the following personnel.

CAREGIVERS

When persons with acute mental illness are first brought in contact with a doctor, informed consent is usually first sought from their caregiver, as the patient is not in an appropriate mind frame to give one himself or herself. Caregivers report that when the situation with a patient deteriorates to a point when they cannot be managed at home, usually when they start disturbing their relatives' night time sleep, the caregivers feel troubled by the patient's symptoms. They then feel compelled to bring the patient to the hospital and stabilise the patient's symptoms. They usually express satisfaction with getting psychotropic medication, particularly when the symptoms that caused the patient to stay awake during the night disappear. Thus, the need of medication in an effort to control symptoms of psychiatric disorders may be frustrating to the patient and caregiver if not controlled.

Unfortunately, in most cases, a lack of knowledge of psychiatric disorders and the importance of professional treatment among caregivers creates a delay in bringing patients to required medical aid and also providing much-needed financial support to patients. With advancing times, the burden of care for persons with psychiatric disorders has shifted from hospitals to families, resulting in a significant cost for the caregiver in emotional and financial terms. Although there is no agreement on whether a specific cluster of psychiatric symptoms has the most impact on a caregiver's burden of care, there is agreement that the more severe the symptoms, the larger the burden felt by the caregiver.

In such cases, strong social support and psychoeducation provided by medical professionals to patients' families and the community help train them in the following duties:

1. Monitoring of medication
2. Strategies to promote medication adherence
3. The importance of family and cultural values inculcated by caregivers in their patient relatives
4. Advocates for services and financial and emotional support to patients

Families of psychiatric patients are a primary source of home care and support for older relatives and people with serious mental illness. They contribute services that would otherwise cost hundreds of billions of rupees annually if purchased independently. Among the benefits provided to patients by their caregivers, the caregivers themselves gain feelings of gratification, love, and pride.

It is suggested that training programs in which mental health professionals and caregivers jointly learn the best ways to work together may be valuable. Caregivers need to be accepted and treated as active partners in patient care and rehabilitation. As a supportive gesture, the burden on the caregivers of people with mental illness can be alleviated with long-term rehabilitation and care.

SOCIAL HEALTH CARE WORKERS

It is believed that the social work tradition is to help psychiatric patients take charge of their own lives and strive for new and improved levels of mental health satisfaction and functioning. With the advancements seen in technology and management of psychiatric disorders, various considerations have to be kept in mind while defining the role of various healthcare professionals in the multidisciplinary treating team. Social workers, who are also considered healthcare professionals, aid in the management of psychiatric patients in myriad ways. Social workers, especially those tending to psychiatric patients, need to understand and address the concerns of their patients who are taking medications. Many social work educators believe that medication training needs to be incorporated into the curriculum provided by social work programs at both the graduate and undergraduate levels.

Among the various services provided by social workers for patients in the community, one of the most prominent is to utilise their professional knowledge of medication dosing. Social workers are meant to be trained in technical terms such as medication half-life, drug potency, the therapeutic index, and the building of drug tolerance. Knowledge of concepts like therapeutic index holds tremendous value, as it measures the relative toxicity or safety of a medication being taken by a patient. It is extremely important for social workers to know the difference between being biomedically equivalent and therapeutically equivalent and to clarify this to their patients. Many times, patients come with doubts, such as the medication not tasting the same, being a different colour when dissolved, and so forth. Concepts like medication fringes should be familiar to social workers in these cases.

There is a huge arena of medication errors which can be dealt with by social workers. These areas include:

1. Reading and writing prescription errors
2. Illegible handwriting
3. Improper transcription
4. Inaccurate dosage calculation
5. Inappropriate abbreviations used in prescribing
6. Labelling errors

Social workers can also be intimately involved in the area of medication compliance. Lack of compliance serves as a great source of medication errors and vice versa. In many cases complex drug regimens or ambiguity in dosing medications can lead to errors and thus medication non-compliance. Here social workers can help in the following ways:

1. They can help in recognising and reporting medication errors
2. They should spend quality time with the patient and ask about and monitor client responses to the medications that they are prescribed, particularly noting side-effects.

3. They can help with educating the client and family members about all aspects and considerations that should be noted when using medications. When a question is asked that the social worker cannot answer accurately, the information should be sought and provided as soon as possible.
4. They can and should refer patients to concerned medical professionals whenever they are approached with a doubt beyond their working capacity. For example, if an anti-anxiety drug (benzodiazepine) is given in high doses over a long period of time and then abruptly discontinued, this can induce seizures. In such cases, it is best for social workers to refer patients to the doctor and not handle medication management by themselves.
5. Taking a very common example, a problem commonly noted in the field by social workers is that some patients are not aware of actual pill taking behaviours. So instead of swallowing an extended-release capsule or tablet, some patients might actually chew on it, thus defeating the entire purpose of consuming extended-release tablets. It is basic information like this dispensed by social workers which makes them an integral part of the multidisciplinary team.
6. Another aspect of their job entails identifying patients with pill-seeking behaviour, which as a concept is different from actual pill-taking behaviour. The psychological directives behind such behaviour are usually to control behavioural symptoms or bring relief in some manner, which might be counterproductive to their illness. Awareness of such phenomena highlights such patients for social workers and brings them help faster than independent treatment seeking.
7. Careful documentation is essential in a social workers' job profile. Most individuals, particularly those who have taken multiple medications, have trouble remembering. It is important to be supportive and keep careful records and documentation that supports the provision of care. It is predicted that with the crunch and blurring of roles in managed care, social workers, along with the other disciplines, will be held accountable for this very important responsibility.

Thus, the more well informed professional social workers are, the more involved they can be with medication regimens and also prevent potential problems. Though it may seem inconsequential, educating patients about basic facts of medications can be vital from a patient's perspective. There is considerable evidence that social work and other forms of psychosocial interventions can assist individuals who suffer from behavioural, affective, or intellectual problems.

NURSES

Irrespective of their role and expertise, general psychiatric nurses are frontline healthcare professionals who encounter both individuals seeking treatment for mental health issues and those who have troubling mental health symptoms but are not overtly seeking assistance and are brought by caregivers or family members. This places them in a prime position, along with their primary care medical colleagues, to improve access and service delivery around mental health. However, this does not imply that all general psychiatry nurses need to become mental health specialists but is a preferred option for enhanced services. Mental health nursing is a specialist practice that requires specific qualifications and expertise, and it does help all nurses to possess knowledge and skills in mental health assessment, care, and treatment appropriate to their practice setting and in alignment with their scope of practice. Such preparation is currently provided within undergraduate nursing programs.

Nurses can even help in administering depot preparations that need to be administered once a month to patients who cannot travel to a psychiatrist. This could improve compliance with medication, as patients can regularly receive medications.

Patients tend to show immense satisfaction with nurses' intervention, and therefore specialist mental health nurses have an important role to play in the care of those with mental illness and have been demonstrated to contribute to improvements in a range of outcomes. Unfortunately, in many jurisdictions, they are simply not sufficiently available within primary care, and thus general nurses are required to manage the increasing number of people presenting to general practice with mental illness and mental health issues.

PHARMACISTS

A role often undefined and thus not appreciated enough is that of pharmacists who are accessible, knowledgeable, and equipped to provide mental health promotion along with care for the patient in the community. Pharmacists are trained in providing improved access to healthcare medication management and can relay the mental health needs of patients in a guided manner. The role of pharmacists has varied from educator to medication provider to consultant on occasion for generations. To reduce the burden of mental health disorders by addressing medication management, pharmacists are well placed in the mental healthcare spectrum to enhance services, as most of the management of psychiatric disorders rests on medications. Pharmacists are easily accessible healthcare professionals, trusted by the general public, and detached from the stigma associated with psychiatric disorders and have regular interactions with consumers who suffer acute mental illness.

Indispensable services which are provided by pharmacists include:

1. Medication counselling: They can provide information on how, when, and at what doses to take medications to patients and their caregivers. This practise has been shown to increase adherence to medications, especially antidepressants and antipsychotic medications, and to add to the convenience of the patient, this service is easily manageable at the community level. It has also been shown to reduce the number of hospitalisations and emergency visits to the hospital.
2. Transition periods: Scenarios where the patient moves from acute to maintenance management or vice versa tend to be periods of instability and thus require team efforts to optimise care. In such cases, the pharmacist can act as a buffer and lessen the impact by easing medication guidelines and promoting interdisciplinary services, documentation, and follow-ups of patients to their respective psychiatrists.
3. Recommendations and references: Pharmacists, during contact with patients, can refer them to well-matched counselling services. They can also refer patients to appropriate nutritionists, physiotherapists, or sleep therapists, among other services. As one of the most accessible health professionals, pharmacists could assist at-risk groups (postpartum women, geriatric patients, teenagers, etc.) in visiting a psychiatrist.
4. Drug-related problems: Pharmacists are trained to identify, solve, or refer and prevent various drug-related problems, thus improving patient quality of life.

While dealing with psychiatric patients, the pharmacist should keep the following things in mind:

- Play a dominant role during the conversation
- Apply the appropriate tone of voice
- Use simple and short sentences and body language

- Avoid discussing several issues simultaneously
- Demonstrate empathy

Bibliography

1. Iseselo MK, Ambikile JS. Medication challenges for patients with severe mental illness: Experience and views of patients, caregivers and mental health care workers in Dar es Salaam, Tanzania. *International Journal of Mental Health Systems.* 2017 Dec;11(1):1–2.
2. Griffith TH. Caregiver views on medication treatment for persons with schizophrenia in a cultural context. Dissertation, University of Penn, USA.
3. Kamusheva M, Ignatova D, Golda A, Skowron A. The potential role of the pharmacist in supporting patients with depression: A literature-based point of view. *Integrated Pharmacy Research & Practice.* 2020;9:49.
4. Mohiuddin AK. Psychiatric pharmacy: New role of pharmacists in mental health. *J Psychiatry Mental Disord.* 2019;4(1):1010.
5. Bentley KJ, Walsh J, Farmer RL. Social work roles and activities regarding psychiatric medication: Results of a national survey. *Social Work.* 2005 Oct 1;50(4):295–303.
6. Dziegielewski SF. *Psychopharmacology and social work practice: Introduction.* UK: Routledge.
7. Muir-Cochrane EC. The role of the community mental health nurse in the administration of depot neuroleptic medication: 'Not just the needle nurse!'. *International Journal of Nursing Practice.* 1998 Dec;4(4):254–260.
8. Hemingway S. Mental health nurses' medicines management role: A qualitative content analysis. *Nurse Prescribing.* 2016 Feb 2;14(2):84–91.

41
Chronic Mental Illness and Experience of the Richmond Fellowship Programme

S. Kalyanasundaram, Prathiksha Shukla and Lata Hemchand

Introduction	442
The Richmond Fellowship Society (India), Bangalore	443
Asha – Halfway Home	444
Jyothi, Long Stay Home	445
Chetana – Day Care Centre	445
Green Skilling Activity	445
Rehabilitation	448
Vocational Rehabilitation	449
Psychological Interventions	451
Rehabilitation Components	452
Individual-Centred Interventions	*452*
Family-Centred Interventions	*452*
Community-Centred Interventions	*453*
Restoring Dignity	453
Challenges Ahead	454
Registration and Other Legal Formalities	454
Conclusion	455

INTRODUCTION

It is estimated that around 10% of the population at any point in time suffers from psychiatric illnesses of varying severity. About 10% of the population in the world has some form of mental disability, and 1% has severe form of mental disorders with disability. The recent development in mental health services in India is the community care approach. Epidemiological surveys in India showed the prevalence of psychiatric disorder varying from 9.5 to 370/1000 population [1]. These conditions cover the entire lifespan of a suffering individual and are very varied. They include problems such as anxiety, phobias, obsessive-compulsive disorders, various kinds of stress reactions (notably post-traumatic stress disorder or PTSD), developmental disorders, mental retardation, substance abuse and addiction, dementia, mood disorders, personality disorders, and various psychotic illnesses such as delusional disorders and schizophrenia.

Most psychiatric illnesses strike when the individual is between 15 and 35 years of age. The illness has long-term implications, as it affects the person during the most productive phase of his/her life and causes interference either in learning of skills or in terms of loss of opportunities for utilizing the skills acquired.

Psychiatric illnesses are disabling conditions where the disability is invisible and spans several areas of living such as cognitive functioning, interpersonal relations, work, communication, and so on. The disabilities often are in several of these domains and may fluctuate depending on the course of the disorder (may be episodic, fluctuating, chronic, progressive, etc.). The process of rehabilitation addresses these deficits through a variety of medical and psychosocial interventions, which are individual, family, and community based.

Psychiatric illnesses are often misunderstood. The more severe forms of these illnesses, like schizophrenia, frequently run a chronic course, and most individuals are left battling residual deficits like lack of motivation and interest, social withdrawal, poor attention and concentration, and poor cognitive skills and retaining new skills in addition to problems in judgement.

A lot of ongoing research seeks to demystify this condition, influenced by myriad biological, psychological, and social factors. The biological basis of schizophrenia has been investigated by neuropathological, neurochemical, and imaging studies. There is also increasing evidence that it is a developmental disorder and that some persons are more vulnerable to developing it. MRI studies have shown differences in brain volumes, and microscopic examinations have pointed to neuronal dysconnectivity in persons with schizophrenia [2,3]. It is likely that highly specific changes in brain structure and function occur with schizophrenia.

Biological factors notwithstanding, the psychosocial aspects of schizophrenia continue to exert enormous influence on various aspects of treatment and rehabilitation and perhaps even on the course and outcome of this disorder.

The Richmond Fellowship Society (India), Bangalore

The Richmond Fellowship Society (RFS) was started in the year 1959 in the United Kingdom by Ms. Elly Jansen, and today RF organizations are established in more than 30 countries, providing effective rehabilitation services to people recovering from severe mental health problems. The Richmond Fellowship is the world's largest network of mental health service providers.

Founded in Bangalore in 1986, Richmond Fellowship Society (India), is a non-governmental organisation working in psychosocial rehabilitation for those suffering from chronic mental illness. The Richmond Fellowship Society (India) RFS(I) is also a not-for-profit organization and a registered society under the Societies' Registration Act (1860) for a charity that rehabilitates the mentally ill, espouses their cause, and trains individuals in psychosocial rehabilitation.

The RFS (India) is one of the founder members of the Richmond Fellowship Asia Pacific Forum (RF ASPAC), started in the year 1993, that comprises RF facilities in Australia, New Zealand, Hong Kong, India, Nepal, and Sri Lanka.

The Fellowship grew from strength to strength under the vigilant, persuasive nurturing and watchful eyes of Ms Elly Jansen, the founder of RF Worldwide, who was bestowed the Order of the British Empire (OBE). Dr G. N. Narayana Reddy and the late Dr S. M. Channabasavanna, both former directors of NIMHANS, Bangalore, and the late M. M. Krishnamurthy and Dr. Prakash Appaya were some of the people who were responsible for starting the Richmond Fellowship in India at Bangalore. This premier NGO in the field of psychosocial rehabilitation celebrated its silver jubilee in July 2011. Dr. S. Kalyanasundaram has been its secretary and hon. CEO for more than 25 years. He, along with a set of dedicated staff, both administrative and professional, have nurtured this organization over the last three decades and more. His dynamic leadership in the field of psychosocial rehabilitation is widely recognized.

RFS (I) has four branches in the country, with two in Karnataka: Bangalore, Delhi, Lucknow, and Sidlaghatta (Chickballapur district in Karnataka) The latter caters to a rural population and provides free consultations and medicine through its monthly mental health camps.

The Bangalore branch of the Fellowship runs the following facilities:

1. Halfway home – Asha for 21 residents (both men and women)
2. Long-stay home – Jyothi for 17 residents (men and women)
3. Day care centre with vocational training – Chetana for 50 clients

The Bangalore Branch has provided rehabilitation services to 1225 clients at our residential and day care centres to date. All three centres provide treatment and support to adults battling chronic mental illnesses such as schizophrenia, schizophrenia with other psychosis, bipolar affective disorder, obsessive compulsive disorder, autism spectrum disorders, and attention deficit hyperactivity disorder (ADHD) and persons with intellectual disabilities. The residents re-learn personal and social skills in a therapeutic environment. In addition, individual and family counselling services are provided. The therapeutic community offers a safe and friendly environment for personal growth and an opportunity to regain self-respect. The Fellowship also offers respite care on a case-to-case basis.

RFS (I) is also India's only NGO that has pioneered exclusive education in the field of psychosocial rehabilitation. It offers a 2-year master's degree in psychosocial rehabilitation and counselling through the Richmond Fellowship Post-Graduate College for PSR, Bangalore (RFPG College), started in 1999, and was affiliated with the Rajiv Gandhi University for Health Sciences, Karnataka. The course was recognised by the Rehabilitation Council of India (RCI) and accredited by the National Assessment and Accreditation Council (NAAC) and under Section 2(f) of the UGC Act. The library and information service of the college houses an enviable collection of books, periodicals, and teaching aids, used extensively not only by the students and staff and by all those who are interested in psychiatric rehabilitation. Due to financial difficulties, the college had to be closed in 2015. Currently, the Fellowship is planning to offer short-term training in PSR to students across the country.

In addition, the Fellowship trains students coming from various educational institutions/hospitals in psychosocial rehabilitation. Post-graduate students studying for medical psychiatric social work/clinical psychology from different universities from India and abroad are posted at RF facilities for block placement/internship and provided 'hands on' training in addition to providing the theorical framework.

ASHA – HALFWAY HOME

Asha runs a comprehensive programme of activities designed to help residents participate in the running of the household to develop social and practical skills. The major areas of rehabilitation programs are:

1. To provide a structured lifestyle
2. Personal hygiene (activities of daily living)
3. Social/independent living skills
4. Medication compliance and insight facilitation

5. Communication and interpersonal relationships
6. Productive utilisation of time and leisure time activities

Based on the success of Asha, RFS – Bangalore branch started a group home, Jyothi, in 1995 for residents who have successfully completed their rehabilitation programme at Asha. The need for such a home was felt by the families who have experienced the benefit their wards have achieved after spending some quality time at our halfway home.

The residents usually stay in this facility anywhere between 12 and 18 months, after which they go home to be with their respective families.

JYOTHI, LONG STAY HOME

The group home Jyothi provides accommodation for people who suffer from severe mental illness but can live more independently with minimal support from mental health professionals. Residents are encouraged to be more independent and to occupy themselves in their areas of interest, which can possibly help them to be economically independent, to some extent. Apart from this, certain group activities like community meetings, group therapy, art therapy, movement therapy, planned recreation, and pocket money distribution are part of the schedule.

The critical thing is that the families and the staff have close collaboration, and we have been conducting yearly meetings with all the families where the residents and the staff meet and interact with all the families. The governing council members also participate in these meetings.

Many residents have spent a little over 25 years in this long stay facility, and all of them see this as their 'home' where there is a great camaraderie and warmth all around.

CHETANA – DAY CARE CENTRE

This was started in the year 1997. This centre also provides vocational training and psychosocial rehabilitation services for clients from Bangalore city. Residents of Asha and Jyothi also attend this facility to learn vocational skills. In addition, clients also learn to develop healthy work habits. A sheltered workshop is provided for those who cannot find employment outside. Chetana can accommodate up to 50 people. Clients suffering from schizophrenia, affective disorders, chronic epilepsy, and mild to moderate intellectual disability with behavioural problems seek help here.

Spending time at the day care and vocational training centre enables persons with disabilities to overcome barriers to accessing or maintaining work and/or the ability to return to work. Clients are given individualized attention by vocational instructors as well as trained mental health professionals. Other activities include planned recreation, games, art and craft activity, basic arithmetic classes (based on need), and individual counselling.

GREEN SKILLING ACTIVITY

One kind of innovative and special training we offer our clients at the day care centre is green skilling activity. The green skill project involves recycling discarded flowers from nearby temples, marriage halls, and other similar places/events into eco-friendly Holi colours. The process involved is as follows: segregating and cutting, drying petals, grinding dried petals, mixing, refining, and packaging. The clients are assigned work per their aptitude and ability. The project is being carried out in the urban community setting of the day care centre. Thirty clients consisting of those with severe mental illness and some with intellectual disability participate in this activity.

Table 41.1 Work done in the tailoring and printing unit at the centre.

Tailoring unit
1. Handmade paper greeting cards
2. Handkerchiefs, bookmarks
3. Purses/bags
4. Complimentary cards
5. Fridge magnets
6. Tab/mobile pouches
7. AEmbroidered tablecloths
8. Bead earrings
9. Kundan rangoli
10. Also take orders for stitching churidar, blouses, and alteration

File unit
1. Making paper files – for office use/conferences, and so on
2. Manual screen printing for visiting cards, bill books, prescription pads, wedding and other invitation cards, and so on

Printing unit
1. Paper/cardboard folders
2. Printing orders for letterheads, visiting cards, invitations, bill/receipt/voucher books
3. Paper and cloth bags
4. Envelopes (white/brown)
5. Gift/fancy envelopes
6. Medicine covers
7. Book binding
8. Pen stand making
9. Spiral binding

Paper cup unit
1. Coffee/tea paper cups: 110 ml, 150 ml, 210 ml

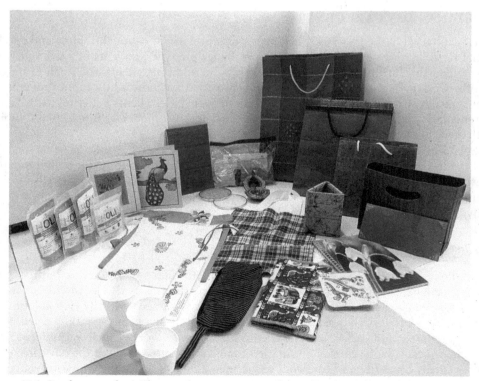

Figure 41.1 Products made at Chetana day care centre and vocational training.

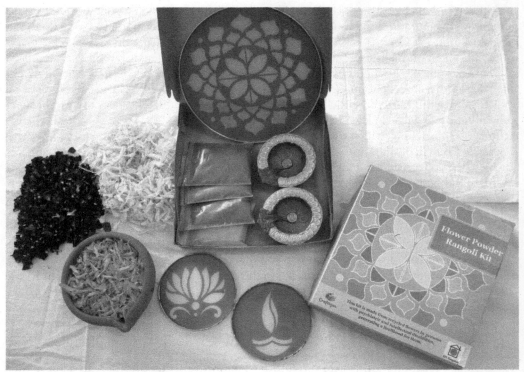

Figure 41.2 Green skilling products.

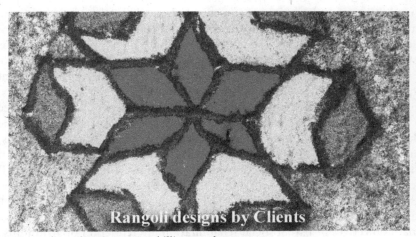

Figure 41.3 Rangoli made using green skilling products.

Staff members underwent training with Craftizen Foundation, our technical partner, involved with research and development. The training began in April 2016, with 2 days of training fortnightly for a period of 4 months. The clients started working with the flowers soon after the training, and the first successful production came out in March 2018.

Flowers being a large part of festivals in India, we as a community are a great consumer of flowers. After the festival, these flowers are dumped in water bodies, resulting in pollution or are allowed to rot. The green skill project is a novel initiative to address these concerns.

The clients engaged in this project have shown improvement in motor skills and social skills, attention, concentration, and motivation. There is a reduction in relapse, and they have shown a positive outlook towards life. The families of the clients reported a decrease in care givers' burden both emotionally and financially. There is significant difference in the pre- and post-assessment done on the clients using following scales: Indian Disability Evaluation and Assessment Scale, Social Occupational Functioning Scale, and Positive and Negative Symptoms Scale.

RFS Bangalore started the Richmond Fellowship Post Graduate College for psychosocial rehabilitation (RF PG College) in 1999. The college offered an M.Sc. in psychosocial rehabilitation and counselling, which was recognised by the government of Karnataka and the Rehabilitation Council of India and affiliated with the Rajiv Gandhi University of Health Sciences. In 2003, the college signed a memorandum of understanding with the National Institute of Mental Health and Neurosciences, Bengaluru (NIMHANS), for the mutual benefit of both parties in the field of psychiatric rehabilitation and for academic pursuits.

The M.Sc. course was designed to impart, through practical hands-on training, including essential counselling skills, the core skills necessary for mental health practitioners. The curriculum also exposed the students to research practices. Students were required, in their second year, to write dissertations on relevant mental health topics.

However, unforeseen circumstances led to the closure of the college in the academic year 2015. Nevertheless, the research and training that the college offered are guided through the research wing of our Fellowship.

REHABILITATION

Psychosocial rehabilitation is care given to persons with mental disorders to achieve their optimum level of social and psychological functioning and is an ongoing process. It should ideally begin with the first contact with a mental health professional (usually a psychiatrist) and is done using a multidisciplinary team approach involving the psychiatrist, clinical psychologist, psychiatric social worker, psychiatric nurse, occupational therapist, and rehabilitation professionals with different and tailor-made methods being adopted to achieve the goal. Therapists and families should ideally become partners in the care of the disabled. Family-related factors are particularly critical. This is of greater relevance in many countries, like India, where over 90% of the chronically mentally ill live with their families [2].

Rehabilitation involves helping the individual go from being a 'patient' to becoming a 'person'. This will be possible only when an individually tailored, integrated, and holistic approach with tested intervention strategies is adopted. Psychiatric rehabilitation is an active treatment involving medication and psychosocial interventions. Rehabilitation aims at getting the individual to lead as functional and meaningful a life as is possible. Therefore, while the focus is on reducing the disability, the environment may also have to be suitably modified to meet the individual's needs. The various settings in rehabilitation, therefore, must cater to these different needs.

The main objectives of psychosocial rehabilitation are reduction of symptoms, improving social and vocational skills, strengthening social support, reducing discrimination and stigma, and bringing about consumer empowerment.

The main goals of psychosocial rehabilitation are to improve/enhance the following:

- Medical management
- Personal hygiene/self-care
- Interpersonal relationships
- Money management
- Work habits
- Leisure activities

- Time management
- Family involvement and therapy
- Home management skills
- Crisis management skills
- Social skills
- Resource mobilization
- Self-esteem
- Motivation

VOCATIONAL REHABILITATION

The aim of vocational rehabilitation is to provide meaningful and constructive activities for the clients so that they have a work routine. It helps in building vocational skills and in improving the self-esteem of clients. As mentioned earlier, the clients alternate between the four different units, which are functional at the Chetana day care centre: the file-making unit, paper cup-making unit, tailoring and embroidery unit, and printing unit. There is also a computer unit, which helps clients develop their computer skills.

Green skilling activity, which has started in the last couple of years, has had a beneficial effect on the overall mental health of clients.

The figures demonstrate some of the work done by the clients at RFS.

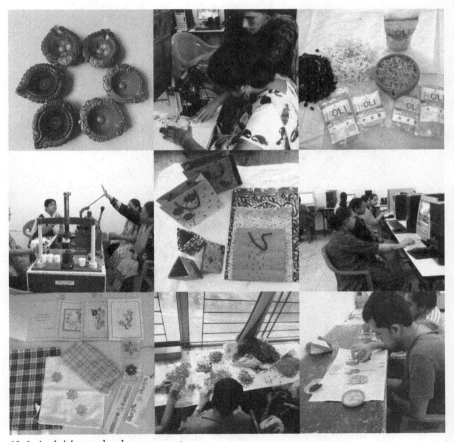

Figure 41.4 Activities at the day care centre.

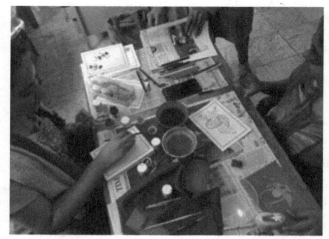

Figure 41.5 Artwork and painting.

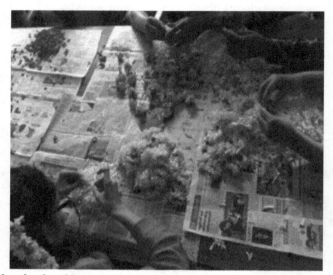

Figure 41.6 Floral garland making.

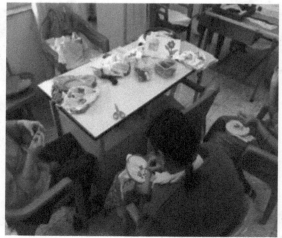

Figure 41.7 Craft work in action.

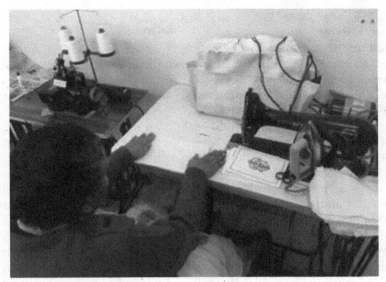
Figure 41.8 Sewing work done by patients.

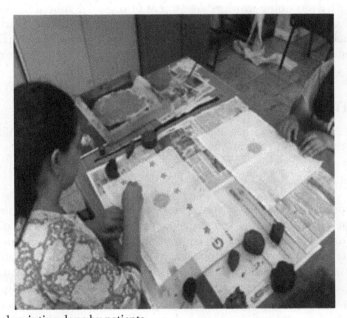
Figure 41.9 Block painting done by patients.

PSYCHOLOGICAL INTERVENTIONS

The overall goals of psychological therapies are to ensure normalization of the patient to the extent possible and optimize patients' functioning through multi-disciplinary and multi-faceted methods. Behaviour modification is an approach based on principles of learning theories and behaviour therapy. It aims at restoring the patient's functioning in specific areas. Paul and Lentz (1977) showed that psycho-social interventions in the form of social learning therapy showed significant improvements in self-care, interpersonal skills, and reduction in bizarre behaviour. Behaviour therapy has made a significant contribution to assessment and understanding of the problem. Behavioural analysis gives a clear framework to formulate a treatment plan [4].

At RFS facilities, behaviour modification techniques such as behavioural contracting and reinforcement schedules are used frequently to help clients develop vocational skills. The use of these interventions is decided on a case-by-case basis. These techniques help in controlling negative behaviours such as anger outbursts, poor personal hygiene, and poor grooming. The emphasis on developing social skills for the clients is one of the key areas of work at the facilities. A social skills training program is held as a group activity every week, which helps clients in their interpersonal interactions within the facility and with their family members.

Some path-breaking work in cognitive deficits in schizophrenia has emerged with different cognitive remediation measures. It is a well-established fact that cognitive impairment in schizophrenia interferes with all aspects of functioning of persons suffering from schizophrenia. The individual's ability to be gainfully employed and important functions like social cognition and the ability to process information are affected. Cognitive deficits do not respond well to the anti-psychotic treatments currently in use. Cognitive enhancement therapy and cognitive retraining methods have been found to be consistently effective. Patients with deficits in attention and memory have shown significant improvements on their scores on neuropsychological tests (Bentall 1990 and Morrison 2004) [5]. Presently, research in cognitive retraining is focused on developing computer-based programs. The process of cognitive retraining involves assessment of cognitive functions, goal setting, and applying appropriate cognitive exercise to improve specific functions. Since many of our clients at RFS facilities suffer from attentional deficits, various attention-enhancing exercises are regularly conducted. Memory games are also used by the staff with those clients who are in need and are cooperative to follow the instructions.

REHABILITATION COMPONENTS

The psychosocial interventions that make up the rehabilitation process could be individual centred, family centred, and community centred.

Individual-Centred Interventions

The main components of client-centred interventions are medication compliance, individual/group therapy, social skills training, independent living skills, vocational training, cognitive retraining, behaviour therapy, community living, and leisure time management. Psychosocial interventions minimise impairment and disability through better compliance with medication and improve role functioning. This will result in better participation in the community, thereby reducing the stigma related to having a severe mental illness. Supportive therapy techniques are used frequently at the facilities and help the clients recognize their own strengths and develop them. Problem-solving skills and milieu therapy are some of the other interventions that are used to optimize the functioning of clients.

Family-Centred Interventions

The main components of family-centred interventions are psychoeducation, counselling, supportive therapy, coping skills, problem solving, crisis management, resource mobilization, and organization of self-help groups. Advocacy, creating awareness of their rights, providing access to information such as schemes and benefits available to disabled individuals, and organizing lobbying groups to influence policymaking are interventions that help foster collaborative and lasting partnerships between professionals and family members.

The families need a lot of support to cope with the burden of care of a person with severe mental illness. Interventions with families include psychoeducation, coping with aggressive or uncooperative behaviour of the client, relapse prevention, and dealing with their own negative emotions. It is also prudent to involve the families in the rehabilitation process. Teaching them to cope with the deficits that the clients may continue to exhibit post-discharge is a case in point. The skills that staff use to help the residents/clients may need to be taught to the family members so that they will be able to use them when appropriate.

Community-Centred Interventions

Community-based interventions in PSR for chronic mental illness in a residential setting like a halfway home have some advantages. One such approach which has proved highly effective is the therapeutic community approach. Therapeutic communities (TC) are small, cohesive communities based on ideas of collective responsibility, citizenship, and empowerment. They are deliberately structured in a way that encourages personal responsibility and avoids unhelpful dependency on professionals. In a TC, the day-to-day experience of living and working together is as important as formal therapy, and the community is structured in such a way as to maximize opportunities for 'the living – learning experience' (Campling, 2001) [6]. The work in a TC rests upon the core values of attachment, containment, respect, communication, interdependence, relationships, participation, process, balance, and responsibility (Association of Therapeutic Communities, 2009) [7]. These humanitarian values of a TC make it an ideal setting for remedial work with persons with severe mental illness. Restoring dignity is vital to the rehabilitation and recovery process (Kalyanasundaram and Sekhar, 2012) [8]. In India, the work done at the Richmond Fellowship Society (India) at the halfway home in Bangalore is worthy of mention in this regard. The results of an evaluative study conducted in this facility convincingly proved its efficacy (Chowdhury et al., 2011) [9].

The main components of community-based interventions are creating awareness, involving communities, resource mobilization, advocacy, empowerment, reduction of stigma, and networking and outreach programs. These can be achieved through the combined efforts of all stakeholders, including the agency, and making most use of the local political mechanisms. Involving and enlisting the support of local village leaders, elders, and other significant persons in rural areas will go a long way in achieving the agency's goal.

RESTORING DIGNITY

For my colleagues everywhere in Richmond Fellowship Society, helping restore a client's dignity means maintaining and building on the dignity that is our own. In our work, this means providing clients and their families the best help we can offer, in the best way possible. In the therapist's role, it means practicing counselling skills, including maintaining professional and personal boundaries, keeping one's personal dignity when one is faced with socially inappropriate behaviour, and being directive when that is called for.

As surrogate caregivers, it means that we double as nurses. When seeking employment options for clients, it means advocacy. When raising funds for our programmes, it means asking for financial and other support without losing our own personal dignity. It means, in a word, rediscovering the dignity of the trusted servant – something that has many times been amply rewarded by the smiles of relief, happiness, and satisfaction. We at RFS Bangalore find the clients and their families a great gift in understanding our own transformation.

In fact, at Richmond Fellowship, democratisation and equality are two cornerstones in the approach followed, known as the therapeutic community. In the TC approach, everything possible is done to help the client overcome his or her psychological disturbance and disability. Issues with which the client is struggling are discussed in a democratic manner between the therapist or rehabilitation professional and the client to arrive at effective alternatives from which the client chooses the one that works best for them, albeit with the guidance provided by the rehab team. Neither the therapist nor the rehabilitation professional tells the client what to do. Instead, the clients assume their share of responsibility for recovery alongside the therapist or rehabilitation professional, who acts as a role model for the client.

CHALLENGES AHEAD

In India, psychosocial rehabilitation, although not a recent development, is available only in certain parts of the country This is an important component of comprehensive management, and unfortunately many states in India lack such rehabilitation programmes. Poor awareness, inadequate manpower, and inadequate facilities are some of the reasons for this. The Richmond fellowship in Bangalore, which has vast experience in training people in psychosocial rehabilitation and counselling, is keen to provide such training for those interested to work in this exciting specialty.

The situation in India reflects the context of mental healthcare in several developing countries.

- Many developing countries have established national mental health programmes. However, these programmes have not been implemented on a mass scale. The ground reality in developing countries has resulted in the absence of even basic care related to mental illness. Despite their honourable intent, most programs fall far below their objectives, end prematurely, or exist only on paper.
- Paralleling the problems in rehabilitation in third-world countries, rehabilitation efforts in India too are plagued by a lack of financial resources, both at the micro level of the individual patient and the family, as well as the agency level. The budgetary allocation to healthcare and specifically mental healthcare should be substantially raised if we need to address their concerns realistically.
- Non-affordability of psychiatric medications and care, lack of accurate information on medicine usage causing discontinuation of medication, and subsequent relapse of the illness are some of the common concerns faced by many. Due to financial difficulties, patients drop out of care, and this in turn results in further disability.

Mental healthcare in India is heavily concentrated in urban areas and in certain pockets of the country with respect to facilities, manpower, and financial support. This rural-urban imbalance greatly restricts access to mental healthcare and rehabilitation for many people who would benefit from such intervention.

REGISTRATION AND OTHER LEGAL FORMALITIES

All rehabilitation facilities must be registered and, per The Mental Health Care Act of 2017, should get a license from competent authorities [10]. As the clients get older and their parents are unable to continue with their role as primary caregivers due to their age, adequate precautions must be taken to monitor their physical health. Alternative arrangements must be in place for another legal guardian to look after the interest of the clients. Proper legal documentation with the help of a lawyer well versed in these matters should be consulted to safeguard the interest of the clients.

- The lack of job opportunities for recovered individuals also makes rehabilitation efforts less effective.
- Sometimes societal insensitivity, stigma, and misconceptions about mental illnesses and expressed emotions in a family are responsible for the re-emergence of the psychiatric symptoms.
- In some cases, prolonged stay in hospitals also interferes in rehabilitation, because this itself may produce the secondary negative symptoms in a patient.
- Difficulties also arise due to the lack of trained staff and psychiatrists. In a country like India, with over 1.3 billion people, at least 13 million suffer from schizophrenia. Of these, nearly one-third would require active psychosocial rehabilitation. We have only around 7000 psychiatrists and not more than 2000 clinical psychologists and psychiatric social workers, and around 1000 trained psychiatric nurses. It is evident that the numbers of professionals available are woefully inadequate to meet the need.
- Burnout among mental health professionals causes rapid turnover of the staff, and the agency needs to make repeated investments in training new staff. This can be a drain on the agency's already scarce resource base.
- Bureaucratic hurdles also slow down the process of rehabilitation in terms of delays in approval and release of funds, licensing, altering policies and legislations to make it more relevant, procedures for accessing due benefits such as pensions, grants, financial assistance, and so on which are not user friendly.
- Many psychiatrists do not associate themselves with working in psychiatric rehabilitation. There is lack of enthusiasm among these professionals about the need for rehabilitation in chronic mental illness.
- Lack of job opportunities for persons recovering from mental illness is also an additional handicap.

Employment provides not only a monetary recompense but also 'latent' benefits – non-financial gains to the worker which include social identity and status, social contacts and support, a means of structuring and occupying time, activity and involvement, and a sense of personal achievement. Social isolation is often particularly problematic for people who experience mental health problems, and work is effective in increasing social networks Studies show a clear interest in work and employment activities among users of psychiatric services, with up to 90% of users wishing to go into (or back to) work. Given the high rates of unemployment in the general population, creating jobs for recovering individuals is an uphill task. People with mental illness are sensitive to the negative effects of unemployment and the loss of structure, purpose, and identity which it brings (Sheth 2005) [11].

Lack of a job and the ensuing financial crisis cause tremendous stress which can cause relapse of symptoms. This in turn may impede ongoing psychosocial rehabilitation efforts.

CONCLUSION

Without a change in the current emphasis and direction, community care for mental illness in the developing world will remain good intentions only. There is a need for innovative approaches that utilize the available resources to ensure that healthcare reaches the population.

To sum up, mental illnesses will assume a gigantic proportion in the coming years. Governments must deploy more resources to tackle illnesses early and rehabilitate patients. Rehabilitation processes should aim not only at the individual but also the family and the community. The government, with its available financial resources but inadequate staff to cater to the needs of the chronic mentally ill, should be willing to partner with NGOs working in these areas to create a viable model of public-private partnerships. This initiative will then address the needs of the clients and their families satisfactorily.

References

1. Kumar, S.G., Premarajan, K.C., Kattimani, S., and Kar, S.S. Epidemiology of mental disability using Indian Disability Evaluation Assessment Scale among general population in an urban area of Puducherry, India. Jan–Mar 2018: www.ncbi.nlm.nih.gov/pmc/articles/PMC5820810/#ref3
2. Thara, R., Padmavathi, R., Srinivasan, T.N. Focus on psychiatry in India. *BJP*. 2004;184(4):366–373.
3. James, S., et al. Demand for access to and use of community mental health care: Lessons from a demonstration project in India and Pakistan. *IJSP*. 2002;48(3):163–176.
4. Paul, G.L. and Lenz, R.J. *Psychosocial treatment of chronic mental patients: Milieu Vs Social learning programs*. Harvard, MA: Harvard University Press. 1977.
5. Bentall, R.P. and Young, H.F. Sensible-hypothesis-testing in deluded, depressed and normal subjects. *British Journal of Psychiatry*. 1996;168:372–375.
6. Campling, P. Therapeutic communities. *Advances in Psychiatric Treatment*. 2001;7:365–372.
7. The Association of Therapeutic Communities. What is a TC? 2009: www.therapeuticcommunities.com
8. Kalyanasundaram, S. and Sekhar, N. Creating supportive communities in mental health: The RFS (I) experience in Bangalore, India. 2012.
9. Chowdhury, R., Dharitri, R., Kalyanasundaram, S., and Rao, N.S.N. Efficacy of psychosocial rehabilitation program: The RFS experience. *Indian Journal of Psychiatry*. 2011;53:45–8.
10. The Gazette of India: Published Authority, Ministry of Law and Justice: http://egazette.nic.in/WriteReadData/2017/175248.pdf
11. Sheth, HC. Common problems in psychosocial rehabilitation. *IJPSR*. 2005;10(1):53–60.

42
Innovative Community Mental Health Approaches From Across the Globe

Pragya Lodha

Introduction	457
What Encompasses Community Mental Health?	458
Task Sharing in Community Mental Health	458
Key Approaches to Facilitate Task Sharing in Innovative Community Mental Health Care	459
Need for Innovations in Community Mental Health	460
Innovations in Community Mental Health: Learning From Model Examples	462
Africa Mental Health Foundation in Kenya	462
The Friendship Bench in Zimbabwe	462
Frugal Innovations for Promoting Mental Health Among Adults and Children in Vietnam	462
Conclusion	462

INTRODUCTION

Community mental healthcare comprises principles and practices to promote mental health for a local population. The various components of community mental healthcare include a) addressing population needs in ways that are accessible and acceptable; b) building on the goals and strengths of people who experience mental illnesses; c) promoting a wide network of support, services and resources of adequate capacity; and d) emphasising services that are both evidence based and recovery oriented [Mueser 2011]. Community mental healthcare is essential in order to meet the unmet needs for affordable care, lack of access to care and insufficient healthcare provision through hospital-based infrastructures. The burden of mental disorders continues to grow, contributing to significant morbidity and disability. Major ramifications are also seen in social and human rights and economic grounds as well. With the increasing burden and widening treatment gap, there is a need for traditional mental healthcare to integrate with innovative community mental healthcare, which will allow greater reach. Though community mental healthcare facilities make healthcare affordable and accessible, especially among low- and middle-income countries (LMICs), it is not the sole healthcare-providing stakeholder. A balance of community as well as hospital-based facilities is needed to ensure optimal mental healthcare provision.

WHAT ENCOMPASSES COMMUNITY MENTAL HEALTH?

Community mental healthcare intervention is better provided as out-patient services and generally provides services at the community and population level. Interventions at the population level include interventions like legislation, regulations and public information campaigns, whereas those at community level address schools, workplaces and neighbourhoods/community groups [Wahlbeck 2015]. Some examples of population-level interventions include reducing demand for alcohol use by setting age limits for alcohol consumption and enforcing blood alcohol limits for drivers, child protection laws, regulations to restrict access to means of self-harm/suicide and search engine optimisation to show suicide prevention helplines when one searches for means to attempt suicide. Interventions at the community level look like mental health awareness programmes, mental health first aid for communities, suicide identification and training programmes, identifying children with behavioural and emotional concerns in classrooms and parenting programmes for parents with young children and adolescents.

One of the purposes to have community mental health is to provide for cost-effective treatments, thus making mental healthcare affordable and accessible to the masses, especially those who are on the lower rungs of the socio-economic ladder. Community mental healthcare looks at 'task sharing' or 'task shifting', which involves allocation of duties to non-specialised staff that were reserved for psychiatrists and mental health professionals [McPake and Mensah 2008]. These non-specialised staff are referred to as lay or community mental health workers who generally require rigorous training and continuous supervision. These are individuals who generally have a rich understanding of the socio-cultural context [Balaji et al. 2012]. The efficacy of task sharing has been demonstrated in LMICs. This model uses a stepped care approach where various steps or levels of healthcare are involved; the most intensive care is reserved for the most severe cases. The purpose is to ensure that everyone gets a basic level of care, and those requiring the next level of care get that. For instance, not everyone may need medical care and may also benefit from psychoeducation, counselling or psychotherapy. Though it isn't easy to integrate community mental health with primary healthcare, a diligent process for the same can help address local communities effectively, make mental healthcare available to many and ensure socio-cultural aspects of care.

TASK SHARING IN COMMUNITY MENTAL HEALTH

Task sharing or task shifting is a concept that is core to community mental health. Task sharing in mental health involves the training of non-specialist health workers (NSHW) to deliver mental healthcare that usually entails brief and low-intensity psychological interventions. NSHW is more like an umbrella term used for individuals who have little or no prior formal training in delivering mental healthcare and have been known by several names in different countries/regions, such as community health workers, community mental health workers, lay health workers, lay counsellors, midwives, nurses, village heath workers, paraprofessionals, religious and traditional healers and many more [Lehmann and Sanders 2007]. Task sharing in community health has shown promising and effective results over a period of time. As a medium of care in mental health, task sharing has existed since the 1970s, beginning with the notion of non-specialist delivery of psychotropic medications in global health [Harding and Chrusciel 1975]. Evidence for the efficacy of NSHW in delivering mental healthcare and support exists over a continuum of roles and tasks and for a range of mental health problems, particularly common mental disorders such as depression and anxiety. Salient to note is the success of NSHW-delivered psychosocial and psychological interventions including delivery of evidence based practices of cognitive behavioural therapy

(CBT) and interpersonal therapy (IPT) as part of global mental health [Whitley 2015] The clinical efficacy, cost friendliness and health system–strengthening components of NSHW-delivered mental healthcare for a range of mental health conditions have been established [Raviola et al. 2019].

KEY APPROACHES TO FACILITATE TASK SHARING IN INNOVATIVE COMMUNITY MENTAL HEALTH CARE

Task sharing in community mental health practices can be facilitated multifariously; some successful evidence-based strategies include:

1. Balanced care model: it is an evidence-based, systematic and flexible approach to planning treatment and care for people living with mental disorders. A balanced care model accounts for gaps in resources and bridges different health delivery platforms. There is a shared responsibility for care among NSHWs, and the role of NSHWs is informed by evidence-based and best practices. A balanced care model develops an interconnected network between primary healthcare facilities, healthcare providers, peer support groups, patients, NSHWs and technology-driven healthcare.
2. Collaborative care: Also referred to as integrative care, this is defined as health services that are managed and delivered such that people receive a continuum of health promotion, disease prevention, diagnosis, treatment, disease management, rehabilitation and palliative care services coordinated across the different levels and sites of care within and beyond the health sector and, according to their needs, throughout the life course [Thornicroft et al. 2019]. Research evidence has shown the success of collaborative care in several dimensions of care and pointed out some key components such as population-based care for specific disorders that prioritises screening, treatment and tracking of outcomes; self-care support including psychoeducation of family and patient about illness and treatments; self-monitoring and adherence support skills; and many others [Kroenke and Unutzer 2017].
3. Training and supervision: One of the challenges and areas of improvisation in the global health network has been sustained training and supervision of NSHWs in provision of mental healthcare with attention to core competencies. Training, supervision, competency assessment and certification are essential to practices of mental healthcare provision as NSHWs, ensuring regular and effective care delivery is underpinned with sustained and rigorous training/supervision.
4. Trans-diagnostic interventions: An integrated care system with NSHWs receiving training and supervision is comprehensive with diagnostic and transdiagnostic tools that can ensure early identification of problems as well discreetly recognising cases and non-cases, a staged approach that addresses problems dimensionally and diagnostically while recognising the opportunity for early intervention across wellness, distress, illness and recurrent illness. This is helpful at a primary care level, as NSHWs can identify less severe problems and address them. This allows planners to identify specific skills for NSHWs, which can include mental health promotion, self-care, community outreach activities, psychoeducation, providing social support, early screening and providing basic psychological intervention. Some resources like enhancing assessment of common therapeutic factors (ENACT), reducing stigma among healthcare providers to improve mental health services (RESHAPE) and the Improving Access to Psychological Therapies (IAPT) Programme are models that have been successfully tried and tested [Clark et al. 2018; Kohrt et al. 2015]. Resources can also then be spent in training NSHWs for these skills to build sustainable efficacy.

5. Digital innovations: use of digital technologies such as mobile applications, teleservices and internet/web platforms can be far reaching from screening, diagnosis, treatment, treatment, care by NSHWs, training and supervision of NSHWs, data management and other administrative tasks as well as care provision through online therapies, self-care, psychoeducation and awareness, peer support and internet and social media interventions [Patel et al. 2018].

NEED FOR INNOVATIONS IN COMMUNITY MENTAL HEALTH

The amount of the health budget allocated to mental health is considerably low; it accounts for less than 2% in LMICs [Semrau et al. 2015]. This is proportionate to the increase in mental health burden, accounting for disability-adjusted life years, years of life lost due to premature mortality and years lost due to disability for people living with mental health conditions. To understand the need for innovation in community mental healthcare, it is essential to understand the reasons for investing in mental health [Patel et al. 2013].

1. Promote human rights and inclusion: People with mental health problems are more likely than others to experience social exclusion, violent victimisation and human rights abuse.
2. Reduce the human impact of mental health problems: Mental health problems lead to extremely distressing symptoms for the affected person and burden for family members. In addition, they are closely associated with physical health problems. There is a high level of co-existence of noncommunicable diseases and mental health problems which compromises treatment and prevention efforts.
3. Prevent premature deaths: People with severe mental health problems die up to 20 years earlier than people without mental health problems, even in high-income countries. Excess mortality is due to suicide and unhealthy lifestyles such as high smoking rates, poor physical health and poorer physical healthcare for people with mental health problems.
4. Reduce economic burden: lost productivity and income are the consequences of untreated mental health problems that result in trillions of dollars being lost every year at a national level.
5. Reduce poverty and social disadvantage: Poverty, social disadvantage and mental health problems are intimately related to one another.
6. Put knowledge of cost-effective treatments into practice: The treatment of mental health problems is as cost effective as other health treatments.

Theories suggest that the need for innovations in healthcare is to make the system holistic. Innovations help identify barriers and loopholes and act to have bridging capacities for unmet needs in healthcare. Innovation can be invited at multiple levels of infrastructure, organisation, care provision, research and policy. Innovation in mental health can provide for:

- Cost-effective and accessible solutions
- Social advantages and inclusion
- Dignity for human rights
- Framework to approach global mental health
- Best practices and evidence-based practices
- Developmental, integrative and holistic approach to health

Innovations in community mental health have the potential to up-scale mental health practices at a universal level and help troubleshoot problems at community level. There are myriad innovations in the field of mental health. Inspired by work in India, innovations can be placed into five categories: a) quality improvement of mental health programmes, b) community-based mental health programmes, c) non-specialist care programmes, d) mobile technology-based mental health programmes and e) tele-technology-based mental health programmes [Pandya et al. 2020].

1. Quality improvement of mental health programmes: quality improvement of mental health programmes refers to the overall qualitative improvement of the programme as well as the human rights condition of the patients accessing healthcare services. This can be achieved by involving multiple stakeholders in delivering healthcare, ensuring early intervention with adherence management and psychosocial care and developing a collaborative care model. A collaborative care model that comprises psychosocial services, non-specialist care and specialist services for making mental health services available at the community and primary healthcare level has been found acceptable and effective in reducing treatment gaps, improving treatment adherence and bringing quicker rehabilitation of mentally ill patients in their family and the society [van Ginneken et al. 2017].
2. Community-based mental health programmes: in conjunction with hospital-based/facility-based care provision, community-based mental health programmes usually entail psychoeducation, adherence management, psychosocial rehabilitation, support for livelihood and referrals. Such initiatives have shown benefits like decreasing the patient's disability, the burden on the family and the costs incurred by the family [Thara et al. 2008].
3. Non-specialist care programmes: these programmes are those run by community mental health workers, lay counsellors, non-specialist health workers, members of self-help groups and community champions. Such a low-cost skill transfer-based contextual mental health service delivery model have been found feasible, acceptable and cost effective, with several beneficial outcomes such as efficacious mental health services in rural and remote areas, increased adherence, follow-ups and reduced disability [Mendenhall et al. 2014].
4. Mobile-technology–based mental health programmes: Mobile technology has the potential to upscale and integrate mental health services with primary healthcare. The digitalisation of services has had an impact on healthcare systems as well, creating possibilities to bring health services to mobile. Examples of use of mobile healthcare in rural India have shown the use of mobile technology by non-specialist community mental health workers for screening, management and referral services and has led to reduced cost of service delivery. There is scope for LMICs and other low-resource areas to benefit immensely from digital technology-based mental health interventions (diagnosis, treatment and prevention) with online, text messaging and telephone support [Naslund et al. 2017].
5. Tele-technology-based mental health programmes: Tele–mental health (tele-psychiatry and tele-psychotherapy) are on the rise. The efficacy of tele-mental health has been shown in two areas, consultation, training and education of staff members and early detection and treatment of mental health problems. With the era of digitalisation, tele-psychiatry and tele–mental health are growing in order to be more effective for a greater number of people. Tele–mental health has made consultations possible through video conferencing and booking appointments online, and therapeutic exercises have become available on mobile applications, and psychotherapy has also found online platforms [Hubley et al. 2016].

INNOVATIONS IN COMMUNITY MENTAL HEALTH: LEARNING FROM MODEL EXAMPLES

Africa Mental Health Foundation in Kenya

An innovative model was set up integrate traditional healers, faith healers and community health workers to detect mental illnesses. The Africa Mental Health Foundation (AMFH) invested to build its referral networks and expand its integration of mental health into existing public and community health services by training formal (nurses, clinical officers) and informal (traditional healers, faith healers) healthcare providers. This model was implemented in Kenya. This approach integrates the informal and formal sectors, building synergies by enhancing communication and shared practices. This innovation helped Kenya build a society of community health workers in addition to formal healthcare providers, of whom there were only 500 for a population of 40 million with a high prevalence of mental illnesses.

The Friendship Bench in Zimbabwe

The Friendship Bench deployed grandmothers as lay community health workers. These grandmothers, or grannies, were middle-aged or older women with little or no education who could earn a small stipend doing community mental health work. These grannies take 4 weeks to learn what depression is and identify it using a simple questionnaire and were taught the basics of cognitive behaviour therapy to use as problem-solving therapy. Zimbabwe had 15 psychiatrists for 1.5 million people; this innovation helped significantly reduce the gap. These grannies deliver service in a safe and comfortable environment on actual benches in open clinic grounds. Patients referred to the benches by clinicians receive up to six counselling sessions (45 minutes each), including one home visit and, in some cases, referral to other health or social services. Specialist support is available via mobile phones and tablets.

Frugal Innovations for Promoting Mental Health Among Adults and Children in Vietnam

Making the most of scarce resources (through frugal innovations) trains community health workers to treat depression and anxiety and provides telephone-based coaching/guidance and support to families of children with behavioural and emotional difficulties. Vietnam has 2 psychiatrists for 100,000 individuals. A project led by the Centre for Applied Research in Mental Health and Addictions (CARMHA) at Simon Fraser University's Faculty of Health Sciences aims to bridge the gap in two low-cost manners: training community health workers to treat adults suffering from depression and anxiety and providing telephone-based coaching as well as support to families of children with behavioural and emotional difficulties.

These are some of several innovative community mental health ideas that have been implemented across the world and benefited thousands of individuals by making community mental healthcare accessible. Similarly, there have been several individual projects that have also been implemented at local regional levels and funded by independent and governmental bodies, for instance, computer skills for people with dementia, mental health self-help kits, therapeutic use of animation with children, working with traumatised refugees and asylum seekers and taking theatre skills into secure mental health units [Brooks et al. 2011].

CONCLUSION

Innovations in community mental health are the way forward to bridge treatment gaps and make mental healthcare affordable and accessible to a larger community of individuals. It is a potential way to address global mental health by upscaling existing mental health interventions, taking from the successes of innovative community mental health models of different parts of the world. Non-specialist health workers or community health workers play a crucial role in exponentially increasing the reach of mental health services to those from remote and low-resource areas. The most benefitted are from the LMICs. Responsible task sharing is the way NSHWs can grow and serve to reduce the existing width of the treatment gap.

Bibliography

1. Clark, D. M., Canvin, L., Green, J., Layard, R., Pilling, S., & Janecka, M. (2018). Transparency about the outcomes of mental health services (IAPT approach): An analysis of public data. *The Lancet*, *391*(10121), 679–686.
2. Balaji, M., Chatterjee, S., Koschorke, M., Rangaswamy, T., Chavan, A., Dabholkar, H., . . . Patel, V. (2012). The development of a lay health worker delivered collaborative community based intervention for people with schizophrenia in India. *BMC Health Services Research*, *12*(1), 1–12.
3. Brooks, H., Pilgrim, D., & Rogers, A. (2011). Innovation in mental health services: What are the key components of success? *Implementation Science*, *6*(1), 1–10.
4. Harding, T. W., & Chrusciel, T. L. (1975). The use of psychotropic drugs in developing countries. *Bulletin of the World Health Organization*, *52*(3), 359.
5. Hubley, S., Lynch, S. B., Schneck, C., Thomas, M., & Shore, J. (2016). Review of key telepsychiatry outcomes. *World Journal of Psychiatry*, *6*(2), 269.
6. Kohrt, B. A., Jordans, M. J., Rai, S., Shrestha, P., Luitel, N. P., Ramaiya, M. K., . . . Patel, V. (2015). Therapist competence in global mental health: Development of the ENhancing Assessment of Common Therapeutic factors (ENACT) rating scale. *Behaviour Research and Therapy*, *69*, 11–21.
7. Kroenke, K., & Unutzer, J. (2017). Closing the false divide: Sustainable approaches to integrating mental health services into primary care. *Journal of General Internal Medicine*, *32*(4), 404–410.
8. Lehmann U, Sanders D. Community health workers: What do we know about them? The state of the evidence on programmes, activities, costs an impact on health outcomes of using community health workers [Internet].World Health Organization; 2007 [cited 2018Dec 17]. www.hrhresourcecenter.org/node/1587.html
9. McPake, B., & Mensah, K. (2008). Task shifting in health care in resource-poor countries. *Lancet*, *372*(9642), 870–871.
10. Mendenhall, E., De Silva, M. J., Hanlon, C., Petersen, I., Shidhaye, R., Jordans, M., . . . Lund, C. (2014). Acceptability and feasibility of using non-specialist health workers to deliver mental health care: Stakeholder perceptions from the PRIME district sites in Ethiopia, India, Nepal, South Africa, and Uganda. *Social Science & Medicine*, *118*, 33–42.
11. Mueser, K. T. (2011). *Oxford textbook of community mental health*. Oxford: Oxford University Press.
12. Naslund, J. A., Aschbrenner, K. A., Araya, R., Marsch, L. A., Unützer, J., Patel, V., & Bartels, S. J. (2017). Digital technology for treating and preventing mental disorders in low-income and middle-income countries: A narrative review of the literature. *The Lancet Psychiatry*, *4*(6), 486–500.
13. Pandya, A., Shah, K., Chauhan, A., & Saha, S. (2020). Innovative mental health initiatives in India: A scope for strengthening primary healthcare services. *Journal of Family Medicine and Primary Care*, *9*(2), 502.
14. Patel, V., & Saxena, S. (2014). Transforming lives, enhancing communities: Innovations in global mental health. *New England Journal of Medicine*, *370*(6), 498–501.
15. Patel, V., Saxena, S., Lund, C., Thornicroft, G., Baingana, F., Bolton, P., . . . UnÜtzer, J. (2018). The Lancet Commission on global mental health and sustainable development. *The Lancet*, *392*(10157), 1553–1598.
16. Raviola, G., Naslund, J. A., Smith, S. L., & Patel, V. (2019). Innovative models in mental health delivery systems: Task sharing care with non-specialist providers to close the mental health treatment gap. *Current Psychiatry Reports*, *21*(6), 1–13.
17. Semrau, M., Alem, A., Ayuso-Mateos, J. L., Chisholm, D., Gureje, O., Hanlon, C., . . . Thornicroft, G. (2019). Strengthening mental health systems in low-and middle-income countries: Recommendations from the Emerald programme. *BJPsych Open*, *5*(5).
18. Thara, R., Padmavati, R., Aynkran, J. R., & John, S. (2008). Community mental health in India: A rethink. *International Journal of Mental Health Systems*, *2*(1), 1–7.
19. Thornicroft, G., Ahuja, S., Barber, S., Chisholm, D., Collins, P. Y., Docrat, S., . . . Zhang, S. (2019). Integrated care for people with long-term mental and physical health conditions in low-income and middle-income countries. *The Lancet Psychiatry*, *6*(2), 174–186.

20. van Ginneken, N., Maheedhariah, M. S., Ghani, S., Ramakrishna, J., Raja, A., & Patel, V. (2017). Human resources and models of mental healthcare integration into primary and community care in India: Case studies of 72 programmes. *PloS One, 12*(6), e0178954.
21. Wahlbeck, K. (2015). Public mental health: The time is ripe for translation of evidence into practice. *World Psychiatry, 14*(1), 36–42.
22. Whitley, R. (2015). Global mental health: Concepts, conflicts and controversies. *Epidemiology and Psychiatric Sciences, 24*(4), 285–291.

43
Optimizing Patient Care in Psychiatry – Child and Adolescent Psychiatry

Anweshak Das and Jayashree Das

Introduction	465
The Developing Brain	466
Mental Health Issues in Children and Adolescents	466
Consequences of Childhood Mental Disorders	467
Barriers in Treatment of Childhood Mental Disorders	467
How to Optimize Treatment and Care in Child and Adolescent Psychiatry	468
Conclusion	472

INTRODUCTION

Globally 1.2 billion adolescents aged 10–19 years today make up 16% of the world's population [1]. Children aged between 0 and 14 years of age contribute to 26% of the world population [2]. A WHO report stated that in some countries, adolescents make up a quarter of the population; in fact, the number of adolescents is expected to rise through 2050, particularly in low- and middle-income countries (LMICs) [3]. Children and adolescents are the future of a nation. They are one of the strongest assets of any society and can contribute enormously to the development of a society and community. The transition from child to adolescent is one of the most challenging and critical periods in any person's life. A plethora of physical, emotional and neurocognitive changes take place during this transition period. For the betterment of any society or any nation, it is of utmost importance that it give particular attention to the health of its child and adolescent population. Health is not only the physical dimension; it should also encompass mental health and emotional wellbeing. Mental health conditions have long been identified as a leading cause of disability in children and adolescents. Over the globe, childhood and adolescent mental health issues are quite common and are in fact on the rise. Mental health issues are among the foremost contributors to the global burden of disease [4]. Children's mental health problems are among the leading causes of disability for children and adolescents and are among global health advocates' highest priorities [5][6][7]. Global figures report that 10–20% of adolescents experience mental health conditions. But the bitter fact is that many of them are underreported, underdiagnosed and undertreated [8]. Fifty percent of children and adolescents develop mental disorders before 14 years of age and 75% by 25 years [9][10]. It is further reported that one-quarter of disability-adjusted life years (DALYs) for mental and substance use disorder occur in the adolescent age group [11].

DOI: 10.4324/9780429030260-47

THE DEVELOPING BRAIN

"When it comes to building the human brain, nature supplies the construction materials and nurture serves as the architect that puts them together" (Kotulak, 1997) [12]. The human brain is born remarkably unfinished. The trillions of neurons are not wired up in the perfect way when a child is born; instead the experiences of life and the effect of the environment determine the wiring of our neurons. Of course genetics and neurobiology play a role, but we cannot underestimate the impact environment plays in the development of the personality and character of any individual. The number of brain cells is the same in children and adults. The only difference is how they are connected. For proper wiring and connection of the neurons, the brain requires a positive and loving environment, without which the brain will struggle to develop normally throughout childhood. The local environment refines one's brain. Without an environment with emotional care and cognitive stimulation, the human brain cannot develop. It is reported in many studies that if a child is exposed to a negative environment, the brain can often recover; once the child is transferred to safe and loving environment, recovery occurs. The younger a child is removed, the better the recovery. A loving and nurturing environment plays a critical role in the developing child brain. Hormones in our body cause obvious physical changes as we take on the appearance of adults, but out of sight, our brains are undergoing enormous changes. Everything you have experienced has altered the physical structure of your brain [13]. In a way, most childhood psychopathologies and childhood mental disorders develop because of negative, pessimistic environmental influences on the developing brain. Childhood trauma, neglect, sexual and physical abuse, bullying, mental disorders in parents, broken families, dysfunctional families, inhumane living conditions, displacement in childhood, children exposed to war and conflict and so on are some of the negative environmental issues that lead to many of the mental health issues in children.

MENTAL HEALTH ISSUES IN CHILDREN AND ADOLESCENTS

The World Health Organization has reported that mental health disorders are one of the leading causes of disability worldwide. Three of the ten leading causes of disability in people between the ages of 15 and 44 are mental disorders [9][14]. The prevalence and pattern of mental and behavioral disorders show a gradual change from children to adolescence [8]. One in six people with mental disorders are aged 10–19 years. Mental health conditions account for 16% of the global burden of disease and injury in people aged 10–19 years [15]. From childhood to adolescence, the prevalence rate increase from 1–2% to 10–20% [16]. The magnitude of mental disorders in children and adolescents varies in different countries [17]. This variation across different countries can be attributed to differences in genetic vulnerability, lack of data due to inadequate research in the area, socio-cultural issues, gender roles, educational level, differences in policy and advocacy systems, economy or financial issues and so on [17][18]. Commonly seen disorders in the childhood and adolescent age group are mood disorders, anxiety disorders, behavior disorders and substance use disorders [19]. Globally, depression is one of the leading causes of illness and disability among adolescents [15]. Among 15–19-year olds, self-harm or suicide is third leading cause of death and DALYs lost [20]. Nearly 90% of the world's adolescents live in low- or middle-income countries, and more than 90% of adolescent suicides are among adolescents living in those countries [15]. Neurodevelopmental disorders like ADHD, intellectual disability and autism are also commonly found in children. Increased access to and use of technology has led to an alarming rise in internet addiction, gambling disorders and game addiction, particularly in the adolescent age group. Children and adolescents are especially vulnerable to sexual violence, which has a clear association with detrimental mental health [15]. Anxiety is the ninth leading cause for adolescents aged 15–19 years and sixth for those aged 10–14 years. Somatic symptoms are very often associated with emotional disorders. Childhood behavioral disorders are the 2nd leading cause of disease burden in young adolescents aged 10–14 years and the 11th leading cause among older adolescents aged 15–19 years. Childhood behavioral disorders like oppositional defiant disorder and conduct disorder are associated with irritability, aggression and mood swings. Eating disorders commonly emerge during adolescence and young adulthood. Eating disorders affect females more commonly than males. Psychosis most commonly and classically emerges in late adolescence or early adulthood. Many risk-taking behaviors such as substance use or sexual risk taking start during adolescence. Globally, the prevalence of binge drinking among adolescents aged 15–19 years was 13.6% in 2016, with males most at risk. The use of tobacco, cannabis and other drugs is another concern. In 2016, based on data available from 130 countries, it was estimated that 5.6% of 15–16-year-olds had used cannabis at least once in the preceding year [15].

CONSEQUENCES OF CHILDHOOD MENTAL DISORDERS

Childhood mental disorders are a global public health concern [21]. Mental health problems cause significant distress to the child, parents, family and the entire community or society. Mental health problems in children often lead to lifelong impairment. Most mental health conditions worsen if not treated as the brain's development continues to be assaulted by negative influences. Mental disorders in childhood can have a detrimental effect on brain development as it hinders the neurobiological, emotional and cognitive development in a child [21]. Ultimately all of these will have tremendous negative social, educational, occupational and economic consequences. These issues make the development and implementation of child mental health initiatives imperative. Early detection and intervention can go a long way in preventing most childhood mental disorders.

BARRIERS IN TREATMENT OF CHILDHOOD MENTAL DISORDERS

The 1989 United Nations Convention on the Rights of the Child commits countries to "ensure that all children have the right to develop physically and mentally to their full potential, to express their opinions freely and to be protected against all forms of abuse and exploitation". The World Health Organization has stated that mental health and emotional wellbeing are basic human rights and need to be protected for children to thrive. Positive mental health and emotional wellbeing in children and adolescents facilitates improved adult productivity and economic stability. But in spite of all the scientific and technological advancement, improved knowledge about the subject, improved research methodologies and better diagnostic procedures there still remains a gap in treatment or some factors acting as barriers in treatment delivery in childhood and adolescent mental health disorders. Less than two-thirds of young people with mental health problems and their families access any professional help. Globally, studies report only 25–35% of affected children and adolescents accessing treatment [22] [23]. These barriers are greater in LMICs. Barriers in treatment are still found in Western countries as well, but the reasons differ from LMICs.

Mostly in western countries, there is a lack of proper referrals from the general practitioners. Although general practitioners are a bridge between patients and specialists, they have difficulty in identifying and managing mental health problems. Most general practitioners lack proper training, skills and knowledge about mental illness and some of them also lack confidence in diagnosing mental disorders. Many times, patients also fear confidentiality issues with general practitioners [22]. Patient-related issues also act as an obstacle in treatment delivery. Many children and adolescents will refuse to accept their problems and at times will try to solve their problem on their own. Many report a lack of confidence in their doctors. Many studies report that children and adolescents are more likely to seek help if they feel respected and if they feel that they are listened and are being cared for [23]. In LMICs, due to poor educational levels and sociocultural beliefs, potent factors acting as barriers are stigma, embarrassment and negative public opinion [23]. Other factors common in most of these countries are lack of time, lack of logistic support, cost and financial issues, lack of proper policies and proper child guidelines, gender and ethnicity issues, cultural beliefs, lack of availability of professionals and so on [23][24]. Lack of parental and family support play a major role in help-seeking behavior. Failure to understand the child's problem and lack of ability to recognize the problem behavior in the child are some of the issues [24].

HOW TO OPTIMIZE TREATMENT AND CARE IN CHILD AND ADOLESCENT PSYCHIATRY

As already stated, the highest priority should be given to address the emotional wellbeing of children and adolescents. It is crucial to emphasize both preventive and therapeutic measures by respecting the rights of children in line with the United Nations Convention on the Rights of the Child. Keeping in mind the biopsychosocial dimension of mental illness, in optimizing care for children and adolescent psychiatry, apart from biological or neuropsychiatric dimensions, the social dimension should also be focused on, which includes parents, family, peers, advocacy groups, policy makers, primary care systems, training programs and service delivery system [8]. The World Health Organization's Atlas of Child and Adolescent Mental Health Resources states that fewer than 33% of the countries have proper child mental health policies and working guidelines [25]. To reduce this gap in services, the WHO's mental health Gap Action Programme (mhGAP) has provided guidelines for general practitioners/non-specialists to enable them to better identify and support priority mental health conditions, particularly in lower-resourced settings [15][17][25]. One of the potent dimensions of mhGAP is to develop management guidelines to recognize, identify and prioritize mental disorders and most importantly to scale up services for people with mental disorders, including children. One very important observation noted globally is that in comparison with other pediatric disorders, pediatric psychiatric disorders have always needed attention and prioritization from policy makers and advocacy groups [26]. Throughout the world, there are lots of gaps and challenges in child and adolescent psychiatry, and taking these into account, the WHO argued there is an urgent need to take steps in strengthening the mental health system for children and adolescents. Along with the WHO, the same concerns have been voiced by Child and Adolescent Psychiatry of the World Psychiatric Association (WPA CAP), the International Association for Child and Adolescent Psychiatry and Allied Professions (IACAPAP) and the World Association for Infant Mental Health (WAIMH). The concept of global mental health for children and adolescents has gained a lot of attention in the last two decades for optimization of child and adolescent mental healthcare. Through this, sincere efforts have been put into training of primary healthcare physicians and workers, improving out patient department and in patient department services, developing evidence-based pharmacological treatments, ensuring the availability of mental health service professionals, parent and teacher training to identify subtle signs and raising community awareness programs to ward off stigma [17][25][27]. Although substantial gains have been made in some areas, many feel that these global health initiatives still are in the infancy stage, lack proper coordination, lack evaluation, lack logistical support and so on. Some of the critical factors for optimizing patient care in child and adolescent psychiatry are listed in the following.

Increasing number of professionals in child and adolescent psychiatry: Worldwide, there are a very few child and adolescent psychiatrists; in high-income countries, the number of child psychiatrists is 1.19 per 100,000 youth, but in low- and middle-income countries, the number is less than 0.1 per 100,000 population [28]. On the other hand, the demand for these professionals is increasing day by day. The lack of resources can be attributed to various factors like time needed to complete a specialization in child psychiatry after doing post-graduation in psychiatry, low availability of seats/post in child psychiatry courses (absent in some of the LMICs), financial factors and poor policy-making strategies neglecting child and adolescent mental health. Some strategies for increasing the workforce may be increasing the number of posts/seats in this area, courses in various institutions, more attractive options for both undergraduate and postgraduate trainees, ensuring the expansion of training positions, attractive financial compensation for professionals working in this area and so on. Focus should also be placed on increasing the other professionals in this area like clinical psychologists, psychiatric social workers, occupational therapists, speech therapists and so on. The goal is to build a multi-disciplinary team of service providers working in a community mental health clinic or child psychiatry outpatient service for the greater benefit of the child.

Primary physicians and primary healthcare workers: More emphasis should be placed on training primary physicians and primary healthcare workers in the area of child and adolescent mental health. They should be given the knowledge and skills to identify and diagnose mental disorders in children so that they become confident and competent enough to refer them to specialists. Also, policies must be made for a better and swifter referral system between primary workers and physicians, particularly in the LMICs, so that there is no delay in treatment delivery. As stated earlier in the chapter, early intervention can go a long way in ameliorating the long-term negative consequences. The Extension for Community Healthcare Outcomes (ECHO) project emphasizes patient-based/real-time education (via team meetings and phone and video-teleconferenced consultations) in order to improve the mental health competencies of primary care providers. Primary physicians and workers can also take an advantage of digital health interventions (DHIs) to increase access to services [27][29]. Another important area that needs to be addressed is the distance between service centers/hospitals, particularly in LMICs. Most of the hospitals and specialist centers are in far-flung areas or in urban settings, which in a way decreases the motivation to seek help.

Liaison with other health professionals: Like primary care workers, doctors or health professionals from other specialties should be made aware of child and adolescent psychiatric issues. Pediatricians, physicians, pediatric surgeons, endocrinologists and dieticians closely work with this age group. Improved liaison, proper referrals and coordination between psychiatrist and other specialties should be stressed.

Multisectoral collaboration: For the proper optimization for patient care in child and adolescent psychiatry, multisectoral collaboration is necessary. It is not only health professionals who deal with these issues. A collaborative and coordinated effort of various sectors is instrumental in bringing changes. These will include policy makers, advocacy groups, human rights departments, volunteer organizations, NGOs, parent support groups and so on. The World Psychiatric Association in collaboration with the WHO and the International Association for Child and Adolescent Psychiatry developed a manual public education campaign, and effectiveness in nine countries (Armenia, Azerbaijan, Brazil, China, Egypt, Georgia, Israel, Russia and Uganda) has been found. The intervention package was aimed for use in a variety of targets, including policy-makers, teachers, parents and children themselves. It had effects on respondent's knowledge of mental illness, confidence in their own awareness and also in improving self-reported willingness to seek healthcare services in case of mental illness [17]. Strategic action plans for child and adolescent mental health are a high priority. The main concept behind this is to create a conscious awareness that child adolescent mental health issues are global public health issues and should be among the top priorities in health policy guidelines. More economic and financial grants, particularly in the LMICs, should be allocated in this area for improved service delivery. In India, only 0.06% of the total national health budget is allocated to mental health, which is even lower than the average mental health budget in low-income countries, which is around 1.5% to 2.7%. In western countries, it is around 6% of the total health budget. This will be possible with a committed and dynamic bunch of policy makers. Multisector mental health policy is best characterized by a holistic, evidence-based approach to identify and treat mental disorders, with specific emphasis on prevention, early intervention in high-risk categories and rehabilitation for recovering patients. Strategic program implementation should be done after problem identification and proper evaluation. Scope for reevaluation and revision of programs and policies should also be kept in mind [27][30][31]. Policies and programs should aim to provide comprehensive, integrated and responsive mental health and social care services to children and adolescents [30]. All policies and framework should be concrete, taking into account the sociopolitical background of the patient. Also, policies should be in accordance with the United Nations Convention on the Rights of the Child. It guarantees children the full range of human rights and sets international standards for the rights of the individual child. At the community level, civil societies, human rights organizations and NGOs should strive to diminish the negative effects of stigma attached to mental illness through community care services. Stigma and discrimination, particularly in the LMICs, are still huge barriers in optimizing patient care. They lead to underreporting of cases as well as delayed treatment-seeking behaviors, which has long-term negative effects [32]

Research in child and adolescent psychiatry: In the last few decades, research in psychiatry has developed by leaps and bounds. From genetics, neurobiology and treatment targets to developmental and cognitive psychology, newer perspectives have sprung up. Child psychiatry is definitely not lagging behind. Broad areas of research should have great promise for translating science into practice. Importance should be given to more longitudinal studies, better surveys, robust cohort studies and ethical clinical trials [27]. This will help with better understanding of childhood psychopathology, diagnosis and treatment. Research and newer innovations in genetics like epigenetics, gene expression studies, neuroimaging studies and neurobiological discoveries will place us in a better position and enhance our skills to better understand childhood psychopathologies and elucidate the etiologic understanding of disorders and phenotypes.

Diagnosis classification and treatment: Although classificatory systems are helpful in diagnosing a disorder, many times, psychiatrists face criticism for overdiagnosing a child's problems and also for unnecessary use of medications for treating problems in a child. There is always an enigma in child and adolescent psychiatric diagnosis. Diagnosing children with psychiatric disorders is even more problematic and potentially harmful than diagnosing adults. There is no consensus in the medical community about what behaviors constitute a particular "disorder." One psychiatrist might diagnose a child with ADHD, another might say that the same child has oppositional defiant disorder (ODD) and a third doctor might diagnose the child with bipolar disorder. Psychiatric diagnoses have been expanded to include normal childhood behaviors because adult behavior standards are being imposed on children. There is a world of difference between what normal behavior in a child is and what normal behavior in an adult is. Temper tantrums and swift changes of mood, for example, are not considered normal in adults. The DSM-5 and coming ICD 11 place importance on categorical diagnosis, which has its own pitfalls [27]. Many countries give a growing consensus and importance to the dimensional approach rather than categorical diagnosis. For better optimization and care in children and adolescents, the classificatory system should be more reliable, valid and sensitive. The cultural and social context should be kept in mind. Neuroscience certainly holds great promise for increasing our understanding of psychopathology, but sociocultural contexts must not be minimized. Mental health and illness are inherently multilevel, multicausal phenomena that require integrated frameworks linking different levels of research — for example, psycho-physiological, socio-physiological, psychosocial and neurobiological. Also, a conscious effort must be made to understand the balance between beneficial effects of medicines and the need to provide rational care [33]. Many professionals still vouch for psychosocial intervention as initial treatment strategies. But, again, this is an area of debate. Institutional care, particularly below the age of 5, poses a risk which should be avoided [27]. Newer technologies like optogenetics, drugs targeting metabolomics and inflammatory circuits and nootropic drugs are being developed to optimize patient care in child and adolescent psychiatry [27]. From a psychological perspective, apart from conventional psychotherapies and behavioral therapies, play therapy, pet therapy, art therapy and so on are being increasingly used to optimize child care. But to have a salutary impact, all of these should be scientifically backed and evidence based, directed at specific symptoms, disorders and developmental stages [27].

Role of parents and teachers: Parents, teachers and educational institutions are pillars of strength for children or adolescents. They can play an instrumental role in prevention as well as early intervention in child mental health issues. When adolescents believe they have the necessary resources to deal with difficulties, they are more likely to make wise choices. If, on the other hand, they feel that they cannot face a problem, they may make poor choices. When a coping mechanism fails and an adolescent cannot adjust to the growing demands or challenges, emotional tension and stress creep up in an adolescent's life. The most common way to release tension from any stressor is anger, and anger is most often expressed by aggression. Aggression in any form, if present, or its manifestations are linked to various psychosocial maladjustments or mental disorders and negatively associated with prosocial behavior and adaptive social functioning, especially during adolescence [34]. It may also be a red flag for development of mental disorders. Over the past half-century, there has been a significant increase in the rates of anxiety and depression in children and adolescents. Reports have suggested that most of the good virtues like empathy, compassion and sympathy have somehow become unknown in today's society. Important factors that buffer this aggression and help in prevention of most childhood common mental disorders are empathy and resilience, which can be acquired through social emotional learning skills and life skills training. The parenting style plays a significant role in development of empathy. The authoritative style of parenting is reported to be best suited for empathy development. Maternal warmth has been found to be an important factor in promoting empathy development. Studies reported that parents who were observed to display more warmth toward their children during a variety of interactions in their home tended to have more empathic children [35]. Parents who provide a model for being sensitive to others' needs and emotions through harmonious interactions with their child and talking about emotions with their child are most likely to have more empathic children. A secure, loving and trusting relationship with parents, peers and teachers is the key to empathy and resilience development. Promoting empathy education in schools through various programs helps a lot. Social emotional learning is a new wave today in western countries. Social emotional learning helps in the development of social skills, empathy, problem-solving abilities, anger management, coping skills and critical thinking. Studies have reported that social emotional learning skills help in a significant way to bring down the aggression level in children and adolescents. Parent skill development workshops to deal with problems in children are being organized at the community level [17]. Globally, school mental health programs are gaining support. These programs mainly stress developing students' EQ through social emotional learning skills and life skill education programs [36][37][38]. Increased stress and fracturing of today's lifestyles make it imperative that schools partner with parents to help children thrive. Childhood mental health disorders can be difficult to recognize, are often undiagnosed or misinterpreted and may be overlooked or treated as simple misbehavior. Informed/trained school staff who recognize early symptoms can help a child and family move toward appropriate treatment. Educators can initiate protective factors that help establish a child's long-term capacity for positive behavior, social competency, academic achievement and most importantly emotional well-being. School-based and school-linked programs have been developed for purposes of early intervention, crisis intervention and prevention, treatment and promotion of positive social and emotional development. Task-shifting exercises train teachers to take up roles relating to the identification, initial treatment and referral of children and adolescents with mental illnesses. A protocol for a cluster-randomized intervention where early childhood teachers would be trained to deliver behavioral management interventions to children has also been developed in some countries [17]. NIMHANS in India runs initiatives such as school health programs, teacher orientation programs, student enrichment programs, and school-based campaigns to increase awareness about psychosocial disorders, understanding oneself and improving interpersonal relationships with peers and teachers [31]. Adolescent health programs are being organized at the community level as part of school and college mental health programs. This aims at building a healthy lifestyle for a healthy mind. It stresses drug awareness activities, sex education, life skill training, yoga, meditation, mindfulness activities, exercise and proper nutrition. This forms a part of preventive policies for mental illness and also for the development of emotional wellbeing in adolescents [8][17].

CONCLUSION

Children and adolescents are the most precious asset of any nation. The early formative years of any child, as well as the adolescent phase, are the most important period for prevention of any mental illness. The utmost care both physically and emotionally should be given to all children and adolescents. This calls for a collective responsibility in a holistic and integrated manner from all sections of society, including the parents. A multipronged approach from different working professionals is needed for optimization of care in child and adolescent mental health. The future of society and communities is in the hands of our children. Prevention, early identification and diagnosis, evidence-based treatment, an available workforce, a better referral system and easy accessibility to service providers, along with community involvement and life skill training can play a pivotal role in optimizing care and treatment in childhood mental disorders.

References

1. www.data.unicef.org
2. www.unfpa.org
3. www.who.inc. Adolescent Health, the Missing Population in Universal Health Coverage.

4. Kilian R, Losert C, Park A, McDaid D, Knapp M. Cost-effectiveness analysis in child and adolescent mental health problems: An updated review of literature. *International Journal of Mental Health Promotion.* 2010;12(4):45–57.
5. Mathers CD, Loncar D. Projections of global mortality and burden of disease from 2002 to 2030. *PLOS Medicine.* 2006;3(11):2011–2030.
6. World Health Organization. *The global burden of disease: 2004 update.* Report for World Health Organization, Geneva. 2008.
7. Collins PY, Patel V, Joestl SS. Grand challenges in global mental health. *Nature.* 2011;475:27–30.
8. Naresh Nebhinani, Jain S. Guest editorial, adolescent mental health: Issues, challenges, and solutions. *Annals of Indian Psychiatry.* June 8, 2019.
9. Kessler RC, et al. Age of onset of mental disorders: A review of recent literature. *Current Opinion Psychiatry.* 2007;20(4):359–364.
10. Kessler RC, et al. Lifetime prevalence and age-of-onset distributions of DSM-IV disorders in the National Co morbidity Survey Replication. *Archive of General Psychiatry.* 2005;62(6):593–602.
11. Global Burden of Disease Collaborative Network. *Global burden of disease study 2016 (GBD 2016) results Seattle.* Institute for Health Metrics and Evaluation, Seattle. 2017.
12. Minnesota Association for Children's Mental Health. *Unlocking the mysteries of children's mental health: An introduction for future teachers.* Rev Ed., St. Paul, Mumbai, India. 2004.
13. David Eagleman. The Brain, the story of you. 2015.
14. Murray C, Lopez A. *World health report 2002: Reducing risks, promoting healthy life.* World Health Organization, Geneva, Switzerland. 2002.
15. www.who.int/news-room/fact-sheets/detail/adolescent-mental-health
16. Malhotra S, Chakrabarti S. *Developments in psychiatry in India.* Springer India, New Delhi. 2015.
17. Rajesh Sagar, Vijay Krishnan. Preventive psychiatry for children and adolescents. *Indian Journal of Social Psychiatry.* 2017;33:118–122.
18. Whiteford HA, Degenhardt L, Rehm J, Baxter AJ, Ferrari AJ, others. Global burden of disease attributable to mental and substance use disorders: Findings from the global burden of disease study 2010. *The Lancet.* 2013;382:1575–1586.
19. Merikangas KR, Nakamura EF, Kessler RC. Epidemiology of mental disorders in children and adolescents. *Dialogues Clinical Neurosciences.* 2009;11:7–20.
20. WHO. Global Accelerated Action for the Health of Adolescents (AAHA). Guidance to Support Country Implementation. 2017.
21. Reem M. Ghandour et al. prevalence and treatment of depression, anxiety, and conduct problems in US children. *Journal of Pediatrics.* 2019 Mar;206:256–267.e3.
22. O'Brien D, Harvey K, Howse J, et al. Barriers to managing child and adolescent mental health problems: A systematic review of primary care practitioners' perceptions. *British Journal of General Practitioners.* 2016;66:e693–e707.
23. Creswell, C, et al. Why do children and adolescents (not) seek and access professional help for their mental health problems? A systematic review of quantitative and qualitative studies. *European Child & Adolescent Psychiatry.* 2020 Jan 21. doi: 10.1007/s00787-019-01469-4
24. Barriers in Accessing Child Mental Health Services for Parents and Caregivers Lauren Kizaur St. Catherine University. https://sophia.stkate.edu/msw_papers
25. Mental, Neurological, and Substance Use Disorders: Disease Control Priorities, Third Edition (Volume 4). James G Scott et al. Childhood Mental and Developmental Disorders. Chapter 82016 Mar 14.
26. Lu C, Li Z, Patel V. Global child and adolescent mental health: The orphan of development assistance for health. *PLoS Medicine.* 2018;15(3):e1002524.
27. Skokauskas, N, et al. Shaping the future of child and adolescent psychiatry. *Child Adolescent Psychiatry Mental Health.* 2019;13:19.
28. World Health, O, et al. *Mental health atlas.* WHO, Geneva, Switzerland. 2017.
29. Mehrotra K, et al. Effectiveness of NIMHANS ECHO blended tele-mentoring model on Integrated Mental Health and Addiction for counsellors in rural and underserved districts of Chhattisgarh, India. *Asian Journal of Psychiatry.* 2018;36:123–127.
30. World Health Organization. *Mental health action plan 2013–2020.* World Health Organization (WHO), Geneva. 2013.
31. Md Mahbub Hossain, et al. Improving child and adolescent mental health in India: Status, services, policies, and way forward. *Indian Journal of Psychiatry.* 2019;61:415–419.
32. Shidhaye R, Kermode M. Stigma and discrimination as a barrier to mental health service utilization in India. *International Health.* 2013;5:68.

33. Martin, A, Bloch, MH, Volkmar, FR. *Lewis textbook of psychiatry*. 5th edition. American Psychiatric Press, New York, USA. 2018.
34. Anderson Craig A. and Bushman Brad A. Human Aggression, Department of Psychology, Iowa State University, Ames, Iowa 50011–3180.
35. Robinson JL, Zahn-Waxler C, Emde RN. Patterns of development in early empathic behavior: Environmental and child constitutional influences. *Social Development*. 1994;3:124–145.
36. Gueldner BA, Merrell KW. Evaluation of a social-emotional learning intervention using performance feedback to teachers in a structured consultation model. *Journal of Educational and Psychological Consultation*. 2011;21:1–27.
37. Harlacher JE, Merrell KW. Social and emotional learning as a universal level of student support: Evaluating the follow-up effect of strong kids on social and emotional outcomes. *Journal of Applied School Psychology*. 2010;26:212–229.
38. Isava DM. An investigation of the impact of a social-emotional learning curriculum on problem symptoms and knowledge gains among adolescents in a residential treatment center. Unpublished doctoral dissertation, University of Oregon, 2006.

44
Community Psychiatry – the Argentina Experience

Eric H. Wainwright and Gustavo E. Tafet

Addiction Treatment 478
Child and Adolescent Care 478
Psychiatric Care in Elderly Patients 479
Family or Domestic Violence 479

The World Health Organization (WHO) authorities highlight that among the most prevalent problems with the greatest impact on the health of the population are depression, psychosis, drug and alcohol abuse, suicide and different forms of violence. We often see that efficient, timely, comprehensive and continuous health coverage is not usually guaranteed in local care processes.

Problems related to mental health are relevant in public health, representing 22% of the total burden of disease in Latin America and the Caribbean, and this trend is currently increasing.[1]

These events generate significant subjective suffering, with severe consequences to the economy and productivity of people and communities and invalidating effects on the social environment, contributing to increasing morbidity, disability and premature mortality (Pan American Health Organization, 2014; World Health Organization, 2017). Different international organizations agree that depression, psychosis, problematic substance use, suicide and different forms of violence have the greatest impact on the health of the population (PAHO, 2014; WHO, 2017).[2]

Historically, Argentina has guaranteed the right to health. Frequently, access to care is not adequate; if real and timely coverage is not guaranteed, with comprehensiveness and continuity of care processes, including articulated health networks that guarantee a comprehensive health system, including the promotion of increasing levels of autonomy, this guarantee will not be fulfilled.[2]

In 2009, the director of the Department of Mental Health and Substance Abuse of the World Health Organization, Benedetto Saraceno, pointed out that 450 million people suffer from severe mental disorders such as schizophrenia and bipolar or other affective disorders in the world, and 24 million of them remain hospitalized in psychiatric hospitals.[1]

He clarified that it is not possible to simply go from a hospital-centered model to a primary care model, particularly as most non-hospitalized patients don't currently have access to adequate treatment.

The existence of functional specialized services that allow a process of adequate supervision and attendance of patients is essential.[1]

The gap between people with mental health problems who receive adequate treatment and those who do not is significant. It has been estimated that in developed and developing countries, more than half of the people suffering mental illness do not have access to adequate treatment. Therefore, increasing the coverage of care continues to be an urgent problem, particularly in developing countries. Approximately 450 million people in the world suffer from diseases such as depression, schizophrenia, dementia or the abuse of alcohol and illicit substances. There are also about a million suicides per year.[3]

The secretary of government of health exercises the role of sanitary stewardship in the country and promotes universal health coverage as a central policy.[2]

Universal health coverage (UHC) has as one of its tactics, the "Family and Community Health Strategy" (ESFC), with an important territorial component in the first level of care that proposes the integration of the health system at the community level. This strategy defines a care model in which the population is nominalized and geo-referenced and in which family and community health teams are responsible for the care processes. With this care model, an attempt is made to achieve comprehensive quality.[2]

In 1990, the countries of Latin America signed the Declaration of Caracas, a document that indicates that the resources, care and treatment for people with mental disorders must safeguard personal dignity and human and civil rights. The agreement establishes the restructuring of psychiatric care, promoting the development of community-based mental health services; that is, end the stigmatization of people with mental disorders and promote their full social reintegration.[1]

In the poorest countries, we estimate that up to 75% do not receive any type of treatment. In addition to this, patients require more efficient access to quality treatments.[3]

Mental health processes are determined by historical, socio-economic, cultural, biological and psychological components, the preservation and improvement of which require a dynamic of social construction linked to the conception of human and social rights of every person.

The National Law on Mental Health No. 26,657 and the National Law on Patient Rights No. 26,529 are regulations that guarantee the right of all people to effective and timely mental healthcare; particularly those with mental illness are recognized as subjects of law, and the law proposes a modality of community approach for their treatment.[2]

In Argentina, in both laws previously mentioned, "mental health is recognized as a process determined by historical, socio-economic, cultural, biological and psychological components, whose preservation and improvement implies a dynamic of social construction linked to the realization of human rights and social problems of every person"; therefore, any problem that implies subjective suffering in the system user is susceptible to attention in the mental health service. The model is based on the promotion of health and psychosocial care, prevention, care and rehabilitation. A community-based, comprehensive, interdisciplinary and intersectoral approach is focused on people that understands the complexity of the processes of health – disease – care – continuity of care in the territorial area where people live their daily lives. Thus, it is assumed that mental health problems are complex and multidimensional and take place in the social framework, which is not, generally, optimal.[2]

The community approach model entails the implementation of a "community-based mental health network", integrated with general health services and with intersectoral articulation. This model is prescribed for the three subsectors of the health system and implies the development of different providers functioning in a network: interdisciplinary mental health teams in primary care centers; mental health services in general hospitals, sanatoriums and hospitals; polyclinics (with outpatient care, 24-hour emergency approach, specialist referral and hospitalization); community day centers; day and night hospitals; different modalities of socio-laboral inclusion; and housing devices with different levels of support (art and mental health, among others).[2]

Before consulting a specialist for psychiatric symptoms, it is usual for patients to visit a general practitioner, who, given the appropriate conditions, may try some initial treatment, prior to referral to the mental health specialist, who would be in charge of carrying out the appropriate treatment. Sometimes this referral may be ignored, such as in mild disorders, such as anxiety or insomnia, which may be managed in primary care; otherwise, they are referred to other specialized treatment alternatives.[3]

There are diseases whose importance is measured by the disability they produce. In some, such as suicide, traffic accidents due to alcohol, homicides associated with addictions and the early death of vulnerable people due to severe mental retardation or schizophrenia, mortality also plays an important role.[3]

If a patient becomes acutely ill and cannot be managed on an outpatient basis and this occurs in the public healthcare system, the patient is transferred to the emergency area. If the condition cannot be stabilized on an outpatient basis, referral to the psychiatric emergency of a general hospital is required. Unfortunately, to date, there are few beds available for this modality, and patients may require a referral to a specialized hospital.[6]

Emergency treatment usually begins in the emergency room, where interdisciplinary attention to mental health emergencies is covered 24 hours, 7 days a week, with teams usually consisting of:

1. psychiatrist
2. psychologist
3. social worker
4. nurse with training in mental health

If the patient is refractory to the treatments described, or in the case of judicialized cases, they may require hospitalization in one of the open door interdisciplinary specialized psychiatric hospitals, where patients enter the emergency ward and are treated by the interdisciplinary team described previously. Here, the patient receives the required treatment of variable duration, according to his needs, in the charge of an interdisciplinary team, in some cases including: occupational therapists, therapeutic companions, legal advisors and other specialists as necessary in some hospitals.[8]

The objective of this network is to guarantee correct access to health in view of the social inclusion of people with mental illness. This system aims to avoid chronic use and stigmatization and preserve and optimize the social and work networks of each user and each system, as well as achieving adequate care for the entire population at risk. All these levels are characterized by services with flexible approach criteria in accordance with the community's problems.[3]

Once the condition has stabilized, the patient may require intermediate levels of support such as a day hospital (day care facility), a halfway house, therapeutic companion or specialized workshops.

In the case of patients from the private sector, the procedure follows similar steps, the ideal being not to occupy resources from the public system but to enter the circuit of their health coverage, either in Social Security, generally starting with a general practitioner, who defines the treatment modality (mild cases) and the necessity of a referral to the specialist's office (more severe cases), who in turn will define the next steps, such as entering a private mental health institution, where the modality and duration of hospitalization will be defined by the in-house team.

Once the condition has stabilized, the patient may require intermediate levels of support, such as a day hospital, a halfway house or therapeutic companion, which are set up through the user's health provider company.

The follow-up to stabilization is initially in the intervening psychiatric center, with gradual independence, in case of longer hospitalizations, by means of incremental leave permits, visit allowances or permits; through the establishments already described; or, generally, outpatient follow-up, depending on the social support available. In the most severe cases, it will need to be more intense. A community center may be required, where a team of psychiatrists, psychologists, nurses, social workers and specialized occupational therapists provide the necessary therapies, making home visits; in addition, a halfway house or protected work environment (cooperative) may be required according to the needs of the patient.[3]

In milder cases, or in which the integrity of the work or social network has not been lost, the patient can be followed on an outpatient basis.

In general, both systems are seen to function in a similar way, with greater differences in social support.

ADDICTION TREATMENT

In Argentina, there are a great variety of private institutions that are dedicated to the treatment of patients who abuse psychoactive substances who may access them through private or semi-private health systems or through private funding.[7]

On behalf of the state, two basic strategies are followed, which are not currently coordinated: On the one hand, there is primary care in public hospitals where non-residential treatments are generally performed (there is an exception where detoxification treatments are performed), mainly through psychological approaches and the National Center for Social Rehabilitation (CENARESO) that provides both outpatient and residential treatments. On the other hand, the Programming Office for the Prevention of Drug Addiction and the Fight against Drug Trafficking (SEDRONAR) offers outpatient and residential treatments in specialized institutions, most of which can be classified in the therapeutic community modality. As defined previously, both these institutions follow different conceptions of the pathological process and do not work in coordination.[7]

Therapeutic communities (TCs), modeled on previous psychiatric experiences, began as little more than basic care units motivationally oriented towards abstinence. Currently, the institutions that provide this type of treatment have incorporated day hospital and outpatient treatments. Today, almost all TCs are made up of a mixed staff of trained professionals and non-professionals (generally recovered addicts who have extensive experience in treating other addicts and managing these types of groups).

CHILD AND ADOLESCENT CARE

The demand for care of children with severe mental disorders has increased in recent years; care being provided by the state, resources in this area have proven insufficient. There are two functional public institutions, giving a specific response to children in this situation. Their capacity is usually at its maximum, functioning with long waiting lists.[5]

In these institutions, staff frequently lack training and do not work in an interdisciplinary fashion, and there are insufficient child and adolescent psychiatrists. The private sector is characterized by a better functioning in this basic area of mental health of children and adults with special needs.[6]

The scarcity of resources means that this vulnerable population is being served only partially.

PSYCHIATRIC CARE IN ELDERLY PATIENTS

The demand for care of elderly patients with mental disorders has also increased in recent years, following the population aging curve in Argentina. These elements evolve in parallel with the other countries in the region.

Currently, the specialized care response provided by the state subsector has proven insufficient. The state welfare system is the main provider of psychiatric care for individuals who are outside the productive sector.[8]

Much of the burden of maintaining the well-being of this population falls on privately hired caregivers or therapeutic companions, frequently personnel with varying degrees of training (requirements are basic). This is heavily dependent on family resources.

The medical treatment of this population with multiple comorbidities is carried out by general practitioners, clinicians, geriatricians, neurologists and/or psychiatrists, depending on the resources available.

Currently the needs of this vulnerable population are partially covered.

FAMILY OR DOMESTIC VIOLENCE

In the health sector of the government of the City of Buenos Aires, there is a Network of Abuse and Violence in which a large part of the city's hospitals participate. It deals primarily with violence against women and minors, and, in addition to the links it maintains within the area, it is related to the School Network for Violence Prevention, dependent on the Ministry of Education of the same jurisdiction.

The care offered by the institutions, including healthcare centers, may include psychological care and counseling, telephone assistance or advice, mutual aid or self-help groups, legal advice, legal sponsorship and shelter homes. The only institution currently including all these services is the Women's Office of the government of the City of Buenos Aires; the other alternatives vary in terms of the services offered, including psychological assistance, mutual aid groups and legal advice. Other related institutions generally provide information for prevention in educational institutions.[4]

Currently, the needs of this population are partially covered, in large part due to the lack of coordination between the institutions in the area.[7]

References

1. PAHO 07/09/2009 "Hospitales psiquiátricos nunca más" in: www.paho.org/arg/index.php?option=com_content&view=article&id=350:hospitales-psiquiatricos-nunca-mas&Itemid=269
2. Lic. N. Fuensalida, Lic. A. Pasquale, Lic. G. Castro Ferro, Dr. A. Brain, Lic. S. Sosa, Dr. A. Zanatta Dec 2018 "Recomendaciones para la red integrada en salud mental con base en la comunidad" in: *Abordaje de la Salud Mental en Hospitales Generales. Dirección Nacional de Salud Mental y Adicciones* 0000001388cnt-2018–12_
3. F. Kzubaj sept 2009 "Psiquiatría/El porcentaje es aún mayor en los países pobres. El 50% no accede a los tratamientos" in: www.lanacion.com.ar/ciencia/el-50-no-accede-a-los-tratamientos-nid 1170931
4. M. Arriagada, L. Ceriani, V. Monópoli. 2013 *Políticas públicas en salud mental: de un paradigma tutelar a uno de derechos humanos/compilado por Malena Arriagada*. Leticia Ceriani; Valeria Monópoli. – 1a ed. – Buenos Aires: Ministerio de Justicia y Derechos Humanos de la Nación. Secretaría de Derechos Humanos, 2013.
5. PAHO/OPSnov 1998 "Perfil de los Sistemas y Servicios de Salud de Argentina. Iniciativa Regional de Reforma del Sector de la Salud en América Latina y el Caribe" in: Área de Desarrollo Estratégico de la Salud Unidad de Políticas y Sistemas de Salud, Organización Panamericana de la Salud, nov 1998.

6. WHO 2003 "LA SALUD MENTAL EN LAS EMERGENCIAS" in WHO/MSD/MER/03.01 Departamento de Salud Mental y Toxicomanías Organización Mundial de la Salud, Ginebra: www.who.int/mental_health/resources/mhe.pdf
7. www.pagina12.com.ar/diario/sociedad/3-131212-2009-09-05.html
8. www.lanacion.com.ar/nota.asp?nota_id=1170931

45
Optimising Assessment Using the House Tree Person Test

Pragya Lodha and Avinash De Sousa

Introduction 481
The House Tree Person Test: An Indian Perspective 481

INTRODUCTION

The House Tree Person Test: An Indian Perspective

Drawings came before writing. Palaeolithic humans learnt to draw stick figures on walls and stone before they learnt to write. The history of drawing is as old as that of humankind. Though drawing has evolved over the centuries in form and style, it continues to be an effective communicative tool, allowing people to express themselves. Drawings have also been recognised as one of the most important forms of communication where language is limited or could not be used. The House Tree Person Test is a projective, free-hand drawing technique that assesses the developmental maturity, personality and emotional characteristics of an individual. John Buck (1948), the developers of the House Tree Person (HTP) Test, believed that artistic creativity represented a stream of personality characteristics that flowed into graphic art. Buck (1948) believed that subjects objectified unconscious difficulties by sketching the inner image of primary processes as 'drawings'. He also believed that the content and quality of the test are not attributable to the stimulus itself; instead they are rooted in the individual's basic personality organisation. The objects of the house, tree, and person were chosen because they were familiar items or concepts even to very young children, were often welcomed by inhibited and guarded individuals, and appeared to stimulate more revealing verbalisations than did other items. Buck also mentions in his original paper that the drawing of the house, tree, and person, in linearity, elicits emotions of the person that ultimately lead to understanding his underlying affective states (Buck 1948).

The HTP test also enables us to detect makers of intellectual and neurological functioning, along with indicators of probable organic brain damage. With a renewed interest in drawing tests, it is better recognised that the HTP is one of the least challenging psychological tests and can be administered to children from 3 years up to adults over 80 years. It is a test that can be used easily with children, young populations, adults, and geriatric populations. The HTP test serves as a great-rapport building test for young children, for patients who may be uncomfortable initiating dialogue, and for those who are illiterate. It is a test that serves as a marker of psychotherapeutic treatment, showing changes in personality and emotional organisation, cognitive styles, and shift in moods. The HTP is also used as a marker of progress in occupational therapy. Overall, the test can be suggestive of prognostic value in a patient suffering from a psychological disorder. Though the HTP is a robust test to assess psychopathology, it can also be administered to healthy individuals (without indicators of psychopathology) as a marker to judge personality in general.

Overall, the HTP involves:

1. Clinician giving instructions to the patient to draw a house, tree, and person.
2. Clinician makes a note of non-verbal demeanour of the patient as part of the test taking behaviour.
3. Clinician asks questions, and patient describes drawings of house, tree, and person.
4. Scoring of the HTP protocol on the basis of various elements of the house, tree, and person.
5. Drawing interpretation based on the manual.

Drawing, as an art, focuses on the 'line' quality and, looking at figure drawings comprehensively, it is observed that drawings differ across cultures, sub-cultures, and socio-demographic regions. Drawings are a function of culture and thus are influenced by determinants of socio-cultural background of an individual, language, and teaching style as well as socio-political and economic demographic variables. Thus, any projective test, including the HTP, is interpreted in the contextual framework of variables like age, sex, and cultural and sub-cultural background of the person. Drawings are also known to vary as a function of geographic shift, especially as cultures also present with differing local norms and colloquial practices from one region to another. Putting House Tree Person in the Indian context, it is crucial to consider how the various characteristics of the drawings change from patient to patient. Several underpinnings and interpretive elements are either not applicable to house, tree, and person drawings made by Indian patients, or characteristics are missing in the international House Tree Person manual that hold value of significance in the Indian context. This chapter reviews the current testing practices in India and elucidates the need for local scoring and interpretive norms for evaluating the House Tree Person test to best understand the clinical and psychopathological underpinnings of Indian patients.

Buck (1948) assumes that patients objectify the unconscious conflicts by drawing the inner images of primary processes. Buck also explains that when an individual draws a house, tree, and person, it leads to eliciting emotions in an individual which are a determinant of the underlying affectional states. As the House Tree Person test stems from Goodenough's Scale of Intellectual Assessment, Buck has also contributed a quantitative scoring system for HTP along with a sign method of scoring. However, most clinicians and researchers evaluate the drawings impressionistically as opposed to using the scoring systems developed by John Buck for quantitative scoring. Psychologists understand that there is no single interpretation that is adequate for any drawing sign. For example, Hammer discusses that for some patients, a chimney may be a phallic symbol, whereas for some, it may be an essential part of the house.

Drawings tests are often labelled culture-free tests; however, it is not so. There is cultural loading in the way drawings are made and interpretation is carried. Thus, it can be better labelled a culture-fair test that allows the administration of the test across various cultures with little or no hindrance in the administration phase. However, it is important for clinicians and early career researchers to be aware that the scoring (if deployed) and interpretation of the House Tree Person test are appropriately completed only within the socio-cultural context of the individual. The drawings made in the HTP are also a function of the artistic skills honed by an individual along with their professional occupation. For example, the drawing of someone who is a professional artist will be far superior in quality to that of someone who is a businessman. Often, some patients do express happiness while taking the drawing test, mentioning that they always wanted to take up drawing. Some children and adults, though not in an artistic profession, still produce superior quality as a result of their interest/passion for art. It is essential to enquire whether art is an interest/hobby/profession for the person before the interpretation proceeds. Additionally, there may be certain drawing characteristics that shall henceforth become normative; for example, a shaded figure drawn by a sketch artist will have to be interpreted with caution.

To date, there has been no effort to Indianise the scoring and interpretation of the HTP in order to enhance the test findings and better understand the personality and emotional organisation along with possible psychopathology of the patient enmeshed in the Indian cultural framework. Developed in 1948, the test was last updated in 1969. Since then, various scoring systems have been developed. The difference in scoring systems shows the difference in the approach of the clinician in the interpretation process. Apart from the scoring systems, variants like the Synthetic HTP and Kinetic HTP have also been developed; nevertheless, HTP continues to be a frequent choice of projective drawing test.

India is a land of diverse cultures, traditions, and ethnicities. With 29 states and 7 union territories, every geographic boundary comes with cultural variation. House Tree Person, being culture fair, is easily administered across states and across rural, semi-urban, and urban areas; however, as clinicians, we see various changes in the way the figures are drawn and described. The following sections shall focus on Indian characteristics of drawings, important as an interpretation element of the HTP test. The findings are based on the experience of two Mumbai-based Indian clinicians, AD and PL, who deployed a qualitative appraisal of structural analysis of interpretation of the HTP figures that considers the structural and content variables (drawings and description of the house, tree, and person). This is based on the experience of having analysed HTP drawings of around 300 patients in their clinical practice. Some changes will be discussed as a resultant to globalisation, whereas some specific features shall be discussed in the Indian context.

A change that we observe as clinicians in practice is understood as a result of globalisation and technological evolution. It must also be remembered that the drawings and descriptions of drawings of HTP are a 'projection' of either the real-life scenario of the patient's life or of a life that the patient desires. Differences are also noted, keeping in mind whether the patient is from a rural or urban background, along with some of the other influential sociodemographic factors, such as economic status, gender, values/beliefs, cultural practices, exposure to education, intellectual level, family dynamics, and developmental course as a person.

It is important to delineate the specificities of these characteristics of drawings in order to understand the socio-cultural relevance which is normative given the background of the patient but would have otherwise been mistaken for psychopathological interpretation. There are specific characteristics of the house in drawings that we have particularly observed in the drawings of Indian patients:

- Thatched houses or hut-like houses which are usually drawn by patients living in rural or semi-urban areas. Here, the shading to indicate thatch may not have a psychopathological indication. However, heavy pencil pressure or excess shading would thus be contraindicated for anxiety. It is interesting if patients living in urban houses draw thatched houses and huts, as we may have to enquire about the need for such a house and whether there was any psychopathological marker related to events that may have

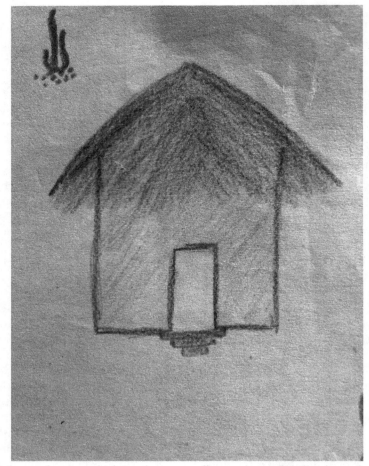

Figure 45.1 A house drawing which is a hut, generally seen in rural India, drawn by a 13-year-old male.

happened in the rural area or the native place going back to their childhood. Shading is often seen in patients, as shading is often taught in basic drawing to enhance the quality of the drawing.

- Patients may also describe their houses as located in villages, as they identify with their native houses, which are usually located in village settings. Another common practice for patients from rural India would be to make a farmland near the house or draw tied cattle (cows/goats/buffaloes) along with a cattle shed near the house, as that is what a common household in rural areas looks like. This may not classify for free-floating anxiety, as often the cattle, cattle shed, and farmlands are thought of as part of the house. Stress related to property issues, distribution of land, wills, assets, and property disputes is very common in India, more so when rural property is present while the person stays and works in the city. Family disputes and interpersonal issues that arise out of property disputes may also be reflected when land or livestock is drawn by patients and must be enquired into. Animals and land have a very special symbolic significance in Indian patients, as they represent power and wealth. The cow is also worshipped, and sometimes religious conflicts may be subconsciously projected in animal

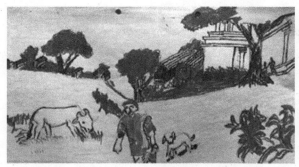

Figure 45.2 Integrated House Tree Person showing a farmer, his farmland, and cattle, drawn by a 16-year-old female.

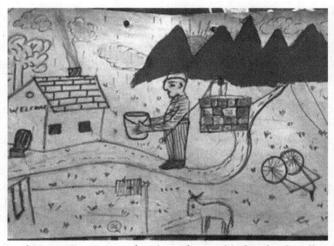

Figure 45.3 Integrated House Tree Person showing a farmer, his farmland, well, and cattle, drawn by a 14-year-old female.

drawings near the house. Drawing two animals of the same breed may even project a sibling rivalry or interpersonal marital issue. The presence of only animal figures in the absence of human drawing may be an indicator of deviation from reality or a psychotic process. Dead animals drawn may indicate loss of self-esteem and guilt, loss of property, or being cheated by ones the patient trusted.

- Another common characteristic that may be found in the rural households would be patients drawing cow-dung cakes in the courtyard area of the yard of the house. This may not be a psychopathological marker, as often the yards or front porches are made of cow dung to keep away infections. Cow dung is considered sacred, and this may be a marker of the level of religiosity of the patient. Orderliness in the arrangement of the cow dung and lot of precision used may be a marker of anal traits and obsessiveness. The religious background plays a role, as this may be seen more in Hindu patients. In India, burning cow dung cakes is a common method to get rid of mosquitoes.
- A common practice for urban people is to now draw flats that may not have a roof, as they themselves live in flats and identify with that as a house. In such a drawing, the roof is generally missing – it can be considered a ceiling, in this these cases, and can be interpreted for concerns of pathology. It is also common for patients to draw towers

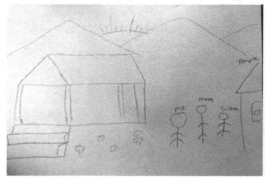

Figure 45.5 Drawing of house showing entire family and temple structure along with house and family, drawn by an 18-year-old female.

and buildings for those who are used to living in or being exposed to skyscrapers or those who have always yearned to live in one of them. It is not uncommon not to have doors and just windows as buildings and towers may be drawn.
- Temples, churches, and mosques being drawn are a common religious symbol that patients who identify with their respective religions may draw. Drawing the *om* (Hindu religious symbol) temple flag, the cross (Christian religious symbol), a crucifix, or a crescent moon with star (Islamic religious symbol) on the house is also an indicator of religious faith/belief, which is normative. Multiple symbols being drawn and detailed description being given of religious practice are markers of obsessive concerns around religion, hyper-religiosity, or religious trauma and caste-based discrimination, which is very common in India. Couples with mixed marriages (marriage between partners belonging to ideologically opposite religions) may have its own interpersonal issues, along with societal stigma, and may be indicated by drawing multiple religious symbols or symbols of those specific religions. Religious segregation and abandonment by the community is also common when a patient suffers from mental illness and may be expressed by these drawings. A patient who has been subjected to religious rituals at a temple or mosque like exorcism rituals to treat mental illness by those believing it to be demonic possession may also draw these symbols.
- It may be common for patients to not draw an attic, as it is not a common part of the household in Indian settings and thus should be excused for interpretation. However, interestingly, some patients do draw the attic; on inquiry, they report identifying with or being desirous of houses from the West, or sometimes it is referred to as a room where no one goes or where the patient likes to be. This then would be suggestive of depressive themes or isolation from the family, low self-esteem, or kinship conflicts. It is essential to probe an attic drawn on roof, which may be suggestive of manic tendencies/grandiose energy or engagement in a fantastical world. Attics may indicate a need to withdraw or remain in isolation and the need for warmth and security or personal space reflected by many patients. Many patients may not have personal space, as they live in overcrowded houses. There is a need for enquiry into rejections from universities abroad when an attic is drawn, as this is a common cause of depression and disappointment seen in Indian patients.
- Likewise, chimneys being drawn may also not be common. It would be expected for Indian patients not to draw chimneys, and thus an absence of chimney may not necessarily suggest lack of psychological warmth or castration fears. The presence of a

chimney on houses should definitely be questioned. Chimneys may be a phallic symbol and indicate the need for an emotional outlet, while patients with sexual inadequacy and erectile issues may also draw chimneys. Sexual longing and pent-up libido or emotion may be indicated when a fuming chimney is drawn. Repressed emotions must be enquired into in psychotherapy sessions when an Indian patient draws a chimney.

- Often curtains may not be drawn on the windows, as it is again not a very common sign noted in rural Indian households. However, curtains may be drawn on doors, as it is a common practice in semi-urban or rural places where often people may simply have a curtain as the door instead of an actual door. Nevertheless, one must probe for sexual relationships or incestual relationships in such cases. The need for privacy and sexual abuse must also be enquired into. Sexual guilt and shame may be asked for along with need for privacy and isolation. Closed curtains may also indicate a lack of trust in others. Excessive detailing on the design of the curtain may be an indication of obsessiveness. Specific symbols drawn on the curtain must be enquired into.
- It would be interesting to question the protocol if patients draw fireplace in the house, as fireplaces are not a part of Indian households and would hold importance for interpretation in the protocol. Fireplaces drawn in the Indian context are a marker of interpersonal conflict within the family. Fireplaces indicate aggression and need for warmth. They are also a symbol of aggression and anger. Patients who live in warm climates, like in India, drawing fireplaces may indicate love needs, longing, and sexual frustration. Marital issues may be reflected in a fireplace, as in Indian customs, marriage rituals involve fire.
- What is also commonly seen in protocols is that patients may draw cars outside their house. Cars may also be labelled with names of the owners or his/her family members, which is a common practice across the country. Excessive focus on the car indicates material wants and striving for superiority. The car may also be a phallic symbol, and sexual frustration may have to be enquired into. Specific numbers on the number plates may have to be asked about. A history of trauma in the form of a vehicular accident may also sometimes be expressed as a car.
- Sometimes patients also draw the insides of the house where they will describe the kitchen, hall, and rooms of the house. It is common to note fixed gender roles depicted like mothers drawn cooking in the house and children seen playing, and the father will be seated in the hall. Often female patients tend to draw the interiors of the house, and it is likely for them to describe it as a house as they have always aspired to maintain that

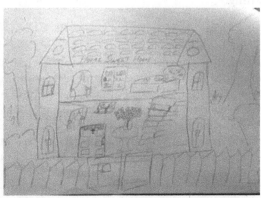

Figure 45.6 Drawing of house showing interiors of the house as desired by the patient, with a cross symbol on the door, drawn by a 34-year-old female.

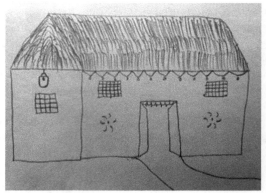

Figure 45.7 Drawing of house decorated with *torans* and *rangoli*, drawn by a 49-year-old female.

way or yearned to own. Do enquire if patients draw a bathroom or corridor or rooms that are generally not drawn in the house. Bathrooms may be an indicator of either sexual abuse or obsessiveness, and kitchens and food may be an indicator of maternal longings, maternal overprotection, focus on food, and eating and feeding issues. The kitchen may also be drawn in mother-in-law/daughter-in law strife, which is very common in Indian settings. The kitchen is a place where the woman feels in complete control of the house, and excessive dominance in the house or lack of dominance and submissiveness with a need for dominance may be expressed drawing the kitchen.

- A lot of female Indian patients decorate the house with *toran* (a string of flowers or beads or other décor in the shape of an archway; it may sometimes also be an archway architecture), or *rangoli* (traditional Indian art form using coloured powder or sand to decorate the floor, courtyard, or flat surface), which is culturally symbolic décor in Indian houses and usually used during auspicious occasions. *Torans* and *rangolis* also differ in style and use across states in India. These being part of the house generally don't confer a psychopathological interpretation but simply are reflective of belief in cultural practices followed by the patient. The type and symbols drawn in the toran or rangoli may be reflected upon if indicative of anything specific.

The second element is the tree, and similarly, there are several aspects of the tree that are unique to the Indian setting:

- Drawing a mango, peepal, coconut, or palm tree is common, as these are common references to trees for Indian patients. It is interesting to note how what is 'common' changes from state to state depending upon the topographical regions. People coming from snowy and hilly areas find pine or apple trees common, people coming from desert regions often make cacti or shrubs, and those coming from coastal areas commonly draw palm and coconut trees. The interpretation is made with caution, keeping in mind what is normative for the demographic background of the person. Peepal trees may indicate the presence of ghosts or spirits, as in Indian culture, ghosts are believed to reside in peepal trees, and this may be enquired into. Deep roots of trees indicate family or transgenerational issues, which are very common in India. Excess cacti drawn by Indian patients may indicate the symbolic nature of pricking or hurt felt by a patient. The rose may symbolise love. The patient and his love for gardening may also be a reason for drawing specific plants if any.

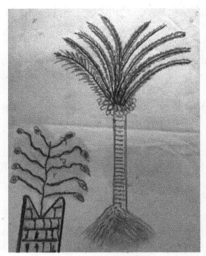

Figure 45.8 Drawing of tree as *tulsi* and palm tree, drawn by a 29-year-old male.

- It is still common for Indian patients to draw a *tulsi* (basil) plant, as it has cultural and religious significance. This plant is frequently found drawn in the courtyards or somewhere on the windowsill of flats and is regarded as an auspicious plant that people pray to. Only the *tulsi* plant being drawn is a marker of strict belief in religious practices. It may also indicate a need for redemption for wrongdoing, excessive shame and guilt, sexual guilt, harsh punitive parenting, physical punishment in childhood, and oedipal conflicts. The God complex as described by Jung may be seen in these patients. The *tulsi* plant, while sacred, may be symbolic of the vagina and menstrual issues in Indian patients, as many women in India due to religious customs are deprived of worship and prayer in temples during menstruation. The *tulsi* being drawn may reflect a masculine protest per Adlerian concepts.
- Patients also make a banyan or a *neem* (Indian lilac) tree with threads around it because these two trees are considered auspicious and prayed to. The neem tree may indicate guilt and a need for purification. Patients with psychosomatic skin disorders like psoriasis and eczema may draw a neem tree. Menstrual guilt may also be reflected in a neem tree. Gulmohar trees are also frequently drawn by Indian patients.
- Rose and lotus are common flowers reported by patients in India. The rose is considered a symbol of balance. It expresses promise, new beginnings, and hope. Its thorns represent defence, physicality, loss, and thoughtlessness. The rose may also be a religious symbol of Jesus, who agreed to be crowned with thorns. The colour of the rose drawn may be enquired into and may be indicative of the emotion at hand. The lotus flower symbolises the power of psychological resistance as the ability to transform adversity into potential. The lotus flower can be a magnificent metaphor for how there are people capable of folding pain up and unfolding it later in the form of serenity, self-control, and persistence.
- Coconuts are commonly drawn by Indian patients, and coconut water symbolises cleansing. A cracked coconut may show annihilation of the egoism of a person. The concept of teachers teaching under a tree or old people sitting under a tree can be reported, as it is a common Indian practice. Strict punishment in childhood by a teacher or abuse may be enquired into. The presence of a good teacher as a father or mother figure may also be a reason for drawing this. Problems in education, disrupted

education, incomplete education, and bullying may be enquired into. Educational aspirations may be another reason for drawing this.
- Patients who are religious may also make some threads around a tree, which is usually a religious practice. These threads are indicative of needs and wants and yearnings that are unfulfilled desires of the patients and must be enquired into.

The last element of the HTP is the person, and the following are specific Indian aspects of this:

- It is not uncommon to see some children and young adults draw the 'person' figure with a mobile phone, which invariably indicates current lifestyle changes, suggesting the rampant growth in use of smartphones. Another variant with globalisation is also seen in the nature of clothing assigned to the person. It is common to note person drawings of boys and girls wearing distressed jeans and tank tops and ornamented with current trending accessories. A further observation is also that the distinct male and female clothing has blurred with greater uniformity of dressing across genders. Sometimes brands of the phones may be specified if the focus is on the phone and yearning in that direction.
- Often female patients draw females with Indianised dressing, adorning *saris* and *salwar kameez*, whereas males may draw persons wearing attire like the *kurta pyjama* or *dhoti*. These are traditionally common attire in the Indian community and should be considered in the cultural framework. Dressing grossly differently from that worn by the patient must be enquired into, and issues related to identification with certain figures may be sought.
- The person figure is also drawn with characteristics like accessories. Females tend to draw *mangalsutra* (necklace which is a symbol of being married), *bindi* (a black rounded stick-on worn on the forehead), bangles and *sindoor* (generally a red powder put in the midline of hair which is a symbol of being married), whereas males draw a

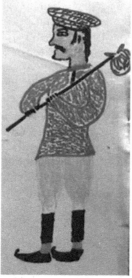

Figure 45.9 Drawing of person as a male wearing *dhoti*, *kurta*, and *mojdi* (traditional footwear in India), drawn by a 19-year-old male.

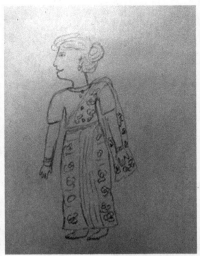

Figure 45.10 Drawing of person as a female wearing *sari*, bangles, and *bindi*, drawn by a 34-year-old female.

turban on the male person, which is a common symbol made by patients who identify with the pertinent socio-religious community. Persons from the Sikh community also draw a *kirpan*, which is a small dagger tied to the waist and is considered a must-have as part of identifying with the Sikh community. These drawings would be an important consideration to include the identification with socio-religious components. The *bindi* can symbolise many aspects of the Hindu culture, but from the beginning, it has always been a red dot worn on the forehead, most commonly to represent a married woman. The *bindi* is also said to be the third eye (aggression) in Hindu religion, and it can be used to ward off bad luck. The word *mangal* means auspicious, and *sutra* means thread – together *mangalsutra* means an auspicious thread uniting the souls. The groom ties the auspicious thread around the bride's neck on the day of their holy nuptial to indicate that their relationship will be as auspicious as the thread. A focus on this may be an indicator of marital strife. The *sindoor* is a symbol of female energy and sexual vitality and must be enquired into when drawn. The *kirpan* is a sword or small dagger, originating from the Indian subcontinent, carried by Sikhs. The Punjabi word *kirpan* has its roots in *kirpa*, meaning mercy, grace, compassion, or kindness, and religious themes must be enquired into.

- Patients who are religious may also show religious pendants, certain religious equipment like the *mala* (string of beads used while praying), or *trishool* (a fork-shaped symbol carried by one of the Hindu gods) being carried by the person. The *trishool* is polyvalent and is an aggressive symbol and also represents the conglomeration of the past, present, and future of the individual. It may at times be a symbol of strength and masculinity.
- The person, most likely the female, may also be holding kitchen accessories like a spoon or cooking utensil, which is a symbol of the gender roles specified by culture. Another variant reflective of the rural areas is women carrying pots.
- It may also be a common practice for person figures to be shown in a praying posture, which may further be indicative of religious beliefs that may be further reflective of adaptive attitudes, obedience, or obsessive religious beliefs/practices.
- The person may also be drawn with a *tilak* on the forehead, which is another religious symbol that is usually indicative of strong beliefs in religion (Hindu). The space between

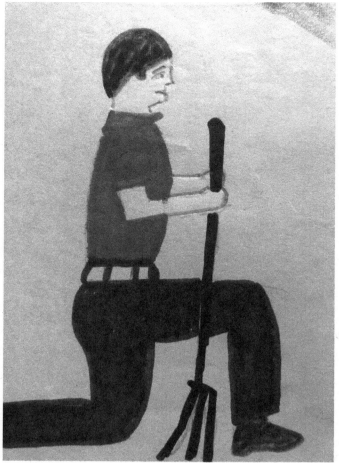

Figure 45.11 Drawing of person as a male holding *trishool*, drawn by a 17-year-old male.

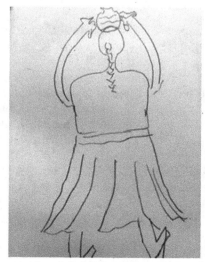

Figure 45.12 Drawing of person as a female holding earthen pots (*matkas*), drawn by 29-year-old male.

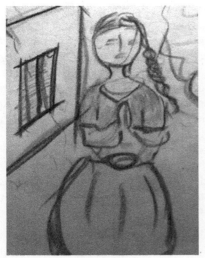 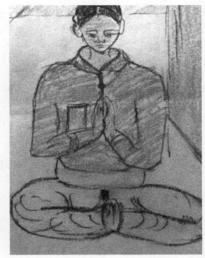

Figure 45.13 and **45.14** Two drawings of a person, one female and one male, folding their hands in a position of praying, drawn by a 15-year-old male and 17-year-old male.

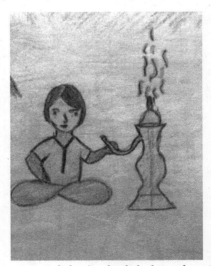

Figure 45.15 Drawing of person as a male having *hookah*, drawn by a 19-year-old male.

the eyebrows is associated with intuition. The forehead signifies spirituality. So, when a long tilak is put, it is indicative of the individual's thoughts towards spirituality.
- The size and shape of the trunk of the body may also vary as drawn by Indian patients, as the physiological makeup varies in the Indian subcontinent.
- Patients may also draw the person wearing slippers and sandals, which are commonly seen footwear in the Indian scenario. The term "en-clothed cognition" is being used to describe the systematic influence that clothes have on a wearer's psyche. Sandals are a risk-free way to express individuality, nonconformity, trendiness, or youthfulness.
- Traditionally, it is common practice to see patients from a rural background draw males with a *hookah*, which has been a part of the normative traditional rural life.

- The show of umbilicus on drawn female figures may also be a common practice by Indian patients and should not be interpreted as for the transparency category of interpretation. The show of cleavage or the bosom, which is uncommon in Indian female figures, must be explored for sexual themes and extramarital affairs as well as sexual inadequacy and body image issues.
- Human figures may also be drawn holding mobile phones, which would generally be accepted given the normalcy of smartphones as part of everyone's life (it would generally be expected in the younger population to draw these). The same holds true for iPads and laptops.

The previous points show the relevance and dire need to have an Indianisation of the test in order to interpret the psychopathological underpinnings and personality variables in the framework of socio-cultural-religious factors that play a crucial role in the bio-psycho-social development of the individual.

Bibliography

Buck JN. (1948). The H-T-P test. *Journal of Clinical Psychology*. 4(2):151–159.

46
Challenges in Patient Care in the Aftermath of an Epidemic and Pandemic

Efi Tsomaka and Konstantinos N. Fountoulakis

Introduction	495
Mental Health During Outbreaks	496
Characteristics of Outbreaks	*496*
Mental Health During and in the Aftermath of an Outbreak	*496*
Risk Factors and Vulnerable Populations	*498*
Prevention and Intervention	501
Prevention	*501*
Intervention	*503*
Future Challenges	507
Social Support and Safety	*507*
Telepsychiatry	*507*
Conclusion	508

INTRODUCTION

Pandemics and epidemics have occupied human attention for centuries, since the Ten Plagues of Egypt and the Athenian plague of 430 B.C. [1]. Apart from the effect on somatic health, outbreaks have a profound effect on the social structure and the economy. Mental health is also affected, either primary or secondary, because of the overall burden. However, since there is little opportunity to explore scientifically the consequences of such events, our knowledge on this matter is limited. Exceptions are the study of HIV pandemics, seasonal flus and the recent outbreaks of SARS [2], EBOLA [3], ZIKA [4] and MERS [5] viral infections.

The last real pandemic known until recently was Spanish flu about a century ago. During the writing of this chapter there is another pandemic occurring worldwide, COVID-19. COVID-19 was labeled a pandemic by WHO on 11 March of 2020. The concerns that will be analyzed are a highly topical issue of modern societies. The subspecialties of psychiatry usually preoccupied with pandemics and epidemics are liaison psychiatry and disaster psychiatry. To approach the topic, we are going to draw on the research done in the recent outbreaks and from other disasters to speculate on the challenges in the aftermath of a pandemic for psychiatric patients in the community.

DOI: 10.4324/9780429030260-50

MENTAL HEALTH DURING OUTBREAKS

Characteristics of Outbreaks

Outbreaks manifest a number of special characteristics which predispose the population to experience distress and even full-blown mental disorders. These characteristics distinguish outbreaks from other mass disasters.

- Information flow: As in other disasters [6], people are informed of a new outbreak from mass media, just as happened with COVID-19. As time passes, information could be both relieving or stressing by itself, depending on the loading and the way of presenting.
- Pattern of the disaster: Epidemics follow a certain epidemiological model, and consequently there is time for society to prepare, plan and program the interventions needed during and after an outbreak. On the other hand, the particular model varies considerably from outbreak to outbreak, and often much time is needed to obtain sufficient information.
- Uncertainty: A common characteristic among disasters is the disruption of feeling of safety. In pandemics, as in bioterrorism [7, 8], there is the uncertainty of whether someone is infected and the health outcome from his/hers infection, especially when we are talking about a new outbreak [7] [9, 10].
- Emergency measures: Another characteristic that distinguishes pandemics are the mandatory measures [11–14] that are usually decided upon for public health protection:
- Social distancing.
- Reduction or stoppage of various activities (e.g., schools, factories, celebrations, etc.).
- Measures of personal hygiene and modification of everyday behavior.
- Quarantine, which was first introduced during the Black Death.

Isolation; quarantine; and closure of schools, workplaces and mass gatherings are some of the precautions that may cause emotions of loneliness and psychological trauma, as well as the disruption of social and family support. These measures can affect people already coping with a psychiatric disorder or lead to the appearance of new psychiatric disorders [12, 13, 15]. It is a challenge for community leaders to plan interventions for people with preexisting psychiatric disorders as well as to prepare sufficient services in the community, focusing on the people who will face post-pandemic psychological consequences.

Mental Health During and in the Aftermath of an Outbreak

A lot of people, after disasters, will overwhelm healthcare facilities and hospitals out of fear they might be infected, although there is not a certainty of actual exposure [8], and mass hysteria may be caused [16–19]. Complaining about somatic symptoms is often. Differential diagnosis of these events is of crucial importance to prevent possible exhaustion of healthcare services [20]. Some divide population after disaster to those developing psychiatric disorders or not [21]. Not all people after disaster suffer from psychiatric disorders. Some are just normal responses that will be overcome on their own in the future. This has to be triaged [21–27].

Mental health problems can be intensified because of the fear of reoccurrence of the outbreak, especially until a vaccine has been created or the whole pathophysiological mechanism of the new agent has been explored. Outbreaks, like other disasters, not only create primary victims (those who will be contaminated and live an individual trauma) but also secondary victims, people living in the community and who live a collective trauma [28], as it disrupts the social networks of a community. As already stated, the uncertainty if someone has been infected is also a distressful factor, and it can be a reason to provoke social stigma. SARS was the first infection widely researched, and from studies about HIV, we know that survivors usually cope with anxiety, fear and psychological trauma. Usually after disasters, most people do not need help, but a substantial proportion of the general population will definitely need professional help to cope with:

- Increased levels of distress as a consequence of the general atmosphere and the conditions the outbreak causes. Isolation and incapability of elders to take care of themselves during an outbreak will increase their anxiety. It is interesting that, on the contrary, often disasters provoke positive outcomes, as they give a sense of purpose [29, 30] to individuals.
- The mandatory measures taken during outbreaks sometimes ban travelling all over the world, and that might make substances not available. Inaccessibility to substances may provoke irritation, aggression, illegal acts and family problems such as domestic violence.
- Adjustment disorder with anxiety or depressive affect [31, 32] after becoming ill or after quarantine or as a consequence of distance isolation. Anxiety and depression [33] in relocated elders from nursing house. Many older people might be the bereaved parents of victims who are usually forgotten by the community, as all the burden falls on the spouse and the children of the deceased. More anxiety for elders with more physical problems.
- Increase in unhealthy or health risk behaviors (increase in tobacco or alcohol or substance use, weight gain, etc.) [34–38]. Alcohol abuse problems [27, 39].
- Daily routine changes could put a high burden on the individual or the family, with frequent conflicts, deterioration of relationships or even violent behaviors and accidents.
- Post-traumatic stress disorder (PTSD) could emerge as the most common disorder for disaster survivors [40, 41] [42], healthcare workers, children and the elderly [43, 44].
- A full-blown mental disorder might emerge, including major depression [45], general anxiety disorder, panic disorder, substance abuse [21, 22, 27, 38, 40, 46, 47] or somatization [37], especially for those working in intensive care units [12, 48].
- Women more often face major depression and PTSD, while men face substance abuse often as comorbid conditions with PTSD [37, 49].
- Infections are linked with a number of somatic and neurological disorders, either primary or as a consequence of treatment, including cognitive impairment, delirium, or encephalitis [50] [51], [52–57].
- Mental health problems in the post-disaster phase may sometimes worsen the physical condition of survivors [10, 21, 58, 59], possibly leading to conditions such as heart disease and diabetes [60, 61]. Among the psychiatric disorders that older people face are functional decrease in patients with dementia.
- "Second injury" victims [62]. Survivors of an epidemic may be vulnerable to distant behavior of healthcare personnel, so they might be traumatized for a second time, as though there is a tendency during disasters for people to be eager to help survivors in the immediate aftermath and forget them later.
- Children may feel insecurity and anxiety and may attribute to pandemics magical characteristics, according to their specific developmental stage and may feel frustration from not meeting their needs (toys), suffer from hyperarousal, irritability, sleeplessness [63], symptoms of fear, hyperactivity, withdrawal from friends or refusal to go back to school.
- Children's clinical symptoms may *also* result in a diagnosis of acute stress disorder, posttraumatic stress disorder, other anxiety disorders or depressive disorders. Children also face difficulties expressing their feelings, so PTSD might be subdiagnosed [64].

- Adolescents may engage in risky behavior or tend to complain about physical symptoms; antisocial behavior and drug and alcohol use are also common.
- Patients under supervision in mental healthcare facilities, such as outpatient clinics or clubs, may face anxiety because of the uncertainty of this situation.
- Psychiatric disorders such as OCD may deteriorate.
- People suffering from generalized anxiety disorder or somatization may face distress and overwhelm healthcare facilities.

Risk Factors and Vulnerable Populations

In every disaster, the community has to prepare a plan for special populations that will need further support and may also face psychological problems in the aftermath of an outbreak. Community service must be alert to identify

- per-event dissociation
- rapid heart rate [65, 66]
- re-experiencing and numbing symptoms, as they might be signs of traumatic stress and occurrence of PTSD and depression at later phase [67, 68]
- women are at high risk of developing PTSD and depression
- men are more susceptible to alcohol abuse [21, 69–75]
- people with previous psychiatric history are more vulnerable to PTSD [21, 76–78]

Our goal is to point out these populations and their special needs [79]. The populations more often facing psychological consequences, as stated in several studies, are

- survivors and their families
- first responders (health workers, paramedics)
- patients with preexisting psychiatric disorders
- the elderly and children [33]

Survivors

Survivors having to stay in isolation with no family support and sensory deprivation can also cause further disorientation. Televisits and telecommunication with their families, except for the necessary treatment, are needed. Community workers must also be prepared for persistent problems the survivors may face after their hospitalization, such as persistent respiratory problems.

Healthcare Workers

As in other disasters, first responders tend to experience stress, burnout and fatigue [80]. In all disasters, healthcare workers are exposed [81], but for pandemics, the case is very different. In the aftermath of a pandemic, health workers have to cope with factors that increase their distress, such as

- Stressful emotions during their duty concerning the capacity of special equipment. Experience from Ebola has shown that many healthcare personnel died because of insufficient equipment [82]. The physical and psychological fatigue of wearing heavy equipment and the effort not to be infected and spread the illness also provoke distress.

- The uncertain nature of the new outbreak. What is different in pandemics is that not only the workers are afraid about their health and the possibility of their infection, but they also worry that they may infect their families and loved ones.
- Another stressful situation that health personnel usually have to face is a significant proportion of elder people that may die during an outbreak.
- As stated for other disasters, this population faces more physical problems, and the capacity of the healthcare systems is not adequate.
- Moreover, there are situations in which they reportedly have to decide who will die and who is going to live, adding another stress-inducing factor.
- Staff might change positions during an outbreak: nurses transferred to ICU units, doctors from other specialties may need to work outside their specialty.
- Another issue they have to face is secondary trauma [83]. The empathy of healthcare professionals is usually to blame for secondary exposure to trauma.

Elderly

Knowledge from other disasters has shown that a special population, the elderly, is usually forgotten during the time of crisis. Healthcare personnel tend to forget them [84]. That might also be the case in the aftermath of pandemics [85, 86]. Several studies mention that disorientation caused by disasters can be fatal for the elderly.

In this group, special attention has to be given to special populations, those who:

- live on their own
- face mobility and sensory disabilities
- have pre-existing psychiatric history
- have cognitive impairment

Among the elderly, there are those with mental health problems such as schizophrenia, affective disorders and dementia [87] which make them an even more vulnerable population of high concern. Some elderly may find it difficult to provide their pet companions with food and veterinarian treatment during isolation periods. Future plans have to be made either for shelters or in-house help.

Sometimes older people are more resilient to disaster than younger people [88], maybe because of stressful life events they experienced in the past and managed to cope with. Healthy older people can play a major role after disasters, as they might

- be useful guides for younger people
- act as volunteers, providing a sense of safety, knowledge and possibly raise others' spirits
- be an active part of the group

Children and Adolescents

Children and adolescents are usual victims of disasters [89], and that is due to

- They usually experience disaster for the first time through their parents. It is also thought that adults are responsible for them, but parents do not necessarily maintain the role of caregiver after disasters.
- First responders are reported to forget the special needs of children and adolescents during disasters [90–93].

- Children and adolescents are more vulnerable to psychological trauma due to the sensitive stages of life physical development, although there is a common belief that children are more resilient, because they are younger.
- They tend to face difficulties following instructions and comprehending threats, due to their cognitive development. As a consequence, they may adopt risk behaviors.

Although children and adolescents usually show vulnerability after disasters [92, 94–96], there are not many epidemiological data for the psychological consequences upon them.

Special Populations

Among these, refugees or immigrants might have left their country and experienced psychological trauma in the past [97, 98], and their lives might be already affected. Community leaders should take that into consideration for post-disaster psychological consequences and understand their different languages and cultural traits.

Addiction

During disasters

- the consumption of substances may increase [99]
- substance users are more vulnerable to infection and to pulmonary diseases [100]
- after pandemics, consumption may be decreased, but the withdrawal cases ending up in hospitals may be increased [101, 102]

Other important concerns that occurred during the most recent pandemic of COVID-19 were:

Behavioral addictions: It is also stated that behavioral addictions may deteriorate. The increase of free time because of loss of jobs has increased:

- the use of the internet
- eating disorders
- gambling
- sleep disorders [103–106]

Opioid users. Moreover, opioid users face some specific difficulties:

- the lockdown of the services that provide them with maintenance treatment limits their access to drugs
- withdrawal symptoms may imitate the symptoms of respiratory diseases, preventing them from seeking help for an infection
- loss of appointments with their therapists for de-addiction [107–109]

Patients With Preexisting Psychiatric Disorders

In the aftermath of a pandemic, planning has to be done for patients with preexisting psychiatric disorders in the community. Community and social psychiatry deals with patients in the community. Specialists usually have to face patients with severe psychiatric disorders and socioeconomic problems. During periods of extreme social disruption, stigma and uncertainty, such as in the aftermath of an outbreak, the provision of mental health services in the community is a challenge. People with previous psychiatric disorders or with preexisting personality traits [110, 111] are susceptible to psychological trauma [21, 72, 77, 112–114].

Psychiatric patients may cope with problems regarding compliance with their therapy, and as a result, a relapse may occur. Mental health specialists should be ready to recognize early signs of a relapse. The reason for these is because of:

- the restriction of in-house appointments because of the fear of contagion and because the use of audio and visual communications is preferred during outbreaks
- cognitive impairment of patients that may prevent them from using internet or other web-based interventions and following certain precautions
- the cancellation of scheduled meetings with their doctors
- disruption of transportation, which limits access to medication
- patients with preexisting psychiatric disorders are at high risk of developing physical illness

Some psychiatric patients may experience feelings of mistrust when it comes to visiting medical healthcare facilities, due to fear of possible infection. All facilities in the community should take all necessary precautions, and specialists should try to obtain the trust of the patients.

During an epidemic, residential facilities may need to be evacuated and their residents transferred to areas that are not infected or less infected. Environmental change may provoke distress in the residents, a matter which must draw the attention of workers [115]. Also, even though an evacuation may not be necessary, mandatory public measures may prohibit visits from families to the residents. This lack of family support must be filled with support from the workers in the facilities. If there is not a plan of evacuation or protective measures in case of a pandemic, it is of high priority in the aftermath to create one. In some residential facilities, visits from relatives or home leaves were not allowed and regular monitoring of vital signs was done daily.

PREVENTION AND INTERVENTION

The term community is described in several studies [116, 117]). Community is an organizing unit in which mental health interventions, public health services, social networks and research plans can take place. In the end of a pandemic in which people have assigned hospitalization a stigma and the meaning of contamination, community services and primary healthcare can play a major role in relief. After a pandemic, as in other disasters, social support networks are disrupted [118], and the community faces economic, psychological, social and behavioral problems.

Prevention

Recognition of Community Needs

- primary assessment of the needs of the community. In the aftermath, the response given should be appropriate
- focused interventions on the special needs of the population
- creation of neighborhood-based groups. Groups with common traumas can be organized in the direction of a psychological first aid approach

Planning

- Cooperation of the government, voluntary organizations and community for future planning and the creation of a disaster management plan are of high importance
- Individuals have to be part of disaster management plans [71], as they concern the whole community

- Community members have to be prepared for a pandemic
- Planning for future emergency and medical supplies available in community centers will relieve hospitals in a future outbreak
- Future plans have to be made in case of pandemics for evacuation of residential facilities and planning of transportation. Studies from other disasters have shown that many nursing houses did not have [119] evacuation plans
- Preparation of mental health services for future pandemics. A challenge after pandemics may be the capacity of mental health services, especially after a catastrophic event, because of the shortage of services that already exists

Identification of Leaders

- [120] Community leaders should mobilize available resources [121] One step of intervention after mass trauma is the mobilization of resources [121] and identifying high-risk populations for psychiatric disorders instead of subdiagnostic distress [122].
- A key component of their actions will be to understand community vulnerabilities, resilience and special traits to avoid threats to the function and safety of community. Leaders must understand the needs of a community and induce communication between individuals. Empathy expression and understanding the impact of isolation and quarantine are extremely important.
- Leaders should have an initial priority risk communication [8, 123, 124]. They should cooperate with communication crisis specialists.
- Leaders should promote governmental trust after an outbreak, as it was proven to provoke less distress during the H1N1 outbreak [125]. They should promote safety and trust of the government through social media and accurate information. They should stay connected with social media and guide individuals to further resources so as to relieve their anxiety. They have to deal with rumors and fake news [126, 127].
- They also have to face the loss of members of communities, grief and funeral changes due to mandatory measures.
- The development and practice of future disaster plans will strengthen community resilience.
- Leaders should work with employers to provide motives to their employees during pandemics and acknowledge their distribution during these periods [128], such as monitoring of internet and legislation.
- Leaders should help prepare community services for possible long-term consequences of trauma to individuals. Chronic PTSD was even found 15 years after the World Trade Center attacks.

Research

- The role of the researchers is to assess the interventions applied to the present for future use. This needs to be done carefully, as the survivors of an outbreak might be overwhelmed by surveys.
- Research in pandemics may be educational for understanding bioterrorism disasters [67, 73, 129].
- Research will help the development of practices exclusively for pandemics among other disaster studies.
- Research will also help to approach ethical issues such as confidentiality about patients with telehealth technologies or doctors working outside their specialty in emergency situations.
- During research, leaders should encourage healthcare professionals to document their findings.

Intervention

Property loss, economic devastation, threat to life and social disruption are common outcomes post-disaster. Interventions are usually categorized as primary, secondary and tertiary [130]. The aftermath of an outbreak may follow chronological stages where different interventions can take place. In some studies, the timetable after a disaster is divided:

- in the immediate phase, 0–14 days post-incident
- intermediate, 14 days to 3 months
- later phase, 3 months and later [131]

Different stages in the aftermath need different interventions [77]. Early intervention takes place days after pandemics, intermediate days to weeks and long-term from a month to years.

Interventions for General Population

Training and Education

- Public health campaigns can be created to protect from emotional epidemiology [132] and stigma of survivors, their families and health workers.
- Public education for emergency preparedness and evacuation of nursing houses and other residential facilities should also be planned.
- Education of parents and individuals is necessary to recognize early psychiatric symptoms in other people.
- Education of healthcare workers is important so they can be ready for a future pandemic or reoccurrence of the existent one. Studies in fire fighters have shown that more experienced and trained firefighters experienced less trauma during a disaster [133]. As also stated in studies for parachute jumpers [134] and pilots [135, 136], the more experienced were less anxious. The presence of more experienced personnel in emergency units and hospitals might decrease psychological consequences to healthcare providers.
- Maintaining self-care is very important for healthcare personnel [137]. Creation of materials to provide to patients and healthcare providers will help with self-care. Also, the creation of Plan for Action (PFA) appropriate for pandemics could be useful.
- Education must also be planned to be elderly-centric, so that they learn how to protect and prepare themselves for an upcoming pandemic [138]. Creative art therapies can be provided in community centers. For example, collage therapy is reported to give relief from stress [139]. Music therapy is proven to help people with dementia [140]
- Psych education and coping skills might be useful for first responders. Coping skills may increase the resilience of healthcare professionals, and compassion fatigue can be avoided. Mindfulness and regulation of their emotions are also important.
- Media in the aftermath of a pandemic may play a major role in public education and social safety. Mass media can inform all civilians with up-to-date news on the epidemic and the community services available to them as well as reassuring ways to go back to normal life.
- Community members, individuals and leaders should be educated about the consequences of psychological trauma. Individuals have to regain their trust in medical health facilities.
- The role of the mental health specialist in cooperation with primary care providers is to inform the public about substance abuse problems, especially alcohol, as it is reported to increase, especially among health workers, after epidemics. They should also inform them about nutrition, sleep and exercise and limiting exposure to media [141].

- Disasters usually cause economic impacts such as loss of jobs [22, 142]. That may create anger toward authorities. Techniques for anger management and emotion regulation are vital, as some people might be frustrated by the mandatory measures of governments. They can try to normalize their feelings through exercising, listening to music or talking to their spiritual leader, as stated in studies from other disasters [143].

Education to Erase Stigma

Stigma, xenophobia and racism are common in the aftermath of a pandemic. It is commonly reported that, after disasters, the creation of stereotypes among disaster victims and disaster helpers is usual. The first are seen as weak, and there is a fear of characterizing them as "permanently patients". On the other hand, helpers are seen as "heroes", powerful and unbeatable. This provokes two problems. The first one is that helpers face difficulties adapting to everyday life after the end of an epidemic as well as additional stress to seek help in the aftermath, as they are afraid they will be characterized as weak because of their role [144]. In studies on radiation survivors, we know that we should be very careful not to stigmatize further survivors of epidemics by using psychiatric labels or isolating them because of the usually unknown nature of a new outbreak, as in radiation contamination [145–147]. The HIV experience has shown that another challenge for communities is the confrontation of discrimination from spreading the disease and the stigmatization of ethnic groups[148]. Minority populations might feel distress because of labeling and being singled out after a disaster, as for Muslims after the London bombings [149]. In many communities, there is also s stigma for seeking mental health services. Parents more often seek help for their children but not for themselves. Moreover, healthcare providers might be reluctant to give a psychiatric diagnosis after a pandemic to avoid stigmatization of people.

Interventions necessary to erase stigma are:

- The cooperation of government, political leaders, public health specialists and mental health specialists is essential for the delivery of reliable information and knowledge about the infections.
- Creation of structured websites and free helplines may help to clarify myths and fake news.
- Good use of social media and protection of knowledge through legislation are important.
- The training of healthcare personnel may protect them from stigmatization and also help them promote appropriate information to patients and their families. The diagnosis of psychiatric disorders is extremely important, as it is vital for the planning of community interventions and for individuals to get the appropriate treatment.
- Another way to avoid stigma among the elderly is to ask them to help in research, so that they feel more useful.

Mental health providers should be alert to recognize stress or distress in parents early and aid with family interventions.

Intervention

The role of the community for effective intervention will be to provide individuals with

- Supportive therapy and make them part of their decisions.
- Promote initiatives and try to adopt their previous routine from before the outbreak.

- Psych education to understand the new conditions of their lives and feel less stigmatized [29].
- It is very common for individuals not to seek help after disasters [150, 151]. For the identification of mental health problems, screening tools and mobile apps could be used.
- The organization of teams consisting of psychiatrists, psychologists, nurses, emergency doctors and general practitioners could promote early detection of psychological consequences.
- Some of the interventions that are mentioned to be efficient are based on a cognitive therapy approach [122].
- Interventions should be available for a long period of time.

Interventions in Schools

Schools are another unit of the community that is important early after a pandemic. Strengthening the school system is of great importance. Return to school for children after an epidemic reflects the return to normalcy and life before the outbreak. After an outbreak, children may return to a problematic school environment [79] and may face family problems, such as alcohol abuse of parents, divorce or family financial problems [152].

- Interventions for education of children and family support can take place through the classroom [153, 154]. They can provide support to the families and students.
- In early intervention after a pandemic, it will be a priority for healthcare providers to tend to the reconnection of families and communities.
- It is reported that children in their early years need play therapy to improve trauma consequences after natural disasters.
- The key to efficient future interventions is the identification of psychologically traumatized children [155].

Accommodation Needs

There must be planning for the people who had to relocate and abandon their homes during a pandemic.

- Health workers who could not return to their homes, as members of their families are vulnerable to infection, and also people who had to remain in a foreign country because of quarantine will need accommodation.
- Homeless people need to be sheltered during outbreaks.

Cultural Status

Language, ethnicity and cultural status all need to be taken into account in any intervention strategy [147]. An important factor of every community after disaster is to identify special characteristics of societies and understand their spiritual behavior and religious beliefs. It is essential to identify these special traits and encourage individuals to address their spiritual leaders.

- Due to cultural differences, many populations might not accept mental health problems and the interventions provided [97, 156].
- On the other hand, different values and beliefs among culture may protect from psychological trauma [98, 157].

- Spiritual activity may increase community's resiliency.
- Religion can also contribute to coping with grief for the victims of a pandemic [158, 159].
- Elderly people who may be more reluctant to seek help may be approached through churches or other community groups of which they may be members.

Appropriate Formats

Interventions and future plans have to be in appropriate formats for people with sensory deficits such as loss of hearing or sight. This population might be of high concern in the aftermath, as they may develop further functional impairment.

Vaccination Hesitancy

A basic aspect of public mental health in the aftermath of a pandemic is the vaccination and immunization of the population. Vaccine hesitancy will be a challenge in the aftermath of an outbreak [160]. Multicomponent interventions and motivational interviews will have to be part of psychiatric medical care facilities in the community in cooperation with primary healthcare facilities [161].

Intervention for Patients With Preexisting Psychiatric Disorders

Along with the difficulties psychiatric patients have to cope with, they have to face additional problems during outbreaks, as already stated. The role of the mental health specialist is very important in the aftermath of a pandemic.

Basic Needs

- Sometimes after pandemics, communications and transportation may be disrupted, so it would be useful for medical supplies to be available in advance.
- For patients following treatments such as lithium and clozapine [162], drug level monitoring should follow specific instructions [108, 163–166].
- Prescheduled appointments could be arranged in mental health centers or in other appropriate buildings without people waiting in waiting rooms. Triage of mental health status could also be done for prioritization of their needs.
- Triage through telephone for new mental health cases could be useful.
- The creation of a community mental health team consisting of a psychiatrist, psychologist, nurses and other specialists for the assessment and monitoring of the patients of their community.
- Appointments with families for their support using audiovisual tools could replace on-site appointments.
- The occupation and training of volunteers could be very useful because of the increased mental health needs after a pandemic.

Education in the Community

Education about hygiene measures and public mental health issues should also be provided. Psychiatric patients may find it difficult to comply with the protective measures (wearing masks) and public instructions, due to possibly impaired judgment and risky behaviors. There is a serious educational role for mental healthcare facilities.

Prediction of High-Risk Patients in the Future

The collection of data of the population each community mental health unit is responsible for may be of high priority to assess them and prioritize the needs of the patients. As a consequence, they may recognize those with less probability to comply with their treatment and probable relapse early. People with mobility problems and problematic family environments and those who are isolated without caregivers or facing cognitive and behavioral impairment may find it difficult to use transportation. In-house appointments for those may be necessary.

FUTURE CHALLENGES

Social Support and Safety

The impact of a disaster is usually proportional to the duration of a disaster. Disasters provoke social disruption, and it is the duty of the community to instill feelings of control and efficacy. Social support is very important in post-disaster time [167, 168]. It is reported that highly supportive societies tend to face fewer mental health problems after disasters [169]. This proves the crucial role social support plays in the aftermath of a pandemic. Building community resilience in advance is a priority for community for a future outbreak.

It is also stated that the reinforcement of sense of safety and calm [154, 170] can decrease posttraumatic stress [122, 171, 172]. Another characteristic is the support, compassion and relief from acute psychological distress, a sense of safety that has to be provided to individuals and the community.

Telepsychiatry

The demand in the aftermath for more mental health services because of the shortage of psychiatrists and other specialists also demands the use of digital psychiatry and telepsychiatry. For patients with satisfactory social function, telepsychiatry may be of great importance [173]. It is reported that telemedical services have been used in disasters.

The advantages of telepsychiatry are:

- Digital health can erase the distance between the psychiatrist and the patient. The same can be the case for pandemics.
- The shortage of available mental health services can be ameliorated with the use of telepsychiatry.
- Healthcare teams such as doctors, nurses and social workers can have meetings through telemedicine services.
- Meetings can also be arranged with other departments of hospitals so that psychiatrists can provide consultation and liaison services digitally or psychological support to healthcare providers.
- International intervention may take place as local providers can get in touch with specialists worldwide [174–178].
- That is of high importance, especially for countries with special cultural traits and a shortage of psychiatrists.
- It is a matter of utmost importance that during the epidemic phase, telecommunications be used to monitor therapy and assess the psychiatric medical state of the patients so that, in the aftermath of a pandemic, patients will not feel forgotten [179].

Limitations to the use of telepsychiatry:

- There is a need for personal data and privacy protection.
- Costs associated with the supporting system needed.
- Special training of the healthcare specialists needed. Hospitals could collaborate with organizations that will provide equipment and devices, use the technology already installed or even search for funds.
- Legislation in countries should be regulated and national licenses could be created.
- Limitations to telephone assessments. There are people who do not have access to the internet or smartphones, not only for financial reasons but also because of cognitive difficulties. For example, older people are not familiar with the internet.

CONCLUSION

In recent decades, there seems to be a gradual increase in the occurrence of pandemics. Of all the disasters, outbreaks cause serious socioeconomic and psychological burdens to the individual as they disrupt the basic structures of society. The cooperation of experts and the exploitation of modern technological advances seems necessary to plan preventive schemes to help psychiatric patients and vulnerable populations manage future crises in accordance with the requirements of modern communities.

References

1. Marr, J.S. and C.D. Malloy, *An epidemiologic analysis of the ten plagues of Egypt.* Caduceus, 1996. **12**(1): p. 7–24.
2. Maunder, R., *The experience of the 2003 SARS outbreak as a traumatic stress among frontline healthcare workers in Toronto: Lessons learned.* Philos Trans R Soc Lond B Biol Sci, 2004. **359**(1447): p. 1117–1125.
3. Shultz, J.M., F. Baingana, and Y. Neria, *The 2014 Ebola outbreak and mental health: Current status and recommended response.* JAMA, 2015. **313**(6): p. 567–568.
4. Kindhauser, M., et al., *Zika: The origin and spread of a mosquito-borne virus.* Bulletin of the World Health Organization, 2016. **94**.
5. Lee, S.M., et al., *Psychological impact of the 2015 MERS outbreak on hospital workers and quarantined hemodialysis patients.* Compr Psychiatry, 2018. **87**: p. 123–127.
6. Bertazzi, P.A., *Industrial disasters and epidemiology: A review of recent experiences.* Scand J Work Environ Health, 1989. **15**(2): p. 85–100.
7. Holloway, H.C., et al., *The threat of biological weapons: Prophylaxis and mitigation of psychological and social consequences.* JAMA, 1997. **278**(5): p. 425–427.
8. Norwood, A.E., H.C. Holloway, and R.J. Ursano, *Psychological effects of biological warfare.* Mil Med, 2001. **166**(12 Suppl): p. 27–28.
9. DiGiovanni, C., Jr., *Domestic terrorism with chemical or biological agents: Psychiatric aspects.* Am J Psychiatry, 1999. **156**(10): p. 1500–1505.
10. Benedek, D.M., H.C. Holloway, and S.M. Becker, *Emergency mental health management in bioterrorism events.* Emerg Med Clin North Am, 2002. **20**(2): p. 393–407.
11. Garcovich, S., et al., *Mass quarantine measures in the time of COVID-19 pandemic: Psycho-social implications for chronic skin conditions and a call for qualitative studies.* J Eur Acad Dermatol Venereol, 2020. **34**(7) Jul: p. e293–e294.
12. Rohr, S., et al., *Psychosocial impact of quarantine measures during serious coronavirus outbreaks: A rapid review.* Psychiatr Prax, 2020. **47**(4): p. 179–189.
13. Brooks, S.K., et al., *The psychological impact of quarantine and how to reduce it: Rapid review of the evidence.* Lancet, 2020. **395**(10227): p. 912–920.
14. Tognotti, E., *Lessons from the history of quarantine, from plague to influenza A.* Emerg Infect Dis, 2013. **19**(2): p. 254–259.
15. Johal, S.S., *Psychosocial impacts of quarantine during disease outbreaks and interventions that may help to relieve strain.* N Z Med J, 2009. **122**(1296): p. 47–52.

16. Bartholomew, R.E. and S. Wessely, *Protean nature of mass sociogenic illness: From possessed nuns to chemical and biological terrorism fears.* Br J Psychiatry, 2002. **180**: p. 300–306.
17. Doyle, C.R., et al., *Mass sociogenic illness – real and imaginary.* Vet Hum Toxicol, 2004. **46**(2): p. 93–95.
18. Jones, T.F., *Mass psychogenic illness: Role of the individual physician.* Am Fam Physician, 2000. **62**(12): p. 2649–2653, 2655–2656.
19. Pastel, R.H., *Collective behaviors: Mass panic and outbreaks of multiple unexplained symptoms.* Mil Med, 2001. **166**(12 Suppl): p. 44–46.
20. Rundell, J.R., *Demographics of and diagnoses in operation enduring freedom and operation Iraqi freedom personnel who were psychiatrically evacuated from the theater of operations.* Gen Hosp Psychiatry, 2006. **28**(4): p. 352–356.
21. North, C.S., et al., *Psychiatric disorders among survivors of the Oklahoma City bombing.* JAMA, 1999. **282**(8): p. 755–762.
22. Galea, S., et al., *Psychological sequelae of the September 11 terrorist attacks in New York City.* N Engl J Med, 2002. **346**(13): p. 982–987.
23. Schlenger, W.E., et al., *Psychological reactions to terrorist attacks: Findings from the National Study of Americans' Reactions to September 11.* JAMA, 2002. **288**(5): p. 581–588.
24. Schuster, M.A., et al., *A national survey of stress reactions after the September 11, 2001, terrorist attacks.* N Engl J Med, 2001. **345**(20): p. 1507–1512.
25. Silver, R.C., et al., *Nationwide longitudinal study of psychological responses to September 11.* JAMA, 2002. **288**(10): p. 1235–1244.
26. Galea, S., et al., *An investigation of the psychological effects of the September 11, 2001, attacks on New York City: Developing and implementing research in the acute postdisaster period.* CNS Spectr, 2002. **7**(8): p. 585–587, 593–596.
27. North, C.S., et al., *Psychiatric disorders in rescue workers after the Oklahoma City bombing.* Am J Psychiatry, 2002. **159**(5): p. 857–859.
28. Raveis, V.H., et al., *Enabling a disaster-resilient workforce: Attending to individual stress and collective trauma.* J Nurs Scholarsh, 2017. **49**(6): p. 653–660.
29. Foa, E.B., *Psychosocial treatment of posttraumatic stress disorder.* J Clin Psychiatry, 2000. **61**(Suppl 5): p. 43–48; discussion 49–51.
30. Ursano, R.J., *Posttraumatic stress disorder: The stressor criterion.* J Nerv Ment Dis, 1987. **175**(5): p. 273–275.
31. Liu, X., et al., *Depression after exposure to stressful events: Lessons learned from the severe acute respiratory syndrome epidemic.* Compr Psychiatry, 2012. **53**(1): p. 15–23.
32. Ooi, P.L., S. Lim, and S.K. Chew, *Use of quarantine in the control of SARS in Singapore.* Am J Infect Control, 2005. **33**(5): p. 252–257.
33. Laditka, S.B., et al., *Disaster preparedness for vulnerable persons receiving in-home, long-term care in South Carolina.* Prehosp Disaster Med, 2008. **23**(2): p. 133–142; discussion 143.
34. Saxon, A.J., et al., *Trauma, symptoms of posttraumatic stress disorder, and associated problems among incarcerated veterans.* Psychiatr Serv, 2001. **52**(7): p. 959–964.
35. Jacobsen, L.K., S.M. Southwick, and T.R. Kosten, *Substance use disorders in patients with posttraumatic stress disorder: A review of the literature.* Am J Psychiatry, 2001. **158**(8): p. 1184–1190.
36. Ford, C.V., *Somatization and fashionable diagnoses: Illness as a way of life.* Scand J Work Environ Health, 1997. **23**(Suppl 3): p. 7–16.
37. Shalev, A., A. Bleich, and R.J. Ursano, *Posttraumatic stress disorder: Somatic comorbidity and effort tolerance.* Psychosomatics, 1990. **31**(2): p. 197–203.
38. Vlahov, D., et al., *Increased use of cigarettes, alcohol, and marijuana among Manhattan, New York, residents after the September 11th terrorist attacks.* Am J Epidemiol, 2002. **155**(11): p. 988–996.
39. Wu, K.K., S.K. Chan, and T.M. Ma, *Posttraumatic stress after SARS.* Emerg Infect Dis, 2005. **11**(8): p. 1297–1300.
40. Fullerton, C.S., R.J. Ursano, and L. Wang, *Acute stress disorder, posttraumatic stress disorder, and depression in disaster or rescue workers.* Am J Psychiatry, 2004. **161**(8): p. 1370–1376.
41. Bremner, J.D., *Acute and chronic responses to psychological trauma: Where do we go from here?* Am J Psychiatry, 1999. **156**(3): p. 349–3451.
42. Breslau, N., et al., *The structure of posttraumatic stress disorder: Latent class analysis in 2 community samples.* Arch Gen Psychiatry, 2005. **62**(12): p. 1343–1351.
43. Neal, L.A. and M.C. Rose, *Factitious post traumatic stress disorder: A case report.* Med Sci Law, 1995. **35**(4): p. 352–354.
44. Rauch, S.A., et al., *Posttraumatic stress, depression, and health among older adults in primary care.* Am J Geriatr Psychiatry, 2006. **14**(4): p. 316–324.

45. Miguel-Tobal, J.J., et al., *PTSD and depression after the Madrid March 11 train bombings.* J Trauma Stress, 2006. **19**(1): p. 69–80.
46. Kessler, R.C., et al., *Social consequences of psychiatric disorders, I: Educational attainment.* Am J Psychiatry, 1995. **152**(7): p. 1026–1032.
47. Galea, S., et al., *Posttraumatic stress disorder in Manhattan, New York City, after the September 11th terrorist attacks.* J Urban Health, 2002. **79**(3): p. 340–353.
48. Styra, R., et al., *Impact on health care workers employed in high-risk areas during the Toronto SARS outbreak.* J Psychosom Res, 2008. **64**(2): p. 177–183.
49. Rundell, J.R., et al., *Psychiatric responses to trauma.* Hosp Community Psychiatry, 1989. **40**(1): p. 68–74.
50. Krebs, F.C., et al., *HIV-1-associated central nervous system dysfunction.* Adv Pharmacol, 2000. **49**: p. 315–385.
51. Sherrini, B.A. and T.T. Chong, *Nipah encephalitis – an update.* Med J Malaysia, 2014. **69**(Suppl A): p. 103–111.
52. Meijer, W.J., et al., *Acute influenza virus-associated encephalitis and encephalopathy in adults: A challenging diagnosis.* JMM Case Rep, 2016. **3**(6): p. e005076.
53. Asselman, V., et al., *Central nervous system disorders after starting antiretroviral therapy in South Africa.* AIDS, 2010. **24**(18): p. 2871–2876.
54. Cohen, L.G., et al., *Erythromycin-induced clozapine toxic reaction.* Arch Intern Med, 1996. **156**(6): p. 675–677.
55. Lurie, I., et al., *Antibiotic exposure and the risk for depression, anxiety, or psychosis: A nested case-control study.* J Clin Psychiatry, 2015. **76**(11): p. 1522–1528.
56. Maldonado, J.R., *Acute brain failure: Pathophysiology, diagnosis, management, and sequelae of delirium.* Crit Care Clin, 2017. **33**(3): p. 461–519.
57. Denke, C., et al., *Long-term sequelae of acute respiratory distress syndrome caused by severe community-acquired pneumonia: Delirium-associated cognitive impairment and post-traumatic stress disorder.* J Int Med Res, 2018. **46**(6): p. 2265–2283.
58. Smith, M.W., et al., *The psychosocial challenges of caring for patients with ebola virus disease.* Health Secur, 2017. **15**(1): p. 104–109.
59. Zatzick, D.F., et al., *Posttraumatic concerns: A patient-centered approach to outcome assessment after traumatic physical injury.* Med Care, 2001. **39**(4): p. 327–339.
60. Leor, J. and R.A. Kloner, *The Northridge earthquake as a trigger for acute myocardial infarction.* Am J Cardiol, 1996. **77**(14): p. 1230–1232.
61. Jacobson, A.M., *The psychological care of patients with insulin-dependent diabetes mellitus.* N Engl J Med, 1996. **334**(19): p. 1249–1253.
62. Symonds, M., *Victim responses to terror.* Ann N Y Acad Sci, 1980. **347**: p. 129–136.
63. Kagan, I., et al., *The SARS threat in Israel: One medical center's experience.* J Nurs Adm, 2004. **34**(7–8): p. 318–321.
64. Lai, B.S., et al., *Mother and child reports of hurricane related stressors: Data from a sample of families exposed to hurricane katrina.* Child Youth Care Forum, 2015. **44**(4): p. 549–565.
65. Shalev, A.Y., et al., *Prospective study of posttraumatic stress disorder and depression following trauma.* Am J Psychiatry, 1998. **155**(5): p. 630–637.
66. Shalev, A.Y. and S. Freedman, *PTSD following terrorist attacks: A prospective evaluation.* Am J Psychiatry, 2005. **162**(6): p. 1188–1191.
67. Arata, C.M., et al., *Coping with technological disaster: An application of the conservation of resources model to the Exxon Valdez oil spill.* J Trauma Stress, 2000. **13**(1): p. 23–39.
68. North, C.S., J.D. Weaver, and B.A. Hong, *Roles of psychiatrists on multidisciplinary mental health disaster teams.* Psychiatr Serv, 2001. **52**(4): p. 536–537.
69. Kasl, S.V., R.F. Chisholm, and B. Eskenazi, *The impact of the accident at the Three Mile Island on the behavior and well-being of nuclear workers; Part I: Perceptions and evaluations, behavioral responses, and work-related attitudes and feelings.* Am J Public Health, 1981. **71**(5): p. 472–483.
70. Maes, M., et al., *Epidemiologic and phenomenological aspects of post-traumatic stress disorder: DSM-III-R diagnosis and diagnostic criteria not validated.* Psychiatry Res, 1998. **81**(2): p. 179–193.
71. North, C.S., et al., *Three-year follow-up of survivors of a mass shooting episode.* J Urban Health, 2002. **79**(3): p. 383–391.
72. Weisaeth, L., *An industrial disaster: Disaster behavior and posttraumatic stress reactions.* Tidsskr Nor Laegeforen, 1986. **106**(27): p. 2220–2224.
73. Lopez-Ibor, J.J., Jr., et al., *Psychopathological aspects of the toxic oil syndrome catastrophe.* Br J Psychiatry, 1985. **147**: p. 352–365.

74. Kasl, S.V., R.F. Chisholm, and B. Eskenazi, *The impact of the accident at the Three Mile Island on the behavior and well-being of nuclear workers: Part II: Job tension, psychophysiological symptoms, and indices of distress.* Am J Public Health, 1981. **71**(5): p. 484–495.
75. Moore, F.D., *Metabolism in trauma: The reaction of survival.* Metabolism, 1959. **8**: p. 783–786.
76. Bromet, E., H.C. Schulberg, and L. Dunn, *Reactions of psychiatric patients to the Three Mile Island nuclear accident.* Arch Gen Psychiatry, 1982. **39**(6): p. 725–730.
77. McFarlane, A.C., *The aetiology of post-traumatic morbidity: Predisposing, precipitating and perpetuating factors.* Br J Psychiatry, 1989. **154**: p. 221–228.
78. North, C.S., et al., *Short-term psychopathology in eyewitnesses to mass murder.* Hosp Community Psychiatry, 1989. **40**(12): p. 1293–1295.
79. Madrid, P.A., et al., *Building integrated mental health and medical programs for vulnerable populations post-disaster: Connecting children and families to a medical home.* Prehosp Disaster Med, 2008. **23**(4): p. 314–321.
80. Roberts, A., *Is your state prepared to respond to trauma?* Bull Am Coll Surg, 2003. **88**(12): p. 13–17.
81. Goulia, P., et al., *General hospital staff worries, perceived sufficiency of information and associated psychological distress during the A/H1N1 influenza pandemic.* BMC Infect Dis, 2010. **10**: p. 322.
82. Schreiber, M., et al., *Maximizing the resilience of healthcare workers in multi-hazard events: Lessons from the 2014–2015 ebola response in Africa.* Mil Med, 2019. **184**(Suppl 1): p. 114–120.
83. Figley, C.R., *Compassion fatigue: Psychotherapists' chronic lack of self care.* J Clin Psychol, 2002. **58**(11): p. 1433–1441.
84. Gibson, M.E., *The smallest victims of the "white plague".* Pediatr Nurs, 2006. **32**(1): p. 71–72, 81.
85. Neupert, S.D., et al., *The effects of the Columbia shuttle disaster on the daily lives of older adults: Findings from the VA Normative Aging Study.* Aging Ment Health, 2006. **10**(3): p. 272–281.
86. Yazgan, I.C., C. Dedeoglu, and Y. Yazgan, *Disability and post-traumatic psychopathology in Turkish elderly after a major earthquake.* Int Psychogeriatr, 2006. **18**(1): p. 184–187.
87. Kessler, D., et al., *Cross sectional study of symptom attribution and recognition of depression and anxiety in primary care.* BMJ, 1999. **318**(7181): p. 436–439.
88. Tugade, M.M., B.L. Fredrickson, and L.F. Barrett, *Psychological resilience and positive emotional granularity: Examining the benefits of positive emotions on coping and health.* J Pers, 2004. **72**(6): p. 1161–1190.
89. Belfer, M.L., *Caring for children and adolescents in the aftermath of natural disasters.* Int Rev Psychiatry, 2006. **18**(6): p. 523–528.
90. Terr, L.C., *Psychic trauma in children: Observations following the Chowchilla school-bus kidnapping.* Am J Psychiatry, 1981. **138**(1): p. 14–19.
91. Pynoos, R.S., et al., *Life threat and posttraumatic stress in school-age children.* Arch Gen Psychiatry, 1987. **44**(12): p. 1057–1063.
92. Pynoos, R.S., et al., *Post-traumatic stress reactions in children after the 1988 Armenian earthquake.* Br J Psychiatry, 1993. **163**: p. 239–247.
93. Pfefferbaum, B., et al., *Posttraumatic stress responses in bereaved children after the Oklahoma City bombing.* J Am Acad Child Adolesc Psychiatry, 1999. **38**(11): p. 1372–1379.
94. Shaw, B.A., et al., *Social structural influences on emotional support from parents early in life and adult health status.* Behav Med, 2003. **29**(2): p. 68–79.
95. Pfefferbaum, B.J., *Aspects of exposure in childhood trauma: The stressor criterion.* J Trauma Dissociation, 2005. **6**(2): p. 17–26.
96. Bromet, E.J., et al., *Children's well-being 11 years after the Chornobyl catastrophe.* Arch Gen Psychiatry, 2000. **57**(6): p. 563–571.
97. Silove, D., *The psychosocial effects of torture, mass human rights violations, and refugee trauma: Toward an integrated conceptual framework.* J Nerv Ment Dis, 1999. **187**(4): p. 200–207.
98. Bell, P., et al., *Women, war and trauma: a study description.* Med Arh, 2001. **55**(1 Suppl 1): p. 31–33.
99. Beaudoin, C.E., *Hurricane Katrina: Addictive behavior trends and predictors.* Public Health Rep, 2011. **126**(3): p. 400–409.
100. Schulte, M.T. and Y.I. Hser, *Substance use and associated health conditions throughout the lifespan.* Public Health Rev, 2014. **35**(2).
101. Columb, D., R. Hussain, and C. O'Gara, *Addiction psychiatry and COVID-19: Impact on patients and service provision.* Ir J Psychol Med, 2020: p. 1–5.
102. Ornell, F., et al., *The impact of the COVID-19 pandemic on the mental health of healthcare professionals.* Cad Saude Publica, 2020. **36**(4): p. e00063520.
103. Kiraly, O., et al., *Preventing problematic internet use during the COVID-19 pandemic: Consensus guidance.* Compr Psychiatry, 2020. **100**: p. 152180.

104. King, D.L., et al., *Problematic online gaming and the COVID-19 pandemic.* J Behav Addict, 2020.
105. Hakansson, A., et al., *Gambling during the COVID-19 crisis: A cause for concern?* J Addict Med, 2020. **14**(4): p. e10.
106. Touyz, S., H. Lacey, and P. Hay, *Eating disorders in the time of COVID-19.* J Eat Disord, 2020. **8**: p. 19.
107. Dubey, M.J., et al., *COVID-19 and addiction.* Diabetes Metab Syndr, 2020. **14**(5): p. 817–823.
108. Dubey, S., et al., *Psychosocial impact of COVID-19.* Diabetes Metab Syndr, 2020. **14**(5): p. 779–788.
109. Ornell, F., et al., *The COVID-19 pandemic and its impact on substance use: Implications for prevention and treatment.* Psychiatry Res, 2020. **289**: p. 113096.
110. Breslau, N., et al., *Traumatic events and posttraumatic stress disorder in an urban population of young adults.* Arch Gen Psychiatry, 1991. **48**(3): p. 216–222.
111. Breslau, N., et al., *Trauma and posttraumatic stress disorder in the community: The 1996 detroit area survey of trauma.* Arch Gen Psychiatry, 1998. **55**(7): p. 626–632.
112. Smith, E.M., et al., *Acute postdisaster psychiatric disorders: Identification of persons at risk.* Am J Psychiatry, 1990. **147**(2): p. 202–206.
113. North, C.S. and E.M. Smith, *Post-traumatic stress disorder in disaster survivors.* Compr Ther, 1990. **16**(12): p. 3–9.
114. North, C.S., E.M. Smith, and E.L. Spitznagel, *Posttraumatic stress disorder in survivors of a mass shooting.* Am J Psychiatry, 1994. **151**(1): p. 82–88.
115. Vyas, A., et al., *Influenza outbreak preparedness: Lessons from outbreaks in residential care facilities in 2014.* Commun Dis Intell Q Rep, 2015. **39**(2): p. E204–E207.
116. Cohen, C.I., et al., *The future of community psychiatry.* Community Ment Health J, 2003. **39**(5): p. 459–471.
117. Jewkes, R. and A. Murcott, *Meanings of community.* Soc Sci Med, 1996. **43**(4): p. 555–563.
118. Kaniasty, K., *Social support, interpersonal, and community dynamics following disasters caused by natural hazards.* Curr Opin Psychol, 2020. **32**: p. 105–109.
119. Castle, N.G., *Nursing home evacuation plans.* Am J Public Health, 2008. **98**(7): p. 1235–1240.
120. Norris, F.H., et al., *Community resilience as a metaphor, theory, set of capacities, and strategy for disaster readiness.* Am J Community Psychol, 2008. **41**(1–2): p. 127–1250.
121. Ursano, R.J., et al., *The impact of disasters and their aftermath on mental health.* J Clin Psychiatry, 2006. **67**(1): p. 7–14.
122. Bryant, R.A. and F.G. Njenga, *Cultural sensitivity: Making trauma assessment and treatment plans culturally relevant.* J Clin Psychiatry, 2006. **67**(Suppl 2): p. 74–79.
123. Moscrop, A., *Mass hysteria is seen as main threat from bioweapons.* BMJ, 2001. **323**(7320): p. 1023.
124. Covello, V.T., et al., *Risk communication, the West Nile virus epidemic, and bioterrorism: Responding to the communication challenges posed by the intentional or unintentional release of a pathogen in an urban setting.* J Urban Health, 2001. **78**(2): p. 382–391.
125. Pfefferbaum, B., et al., *The H1N1 crisis: A case study of the integration of mental and behavioral health in public health crises.* Disaster Med Public Health Prep, 2012. **6**(1): p. 67–71.
126. Wood, M.J., *Propagating and debunking conspiracy theories on Twitter during the 2015–2016 zika virus outbreak.* Cyberpsychol Behav Soc Netw, 2018. **21**(8): p. 485–490.
127. Towers, S., et al., *Mass media and the contagion of fear: The case of ebola in America.* PLoS One, 2015. **10**(6): p. e0129179.
128. Tan, W., et al., *Is returning to work during the COVID-19 pandemic stressful? A study on immediate mental health status and psychoneuroimmunity prevention measures of Chinese workforce.* Brain Behav Immun, 2020. **87**: p. 84–92.
129. Bowler, R.M., et al., *Psychological, psychosocial, and psychophysiological sequelae in a community affected by a railroad chemical disaster.* J Trauma Stress, 1994. **7**(4): p. 601–624.
130. Sorenson, S.B., *Preventing traumatic stress: Public health approaches.* J Trauma Stress, 2002. **15**(1): p. 3–7.
131. Shalev, A.Y., R. Tuval-Mashiach, and H. Hadar, *Posttraumatic stress disorder as a result of mass trauma.* J Clin Psychiatry, 2004. **65**(Suppl 1): p. 4–10.
132. Ofri, D., *The emotional epidemiology of H1N1 influenza vaccination.* N Engl J Med, 2009. **361**(27): p. 2594–2595.
133. Hytten, K. and A. Hasle, *Fire fighters: A study of stress and coping.* Acta Psychiatr Scand Suppl, 1989. **355**: p. 50–55.
134. Fenz, W.D. and S. Epstein, *Gradients of physiological arousal in parachutists as a function of an approaching jump.* Psychosom Med, 1967. **29**(1): p. 33–51.
135. Drinkwater, B.L., T. Cleland, and M.M. Flint, *Pilot performance during periods of anticipatory physical threat stress.* Aerosp Med, 1968. **39**(9): p. 994–999.

136. Mefferd, R.B., Jr., et al., *Stress responses as criteria for personnel selection: Baseline study.* Aerosp Med, 1971. **42**(1): p. 42–51.
137. Hyer, K. and L. Rudick, *The effectiveness of personal emergency response systems in meeting the safety monitoring needs of home care clients.* J Nurs Adm, 1994. **24**(6): p. 39–44.
138. Rosenkoetter, M.M., et al., *Disaster evacuation: An exploratory study of older men and women in Georgia and North Carolina.* J Gerontol Nurs, 2007. **33**(12): p. 46–54.
139. Schmitt, B. and L. Frölich, *Creative therapy options for patients with dementia: A systematic review.* Fortschr Neurol Psychiatr, 2007. **75**(12): p. 699–707.
140. Moreno-Morales, C., et al., *Music therapy in the treatment of dementia: A systematic review and meta-analysis.* Front Med (Lausanne), 2020. **7**: p. 160.
141. Pfefferbaum, B., et al., *Television exposure in children after a terrorist incident.* Psychiatry, 2001. **64**(3): p. 202–211.
142. Nandi, A., et al., *Job loss, unemployment, work stress, job satisfaction, and the persistence of posttraumatic stress disorder one year after the September 11 attacks.* J Occup Environ Med, 2004. **46**(10): p. 1057–1064.
143. Crimando, S.M., *The bio-psycho-social consequences of terrorism.* N J Med, 2004. **101**(9 Suppl): p. 84–88; quiz 88–89.
144. Short, D.P., *Hospital role in community health care.* N Z Hosp, 1979. **31**(3): p. 2–3.
145. Shultz, J.M., et al., *The role of fear-related behaviors in the 2013–2016 West Africa ebola virus disease outbreak.* Curr Psychiatry Rep, 2016. **18**(11): p. 104.
146. Faherty, L.J. and C.A. Doubeni, *Unintended consequences of screening for ebola.* Am J Public Health, 2015. **105**(9): p. 1738–1739.
147. Reardon, S., *Ebola's mental-health wounds linger in Africa.* Nature, 2015. **519**(7541): p. 13–14.
148. Griffith, J.L. and B.A. Kohrt, *Managing stigma effectively: What social psychology and social neuroscience can teach us.* Acad Psychiatry, 2016. **40**(2): p. 339–347.
149. Rubin, G.J., et al., *Psychological and behavioural reactions to the bombings in London on 7 July 2005: Cross sectional survey of a representative sample of Londoners.* BMJ, 2005. **331**(7517): p. 606.
150. Ursano, R.J., *Preparedness for SARS, influenza, and bioterrorism.* Psychiatr Serv, 2005. **56**(1): p. 7.
151. Weisaeth, L., *Acute posttraumatic stress: Nonacceptance of early intervention.* J Clin Psychiatry, 2001. **62**(Suppl 17): p. 35–40.
152. Osofsky, H.J., et al., *Factors contributing to mental and physical health care in a disaster-prone environment.* Behav Med, 2015. **41**(3): p. 131–137.
153. McDermott, B.M., et al., *Posttraumatic stress disorder and general psychopathology in children and adolescents following a wildfire disaster.* Can J Psychiatry, 2005. **50**(3): p. 137–143.
154. Harvey, A.G., and R.A. Bryant, *Acute stress disorder: A synthesis and critique.* Psychol Bull, 2002. **128**(6): p. 886–902.
155. Goenjian, A., et al., *Moral development and psychopathological interference in conscience functioning among adolescents after trauma.* J Am Acad Child Adolesc Psychiatry, 1999. **38**(4): p. 376–384.
156. Agusto, F.B., M.I. Teboh-Ewungkem, and A.B. Gumel, *Mathematical assessment of the effect of traditional beliefs and customs on the transmission dynamics of the 2014 Ebola outbreaks.* BMC Med, 2015. **13**: p. 96.
157. Bryant, B., et al., *Psychological consequences of road traffic accidents for children and their mothers.* Psychol Med, 2004. **34**(2): p. 335–346.
158. Walsh, K., et al., *Spiritual beliefs may affect outcome of bereavement: Prospective study.* BMJ, 2002. **324**(7353): p. 1551.
159. Chan, C.L., T.H. Chan, and S.M. Ng, *The Strength-Focused and Meaning-Oriented Approach to Resilience and Transformation (SMART): A body-mind-spirit approach to trauma management.* Soc Work Health Care, 2006. **43**(2–3): p. 9–36.
160. McClure, C.C., J.R. Cataldi, and S.T. O'Leary, *Vaccine hesitancy: Where we are and where we are going.* Clin Ther, 2017. **39**(8): p. 1550–1562.
161. Leask, J., et al., *Communicating with parents about vaccination: A framework for health professionals.* BMC Pediatr, 2012. **12**: p. 154.
162. Raaska, K. and P.J. Neuvonen, *Ciprofloxacin increases serum clozapine and N-desmethylclozapine: A study in patients with schizophrenia.* Eur J Clin Pharmacol, 2000. **56**(8): p. 585–589.
163. Asmundson, G.J.G. and S. Taylor, *How health anxiety influences responses to viral outbreaks like COVID-19: What all decision-makers, health authorities, and health care professionals need to know.* J Anxiety Disord, 2020. **71**: p. 102211.
164. Xiao, C., *A novel approach of consultation on 2019 novel coronavirus (COVID-19)-related psychological and mental problems: Structured letter therapy.* Psychiatry Investig, 2020. **17**(2): p. 175–176.

165. Seminog, O.O. and M.J. Goldacre, *Risk of pneumonia and pneumococcal disease in people with severe mental illness: English record linkage studies.* Thorax, 2013. **68**(2): p. 171–176.
166. Yao, H., J.H. Chen, and Y.F. Xu, *Patients with mental health disorders in the COVID-19 epidemic.* Lancet Psychiatry, 2020. **7**(4): p. e21.
167. Kaniasty, K. and F.H. Norris, *A test of the social support deterioration model in the context of natural disaster.* J Pers Soc Psychol, 1993. **64**(3): p. 395–408.
168. Norris, F.H. and K. Kaniasty, *Received and perceived social support in times of stress: A test of the social support deterioration deterrence model.* J Pers Soc Psychol, 1996. **71**(3): p. 498–511.
169. North, C.S., et al., *Psychosocial adjustment of directly exposed survivors 7 years after the Oklahoma City bombing.* Compr Psychiatry, 2011. **52**(1): p. 1–8.
170. McNally, R.J., R.A. Bryant, and A. Ehlers, *Does early psychological intervention promote recovery from posttraumatic stress?* Psychol Sci Public Interest, 2003. **4**(2): p. 45–79.
171. Charney, D.S., *Psychobiological mechanisms of resilience and vulnerability: Implications for successful adaptation to extreme stress.* Am J Psychiatry, 2004. **161**(2): p. 195–216.
172. McEwen, J., *The new new public health.* Lancet, 1998. **352**(9131): p. 903; author reply 904.
173. Lovejoy, C.A., V. Buch, and M. Maruthappu, *Technology and mental health: The role of artificial intelligence.* Eur Psychiatry, 2019. **55**: p. 1–3.
174. Kannarkat, J.T., N.N. Smith, and S.A. McLeod-Bryant, *Mobilization of telepsychiatry in response to COVID-19-moving toward 21(st) century access to care.* Adm Policy Ment Health, 2020. **47**(4): p. 489–491.
175. Varker, T., et al., *Efficacy of synchronous telepsychology interventions for people with anxiety, depression, posttraumatic stress disorder, and adjustment disorder: A rapid evidence assessment.* Psychol Serv, 2019. **16**(4): p. 621–635.
176. Barnett, M.L., et al., *Trends in telemedicine use in a large commercially insured population, 2005–2017.* JAMA, 2018. **320**(20): p. 2147–2149.
177. Douglas, M.D., et al., *Assessing telemedicine utilization by using medicaid claims data.* Psychiatr Serv, 2017. **68**(2): p. 173–178.
178. Hubley, S., et al., *Review of key telepsychiatry outcomes.* World J Psychiatry, 2016. **6**(2): p. 269–282.
179. Hao, F., et al., *Do psychiatric patients experience more psychiatric symptoms during COVID-19 pandemic and lockdown? A case-control study with service and research implications for immunopsychiatry.* Brain Behav Immun, 2020. **87**: p. 100–106.

47
Optimizing Psychiatric Care Using Functional Neuroimaging

Suvarna Badhe and Avinash De Sousa

Introduction	515
Basics of fMRI	515
Guidelines for Effective Patient Training	516
Guidelines for Effective Scanning	516
Types of fMRI Studies Commonly Used in Psychiatric Diseases	517
Post-Processing Guidelines	517
Advantages of fMRI	*518*
Disadvantages of fMRI	*518*
PET	518
Presentations and Uses of fMRI and PET in Various Psychiatric Diseases	519
Schizophrenia	519
Major Depression	519
Bipolar Disorder	519
PTSD	520
OCD	520
ADHD	520
Substance Abuse	521
Conclusion/Future Clinical Applications of fMRI in Psychiatric Diseases	521

INTRODUCTION

Functional neuroimaging has multiple clinical, pre-surgical and research applications today. In psychiatry it has the potential to provide a better understanding of disease pathology as well as to help in assessing treatment response. In this chapter, we outline the basics of functional MRI (fMRI) and positron emission tomography (PET); provide useful guidelines on achieving an optimal functional study; and share some interesting data on various studies performed on patients with psychiatric diseases such as schizophrenia, major depression, bipolar disorder, post traumatic stress disorder (PTSD), obsessive compulsive disorder (OCD), attention deficit hyperactivity disorder (ADHD) and substance abuse. We also touch on future clinical applications of functional neuroimaging in psychiatric disease.

BASICS OF FMRI

fMRI is a neuroimaging technique used to map neural activity in the brain and spinal cord.

DOI: 10.4324/9780429030260-51

The primary form of fMRI uses blood-oxygen-level-dependent (BOLD) contrast to study brain activity. Oxygenated blood is diamagnetic, which means that it does not interfere with the magnetic field of the machine; hence, an increased intensity/signal is perceived on the scan. Deoxygenated blood is paramagnetic, which implies that it interferes with the magnetic field, and hence a decreased signal is seen on scans. Neural activity induces an increase in cerebral blood flow (CBF) and cerebral blood volume (CBV), which leads to a net increase in cerebral oxygenation in the active regions of the brain. The difference between the signals during activity versus rest is what is measured during conventional fMRI studies. Even at rest, different areas of the brain function at various levels of oxygenation. These can also be recorded using resting-state fMRI scans.

Over the years, we have noticed that by conducting a fMRI scan in a certain manner, we've had consistently better results. We'd like to share these tips with you.

GUIDELINES FOR EFFECTIVE PATIENT TRAINING

Patient training is considered routine; however, often it is the most important step in a fMRI study. To start off, introduce yourself and greet the patient with a smile. Engage in some quick small talk. Make the patient feel comfortable. We've regularly observed that the more comfortable and cooperative the patient is, the better the results of the fMRI study are. Briefly explain how functional MRI works to the patient. Go over each task in a slow and detailed manner. Have the patient explain their understanding of the test to you, and if needed, have them repeat the instructions back to you. For motor tasks, practice the movements with the patient beforehand. Study the patient's history adequately so that you have a better understanding of their psychiatric deficit and can focus on the necessary fMRI paradigms required to help their specific condition. Answer any questions they might have to the best of your ability. If they still seem unsettled, try to accommodate any reasonable requests they may have to make them feel at ease. Reassure the patient that the test will be done keeping their comfort in mind. Prior to the scan, always make sure the patient does not have any metallic objects on their person. Request them to use the restroom before scanning, as ideally its best if their head position remains the same throughout the scan.

GUIDELINES FOR EFFECTIVE SCANNING

Have the patient lie down on the scanning bed with their hands by their side. Place a pillow below their knees if that makes them more comfortable. Place towels beside their head to prevent them from moving their head. Offer them some water if their throat feels parched. This minimizes their need to cough or clear their throat during the scan and cause motion artifacts. Offer them a blanket if they are cold in the scanning room. Instruct them to keep their head as still as possible, especially when the machine is making a loud sound. Give them a response button if required as well as the emergency button. Let them know that if they feel any discomfort, they may press the emergency button and you will come and check in on them immediately. Give them headphones if required or earplugs to partially block the scanner sounds. Let them know that you will intermittently communicate with them through the headphones. For task-based fMRIs, make sure they can see the stimulus screen clearly and completely. Before leaving the room, ask them if they have any questions and reassure them that you are monitoring them closely. Once the scan begins, monitor the patient diligently. If you notice movements, gently instruct them to remain still. If the movement is excessive, stop the scan, have a word with the patient and re-run the paradigm. Spending a few extra minutes making sure that the scan is run properly will reap dividends when it comes to the results, as no amount of post-processing can improve poor baseline data. Performing fMRI scans on children is definitely more challenging than testing adults. As with adults, making them feel comfortable is essential. It might also be beneficial have multiple practice rounds beforehand and prioritize performance of the tasks as compared to focusing on unwanted movements. If they can handle only short scan times, multiple breaks during the study will be beneficial. Tasks with bright colors and interesting pictures might help engage the children better. Resting-state scans can be valuable when task-based scans cannot be performed.

TYPES OF FMRI STUDIES COMMONLY USED IN PSYCHIATRIC DISEASES

Task-based scans: Here we use specific tasks to elicit a response in a particular region of the brain, for example, having the patient read and understand complex sentences, think of antonyms or generate words using a given letter causes activations in the language centers in the frontal, prefrontal and temporal areas of the brain. This activation may be diminished in certain psychiatric illnesses.

Cerebral blood flow: Here the patient is asked to hold their breath for 20–30 s at a time followed by regular breathing. The breath hold causes temporary hypercapnia (increase in CO_2) which in turn causes an increase in CBF, and hence there is increased oxygenation to the entire cerebral cortex, which can be picked up as a robust bold signal.

Resting state: Here the patient is asked to try to clear their mind of any distinctive thoughts and try to attain a relaxed state of mind. They're encouraged to keep their eyes open, stay awake and let their mind wander feely. This scan measures brain activity at a state of relative rest where areas like the default mode network are in use while motor and language centers are inactive.

POST-PROCESSING GUIDELINES

After the fMRI tasks are completed, a regular anatomical MRI is also acquired with their head in the same position. The BOLD data set is then overlaid on to the anatomical scan so as to get the final fMRI image. While adjusting the bold signal during post processing, we should set the threshold to a level such that we are able to remove as much noise (motion, breathing related signal spikes) as possible while still leaving behind relevant bold signal. To confirm if an activation is indeed due to brain activity, we can check the time series graph for that particular area. If the graphical representation of patient data coincides with the ideal waveform for that task, the signal is most likely produced due to neural activity. When processing a resting state study, adjust the frequency to a low level (0.01–0.08 Hz) to reduce signals due to physiological noise such that only the desired bold signal is left behind. In clinical practice, fMRIs are used to aid in diagnosis, understand the origins of various disease symptoms or assist pre-surgical planning. In these cases, a single fMRI scan is generally sufficient. However, in some cases a repeat study might prove useful. When studying the effects of a certain drug or treatment modality, it might be helpful to perform a second scan post-treatment to ascertain the changes, if any, that might be present in brain function and correlate them to the patients' current symptoms or lack thereof. Occasionally a post-surgical fMRI study might be done in prior pre-surgically scanned patients to detect signs of neural plasticity. The most common reason for a repeat study usually is due to an unsatisfactory original study lacking any usable data. It is worth noting that going through the process of a functional scan can be very challenging for some psychiatric patients, and hence it should only be performed or repeated when potential benefits are present.

To further the applications of functional neuroimaging, researchers are carrying out multiple clinical studies and trials. Oftentimes patients need to be recruited to such trials. In this situation, review the details of the study thoroughly and clarify any part of the study that you haven't understood with the principal investigator. When speaking to a subject that fits the study criteria, first ensure that they are adequately prepared for the functional scan that they have come in for. Then proceed to explain the research study to them in simple and easy-to-understand words while still covering all the details. Go over the risks and potential benefits of the study. Make sure to let them know what their data will be used for, if they would need to come back for another scan, if they will be injected with a radio-opaque-dye or if they will be exposed to any radiation (PET). If they respond positively, hand them the consent form. Have them read through it and then take the time to answer any questions they might have. If they decline, respect their decision and proceed with the routine functional scan at hand.

The functional scan results will show multiple-colored activations in different areas of the brain. fMRI changes in psychiatric diseases are not always discernible. In some cases, the bold signal might be too weak to show activation in the desired areas. Some scans might show increased activations in expected or unexpected areas, while in other cases, the scan may look no different than healthy controls. However, cases that show some variation from baseline can help in understanding disease processes and various symptoms and possibly assist in the diagnosis of that particular disease by providing a functional representation of the brain in a disease state. However, it is prudent to keep in mind that neuroimaging studies are purely correlational and do not reveal what is causing the reduction in blood flow. fMRI on its own, without proper correlation to standard psychiatric evaluation, is not useful in clinical practice.

Advantages of fMRI

fMRI is a non-invasive scan and does not require injections of radioactive isotopes like PET or single positron emission computed tomography. It doesn't require any radiation exposure like in X-rays and computed tomography (CT) scans. It produces very high-resolution images. Compared to the traditional questionnaire methods of psychological evaluation, fMRI is more objective, allowing for better understanding of psychiatric disease processes and can help assess treatment effects.

Disadvantages of fMRI

fMRI an expensive study. The BOLD signal is very susceptible to motion; hence the patient has to stay very still, sometimes for long periods of time. It can be hard to distinguish whether the areas of activation are due to neural activity or other physiological functions, motion artifacts and so on. BOLD depends on autoregulation of cerebral blow flow which may be altered due to ischemia, vasospasm, tumors, certain drugs and so on.

PET

Positron emission tomography is a type of nuclear medicine procedure that measures the metabolic activity of body tissues at a cellular level. Radionuclides, such as F-18 (^{18}F-FDG), carbon-11 and oxygen-15, emit positrons. These positrons undergo annihilation with electrons, which results in the release of photons. These annihilation photons, and not positrons, are detected during PET. Combining PET with another form of imaging such as CT or MRI is required, as by itself, PET data has poor anatomical detail. Good anatomical images help in differentiating normal and abnormal radiotracer uptake, thereby increasing accuracy of the study [1]. A variety of psychiatric disorders have been studied using PET. Currently the results of PET scans help in the better understanding of illnesses like schizophrenia, depression, OCD, PTSD and substance abuse.

PRESENTATIONS AND USES OF FMRI AND PET IN VARIOUS PSYCHIATRIC DISEASES

In various psychiatric diseases, fMRI activations in patient studies are compared to activity maps of healthy individuals. Also, by using various different cognitive fMRI tests, we can understand the subtle differences in patient brains and how they perform various functions. By studying PET scans in psychiatric conditions, we can better appreciate the changes in metabolic activity in different brain regions.

SCHIZOPHRENIA

Schizophrenia is a lifelong disease which affects multiple major aspects of life such as education, work, interpersonal relations and self-care. Since we observe deterioration in a variety of neural functions, we can employ multiple types of cognitive fMRI tasks to assess the patient. Commonly used tasks are working memory paradigms, memory encoding and recognition tasks and positive and negative mood evocation tasks. In healthy individuals, these tasks would robustly activate areas in the prefrontal cortex, temporal cortical areas, hippocampus, parahippocampal gyrus, amygdala and basal ganglia. However, in schizophrenia, decreased activation is seen in these areas, with a more pronounced decrease seen in the prefrontal cortex [2]. PET has been used extensively in schizophrenia. Most studies report dysfunction in the frontal, thalamic and hippocampal areas with negative symptoms being correlated to the degree of frontal hypometabolism [3].

MAJOR DEPRESSION

A patient is said to have major depression when they have two or more episodes of major depressive disorder without any episodes of mania. Symptoms are varied, such as loss of interests, deep despair, sleep troubles and feelings of worthlessness, and both fMRI and PET studies have shown multiple areas of the brain with decreased function. It is hypothesized that areas in the limbic system as well as the cortex are affected. There is also thought to be a failure of systems that usually provide a healthy autoregulation of emotion during distressing times [4]. Interestingly, a decreased cerebral blood flow (CBF) and decreased cerebral glucose metabolism (CMRglc) have been observed in the dorsolateral and dorsomedial prefrontal cortex while an increased CBF and CMRglc have been observed in the venterolateral, venteromedial and orbitofrontal cortex as well as the amygdala and insular cortex [5,6]. Another application of fMRI in major depression is studying the changes in bold response pre- and post-treatment. Some studies have shown favorable changes post-treatment; however, more studies are required to correlate this.

BIPOLAR DISORDER

Bipolar disorder is an illness characterized by depressed states and manic episodes in affected individuals. The depressed states are similar to major depression and show similar neural activity as well. The manic state is characterized by symptoms of elevated mood, excessive energy levels and altered thought processes [7]. fMRI studies can be done on patients in depressed states or manic states as well as basal states to compare the changes in brain function. Inconsistencies in activation were observed over the brain hemispheres. In the manic state, increased activation was seen in the right side of the ventral prefrontal cortex, while the depressed state showed a greater increase in signal in the left ventral pre-frontal cortex [8]. This could help us understand brain function during the different mood states as well as their variability as compared to healthy individuals. Working memory also seems to be greatly affected in bipolar patients. Studies comparing working memory tasks in heathy vs bipolar subjects showed significant decrease in signal in the prefrontal cortex in bipolar individuals while in a euthymic state [9]. Strong family history being a significant risk factor for the development of bipolar disorder, several studies have been conducted to compare fMRI activations in this group of subjects. It has been observed that, as compared to controls, children without disorders, born to parents with bipolar disease, showed altered activation in a number of cortical and subcortical areas.

PTSD

PTSD is a disorder which is caused by situations of extreme stress in a person's life such as sexual or physical abuse, car accidents, natural disasters and combat. Common symptoms include flashbacks of the traumatic event, trouble sleeping, intrusive memories, avoidance of traumatic stimuli and social dysfunction. It is observed that there is an exaggeration of fear response in these patients. They tend to have a generalization of danger cues, such that, even with stimuli that may not be dangerous but are associated with past traumatic memories will result in PTSD symptoms [10]. fMRI studies have been done where the patient is shown auditory or visual stimuli which remind them of their past trauma to understand the cause of their altered response. They've shown a greatly increased signal in the amygdala and a decreased signal in the medial prefrontal cortex [11]. Often people with PTSD face memory deficits. This has been observed on fMRI scans as a decreased signal in the hippocampal region as well as reduced hippocampal volume [12]. It is yet to be determined if the stressful event causes reduction in hippocampal volume due to cortisol-induced reduction in brain neurotropic factors or if a congenital smaller hippocampal size predisposes the subject to PTSD [13]. PET studies have also shown hypoactivation of the hippocampus during memory tasks.

OCD

Obsessive-compulsive disorder is a complicated disorder with varied symptoms, the most prominent being obsessive and repetitive thoughts and compulsions to perform certain repetitive behaviors. The patients perform these behaviors to help them cope with daily stresses; however, they usually end up leading to higher levels of distress. Neuroimaging findings in OCD depend on multiple factors. Task-based fMRI studies such as the response inhibition (Go/No-go) task have shown decreased activation in the right thalamus during response inhibition [14]. This positively correlates to traditional literature, which has noted functional and structural abnormalities in the thalamus in OCD subjects. Experiments involving symptom provocation have shown increased activations in the orbito-frontal cortex (OFC) and in the frontal-subcortical circuitry. This supports current theories that dysfunctions in these areas are the cause of many of the symptoms in OCD. Resting state functional studies as well as PET scans in OCD subjects have shown increased CBF and higher metabolism in the OFC. Another study done on OCD patients concurrently having major depression showed reduced CBF to the thalamus, caudate and hippocampal areas as compared to controls or patients with only OCD. Hence, we must be aware of the changes that can occur in patients with only one disease versus those with multiple conditions, as they can alter functional data [15].

ADHD

ADHD is one of the most common neurodevelopmental disorders of childhood. Children with ADHD usually have trouble paying attention and have excessively high levels of impulsivity and hyperactivity. Multiple fMRI studies have been performed on children with ADHD.

Most of them observed reduced activation in the frontal and fronto-striatal networks as compared to controls [16]. In adults, working memory tests have shown decreased activation in the left inferior occipital and cerebellar regions and a 'trend of deactivation' in the right prefrontal cortex possibly suggesting decreased activation in the fronto-cerebellar circuit. Functional connectivity studies which correlate spatially remote neuropsychological events have found significantly lower connectivity in fronto-parietal and fronto-striato-parieto-cerebellar networks in adolescents and adults with ADHD compared to controls [15]. The default mode network (DMN) comprises the medial prefrontal cortex; posterior cingulate; precuneus; and medial, lateral and inferior parietal cortices and is thought to be associated with mental functions during a state of relative rest, such as when the mind is left to wander. Studies showed that adolescents with ADHD were unable to suppress this network during specific tasks as well as having some reduced connectivity in this network. This could explain symptoms of attention deficits and irregular behavioral responses. It is also worth noting that scans performed after administering methylphenidate showed effective suppression of the DMN and better performance. However, further studies are still required to establish the effect of medications on brain activation in ADHD [17].

SUBSTANCE ABUSE

Substance abuse refers to excessive use of a drug in a way that is harmful to oneself or others. Commonly abused substances are alcohol, pain medication and illegal drugs. Most studies that compare fMRI data of patients with a history of moderate to severe substance abuse show some alterations in brain activity as compared to healthy controls. A spatial working memory test performed on alcohol-dependent women demonstrated significantly lower BOLD responses than controls in the right superior, right inferior parietal, right middle frontal, right postcentral and left superior frontal cortical areas [18], while most PET studies report decreased whole-brain metabolism, with the parietal lobe being affected disproportionately [19]. In another study, cocaine-dependent (CD) subjects and non–drug using control subjects underwent fMRI while performing a working memory task. They observed altered brain function in frontal, striatal and thalamic brain regions known to be part of a circuit associated with motor control, reward and cognition in CD subjects [20]. PET studies have shown decreased metabolism [21] in cortical and subcortical structures when cocaine was acutely administered to chronic cocaine users. With cannabis use gaining popularity, it is important to study its effects on brain function. A verbal working memory task and a visuo-auditory selective attention task was performed by moderate frequent cannabis users as well as healthy controls. While both groups performed equally well on the tasks, cannabis users showed altered brain activity in the left superior parietal cortex [22]. fMRI may also be used to predict drug use in the future. However more studies are still required.

CONCLUSION/FUTURE CLINICAL APPLICATIONS OF FMRI IN PSYCHIATRIC DISEASES

Throughout our review, we have seen trends of decreased activity in cortical and subcortical areas in the diseased brain; however, in certain disorders, increased activity is also present in some parts of the brain. Many researchers think that the areas of increased activity are present to compensate for the decreased activations in the traditional areas of function. Currently it is difficult to localize functional deficits in various diseases to a specific brain region. However, with the advent of functional connectivity, we may be able to get a better picture of the connection between various affected areas. In the future we anticipate standardized fMRI tasks which can produce reliable activation patterns in diseased and healthy brains. We also would like to have further studies on new neurotransmitter ligands in PET imaging, which can be used in psychiatric diseases. The hope is that with numerous further studies and more data on neural deficits in various diseases, we can find some useful commonalities which can aid in clinical diagnosis and treatment.

References

1. Kapoor V, McCook BM, Torok FS. An introduction to PET-CT imaging. *RadioGraphics*. 2004;24(2):523–543.
2. Hofer A, Weiss EM, Golaszewski SM, Siedentopf CM, Brinkhoff C, Kremser C, et al. An FMRI study of episodic encoding and recognition of words in patients with schizophrenia in remission. *Am J Psychiatry*. 2003;160(5):911–918.
3. Newberg AB, Moss AS, Monti DA, Alavi A. Positron emission tomography in psychiatric disorders. *Annals of the New York Academy of Sciences*. 2011;1228(1), E13–E25.
4. Mayberg HS. Modulating dysfunctional limbic-cortical circuits in depression: Towards development of brain-based algorithms for diagnosis and optimized treatment. *Br Med Bull*. 2003; 65:193–207.
5. Bench CJ, Friston KJ, Brown RG, Scott LC, Frackowiak RS, Dolan RJ. The anatomy of melancholia-focal abnormalities of cerebral blood flow in major depression. *Psychol Med*. 1992;22(3):607–615.
6. Siegle GJ, Thompson W, Carter CS, Steinhauer SR, Thase ME. Increased amygdala and decreased dorsolateral pre-frontal BOLD responses in unipolar depression: Related and independent features. *Biol Psychiatry*. 2007;61(2):198–209.
7. Habecker EL, Daniels MA, Canu E, Rocca MA, Filippi M, Renshaw PF. fMRI in psychiatric disorders. *fMRI Techniques and Protocols*. 2016, p. 657–697.
8. Blumberg HP, Leung HC, Skudlarski P, Lacadie CM, Fredericks CA, Harris BC, et al. A functional magnetic resonance imaging study of bipolar disorder: State and trait-related dysfunction in ventral prefrontal cortices. *Arch Gen Psychiatry*. 2003;60(6):601–609.
9. Lagopoulos J, Ivanovski B, Malhi GS. An event-related functional MRI study of working memory in euthymic bipolar disorder. *J Psychiatry Neurosci*. 2007;32(3):174–184.
10. Charney DS. Psychobiological mechanisms of resilience and vulnerability: Implications for successful adaptation to extreme stress. *Am J Psychiatry*. 2004;161(2):195–216.
11. Lanius RA, Williamson PC, Densmore M, Boksman K, Gupta MA, Neufeld RW, et al. Neural correlates of traumatic memories in posttraumatic stress disorder: A functional MRI investigation. *Am J Psychiatry*. 2001;158(11):1920–1922.
12. Geuze E, Vermetten E, Bremner JD. MR-based in vivo hippocampal volumetrics: 2. findings in neuropsychiatric disorders. *Mol Psychiatry*. 2005;10(2):160–184.
13. Gilbertson MW, Shenton ME, Ciszewski A, Kasai K, Lasko NB, Orr SP, Pitman RK. Smaller hippocampal volume predicts pathologic vulnerability to psychological trauma. *Nat Neurosci*. 2002;5(11):1242–1247.
14. Roth RM, Saykin AJ, Flashman LA, Pixley HS, West JD, Mamourian AC. Event related functional magnetic resonance imaging of response inhibition in obsessive-compulsive disorder. *Biol Psychiatry*. 2007;62(8):901–909.
15. Saxena S, Brody AL, Ho ML, Alborzian S, Ho MK, Maidment KM, et al. Cerebral metabolism in major depression and obsessive-compulsive disorder occurring separately and concurrently. *Biol Psychiatry*. 2001;50(3):159–170.
16. Cubillo A, Halari R, Ecker C, Giampietro V, Taylor E, Rubia K. Reduced activation and interregional functional connectivity of fronto-striatal networks in adults with childhood Attention-Deficit Hyperactivity Disorder (ADHD) and persisting symptoms during tasks of motor inhibition and cognitive switching. *Journal of Psychiatric Research*. 2010;44(10):629–639.
17. Weyandt L, Swentosky A, Gudmundsdottir BG. Neuroimaging and ADHD: fMRI, PET, DTI findings and methodological limitations. *Developmental Neuropsychology*. 2013;38(4):211–225.
18. Tapert SF, Brown GG, Kindermann SS, Cheung EH, Frank LR, Brown SA. fMRI measurement of brain dysfunction in alcohol-dependent young women. *Alcoholism: Clinical and Experimental Research*. 2001;25(2):236–245.
19. Samson Y, Baron JC, Feline A, et al. Local cere-bral glucose utilization in chronic alcoholics, a positron tomography study. *J. Neurol. Neurosurg. Psychiatr*. 1989;49:1165–1170.
20. Moeller FG, Steinberg JL, Schmitz JM, Ma L, Liu S, Kjome KL, et al. Working memory fMRI activation in cocaine-dependent subjects: Association with treatment response. *Psychiatry Res*. 2010;181(3):174–182.

21. London ED, Cascella NG, Wong DF, et al. Cocaine-induced reduction of glucose utilization in human brain: A study using positron emission tomography and (Fluorine-18)-fluorodeoxyglucose. *Arch. Gen. Psychiatry*. 1990;47:567–574.
22. Jager G, Kahn RS, Van Den Brink W, Van Ree JM, Ramsey NF. Long-term effects of frequent cannabis use on working memory and attention: An fMRI study. *Psychopharmacology*. 2006;185(3):358–368.

48

Personalized Psychiatry of Psychoneurological Diseases
From Theory to Clinical Practice

Regina F. Nasyrova, Nikolay G. Neznanov, Natalia A. Shnayder

Introduction	525
New Approaches to Treatment of Psychoneurological Diseases	526
Pharmacogenetic Testing for Psychiatry and Neurology	526
Algorithm of Personalized Approach to Use of Chlorpromazine	527
Conclusions	533

ABBREVIATIONS

5HT2C – 5-hydroxytryptamine 2C receptor
7-HOCPZ – 7-hydroxy chlorpromazine
ADR – adverse drug reaction
AP – antipsychotic
BBB – blood brain barrier
COMT – catechol-O-methyltransferase
CPIC – Clinical Pharmacogenetics Implementation Consortium
CPZ – chlorpromazine
CPZNO – chlorpromazine nitric oxide
CPZSO – chlorpromazine sulfoxide
CYP – cytochrome 450
CYP1A2 – enzyme 1A2 of cytochrome 450
CYP2B6 – enzyme 2D6 of cytochrome 450
CYP2C19 – enzyme 2C19 of cytochrome 450
CYP2C9 – enzyme 2C9 of cytochrome 450
CYP2D6 – enzyme 2D6 of cytochrome 450
CYP3A4 – enzyme 3A4 of cytochrome 450
Del – deletion
DNA – deoxyribonucleic acid
DPWG – Dutch Pharmacogenetics Working Group
DRD2 – dopaminergic receptor D2
DRD3 – dopaminergic receptor D3
EM – extensive metabolizer
EPM2A – epilepsy, progressive myoclonus type 2A

EPS – extrapyramidal syndrome
EU – European Union
FDA – Food and Drug Administration
HTR2A – 5-hydroxytryptamine 2A receptor
IM – intermediate metabolizer
Ins – insertion
MC4R – melanocortin 4 receptor
PGx – pharmacogenetic testing
PM – poor metabolizer
SLC6A4 – solute carrier family 6 member 4
SNV – single nucleotide variant
UM – ultra-rapid metabolizer
USA – United States of America

INTRODUCTION

Personalized medicine is an approach to providing medical care based on the individual characteristics of patients. This is a new doctrine of modern healthcare based on practical application of new molecular technologies (the so-called "omics": genomics, transcriptomics, proteomics, metabolomics, microbiomics) to improve the estimation of predisposition to diseases (prediction) and their prevention and treatment with the use of interventions, including medicinal therapy and surgery.

Pharmacogenomics is the study of the role of the genome in drug response. Its name (pharmaco- + genomics) reflects its combining of pharmacology and genomics. Pharmacogenomics analyzes how the genetic makeup of an individual affects their response to drugs [1]. It deals with the influence of acquired and inherited genetic variation on drug response in patients by correlating gene expression or single-nucleotide polymorphisms with pharmacokinetics (drug absorption, distribution, metabolism, and elimination) and pharmacodynamics (effects mediated through a drug's biological targets) [2, 3, 4]. The term pharmacogenomics is often used interchangeably with pharmacogenetics. Although both terms relate to drug response based on genetic influences, pharmacogenetics focuses on single drug-gene interactions, while pharmacogenomics encompasses a more genome-wide association approach, incorporating genomics and epigenetics while dealing with the effects of multiple genes on drug response [5, 6, 7].

New biomedical products emerging in the recent years as a result of implementation of the genome research project allow scientists and clinicians to more accurately determine the genetic basis of many neuropsychiatric disorders, to control the predisposition to the development of an increasingly wide range of diseases, and to personalize more effective and safe ways of their treatment and prevention [8]. These include the forefront advances of the burgeoning personalized medicine industry such as deoxyribonucleic acid (DNA) sequencing, proteomic analysis, microarrays, and advances in optics and imaging technologies. Pharmacogenomics seeks to find and characterize correlations between the genotype (genetic profile) and the phenotype (therapeutic response) of a patient in order to develop individual medications and treatment regimens. At the same time, it is generally recognized that the closest to implementation in real clinical practice and most promising technology of personalized medicine is pharmacogenetic testing (PGx).

Significant progress in the treatment of mental and neurological disorders as well as diseases of addiction over the past 50 years has been achieved due to the initial empirical discoveries of the psychotropic properties of certain drugs. Discoveries in pharmacology have revolutionized psychiatric and neurological clinical practice and resulted in unconditional recognition of psychiatry and neurology as independent clinical disciplines adding effective medicinal treatment to other therapeutic interventions. However, a significant problem to face was low predictability of the drug response and serious adverse drug reactions (ADRs) of psychotropic drugs of the first generation that may significantly worsen the quality of life of patients and cause low adherence to drug therapy [8].

NEW APPROACHES TO TREATMENT OF PSYCHONEUROLOGICAL DISEASES

Pharmacogenetics aims to develop rational means to optimize psychopharmacotherapy with respect to the patients' genotype to ensure maximum efficiency with minimal ADRs [9]. Through the utilization of pharmacogenetics, it is hoped that pharmaceutical drug treatments can deviate from what is dubbed the "one-dose-fits-all" approach. Pharmacogenetics also attempts to eliminate the trial-and-error method of prescribing, allowing psychiatrics and neurologists to take into consideration their patient's genes, the functionality of these genes, and how this may affect the efficacy of the patient's current or future treatments (and, where applicable, provide an explanation for the failure of past treatments) of psychoneurological diseases [5, 10, 11]. Such approaches promise the advent of precision medicine and even personalized medicine, in which drugs and drug combinations are optimized for narrow subsets of patients or even for each individual's unique genetic makeup [12, 13].

The recent improvement of the therapeutic process in psychiatry and neurology involves three complementary approaches.

The first approach is to develop biomarkers to identification of patients at high risk of developing ADRs and/or early diagnosis of ADRs. The second seeks to improve the synthesized pharmacologically active molecules, which provides an increase in the drug effectiveness and safety. The third approach involves considering the patient's genotype as a possible marker of the response to a drug in order to confront the extremely difficult prediction of an individual response to a drug making the treatment of mental and neurological disorders a problem area [8].

Whether used to explain a patient's response or lack thereof to a treatment, or act as a predictive tool, these approaches hope to achieve better treatment outcomes, greater efficacy, and minimization of the occurrence of drug toxicities and ADRs. For patients who have a lack of therapeutic response to a treatment, alternative therapies can be prescribed that would best suit their requirements. In order to provide pharmacogenetic recommendations for a given drug, two possible types of input can be used: genotyping or exome or whole genome sequencing [15]. Sequencing provides many more data points, including detection of mutations that prematurely terminate the synthesized protein (early stop codon) [15, 16].

PHARMACOGENETIC TESTING FOR PSYCHIATRY AND NEUROLOGY

In 2004, the Food and Drug Administration (FDA) approved the first pharmacogenetic test, AmpliChip CYP450, which provides information about the patient's genotype by allelic variants of the cytochrome P450 genes (*CYP2D6* and *CYP2C19*). The AmpliChip CYP450 test combines the patented Roshe polymerase chain reaction (PCR) technology and the Affymetrix microchip technology. In December 2004, the Affymetrix Gene Chip System 3000 Dx, which produces AmpliChip CYP450, received FDA approval for diagnostic use. According to PGx results, patients are divided into two phenotypes (extensive and poor metabolizers) depending on the carrier of alleles of three single-nucleotide variants (SNVs) of the *CYP2C19* gene and four phenotypes depending on the carrier of 27 alleles of SNVs (including 7 duplications) of the *CYP2D6* gene. However, the results of PGx obtained using AmpliChip are not sufficient to predict the effectiveness and safety of antipsychotic therapy [17, 18].

A good example of a system for assessing the genetic contribution to the metabolism of drugs is the gene sight psychotropic algorithm, developed by a group of scientists at the Mason Clinic (USA). The test is non-invasive and easy to use: to collect a sample of the patient's DNA, only a scraping of the buccal epithelium is required. The results are provided to the doctor or patient within 36 hours. The gene sight psychotropic algorithm is based on a multi-gene multivariate genetic test that takes into account the features of the genotype, phenotype, and information about the metabolism of drugs. The analysis is performed on 59 allelic variants of eight genes (*CYP1A2, CYP2C9, CYP2C19, CYP3A4, CYP2B6, CYP2D6, HTR2A,* and *SLC6A4*). The information automatically analyzed by the program on the results of the patient's genotyping is provided to the psychiatrist. The gene sight psychotropic algorithm contains a list of antipsychotics and antidepressants, divided into three categories: "use as directed", "use with caution", and "use with increased caution and with more frequent monitoring", as well as additional information that helps the doctor make a decision on the appointment or cancellation of drugs in a particular patient. Thus, this algorithm allows you to make a decision on the appointment of drug therapy without the involvement of a clinical pharmacologist [18, 19].

Another pharmacogenetic test, the gene cept assay, developed in the United States, allows a clinical pharmacologist to easily make a decision about prescribing antipsychotics and antidepressants (www.dynacare.ca). The analysis of the gene cept assay covers a wide range of drugs used in the treatment of various mental disorders, including depression, obsessive-compulsive disorder, schizophrenia, attention deficit hyperactivity disorder, bipolar disorder, and so on. The study is based on allelic variants in 20 genes, including *5HT2C, MC4R, DRD2, COMT,* and genes encoding liver cytochrome P450 isoenzymes. The conclusion is provided to the psychiatrist within 8 working days in the form of a detailed table with recommendations for prescribing drugs for a particular patient [18].

In the Russian practice, to help clinicians, it is necessary to develop a convenient software for decoding the data of PGx; such work is actively carried out at the Center for Personalized Psychiatry and Neurology of V.M. Bekhterev National Medical Research Center for Psychiatry and Neurology (St. Petersburg) [8, 11]. This will allow psychiatrists and neurologists to make their own decisions about the choice of the drug and its dosage regimen without the help of a clinical pharmacologist as an additional expert, as well as to minimize errors in the interpretation of the results of PGx. The development of accessible algorithms and decision-making programs for the interpretation of PGx data will allow the popularization of PGx through quick and easy access to information from both the patient and the attending physician. In addition, PGx can help reduce the cost of drug therapy by reducing the time to select the optimal dose of the drug and the cost of correcting ADRs [18].

ALGORITHM OF PERSONALIZED APPROACH TO USE OF CHLORPROMAZINE

Antipsychotics (APs) are a group of psychotropic drugs for the treatment of mental disorders, in particular schizophrenia. In the mid-1950s, the first AP was synthesized (known as chlorpromazine [CPZ]). This drug has revolutionized the treatment of psychotic disorders. Studies of the properties of CPZ contributed to the widespread use of the drug in psychiatric practice. According to Edward Shorter: "CPZ initiated a revolution in psychiatry comparable to the introduction of penicillin in general medicine" [20]. The use of phenothiazine compounds as AP was the result of research by Henri Marie Laborit, a French army surgeon who was looking for a pharmacological method to prevent surgical shock [21]. That's why CPZ has a weak anticholinergic and strong sympatholytic effect, and it was originally used as an antihistamine drug. Since 1958, other APs began to appear, such as haloperidol, thioproperazine, trifluoperazine, and others. All these drugs, in addition to the antipsychotic effect, caused severe adverse drug reactions in patients, in particular from the neurological system, such as AP-induced extrapyramidal syndrome (EPS). Thus, this group of drugs was called "antipsychotics". It was believed that the severity and incidence of EPS were directly proportional to the therapeutic effect of AP. However, later other drugs began to appear, such as clozapine, olanzapine, risperidone, quetiapine, aripiprazole, amisulpiride, ziprasidone, and so on. They caused AP-induced EPS to a lesser extent, and the antipsychotic effect was more pronounced. Thus, the term "neuroleptics" was called into question, and today the more correct term is "antipsychotics" [22]. Also, due to the differences in drugs in the form of the severity of the antipsychotic effect and the manifestation of AP-induced EPS, they were divided into two groups: first- and second-generation APs. Thus, CPZ belongs to the first-generation APs or typical APs [23]. CPZ is currently used in patients with schizophrenia in Russia. However, in the countries of the European Union (EU), its use has been de facto discontinued since the mid-nineties of the 20th century due to high neurotoxicity and a huge number of ADRs [23].

CPZ has antipsychotic, sedative, and antiemetic effects. The drug weakens or completely eliminates delusions and hallucinations, relieves psychomotor agitation, and reduces anxiety. CPZ is used to treat both psychotic disorders, including schizophrenia, manic bipolar disorder, and amphetamine-induced psychotic disorders [11]. The drug is recognized as the standard by which other APs are assessed [24]. CPZ has antiemetic and hypothermic action and enhances the action of barbiturates, alcohol, and anesthetics [11, 23].

The mechanism of the antipsychotic action of CPZ is associated with the blockade of postsynaptic dopaminergic receptors in the brain mesolimbic structures. The high-affinity antagonism of CPZ to dopaminergic D2 receptors determines not only the therapeutic effect but also the development of EPS [11, 22]. It also has anticholinergic and antihistaminergic effects: dry mouth, blurred vision, retention of urine, anxiety, tremor, weight gain, lowering blood pressure, dizziness, and hyperprolactinemia [23, 25]. It causes a hypotensive effect and disrupts the intracardiac impulse conduction, lengthening the QT interval as adrenergic antagonist. CPZ at low-threshold doses (2.5 mg/kg) increases the concentration of dopamine and norepinephrine metabolites [23, 26]. A correlation has been established between the IC50 values (concentration of half-maximal inhibition) for AP and their clinical activity: the higher the affinity for dopaminergic receptors, the higher the clinical AP efficacy [22]. In addition to the blockade of dopaminergic receptors in the mesolimbic structures of the brain, CPZ has a blocking effect on α adrenergic receptors, capable of binding to cholinergic receptors [27].

CPZ is produced in the form of tablets or pills of 25, 50, and 100 mg and in the form of ampoules of 1, 2, and 5 ml of a 2.5% solution and 5 ml of a 0.5% solution. Also there are tablets of 10 mg for children. CPZ is produced under various trade names; those most often used are Aminazine, Chlorpromazine, and Chlorpromazine hydrochloride. Dosage regimen: small doses – up to 100 mg/day, average therapeutic doses – 200–300 mg/day, large doses – up to 500 mg/day. The bioavailability of CPZ after single oral doses compared with single intramuscular doses ranges from 10% to 69%. CPZ binds to plasma proteins (95–98%) [28].

CPZ is metabolized in the liver, with the formation of a number of active and inactive metabolites. Metabolic pathways of the drug include hydroxylation, conjugation with glucuronic acid, N-oxidation, oxidation of sulfur atoms, and dealkylation. The main metabolites are CPZ N-oxide (CPZNO), CPZ sulfoxide (CPZSO), and free and bound 7-hydroxy CPZ (7-HOCPZ) [29]. Plasma sulfoxide and plasma sulfoxide to CPZ ratios are higher in nonresponder patients than in responders. The serum level of CPZ N-oxide in patients taking the drug for a long time is about half of the level of the drug at the beginning of therapy. A decrease in the level of unchanged CPZ in blood plasma is recorded 2 weeks after oral administration, which is due to the activation of microsomal oxidizing enzymes of the liver and intestines [30]. CPZ is almost completely metabolized in the body, and less than 1% is excreted in the form of an unchanged drug in the urine. Different ratios of conjugated and unconjugated metabolites in urine are observed after intramuscular and oral doses of CPZ, which can explain the effect of "first pass" in the liver after oral administration of the drug [23].

CPZ metabolism is mediated by enzymes of the cytochrome P450 family (CYP). It was found that CPZ is a competitive inhibitor of the enzyme 2D6 of cytochrome P450 (CYP2D6) and to a lesser extent the enzyme CYP1A2. The half-life varies from 2 to 31 hours, but in 80% of cases, it is 6 hours or less. CPZ penetrates the blood-brain barrier (BBB), while the concentration in the brain is higher than in the plasma [11, 23].

CPZ-induced EPS characterized by the occurrence of motor disorders. It is as a result of damage to the basal ganglia and subcortical-thalamic connections. Drug-induced EPS is subdivided into primary and secondary. Among primary EPS, drug-induced parkinsonism is the most common (the leading form of secondary parkinsonism) [22].

Pharmacogenetic markers of CPZ safety are being actively studied. Some pharmacogenetic markers of therapy safety have been established: SNVs of candidate genes for dopaminergic receptors D2 and D3 (*DRD2*, *DRD3*), laforine phosphatase (*EPM2A*), and enzyme 2D6 of CYP 450 (*CYP2D6*) [11].

An association has been established between the carriage of −141C Ins/Del of *DRD2* gene and the risk of schizophrenia [23]. This variant affects the density of dopamine D2 receptors; the carriage of the Del allele leads to a higher density of D2 receptors [31]. In carriers of this polymorphism, low efficiency of AP therapy was established [32]. An *in vitro* study shows that the Del of the −141CIns/Del variant is directly associated with the level of DRD2 expression [33]. However, there are reports of opposite results [34].

The dopamine D3 receptor is predominantly expressed in areas of the limbic and basal ganglia associated with cognitive, emotional, and motor functions. The missense variant in exon 1 of the *DRD3* gene leads to the substitution of serine for glycine (rs6280, Ser9Gly) in the N-terminal extracellular domain of the receptor protein, which leads to a change in the affinity for dopamine. The replacement Gly can increase the density of D3 receptors in some areas of the brain. Patients with a heterozygous Ser/Gly genotype respond better to CPZ therapy. Carriage of the Gly increases the risk of EPS, including AIP, and reduces the effectiveness of CPZ therapy [35].

The *EPM2A* gene encodes laforin phosphatase, a protein involved in the regulation of glycogen metabolism in brain [36]. Andrade and Singh put forward a hypothesis about the possible role of impaired glycogen metabolism in the development of schizophrenia and the response to AP [37]. Patients with the TT genotype (rs1415744) of *EPM2A* gene showed a low efficacy of CPZ therapy compared with patients with CC and CT genotypes [36].

Patient' genotypes are usually categorized into the following predicted phenotypes depending on the carrier of low-functional (partially functioning)/nonfunctional alleles of SNVs of genes encoding enzymes of drug metabolism [11]:

- ultra-rapid metabolizer (UM): patients with substantially increased metabolic activity;
- extensive metabolizer (EM): normal metabolic activity;
- intermediate metabolizer (IM): patients with reduced metabolic activity;
- poor metabolizer (PM): patients with little to no functional metabolic activity.

The two extremes of this spectrum are PMs and UMs. Efficacy of APs is not only based on these metabolic statuses but also the type of drug consumed. Also, drugs can be classified into two main groups: active drugs and prodrugs. Active drugs refers to drugs that are inactivated during metabolism, and prodrugs are inactive until they are metabolized.

For example, the enzyme CYP2D6, also known as debrisoquine hydroxylase (named after the drug that led to its discovery), *CYP2D6* is the most well-known and extensively studied CYP gene [38]. It is a gene of great interest also due to its highly polymorphic nature and involvement in a high number of medication metabolisms (both as a major and minor pathway). More than 100 *CYP2D6* genetic variants have been identified [39]. Both SNVs and polymorphisms in the *CYP2D6* gene (leading to versions of the enzyme with differing levels of metabolic activity) and copy number variants are known. For certain drugs, predominantly metabolized by CYP2D6, these variations can lead to unusually high or low drug concentrations in serum (referred to as PM and UM phenotypes, respectively), thus leading to increased ADRs or reduced efficacy of many APs, including CPZ [11]. The frequency of *CYP2D6* varies geographically, with the highest prevalence of PMs found in east Asia and the lowest prevalence in the Americas [40]. Homozygous and heterozygous carriers of low-functional and non-functional SNVs of *CYP2D6* gene have a high risk of developing CPZ-induced ADRs, including AP-induced EPS [22, 41]. A high incidence of EPS has been shown in patients with schizophrenia with the PM phenotype compared to a group of patients carrying one or more high-functioning SNVs (UM and EM phenotypes) of the *CYP2D6* gene [42]. Similar results were obtained by de Leon et al. (2005): the risk of developing EPS was six times higher in patients with the PM phenotype compared to patients with the EM phenotype [43]. Currently, the prognostic role of 12 low-functional and nonfunctional alleles of SNVs of the *CYP2D6* gene is shown. The carriage of these risk alleles determines the PM phenotype in patients with schizophrenia and requires a personalized approach to the selection of APs (including CPZ) and their dosage in the monotherapy or polytherapy regimen.

The *CYP1A2* gene encodes an enzyme that accounts for approximately 15% of all CYP450 isoenzymes. This enzyme also participates in the metabolism of CPZ. The carriage of high-functioning SNVs of the *CYP1A2* gene in patients with the UM phenotype may be associated with a reduced response to CPZ [11], and SNVs in the same gene associated with reduced enzyme activity were associated with the development of AP-induced EPS. However, the risk of developing CPZ-induced EPS is higher in carriers of low-functional and nonfunctional alleles of SNVs of *CYP2D6* gene [11, 24]. Bakker et al. (2012) analyzed two SNVs (rs2069514 [G/A] and rs762551 [A/C]) of the *CYP1A2* gene and found no statistically significant associations with the risk of EPS in patients with schizophrenia [44].

So, CPZ-induced EPS is a genetically determined neurological ADR to AP therapy for schizophrenia [22]. To date, the most studied candidate genes predisposing the development of CPZ-induced EPS are *DRD2*, *DRD3*, *EPM2A*, and *CYP2D6*. However, the genetics and mechanism of development of this ADR continue to be actively studied [22]. This is important for the development of personalized psychophysiological therapy strategies for schizophrenia and preventive PGx panels [11, 23].

In patients of the first group (A) (low risk of developing CPZ-induced EPS), CPZ should be initiated at moderate therapeutic dosages. In patients of the second group (B) (medium risk of developing CPZ-induced EPS), CPZ can be prescribed in low doses, and in patients of the third group (C) (high risk of developing CPZ-induced EPS), CPZ is contraindicated (Figure 48.1) [23].

Taking into account the pharmacogenetic features of CPZ metabolism associated with the carrier of low-functional and non-functional SNVs of the *CYP2D6* gene, we developed an algorithm for stratification of ADRs risk groups (Table 48.1).

STANDARD STRATEGIES FOR CORRECTING AP-INDUCED EPS [22]

1. Reduction of the dose of the taken AP (for example, CPZ);
2. AP therapy correction:

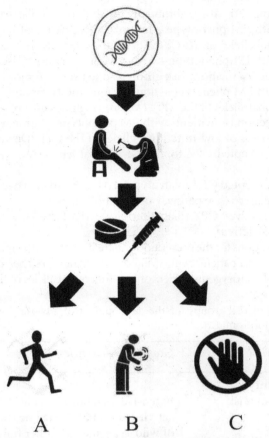

Figure 48.1 Options for the development of ADRs in patients with schizophrenia during chlorpromazine therapy [23].

- changing the accepted AP (for example, CPZ) to another (alternative) one;
- changing the accepted typical AP to an atypical AP;
- changing the received AP to an alternative AP of the same generation but with a lower degree of activity;
- changing of a received AP of the same generation to an AP with an alternative path of metabolism.

3. prescribing medications for the treatment of ADRs (correctors).

PERSONALIZED STRATEGIES FOR PREVENTION AND CORRECTING AP-INDUCED EPS AFTER PGX [22]

1. Refusal to prescribe CPZ to patients with the PM phenotype – heterozygous and homozygous carriers of non-functional alleles of the *CYP2D6* gene (high risk group and very high risk group respectively) (Table 48.1).
2. Reduction of CPZ start dose:
   - to patients with IM phenotype – heterozygous carriers of low-functional alleles of the *CYP2D6* gene (medium risk group) – at 25% of the average daily dose;
   - to patients with PM phenotype – homozygous and compound-heterozygous carriers of low-functional alleles of the *CYP2D6* gene (high risk group) – at 50% of the average daily dose (Table 48.1).

3. Conducting therapeutic drug monitoring of AP in blood plasma:
   - to patients with EM phenotype – homozygous carriers of wild-type allele or other fully functional alleles of the *CYP2D6* gene – one time in 12 months;
   - to patients with IM phenotype – heterozygous carriers of low-functional alleles of the *CYP2D6* gene (medium risk group) – one time in 6 months;
   - to patients with PM phenotype – homozygous and compound-heterozygous carriers of low-functional alleles of the *CYP2D6* gene (high risk group) – one time in 3 months.
4. AP therapy correction (to patients with PM phenotype – homozygous and compound-heterozygous carriers of low-functional alleles of the CYP2D6 gene):
   - changing the accepted CPZ to another typical AP with an alternative pathway of metabolism;
   - changing the accepted CPZ to an atypical AP with an alternative pathway of metabolism with an alternative pathway of metabolism;
   - changing the received CPZ to an alternative AP of the same generation, but with a lower degree of activity.
5. Prescribing medications for the prevention and treatment of CPZ-induced ADRs (for example, EPS correctors) to patients with IM and PM phenotypes (heterozygous and homozygous/compound-heterozygous carriers of low-functional alleles of the *CYP2D6* gene).

Table 48.1 Stratification of risk groups for the development of adverse drug reactions against the background of taking chlorpromazine.

Allele name	ADR risk	Group characteristics
Fully functional variants		
CYP2D6*1 (also known as wild-type)	Low risk	Extensive metabolizers (EMs): normal metabolic activity of CYP2D6 enzyme (homozygous carriers of wild-type allele or other fully functional alleles)
CYP2D6*2		
CYP2D6*39		
CYP2D6*41xN		
Low-functional (partially functioning) variants		
CYP2D6*9	Medium risk	Intermediate metabolizers (IMs): patients with reduced metabolic activity of CYP2D6 enzyme (heterozygous carriers of partially functioning alleles)
CYP2D6*10		
CYP2D6*10xN		
CYP2D6*17	High risk	Poor metabolizer (PM): patients with little to no functional metabolic activity of CYP2D6 enzyme (homozygous carriers or compound-heterozygous carriers of partially functioning alleles)
CYP2D6*29		
CYP2D6*41		
CYP2D6*52		
Non-functional variants		
CYP2D6*2XN	High risk	Poor metabolizer (PM): patients with no functional metabolic activity of CYP2D6 enzyme (heterozygous carriers of non-functional alleles)
CYP2D6*3		
CYP2D6*3A		
CYP2D6*3B	Very high risk (dangerous risk)	Poor metabolizer (PM): patients with no functional metabolic activity of CYP2D6 enzyme (homozygous carriers or compound-heterozygous carriers of non-functional alleles)
CYP2D6*4		
CYP2D6*4F		

Allele name	ADR risk	Group characteristics
CYP2D6*4G		
CYP2D6*4H		
CYP2D6*4xN		
CYP2D6*5		
CYP2D6*6		
CYP2D6*7		
CYP2D6*8		
CYP2D6*11		
CYP2D6*12		
CYP2D6*14		
CYP2D6*15		
CYP2D6*18		
CYP2D6*19		
CYP2D6*20		
CYP2D6*21		
CYP2D6*38		
CYP2D6*40		
CYP2D6*42		
CYP2D6*44		
CYP2D6*56		

CONCLUSIONS

To summarize, PGx is designed to personalize the use of an increasing number of drugs used in the treatment of neuropsychiatric diseases [11]. Currently, the indications for the use of PGx in real clinical practice are the following cases:

- the use of drugs with a large spectrum and significant severity ADRs, usually with a narrow therapeutic range, which are used for a long time (often for life);
- the use of drugs with a large interindividual variation in effectiveness;
- the use of drugs in patients at high risk of ADRs and/or treatment failure, including those with a hereditary history of these effects of specific drugs.

The collection of biological material for PGx in a patient does not require prior preparation. The results of the PGx represent the identified genotypes of the patient for one or more SNVs. As a rule, a clinical pharmacologist or clinician (psychiatrist, neurologist) interprets the results of PGx and formulates recommendations for the choice of the drug (s) and its (their) dosage regimen for a particular patient (person).

Based on the analysis of the results of our own research and literature data, we concluded that PGx in clinical psychiatric and neurological practice in the future will be shown in the following situations:

- patients with a high risk and very high risk of ADRs;
- before prescribing drugs with a narrow therapeutic range;
- before prescribing drugs with a large range of ADRs;
- before prescribing a drug that causes prognostically unfavorable or dangerous ADRs (for example, malignant neuroleptic syndrome, long QT interval and risk of sudden cardiac death, etc.);
- the patient plans to use the drugs for a long time.

Disclosure of pharmacogenetic predictors of psychopharmacotherapy-induced ADRs in the treatment of patients with schizophrenia and other psychiatric/neurological disorders [45–53] may provide a key to developing a strategy for their personalized prevention and therapy in real clinical practice. Taking into account the carriage of SNVs/polymorphisms of the candidate genes associated with a high risk of developing ADRs, therapeutic strategies can be individually changed in each specific clinical case. However, it should be recognized that the question of the genetics of APs-induced ADRs is far from being resolved.

The panel for PGx can be considered suitable for real clinical practice under the following conditions:

1. the presence of a pronounced association between the detected risk allele (alleles) of SNVs of the candidate gene and an unfavorable pharmacological response (development ADRs or insufficient effectiveness of the drug);
2. the detected (usually minor) allele (alleles) of SNVs of the candidate gene must occur in the population with a frequency of at least 1%;
3. the pharmacogenetic panel should have a high sensitivity, specificity, and predictive value of positive and negative results;
4. the algorithm for the use of drugs depending on the results of pharmacogenetic tests needs to be based on the selection of drugs, their dosage regimen, personalized management of a patient, and so on;
5. the advantages of using drugs using the results of a pharmacogenetic panel in comparison with the traditional approach should be proved, including improving the effectiveness and safety of psychopharmacotherapy, as well as clinical and economic profitability.

Currently, there is no doubt that the introduction of PGx in clinical practice is a real path to personalized psychiatry and neurology and, as a result, to improve the effectiveness and safety of pharmacotherapy of psychiatric and neurological diseases. A number of pharmacogenetic panels have already been developed and are being actively implemented in real clinical practice. In addition, the development of genetic microchips is actively underway (microarray-technology), allowing us to identify simultaneously a whole series of risk alleles responsible for changing the pharmacological response.

However, the pace of implementation of pharmacogenetics in real clinical practice cannot be considered satisfactory. A number of problems still need to be solved in order for clinical psychopharmacogenetics to become an applied science and for PGx to become mandatory studies in everyday clinical psychiatric and neurological practice.

Finally, deficits in prescriber knowledge surrounding translating genetic information into clinical action points [54] may also contribute to the poor uptake of testing. Ongoing efforts to collate evidence and information for clinical utilization have been fruitful, and the Pharmacogenomics Knowledgebase provides a repository of pharmacogenomic-based drug dosing clinical guidelines from multiple sources, including the Clinical Pharmacogenetics Implementation Consortium (CPIC) and Dutch Pharmacogenetics Working Group (DPWG) [55].

References

1. Ermak G. Emerging medical technologies. *World Scientific*. 2015;9(1):120–125. ISBN 978-981-4675-80-2.
2. Johnson J.A. Pharmacogenetics: Potential for individualized drug therapy through genetics. *Trends Genet*. 2003;19(11):660–666. doi: 10.1016/j.tig.2003.09.008.
3. Center for Pharmacogenomics and Individualized Therapy. https://pharmacy.unc.edu/event/cpit-seminar/ Retrieved 2014–06–25.
4. Rollinson V., Turner R.M., Pirmohamed M. Pharmacogenomics: An overview. *Pharmacogenetics and Pharmacogenomics*. 2017.
5. Sheffield L.J., Phillimore H.E. Clinical use of pharmacogenomic tests in 2009. *Clin Biochem Rev*. 2009;30(2):55–65. PMC 2702214.
6. Shin J., Kayser S.R., Langaee T.Y. Pharmacogenetics: From discovery to patient care. *Am J Health Syst Pharm*. 2009;66(7):625–637. doi: 10.2146/ajhp080170.
7. Center for Genetics Education. www.genetics.edu.au/.
8. Neznanov N.G. A paradigm shift to treat psychoneurological disorders. *Personalized Psychiatry and Neurology*. 2021;1(1):1–2.
9. Becquemont L. Pharmacogenomics of adverse drug reactions: Practical applications and perspectives. *Pharmacogenomics*. 2009;10(6):961–969. doi: 10.2217/pgs.09.37.
10. Hauser A.S., Chavali S., Masuho I., et al. Pharmacogenomics of GPCR drug targets. *Cell*. 2018;172(1–2):41–54.e19. doi: 10.1016/j.cell.2017.11.033.
11. Clinical psychopharmacogenetics. By Ed.: R.F. Nasyrova, N.G. Neznanov. SPb: DEAN Publishing House, 2019. 405 p. (In Russ).
12. Guidance for Industry Pharmacogenomic Data Submissions. *U.S. Food and Drug Administration*. March 2005. Retrieved 2008–08–27.
13. Squassina A., Manchia M., Manolopoulos V.G., et al. Realities and expectations of pharmacogenomics and personalized medicine: Impact of translating genetic knowledge into clinical practice. *Pharmacogenomics* 2010;11(8):1149–1167. doi: 10.2217/pgs.10.97.
14. Zaza G., Granata S., Tomei P., Gassa A.D., Lupo A. Personalization of the immunosuppressive treatment in renal transplant recipients: The great challenge in "omics" medicine *Int J Mol Sci*. 2015;16(2);4281–4305.
15. Huser V., Cimino J.J. Providing pharmacogenomics clinical decision support using whole genome sequencing data as input: AMIA joint summits on translational science proceedings. *AMIA Joint Summits on Translational Science*. 2013;81. PMID 24303303.
16. Kalow W. Pharmacogenetics and pharmacogenomics: Origin, status, and the hope for personalized medicine. *Pharmacogenomics J*. 2006;6(3):162–165. doi: 10.1038/sj.tpj.6500361.
17. Pouget J.G., Shams T.A., Tiwari A.K., Müller D.J. Pharmacogenetics and outcome with antipsychotic drugs. *Dialogues in Clinical Neuroscience*. 2014;16(4):555–566.
18. Dobrodeeva V.S., Scopin S.D., Nasyrova R.F., Shnayder N.A. Problems and prospects of implementation of pharmacogenetic testing in real clinical practice in the Russian Federation. *Bulletin of Neurology, Psychiatry and Neurosurgery*. 2020;3:6–8. (In Russ). doi: 10.33920/med-01-2003-01.
19. Greden J.F., Parikh S.V., Rothschild A.J., et al. Impact of pharmacogenomics on clinical outcomes in major depressive disorder in the GUIDED trial: A large, patient- and rater-blinded, randomized, controlled study. *Journal of Psychiatric Research*. 2019;111:59–67. doi: 10.1016/j.jpsychires.2019.01.003.
20. Shorter E.A. History of psychiatry. In: *From the era of Asylum to the age of Prozac*. New York: John Wiley & Sons, Inc. 1997.
21. Lopez-Munoz F., Alamo C., Cuenca E., et al. History of the discovery and clinical introduction of chlorpromazine. *Annals of Clinical Psychiatry*. 2005;17(3):113–135. doi: 10.1080/10401230591002002.
22. Shnayder N.A., Vaiman E.E., Neznanov N.G., Nasyrova R.F. *Pharmacogenetics of antipsychotic: Induce extrapyramidal disorders*. SPb: DEAN Publishing House, 2021. 288 p. (In Russ).
23. Vaiman E.E., Novitsky M.A., Nasyrova R.F. Pharmacogenetics of chlorpromazine and its role in the development of antipsychotic-induced parkinsonism. *Personalized Psychiatry and Neurology*. 2021;1(1):11–17.
24. Adams C.E., Awad G.A., Rathbone J., et al. Chlorpromazine versus placebo for schizophrenia. *Cochrane Database of Systematic Reviews*. 2014. doi: 10.1002/14651858.cd000284.pub3.
25. Mi H., Thomas P.D., Ring H.Z., et al. PharmGKB summary. *Pharmacogenetics and Genomics*. 2011;21(6):350–356. doi: 10.1097/FPC.0b013e32833ee605.

26. Carlsson A., Lindqvist, M. Effect of chlorpromazine or haloperidol on formation of 3-methoxytyramine and nor-metanephrine in mouse brain. *Acta Pharmacologica et Toxicologica.* 1963;20(2):140–144. doi: 10.1111/j.1600-0773.1963.tb01730.x.
27. Mailman R., Murthy V. Third generation antipsychotic drugs: Partial agonism or receptor functional selectivity? *Current Pharmaceutical Design.* 2010;16(5):488–501. doi: 10.2174/138161210790361461.
28. Mashkovsky M.D. *Medicines.* 16th edition. Moscow: Novaya Volna, 2005. S. 52, 763. 1200 p. (In Russ).
29. Yeung P.K.F., Hubbard J.W., Korchinski E.D., Midha K.K. Pharmacokinetics of chlorpromazine and key metabolites. *European Journal of Clinical Pharmacology.* 1993;45(6):563–569. doi: 10.1007/bf00315316.
30. Hill M.J., Reynolds G.P. 5-HT2C receptor gene polymorphisms associated with antipsychotic drug action alter promoter activity. *Brain Research.* 2007;1149;14–17. doi: 10.1016/j.brainres.2007.02.038.
31. Ray W.A., Meredith S., Thapa P.B., et al. Antipsychotics and the risk of sudden cardiac death. *Archives General Psychiatry.* 2001;58(12):1161–1167. doi: 10.1001/archpsyc.58.12.116.
32. Wu S., Xing Q., Gao R., et al. Response to chlorpromazine treatment may be associated with polymorphisms of the *DRD2* gene in Chinese schizophrenic patients. *Neuroscience Letters.* 2005;376(1):1–4. doi: 10.1016/j.neulet.2004.11.014.
33. Jönsson E.G., Nöthen M.M., Grünhage F., et al. Polymorphisms in the dopamine D2 receptor gene and their relationships to striatal dopamine receptor density of healthy volunteers. *Molecular Psychiatry.* 1999;4(3):290–296. doi: 10.1038/sj.mp.4000532.
34. Mihara K., Kondo T., Suzuki A., et al. No relationship between−141C Ins/Del polymorphism in the promoter region of dopamine D2 receptor and extrapyramidal adverse effects of selective dopamine D2 antagonists in schizophrenic patients: A preliminary study. *Psychiatry Research.* 2001;101(1):33–38. doi: 10.1016/s0165-1781(00)00247-x.
35. Reynolds G.P., Yao Z., Zhang X., Sun J., Zhang Z. Pharmacogenetics of treatment in first-episode schizophrenia: D3 and 5-HT2C receptor polymorphisms separately associate with positive and negative symptom response. *European Neuropsy-Chopharmacology.* 2005;15(2):143–151. doi:10.1016/j.euroneuro.2004.07.001
36. Porcelli S., Balzarro B., Lee S.-J., et al. PDE7B, NMBR and EPM2A variants and schizophrenia: A case-control and pharmacogenetics study. *Neuropsychobiology.* 2016;73(3):160–168. doi: 10.1159/000445295.
37. Andrade D.M., Turnbull J., Minassian B.A. Lafora disease, seizures and sugars. *Acta Myol.* 2007;26:83–86. PMID: 17915579.
38. Badyal D.K., Dadhich A.P. Cytochrome P450 and drug interactions. *Indian Journal of Pharmacology.* 2001;33:248–259.
39. Ingelman-Sundberg M. Pharmacogenetics of cytochrome P450 and its applications in drug therapy: The past, present and future. *Trends Pharmacol Sci.* 2004;25(4):193–200. doi: 10.1016/j.tips.2004.02.007.
40. Zhou Y., Ingelman-Sundberg M., Lauschke V.M. Worldwide distribution of cytochrome P450 alleles: A meta-analysis of population-scale sequencing projects. *Clinical Pharmacology & Therapeutics.* 2017;102(4):688–700. doi: 10.1002/cpt.690.
41. Ravyn D., Ravyn V., Lowney R., Nasrallah H.A. CYP450 pharmacogenetic treatment strategies for antipsychotics: A review of the evidence. *Schizophr Res.* 2013;149(1–3):1–14. doi: 10.1016/j.schres.2013.06.035
42. Brockmöller J., Kirchheiner J., Schmider J., et al. The impact of the CYP2D6 polymorphism on haloperidol pharmacokinetics and on the outcome of haloperidol treatment. *Clin Pharmacol Ther.* 2002;72(4):438–452. doi: 10.1067/mcp.2002.127494.
43. De Leon J., Susce M.T., Pan R.M., et al. The CYP2D6 poor metabolizer phenotype may be associated with risperidone adverse drug reactions and discontinuation. *J Clin Psychiatry.* 2005 Jan;66(1):15–27. doi: 10.4088/jcp.v66n0103.
44. Bakker P.R., Bakker E., Amin N., van Duijn C.M., et al. Candidate gene-based association study of antipsychotic-induced movement disorders in long-stay psychiatric patients: A prospective study. *PLoS One.* 2012;7(5):e36561. doi: 10.1371/journal.pone.0036561.
45. Dobrodeeva V.S., Shnayder N.A., Mironov K.O., Nasyrova R.F. Pharmacogenetic markers of antipsychotic induce weight gain: System of leptin and neuropeptide Y. V.M. Bekhterev. *Review of Psychiatry and Medical Psychology.* 2021;1:3–10. (In Russ). doi: 10.31363/2313-7053-2021-1-3-10.

46. Bobrova O.P., Shnayder N.A., Petrova M.M. et al. Predicting of fentanyl-associated neurotoxicity in pancreatic cancer with clinical, genetic model. *Experimental and Clinical Gastroenterology.* 2021;(3):136–145. (In Russ). doi: 10.31146/1682-8658-ecg-187-3-136-145.
47. Shnayder N.A., Petrova M.M., Popova T.E., et al. Prospects for the personalized multimodal therapy approach to pain management via action on NO and NOS. *Molecules.* 2021:26:2431. doi: 10.3390/molecules26092431.
48. Shnayder N.A., Petrova M.M., Shesternya P.A., et al. Using pharmacogenetics of direct oral anticoagulants to predict changes in their pharmacokinetics and the risk of adverse drug reactions. *Biomedicines.* 2021;9(5):451. doi: 10.3390/biomedicines9050451.
49. Shnayder N.A., Petrova M.M., Moskaleva P.V., et al. The role of single-nucleotide variants of NOS1, NOS2, and NOS3 genes in the comorbidity of arterial hypertension and tension-type headache. *Molecules.* 2021;26(6):1556. doi: 10.3390/molecules26061556.
50. Bobrova O.P., Zyryanov S.K., Shnayder N.A., Petrova M.M. Predicting opioid therapy safety in pancreatic cancer patients. *Russian Open Medical Journal.* 2020;9(4):e0417. doi: 10.15275/rusomj.2020.0417.
51. Bobrova O.P., Zyryanov S.K., Shnayder N.A., Petrova M.M. Personalized calculator for prediction of opioid: Associated pharmacoresistance in patients with pancreas cancer. *Archiv EuroMedica.* 2020;10(4):20–22. doi: 10.35630/2199-885X/2020/10/4.3.
52. Drokov A.P., Lipatova L.V., Shnayder N.A., Nasyrova R.F. Pharmacogenetics markers for methabolic impairments in treatment with valproic acid. *Neuroscience and Behavioral Physiology.* 2020;50(1):13–19. doi: 10.1007/s11055-019-00861-6.
53. Nasyrova R.F., Moskaleva P.V., Vaiman E.E., et al. Genetics factors of nitric oxid's system in psychoneurological disorders. *International Journal of Molecular Sciences.* 2020;21(5):1604. doi: 10.3390/ijms21051604.
54. Haga S.B., Burke W., Ginsburg G.S. et al. Primary care physicians' knowledge of and experience with pharmacogenetic testing. *Clin Genet.* 2012;82(4):388–394. doi: 10.1111/j.1399-0004.2012.01908.x.
55. Swen J.J., Nijenhuis M., de Boer A., et al. Pharmacogenetics: From bench to byte-an update of guidelines. *Clin Pharmacol Ther.* 2011;89(5):662–673. doi: 10.1038/clpt.2011.34.

49

Exploring fNIRS Potential as an Investigational Tool in Psychiatry

Jitender Jakhar, Debanjan Banerjee, Nand Kumar

Introduction	538
Principles of fNIRS	538
Basic of Near-Infrared Spectroscopy	539
Essential Components of fNIRS System	*539*
NIRS Instrumentation and Brain Oximetry	539
fNIRS Optode Placement	*541*
Validation Study With MRI	541
Comparison of fNIRS With Other Neuroimaging Modalities	541
Application of fNIRS in Psychiatric Disorders	542
Future Directions	543

INTRODUCTION

Functional near-infrared spectroscopy (fNIRS) is a non-invasive, safe, cost-effective, and emerging neuroimaging technology that covers a wide range of participant populations, from infants to the elderly, and translates clinical utility from a laboratory setting into a more realistic everyday clinical environment. In the last 20 years, there has been an exponential increase in the use of several relatively low-cost imaging techniques, including fNIRS as an investigational tool in brain research. In this chapter, we aim to provide a comprehensive understanding of the basic principles, cross-validation work, relative merits, and limitation of fNIRS when compared with other brain imaging modalities and discuss its clinical and future implications on study related to neuropsychiatric conditions.

PRINCIPLES OF FNIRS

The utility of fNIRS as an experimental in-vivo tool for clinical monitoring of tissue hemodynamic status was first described by the pioneering work of Frans Jobsis (1), and since then, this principle has been applied across disorders to study cerebral hemodynamics in both healthy and diseased states. fNIRS is an optical neuroimaging technique that allows the measurement of brain tissue concentration changes of oxygenated (HbO_2) and deoxygenated (HbR) hemoglobin following neuronal activation. In the electromagnetic spectrum of light, near-infrared light is weakly absorbed by the tissues, and this wavelength of light (620–900 nm) is termed an optical window. There is minimal attenuation of this range of light by skull structure (i.e., scalp skin, bony skull, dura mater, and CSF) and substances (i.e., cytochrome oxidase, water, lipid, and melanin). This light travels a few centimeters into the tissue (optical length) and is then reflected back. In tissue, the most dominant chromophore within this optical window is hemoglobin, located in small vessels (<1 mm in diameter). fNIRS cannot detect the changes in hemodynamic status reliably in blood vessels >1 mm because larger blood vessels can completely absorb the light. In particular, HbO_2 and HbR absorb the NIR light differently: HbO_2 absorption is higher for >800 nm; on the contrary, the HbR absorption coefficient is higher for <800 nm (2).

The overarching principle governing the operation of fNIRS systems is that when a brain area is active and involved in the execution of a certain task, the brain's metabolic demand for oxygen and glucose increases, leading to an oversupply in regional cerebral blood flow (rCBF) to meet the increased metabolic demand of the brain, referred to as neurovascular coupling (3). During this coupling, the concentration of HbO_2, HbR, and total Hb alter in the cortical region of the brain, allowing these changes to be detected with impressive temporal resolution. The temporal increase in regional blood flow normally exceeds the local tissue oxygen requirement, resulting in a decrease in HbR in venous blood. Thus, increases in t-Hb and HbO_2 with a decrease in HbR are expected to be observed in activated areas, leading to changes in the intensity of reflected light, which can be estimated by fNIRS. Some studies report that HbR is a better measure of cortical activation changes and preferred to be measured in study. However, contradictory findings have been reported in other studies, suggesting HbO_2 may be a better indicator than HbR and changes in oxy Hb levels are correlated strongly with the BOLD signal of fMRI (2).

In addition to absorption, the NIR light is also scattered when it travels through the biological tissue, and the brain volume measured corresponds to a banana-shaped path between the source and detector. Generally, during a stimulus event, the hemodynamic response reaches a peak at 5 s after the stimulus onset and goes back to its baseline with a certain delay (16 s) from the stimulus onset).

BASIC OF NEAR-INFRARED SPECTROSCOPY

Essential Components of fNIRS System

1. Light source: laser diode or light-emitting diode of near-infrared range
2. Detector: types of available detectors are avalanche photodiode, silicon photodiodes, photomultiplier tubes, and charge-coupled diodes
3. Flexible optic fiber: to carry the NIR light to source and from detector tissue

The detector is generally placed 2–7 cm away from the source. Typical values that ensure sensitivity for hemodynamic changes within the top 2–3 mm of the cortex are 3–4 cm for adult studies and 2–3 cm for infants extending laterally 1 cm, perpendicular to the axis of source-detector spacing. The portion of tissue interrogated by the NIR light is called a channel and is located at the midpoint between the source and the detector

NIRS Instrumentation and Brain Oximetry

Briefly, three different NIRS techniques are used, each based on a specific type of illumination:

1. Continuous measurement (CW) – is based on tissue illumination at constant amplitude and simply measures the light attenuation and amplitude decay through the head. These devices measure changes in intensity at different wavelengths. CW devices can

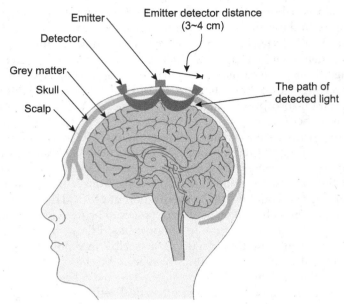

Figure 49.1 What happens in near-infrared spectroscopy.
Source: Image courtesy (4)

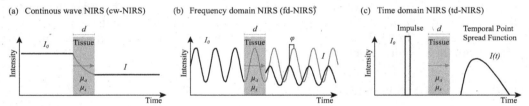

Figure 49.2 Waves and frequency of NIRS.
Source: Image courtesy (5)

provide information on relative concentration changes of HbO_2 and HbR but cannot resolve absolute baseline concentrations, that's why measurements of HbO_2 and HbR start from zero (4).
2. Time-domain (TD) – Illuminate the head in pulses of extremely short duration (picoseconds) and detect the temporal distribution of photon is measured as they leave the tissue, permitting quantification of the baseline hemoglobin concentrations. It provides better spatial resolution and depth discrimination than can be achieved with continuous-wave devices.
3. Frequency domain (FD) – illuminates the head with intensity-modulated light, measuring both attenuation and phase delay. Frequency domain light is continuously shined onto the tissue and its amplitude modulated at frequencies on the order of tens to a hundred megahertz. Amplitude decay and phase shift of the detected light with respect to incident light are measured.

Each of these techniques has unique advantages and disadvantages, but in psychiatric disorders for monitoring the brain function, frequency domain or continuous wave systems are commonly used. In ascending order, CW, FD, and TD-based instruments increase in cost and technological complexity. The quantitation of NIRS parameters depends on the NIRS technology adopted. The most commonly used CW-based instrument measures oxygenation changes in Hb between emitted and detected light calculated using modified Lambert–Beer's law (6).

fNIRS Optode Placement

fNIRS optode placement on the scalp surface is based on the assumption that it will measure the cortical changes during the experiment on the required brain area that is relevant in the study design. The probe set is positioned over different areas of the head, for example, the prefrontal cortex, frontal lobe, parietal lobe, temporal lobe, or pre-supplementary motor areas. The positioning of fNIRS probes over the scalp is similar to the attachment of electroencephalogram (EEG) electrodes on the scalp according to the EEG 10/20 system. However, in actual clinical scenarios, this translation of optode placement into design remains the limiting factor in the research. The MNI (Montreal Neurological Institute) coordinates of the optodes and the measurement points (channels) can be calculated using a probe placement method (7) based on a physical model of the head surface and a 3D digitizing system of ICBM152 (8) (the standard brain template in neuroimaging studies). Recently, the fNIRS optode location decider (fOLD) approach (8) is based on the concept of differential sensitivity from photon transport simulation and compiling the result into a tool box to help in optimal and more precise optode placement. The multi-channel fNIRS tool uses multiple sources and detector probes and can measure brain activity between the probes. Currently, up to 52 channels, 68 channels, and 72 channels were released on the market. More recently, wearable and/or fiberless fNIRS instruments were developed. These devices are based on CW technology, are battery-powered, and usually use LEDs directly coupled to the head. The absence of fiberoptics bundles makes them more lightweight and more robust to movement artifacts. Participants can thus move more naturally with fewer constraints.

VALIDATION STUDY WITH MRI

fNIRS or optical topography or NIR imaging mainly detects changes in optical properties of the human cortex simultaneously from multiple measurement sites, and the results can be displayed either in the form of a map or image over a specific area. The image intensity varies with Hb concentration and is equivalent to the era of BOLD-based functional MRI sequences. Several studies have been conducted to validate and compare the metabolic correlates of neural activity as measured by fNIRS (i.e., increase in HbO_2 and decrease in HbR) with the gold standard measured by fMRI (i.e., the blood oxygenation level-dependent response (9). Positive correlations between the BOLD signal and HbO_2 were found as well as anticorrelation with HbR, showing that fNIRS results are highly consistent with fMRI findings.

COMPARISON OF FNIRS WITH OTHER NEUROIMAGING MODALITIES

As the optical components do not interfere with electromagnetic fields, fNIRS is ideal for multimodal imaging (e.g., fNIRS–fMRI, fNIRS–EEG) to gather more complete information related to neurovascular coupling. There are many merits of fNIRS over other neuroimaging modalities, summarized in Figure 49.3.

fNIRS has some limitations as well. It only measures the change in the relative concentrations of hemoglobin levels but not the absolute values. fNIRS does not give any information

	fNIRS	fMRI	EEG/MEG	PET
Signal	HbO$_2$ HbR	BOLD (HbR)	Electromagnetic	Cerebral blood flow
				Glucose metabolism
Spatial resolution	2-3 cm	0.3 mm voxels	5-9 cm	4 mm
Penetration depth	Brain cortex	Whole head	Brain cortex for EEG/deep structures for MEG	Whole head
Temporal sampling rates	Up to 10 Hz	1- 3 Hz	>1000 Hz	<0.1 Hz
Range of possible tasks	Enormous	Limited	Limited	Limited
Robustness to motion	Very good	Limited	Limited	Limited
Range of possible Participants	Everyone	Limited, can be challenging for children/patients	Everyone	Limited
Sounds	Silent	Very noisy	Silent	Silent
Portability	Yes, for portable systems	None	Yes, for portable EEG systems	None
Cost	Low	High	Low for EEG; high for MEG	High

Figure 49.3 Merits of fNIRS.

Source: Image courtesy: (10)

on the anatomical location of the fNIRS signal. The fNIRS signals are corrupted by signals arising from respiration, cardiac pulsation, blood pressure waves, and motion artifacts. fNIRS can monitor and measure the brain activity of only the superficial cortex, and the depth is limited to 2–3 mm with a very poor spatial resolution (order of 1 cm^2) in comparison to fMRI.

APPLICATION OF FNIRS IN PSYCHIATRIC DISORDERS

Understanding the neural correlates of psychiatric conditions is fundamental in the application of fNIRS, considering that symptoms and behaviors may be caused by particular activation and deactivation patterns of the cerebral cortex when engaged in cognitive tasks and these brain activities can be measured by fNIRS. In 1985–87, fNIRS was used for the first time to monitor cerebral oxygenation in infants. The potential application of fNIRS has been demonstrated in various neurological disorders ranging from multiple sclerosis, traumatic brain injury, Alzheimer's, and parkinsonism to epilepsy. But we will be focused on research studies in psychiatric disorders. Andreas Fallgatter and Masato Fukudahave been the driving force of the application of fNIRS in psychiatry. The first application of fNIRS on subjects affected by psychiatric disorders by using a single-channel system (Okada) was done in 1994 (11) and aimed at finding and qualifying disturbances in inter-hemispheric integration in brain oxygenation changes during a mirror drawing task. These results demonstrated for the first time the usefulness of fNIRS in psychiatry. The majority of the fNIRS studies on schizophrenia have focused on assessing the dysfunctional cortical area possibly responsible for executive dysfunction deficits. PFC hypoactivation during the cognitive task is the most consistent finding, with the exception of a few others, and the possibility of these fNIRS findings has been proposed as a potential biomarker for schizophrenia (12). The verbal fluency task (VFT) is the most commonly investigated task, and other cognitive tasks tried are the

Table 49.1 Major studies of fNIRS.

Author	Disorder	Key findings
Ehlis 2007	Schizophrenia	Verbal fluency tasks generally lead to obvious frontal activation in healthy controls and significantly reduced frontal activation in patients with schizophrenia.
Ehlis 2008	ADHD	During the n-back test, ADHD patients showed reduced task-related increase in the concentration of HbO_2 in ventro-lateral prefrontal cortex.
Nishimura 2009	Panic disorder	HbO_2 changes in left inferior PFC were significantly associated with frequency of panic attacks, whereas HbR changes in the anterior area of the right PFC were significantly associated with the severity of agoraphobia.
Okada 2013	OCD	During the Stroop color-word tasks, HbO_2 changes in the PFC of patients with OCD were significantly smaller than in healthy subjects.
Liu 2014	Major depressive disorder	During the verbal fluency task, hypoactivation in lateral PFC was observed in patients with MDD. Correlation analysis found that HbO_2 concentration exchanges in the bilateral PFC and anteromedial PFC were associated with the severity of depression.

trail making test, tower of London, and Sternberg and Stroop test. In comparison, a study in depression patients also suggests that hypoactivation of the frontotemporal cortex is found both in schizophrenia and depressive disorder, but the initial rise of oxyHb was steeper than subjects with major depressive disorder (13). Another study in ADHD subjects ($n = 13$) when compared with healthy controls ($n = 13$) found a deficit in prefrontal working memory tasks. The results showed that prefrontal activation was significantly lower in those with ADHD relative to controls. There are even attempts in neurorehabilitation patients to screen for depressive symptoms using fNIRS, but the sample size was small to draw conclusions (14). A summary of other fNIRS studies in major disorders is given in Table 49.1.

FUTURE DIRECTIONS

The promise of fNIRS in assisting psychiatric diagnosis led the Japanese Health Ministry to approve fNIRS as an advanced medical technology in 2014. Growth in the fNIRS community is now exponential, with the number of papers published in journals doubling every 3.5 years. For instance, *NeuroImage*, a highly relevant journal for the neuroimaging community, dedicated a special issue to commemorate the first 20 years of fNIRS research in 2014. Future research should particularly focus on understanding the cognitive domain of the brain and further expanding the presently used activation paradigms and cortical regions of interest.

Moreover, the potential of the technique in practical scenarios like neurofeedback during cognitive sessions, aiding in diagnostics, or utility as a potential neural biomarker should be more intensively explored. Current attempts to develop systematic tools for artifact correction and study anatomical and physiological confounds of the fNIRS signal will further pioneer such development. It has the exciting potential to provide more ecologically valid brain-behavior examinations that can clarify many unanswered questions about various disorders.

References

1. Jobsis F. Noninvasive, infrared monitoring of cerebral and myocardial oxygen sufficiency and circulatory parameters. *Science*. 1977 Dec 23;198(4323):1264–1267.
2. Yamashita Y, Maki A, Koizumi H. Wavelength dependence of the precision of noninvasive optical measurement of oxy-, deoxy-, and total-hemoglobin concentration. *Medical Physics*. 2001;28(6):1108–1114.
3. Phillips AA, Chan FH, Zheng MMZ, Krassioukov AV, Ainslie PN. Neurovascular coupling in humans: Physiology, methodological advances and clinical implications. *Journal of Cerebral Blood Flow & Metabolism* [Internet]. 2016 Apr 24 [cited 2019 Nov 11];36(4):647–664. Available from: http://journals.sagepub.com/doi/10.1177/0271678X15617954
4. Naseer N, Hong KS. *fNIRS-based brain-computer interfaces: A review*. Vol. 9, Frontiers in human neuroscience. New York, USA: Frontiers Media S. A.; 2015.
5. Scholkmann F, Kleiser S, Metz AJ, Zimmermann R, Mata Pavia J, Wolf U, et al. *A review on continuous wave functional near-infrared spectroscopy and imaging instrumentation and methodology*. Vol. 85, NeuroImage. New York, USA: Academic Press; 2014. p. 6–27.
6. Baker WB, Parthasarathy AB, Busch DR, Mesquita RC, Greenberg JH, Yodh AG. Modified Beer-Lambert law for blood flow. *Biomedical Optics Express*. 2014 Nov 1;5(11):4053.
7. Cutini S, Scatturin P, Zorzi M. A new method based on ICBM152 head surface for probe placement in multichannel fNIRS. *NeuroImage*. 2011 Jan 15;54(2):919–927.
8. Mazziotta J, Toga A, Evans A, Fox P, Lancaster J, Zilles K, et al. *A probabilistic atlas and reference system for the human brain: International Consortium for Brain Mapping (ICBM)*. Vol. 356, Philosophical transactions of the royal society B: Biological sciences. London, UK: Royal Society; 2001. p. 1293–322.
9. Zimeo Morais GA, Balardin JB, Sato JR. FNIRS Optodes' Location Decider (fOLD): A toolbox for probe arrangement guided by brain regions-of-interest. *Scientific Reports*. 2018 Dec 1;8(1).
10. Pinti P, Tachtsidis I, Hamilton A, Hirsch J, Aichelburg C, Gilbert S, et al. The present and future use of functional near-infrared spectroscopy (fNIRS) for cognitive neuroscience. *Annals of the New York Academy of Sciences* [Internet]. 2018 Aug 7 [cited 2019 Nov 12]; Available from: http://doi.wiley.com/10.1111/nyas.13948
11. Okada F, Tokumitsu Y, Hoshi Y, Tamura M. Impaired interhemispheric integration in brain oxygenation and hemodynamics in schizophrenia. *European Archives of Psychiatry and Clinical Neuroscience* [Internet]. 1994 [cited 2019 Nov 12];244(1):17–25. Available from: www.ncbi.nlm.nih.gov/pubmed/7918697
12. Kumar V, Shivakumar V, Chhabra H, Bose A, Venkatasubramanian G, Gangadhar BN. Functional near infra-red spectroscopy (fNIRS) in schizophrenia: A review. *Asian Journal of Psychiatry* [Internet]. 2017;27(2017):18–31. Available from: http://dx.doi.org/10.1016/j.ajp.2017.02.009
13. Suto T, Fukuda M, Ito M, Uehara T, Mikuni M. Multichannel near-infrared spectroscopy in depression and schizophrenia: Cognitive brain activation study. *Biological Psychiatry*. 2004 Mar 1;55(5):501–511.
14. Zhu Y, Jayagopal JK, Mehta RK, Erraguntla M, Nuamah J, McDonald AD, et al. Classifying major depressive disorder using fNIRS during motor rehabilitation. *IEEE Transactions on Neural Systems and Rehabilitation Engineering* [Internet]. 2020 Apr 1 [cited 2021 May 27];28(4):961–969. Available from: https://pubmed.ncbi.nlm.nih.gov/32054581/

50

Optimising Patient Care in Psychiatry
Psychosocial Rehabilitation

Durva Sail, Chitrita Sengupta Chaki, Avinash De Sousa

Introduction	545
Basic Characteristics of Psychosocial Rehabilitation	546
Populations Which Can Benefit From Psychosocial Rehabilitation	547
Strategies of Psychosocial Rehabilitation	548
Major Components of Psychosocial Rehabilitation	548
Symptomatic Remission	548
Self-Efficacy and Management of Illness	549
Psychotherapeutic Interventions	549
The Role of the Psychiatrist in Rehabilitation	554

INTRODUCTION

Psychosocial rehabilitation is a process that facilitates opportunities for persons with chronic mental illness to reach their optimal level of independent functioning in society and for improving their quality of life.[1,2] Tracing historically, its foundation can be marked as an amendment of the United States Vocational Rehabilitation Act in 1943 through which financial support and vocational rehabilitation services were provided to people with psychiatric disabilities.[3] Interventions facilitating symptom management, social skills training and improving cognitive performance form major components of this act. The concept has evolved from medication compliance and reduced hospitalisation to helping the patient attain independence, employment, meaningful interpersonal relationships, and an improved quality of life,[4] enabling people with mental illness to achieve the highest level of functioning in all domains as well as self-efficacy. Involvement of families and significant other increases program success.[5,6] Psychosocial recovery and rehabilitation are very helpful to foster successful treatment outcomes and community integration and improve functional outcomes, independence, symptomatic remission, meaningful relationships and quality of life.

Five core objectives of psychosocial rehabilitation have been explained by Dhillon and Dollieslager[5] as follows:

- Assess the patient's personal goals in life based on his or her strengths, preferences, abilities and needs, including self-efficacy, autonomy and quality of time with friends and family and how they can be facilitated by inpatient rehabilitation and symptomatic remission.

DOI: 10.4324/9780429030260-54

- Provide health education to the patient and significant others concerning the nature of the psychiatric illness and how medications and psychotherapeutic interventions may be useful in restoring self-control.
- Educate the patient about medication and treatment of adverse effects and the importance of self-monitoring and collaborating with the nurse or other healthcare provider concerning medication and its effect.
- Embrace the patient's culture and needs and collaborate with the family or other community-based resources.
- Engage the patient in decision making regarding appropriate discharge planning to facilitate community integration and plans for residential and other treatment needs.

Basic Characteristics of Psychosocial Rehabilitation

1. **Person-Centred Approach** – psychosocial rehabilitation places great emphasis on maintaining individuality. By acknowledging every person's individuality, all treatment plans are tailored to the individual needs of the patient. There is no standardised treatment for the entire population. It is very important for psychosocial rehabilitation practitioners to understand and respect diversity. Psychosocial rehabilitation is thus a person-centred approach: where the treatment plan is in line with the patient's values, hopes and aspirations.
2. **Environmental Factors** – the patient's environmental factors hold great importance in psychosocial rehabilitation, as either the patient's environment is changed to suit the capacities of the patient or the patient's capacities are adapted to their surrounding setting. Psychosocial rehabilitation thereby focuses on working on the patient's strengths and capacities while simultaneously making environmental modifications. Psychosocial rehabilitation goes beyond direct patient care and extends to adapting social and physical environments to meet the patient's needs.
3. **Building Strengths** – psychosocial rehabilitation's primary focus is building on the patient's strengths so that they can independently live their lives to the greatest extent possible. It works towards self-determination and empowering the patient. Once a patient builds their strengths, they can use those aspects to help reintegrate themselves into society and live purposeful, fulfilling lives.
4. **Integrated Approach** – since psychosocial rehabilitation is multidimensional, it often requires a collaborative effort from multiple professionals like counsellors, psychiatrists, occupational therapists, physiotherapists, outreach workers, social workers, physicians and so on.
5. **Hope** – psychosocial rehabilitation works towards achieving certain individual goals for each patient and is hence a future-oriented approach. A large part of this approach has hope as a crucial component. Hope not only becomes a motivating force but also instils a sense of optimism. Hope helps patients work on themselves and move beyond their illnesses or disabilities and gain back some amount of self-esteem and self-belief. Psychosocial rehabilitation practitioners work with respect towards their patients, with the belief that every individual is capable of making progress.
6. **Ongoing Process** – psychosocial rehabilitation isn't something that happens overnight; it is a continuous ongoing process that happens gradually. As individuals, we are constantly changing, and hence even interventions go through various modifications over different times and different situations.

POPULATIONS WHICH CAN BENEFIT FROM PSYCHOSOCIAL REHABILITATION

1. **People with chronic and severe mental illnesses**
   Living with mental illnesses can be very challenging for people to cope with. Additionally, they have to face a lot of stigma and discrimination. Very often, people with chronic mental illnesses tend to isolate themselves from others. A vast majority of people with mental illnesses also face unemployment. They lack control over their lives, and their self-esteem takes a massive hit. A mental illness can hamper multiple aspects of a person's life, leaving them clueless and confused as to how and where to get help. These people need assistance to regain control over their lives and get reintegrated into society. In these cases, psychosocial rehabilitation is a great way to get help through its multidimensional approach. People suffering with chronic and severe forms of mental illnesses can use psychosocial rehabilitation to improve their quality of life by reaching their optimal level of independent functioning. Through psychosocial rehabilitation, the patient can build on their strengths and feel empowered. The entire rehabilitation process focuses on improving a person's social, cognitive and intellectual skills so that they can lead fulfilling lives.

2. **People with disabilities who need ongoing assistance throughout life**
   In 1996 the World Health Organisation (WHO) developed an international consensus document regarding psychosocial rehabilitation. It stated that psychosocial rehabilitation is a process that facilitates opportunities for individuals to reach their optimal level of independent functioning in the community. It implies both improving individual's competencies and introducing environmental changes in order to create a life of the best quality for people who have experienced a mental disorder, which produces a certain level of disability. Psychosocial rehabilitation aims to provide the optimal level of functioning of individuals and societies, and the minimisation of disabilities and handicaps, stressing individuals' choices about how to live successfully in the community (WHO, 1996). With technology rapidly progressing, there is a lot of external aid that can be given to people with physical disabilities. For example, someone who is blind can use text-to-audio features on a smart phone and can independently work a job. Psychosocial rehabilitation not only teaches the patient coping strategies to deal with their disability and maximise their strengths but also helps adapt the patient's environment to suit their convenience.

3. **People lacking a support system and resources**
   Although awareness about mental health is growing, there is still a long way to go, as a lot of people still attach a lot of stigma to it and consider it a taboo topic. People with mental health–related issues and disabilities often do not get the support and resources that they require. In many cases, families do not encourage visiting mental health professionals, and they look down upon it. This causes mental health problems to progressively get worse, and even if the person decides to get help, they attach a lot of shame and guilt to it. Psychosocial rehabilitation services can help guide people in the right direction through the advice of professionals. Through sound advice and guidance by psychosocial rehabilitators, a person can work on regaining their autonomy and self-confidence. Not only can they work on the mental illness or disability itself, but they can also get help vocationally and get social skills training. If they have a physical disability, there are professionals like occupational therapists or physiotherapists who can help them cope with it. If the person comes from a low economic background, there are many social workers who can help them through initiatives and organisations that are set up to aid underprivileged people via psychosocial rehabilitation.

4. **Geriatric Population**
    a. The geriatric population often need psychosocial rehabilitation, as they face multiple age-related problems. Older people face a lot of physical problems like loss of muscle, lack of energy weakness, weakening of bones and slowing down of bodily movements, and eventually in some cases they need assistance in performing simple day-to-day tasks. Besides physical issues, there are a lot of psychological challenges that come with aging as well. According to the World Health Organisation, dementia and depression are the most prevalent neurological issues in the elderly. Dementia impairs cognitive abilities like memory thinking, problem solving and so on. Old people living with Alzheimer's also eventually find it very hard to manage alone and need 24/7 assistance, as they can't even perform simple tasks like brushing their teeth or eating their food on their own. A comprehensive study was conducted between 2010 and 2017 for a systematic review of psychosocial interventions in dementia.[7] Results showed good evidence that multi-component exercise improves global physical and cognitive functions and daily activities. The study also showed evidence that group-based cognitive stimulation improves cognitive functions, social interactions and general quality of life. It also highlights how people with dementia can improve social integration through group activities.[7]
    b. With all these physical and psychological changes that take place during old age, psychosocial rehabilitation is ideal, as it is a multidimensional approach that covers all aspects of their lives. Not only are physical and cognitive impairments treated, older people are also taught coping strategies and adaptive behaviours. They also build on their strengths and try to stay as independent as possible. Through cognitive stimulating activities, they can sharpen their minds and prevent cognitive decay.

STRATEGIES OF PSYCHOSOCIAL REHABILITATION

There are two basic strategies of psychosocial rehabilitation:

1. Facilitating social skills through training to enhance functional competence of the disabled individual.
2. Modifying the patient's social emotional and physical environment to compensate for continuing disabilities and handicaps.

To reach optimal outcomes, both of these strategies need to be implemented hand in hand.

MAJOR COMPONENTS OF PSYCHOSOCIAL REHABILITATION

Symptomatic remission, self-efficacy and management of illness, psychotherapeutic interventions consisting of intensive case management, skills training, psychoeducation and family therapy and supported employment together contribute to psychosocial rehabilitation.[6,8–11]

Symptomatic Remission

At the beginning, that is, in the acute phase, it is necessary to control positive as well as negative symptoms with an aid of pharmacological interventions and stabilise the patient. Through this approach, symptoms ultimately leading to cognitive and psychosocial deficits associated with schizophrenia and other severe and persistent psychiatric disorders are targeted. As research suggests, integrating these components into psychosocial rehabilitation treatment planning helps patients practice real-life social, vocational and interpersonal skills; enhances their quality of life; and sustains recovery.[12-15]

Self-Efficacy and Management of Illness

Structured interventions that promote self-efficacy, independence, employment, quality interpersonal relationships and a good quality of life form the basis of self-management of illness. It is a crucial step for moving from inpatient to community-based settings. Hence it is expected that patient and family needs must be assessed thoroughly throughout the course of treatment, which will further serve as a guide to treatment planning, helping to facilitate competence in managing symptoms and responsibility for treatment outcomes.

Psychotherapeutic Interventions

1. **Intensive Case Management**
   Coordination, integration and allocation of holistic care within a spectrum of resources is expected in case management. This concept has evolved over the years to overcome deficiencies in community-based mental healthcare and correct fragmented care and lack of continuity of care.[16] The ACT program is a contemporary approach to intensive case management.[16-18] An interdisciplinary community team which includes a case manager, nurse and other providers is assigned patients. ACT team members have lower caseloads than their predecessors. It is composed of coordination of various services and resources that feature outreach and affording in-home services. There is a high staff-to-patient ratio that delivers services when and where needed by the patient, 24 hours a day, 7 days a week.[16-18]

2. **Skill training and rehabilitation**
   The patient's social and functional status often parallel symptom management and cognition. Studies also support that cognitive capabilities and community functioning are strongly related. A comprehensive biopsychosocial assessment and determining the patient's mental and physical health, present and past coping skills, trauma history, quality of interpersonal relationships, strengths, preferences, abilities and needs and readiness for training and rehabilitation is needed.

   A systematic attempt to change the patient's behaviour in a comprehensive array of behavioural, cognitive and functional domains is made with the help of skill development interventions. These cover a wide array of activities such as self care (grooming and personal hygiene), management of the tasks of daily living, peer and other affiliative roles, communication, vocational and employment roles, recreational and leisure skills, the ability to access and public transport and public agencies, coping with residual symptoms and ameliorating cognitive deficits through remediation. Skills training constitutes following independent but closely interwoven areas of skill development. These are: a) social skills training and b) vocational rehabilitation.

   a. Social skills training
   This refers to necessary competencies that allow for optimal social performance. Social skills training employs learning theory principles to facilitate optimal social and community functioning, including activities of daily living, employment, leisure and interpersonal relationships. The premise of social skills training is that it affords the patient opportunities to reach an optimal level of functioning and self-efficacy and reduce relapse. Bellack and Mueser[19] described the following models of social skills training: basic and social problem solving. The basic model involves corrective learning, practiced through various means, including role playing. The social problem-solving

model, such as cognitive remediation, focuses on improving information processing assumed to result in social skills deficits.

A wide variety of social skills training models are available to the contemporary practitioner. However, most of them are designed around a framework which incorporates the following basic principles enumerated by Lieberman.[20]

    i. **Problem definition** The patient's problems should be defined in terms of behavioural deficits and excesses, and appropriate social behaviour must be identified.

    ii. **Inventory of assets** The strengths and capabilities of the patient in a social context should be identified, as they serve as the template on which skill acquisition can be facilitated.

    iii. **Establishing a therapeutic alliance** It is critical for the person involved in a skills training programme to establish a rapport with the patient and appear caring, empathetic and non-judgemental. These attributes in the therapist are essential for forging a therapeutic alliance with the patient.

    iv. **Goal setting** Formulating positive, realistic and attainable goals is the next step in a social skills training programme. These goals are generally identified in consultation with the patient and significant others like family members.

    v. **Behavioural rehearsal** The critical element in the training of social skills is to simulate real-life social situations which are related to the patient's goals and through the process of role play the patient acquires the competence to deal with these situations.

    vi. **Positive reinforcement** Every step in a social skills training programme, from defining attainable goals to carrying out homework assignments, must have a component of positive reinforcement built into it.

    vii. **Shaping** The fundamental principle of shaping is to break down long-term goals into smaller, more easily attainable units and successively reinforce those behaviours required to achieve the subgoals.

    viii. **Prompting** This is a form of directive instruction in which prompts or cues are given to facilitate acquisition of a desired behaviour.

    ix. **Modelling** This is another form of directive instruction in which the therapist demonstrates the specific behavioural component which needs to be acquired.

    x. **Homework and in vivo practice** Homework assignments are necessary to generalise and maintain the specific behavioural skills that have been acquired in the training sessions.

b. **Cognitive remediation:** While the existence of cognitive deficits has been extensively documented in the literature, attempts to go beyond conceptualising and identifying these deficits and offering remediation are a fairly recent phenomenon. The restoration of cognitive functioning, commonly referred to as cognitive remediation or cognitive retraining, is an emerging discipline which receives inputs form the fields of clinical neurospsychology, rehabilitation and behavioural psychology. It is another important aspect of social problem-solving model. We will focus on four basic approaches suggested by Green.[21]

    i. **General stimulation approach:** This approach requires that the patient repeatedly perform tasks in an attempt to remedy a deficiency. Although this approach is practical and commonly used, questions regarding generalisability outside the training situation have not yet received satisfactory answers.

    ii. **Substitution transfer approach:** This approach guides the patients to use alternative strategies for achieving goals and can be used in memory rehabilitation. Use of external aids like checklists and visual imagery as mnemonic devices represent substitution transfer approaches.

iii. **Behavioural learning approaches:** Reinforcement, response cost, modelling and shaping represent some of the behavioural principles used in cognitive retraining. It has been argued that behaviourally oriented remediations are relevant to schizophrenia because of the presence of motivational deficits in this disorder.
iv. **Organisational strategies**: Poor organisation of information is regarded as a core deficit in schizophrenia; hence, interventions that require subjects to organise information more thoroughly could improve several cognitive measure including memory.

c. **Vocational rehabilitation:** It would be appropriate to look at the contemporary conceptual framework of work therapy as a prelude to discussing current approaches in vocational rehabilitation. Work therapy is no longer seen as a means of keeping psychiatrically disabled individuals occupied through structured activity but is conceptualised as a series of proactive measures that enable the psychiatrically disabled individual to function to his or her optimal capacity, either in a competitive environment or in a sheltered but stimulating setting, depending on the preference and disabilities of the target population. This redefinition of work therapy from passive "make work" approach to an "active participatory" work restoration approach has resulted not only in a more comprehensive system of evaluation, training and guidance but also in an extensive array of vocational training and placement options.

The two main paradigms currently dominating the practice of vocational rehabilitation are known as Train and Place and Place and Train.

i. **Train and Place approaches:** Train and place approaches have been the mainstay of psychiatric rehabilitation for over three decades and are based on the vocational potential through a sequence of steps based on the presence of both abilities and disabilities. Jacobs[22] has argued that vocational rehabilitation programmes should be designed as a continuum of services that can be divided into the following seven steps:

a. **Work skills assessment:** This includes an evaluation of both premorbid vocational competence and current level of functioning.

b. **Work adjustment:** The training and skills imparted at this step in the continuum of services are often referred to as prevocational because the emphasis is not on the acquisition specific or technical work skills but on ability of the patient to manage the work environment, get along with coworkers, report for work on time and adjust to the discipline of the work milieu. Most work therapy programmes in India focus primarily on this step of work adjustment, which is commonly referred to as "work habit" skills, because a significant majority of jobs in India fall under the ambit of the unstructured economy where a high degree of specialised training or competence is not required. Additionally there is a paucity of vocational training facilities which impart specialised work skills to people who have psychiatric disabilities. Therefore, equipping disabled individuals with generic work skills rather than specialised work skills is likely to be of greater benefit in economies which have a high unorganised component. It should, however, be pointed out that in urban areas, there is a growing need for vocational rehabilitation facilities to incorporate specialised vocational training programmes in their work therapy curriculum to enable the psychiatrically disabled to enter the organised economy.

c. **Training for specific jobs**: This step involves the learning of skills for specific jobs or preparing the person for a specialised trade.

d. **Sheltered employment:** In a sheltered employment setting, patients are exposed to a simulated work environment that is supportive and cognisant of their disabilities.
e. **Transitional employment:** In this step, although patients are exposed to the realities of competitive workplace, they work under the supervision of a mental health or rehabilitation professional who offers them emotional support and guidance.
f. **Job maintenance:** This represents the goal of vocational rehabilitation, and patients need specific skills and emotional support not only to obtain jobs but also maintain them. In the evaluate, train and place approach, it is not necessary for all patients to progress through all the steps that have been described. Some patients can skip few of the intermediate steps if they possess good premorbid work skills. In the case of severely disabled patients, full employment in competitive settings may not represent a feasible goal, and regular employment in a sheltered setting may represent the optimal vocational potential for these individuals.

ii. **Place and train paradigms:** Exposing patients to the realities of the market place and giving them "on the spot training" is the philosophy of this genre of programmes. Protagonists of this paradigm argue that not only does this approach allow patients to acquire the appropriate skills in real life settings, it also give employers an opportunity to identify the abilities of the patients instead of focusing on the disabilities. It uses the following strategies for implementation.

a. **Job coach:** The job coach is a rehabilitation professional responsible for carrying out on the spot training, supervision and guidance of the disabled person who is working in a competitive employment setting. The job coach is also responsible for liaising with the employers and coworkers of the disabled person to ensure that an environment is created which allows for compensation of handicaps and magnification of the individual's abilities so that the vocational potential of the patient is reached. Although several authors have reported success with this approach, it is exceedingly manpower intensive and can be used only with carefully selected groups of psychiatrically disabled.
b. **Job clubs:** This concept was pioneered in the United States by Azrin and associates[23] and places the primary responsibility of finding a job with the patient. This is in contrast to train and place approaches in which placement in a job represents the final goal of a vocational rehabilitation programme and is therefore a task to be carried out by rehabilitation professionals. In the job club setting, patients are assisted by a Job Club counsellor who teaches employment seeking skills and also encourages and motivates patients to continue with their efforts.
c. **Work cooperatives:** Rehabilitation professionals in Italy and other parts of Europe are the pioneers of the work cooperative movement, which can be regarded as an innovative experiment. There are several hundred work cooperatives in the service industry and small scale manufacturing sector in Italy alone. A work cooperative is formed when both non-disabled and psychiatrically disabled people pool in their resources to set up a joint venture in which they function as employers-cum-workers. The work cooperatives give an opportunity for psychiatrically disabled individuals to work alongside typical people, and there is a high degree of motivation for the psychiatrically disabled to work to their optimum capacity, as they are not just employees, but also part owners of the enterprise. Rehabilitation professionals in

India should actively consider work cooperatives as a vocational rehabilitation option and attempt to replicate the Italian experience. The challenge of experimenting with this new vocational rehabilitation approach is facilitated by the fact that India has considerable expertise with the setting up and management of cooperatives in the farming and dairy sector.

3. **Psychoeducation and Family Therapy:** The global burden of serious psychiatric disorders, such as schizophrenia and bipolar disorder, often extends to the family, culture and community. Efforts to strengthen family- and community-based resources are crucial to successful reintegration into the community and prevention of rehospitalisation. The ACT program has been mentioned as one aspect of this process. Another aspect of the ACT program requires family or significant other involvement. Family involvement is generally acknowledged as a key factor in patient functional outcomes, recovery, and quality of life. We are expected to assess family stressors, perception of symptoms and disorders, coping and learning styles and family strengths, and provide health education that enables family members to understand their loved one's symptoms, ways to manage them and how to facilitate health coping skills. Family stress often manifests as expressed emotion or an index of criticism, overinvolvement and hostility. The expressed emotion and impaired family functioning research demonstrates that when levels of emotion or stress are reduced, so are psychotic relapses.[24,25]

   There are many psychosocial family interventions, including those that begin on inpatient units and continue on an outpatient basis. As with most models, family intervention is an integral part of this training; this particular model for first-episode psychosis is based on Anderson and colleagues'[26] psychoeducation and management teaching model, modified to address the specific needs of younger first-episode patients. A period of engagement, initial crisis resolution, social support and a series of psychoeducation workshops strengthen the patient and family's coping skills and assist them in managing various stressors associated with having a serious and chronic mental disorder. This psychoeducation model was designed for first-episode psychosis, but major components can be modified to meet the needs of most patients experiencing a serious and chronic mental illness.

4. **Supported Employment:** One major aim of psychosocial rehabilitation is to prepare the patient for supported employment.[17,18,27,28] Necessary evaluations for supported employment are conducted by vocational rehabilitation and/or occupational specialists. Major advantages of these programs include helping the patient make person-centred choices based on their strengths, abilities, preferences and needs and shared-decision making and acquire necessary skills to maintain competitive and gainful employment. These programs also offer incentives for patients with severe and chronic psychiatric and substance use disorders to increase their autonomy as recovery or rehabilitation progresses. In addition to benefiting the patient, supported employment adds to the workforce and community. Through structured or supervised workshops and work programs, patients gain a sense of self-worth and independence and develop interpersonal relationships that involve family members and peers. Research studies indicate that a major barrier to supported employment is access despite increasing use. As the patient regains hope and moves through the recovery process and treatment plan continuum, his or her ability to feel confidence and control his or her symptoms often is guided by available resources, absence of substance use disorders, and motivation to stay in treatment.

THE ROLE OF THE PSYCHIATRIST IN REHABILITATION

Cancro[29] considers a psychiatrist well trained if he is able to prescribe psychosocial interventions, such as social skills training, as well as prescribe medication, though this does not indicate individual psychiatrists should be able to do everything single-handedly. However, it is expected that he or she should be able to direct team who will further serve the patients. As we all know, many different competencies are required in psychiatric rehabilitation, making it multidisciplinary.[30] The psychiatrist has a special role in rehabilitation, and the symptom management side effect profile needs close attention, as it can weaken a person's ability to perform his or her social roles and impair vocational rehabilitation. Also, non-compliance with medication taking is one of the most serious problems in the long-term treatment of persons with serious mental illness.[31] Many patients living in the community want to take responsibility for their medication themselves. Training in self-management of medication emphasises patients' autonomy and increases acceptance of and responsibility for treatment.[32] As a matter of course, though young psychiatrists today are very well trained in diagnostic procedures and prescription of medications directed almost exclusively to symptom control, but training is lacking in integrating pharmacological and psychosocial interventions.[33] There are higher chances of confrontation with the negative developments of difficult-to-treat patients who are frequently re-hospitalised in younger psychiatrists. This is possibly one of the reasons it was found in a study that psychiatrists in institutional settings do not hold fewer stereotypes of mentally ill people than the general population, nor do they display a greater willingness to closely interact with mentally ill people.[34] Therefore, it would be beneficial if the community training of young psychiatrists could take priority over hospital-based training. More training opportunities to experience the patients in the "real world" would allow psychiatrists in institutional settings to develop a more positive perspective and better understanding of persons with severe and persistent mental disorders.

References

1. Llewellyn-Beardsley J, Rennick-Egglestone S, Callard F, Crawford P, Farkas M, Hui A, Manley D, McGranahan R, Pollock K, Ramsay A, Sælør KT. Characteristics of mental health recovery narratives: Systematic review and narrative synthesis. *PLoS One*. 2019 Mar 28;14(3):e0214678.
2. Shihabuddeen I, Chandran M. Psychiatric rehabilitation in India: Prioritizing the role of a general hospital psychiatry unit. *Delhi Psychiatry J*. 2011;14:51–53.
3. Sarada Menon M. Psychosocial rehabilitation: Current trends. *Nimhans Journal*. 1996;14:295–306.
4. Drake RE, Goldman HH, Leff HS, Lehman AF, Dixon L, Mueser KT, Torrey WC. Implementing evidence-based practices in routine mental health service settings. *Psychiatric Services*. 2001 Feb;52(2):179–182.
5. Dhillon AS, Dollieslager LP. Rehab rounds: Overcoming barriers to individualized psychosocial rehabilitation in an acute treatment unit of a state hospital. *Psychiatric Services*. 2000 Mar;51(3):313–317.
6. Drake RE, Mercer-McFadden C, Mueser KT, et al. A review of integrated mental health and substance abuse treatment for patients with dual disorders. *Schizophr Bull*. 1998;24:589–608.
7. McDermott O, Charlesworth G, Hogervorst E, Stoner C, Moniz-Cook E, Spector A, Csipke E, Orrell M. Psychosocial interventions for people with dementia: A synthesis of systematic reviews. *Aging & Mental Health*. 2019 Apr 3;23(4):393–403.
8. Hogan F. President's new freedom commission on mental Health, achieving the promise: Transforming mental health care in America. Final report. Rockville, MD: Substance Abuse and Mental Health Services Administration; 2003.
9. United States, Public Health Service, Office of the Surgeon General, Center for Mental Health Services (US), National Institute of Mental Health (US), United States, Substance Abuse, Mental Health Services Administration. Mental health: Culture, race, and ethnicity: A supplement to mental health: A report of the Surgeon General. Department of Health and Human Services, US Public Health Service; 2001.

10. Substance Abuse and Mental Health Services Administration. Leading change: A plan for SAMHSA's roles and actions 2011–2014 executive summary and introduction. Rockville (MD): Substance Abuse and Mental Health Services Administration; 2011. HHS publication No. (SMA) 11–4629 summary.
11. Gaumond P, Whitter M. Access to Recovery (ATR) approaches to recovery-oriented systems of care: Three case studies. *Journal of Drug Addiction, Education, and Eradication.* 2013 Oct 1;9(4):287.
12. Valencia M, Fresán A, Barak Y, Juárez F, Escamilla R, Saracco R. Predicting functional remission in patients with schizophrenia: A cross-sectional study of symptomatic remission, psychosocial remission, functioning, and clinical outcome. *Neuropsychiatric Disease and Treatment.* 2015;11:2339.
13. Brewer WJ, Lambert TJ, Witt K, Dileo J, Duff C, Crlenjak C, McGorry PD, Murphy BP. Intensive case management for high-risk patients with first-episode psychosis: Service model and outcomes. *The Lancet Psychiatry.* 2015 Jan 1;2(1):29–37.
14. Robinson DG, Gallego JA, John M, Petrides G, Hassoun Y, Zhang JP, Lopez L, Braga RJ, Sevy SM, Addington J, Kellner CH. A randomized comparison of aripiprazole and risperidone for the acute treatment of first-episode schizophrenia and related disorders: 3-month outcomes. *Schizophrenia Bulletin.* 2015 Nov 1;41(6):1227–1236.
15. Nakajima S, Takeuchi H, Fervaha G, Plitman E, Chung JK, Caravaggio F, Iwata Y, Mihashi Y, Gerretsen P, Remington G, Mulsant B. Comparative efficacy between clozapine and other atypical antipsychotics on depressive symptoms in patients with schizophrenia: Analysis of the CATIE phase 2E data. *Schizophrenia Research.* 2015 Feb 1;161(2–3):429–433.
16. Mueser KT, Bond GR, Drake RE, Resnick SG. Models of community care for severe mental illness: A review of research on case management. *Schizophrenia Bulletin.* 1998 Jan 1;24(1):37–74.
17. Hengartner MP, Klauser M, Heim G, Passalacqua S, Andreae A, Rössler W, von Wyl A. Introduction of a psychosocial post-discharge intervention program aimed at reducing psychiatric rehospitalization rates and at improving mental health and functioning. *Perspectives in Psychiatric Care.* 2017 Jan;53(1):10–15.
18. Marshall M, Lockwood A. Assertive community treatment for people with severe mental disorders. *Cochrane Database of Systematic Reviews.* 1998(2).
19. Bellack AS, Mueser KT. Psychosocial treatment for schizophrenia. *Schizophrenia Bulletin.* 1993 Jan 1;19(2):317–336.
20. Liberman RP, editor. *Psychiatric rehabilitation of chronic mental patients.* New York: American Psychiatric Pub; 1988.
21. Green MF. Cognitive remediation in schizophrenia: Is it time yet? *American Journal of Psychiatry.* 1993 Feb 1;150:178-.
22. Jacobs HE. Vocational rehabilitation. In: *Psychiatric rehabilitation of chronic mental patients* (Ed.) R.P. Liberman. New York: American Psychiatric Press; 1988.
23. Azrin NH, Philip RA. The job club method for the job handicapped: A comparative outcome study. *Rehabilitation Counseling Bulletin.* 1979 Dec;23(2):144–155.
24. Atadokht A, Hajloo N, Karimi M, Narimani M. The role of family expressed emotion and perceived social support in predicting addiction relapse. *International Journal of High Risk Behaviors & Addiction.* 2015 Mar;4(1).
25. Koutra K, Triliva S, Roumeliotaki T, Basta M, Simos P, Lionis C, Vgontzas AN. Impaired family functioning in psychosis and its relevance to relapse: A two-year follow-up study. *Comprehensive Psychiatry.* 2015 Oct 1;62:1–2.
26. Anderson CM, Reiss DJ, Hogarty GE. *Schizophrenia and the family: A practitioner's guide to psychoeducation and management.* New York: Guilford Press; 1986 May 12.
27. Kinoshita Y, Furukawa TA, Kinoshita K, Honyashiki M, Omori IM, Marshall M, Bond GR, Huxley P, Amano N, Kingdon D. Supported employment for adults with severe mental illness. *Cochrane Database of Systematic Reviews.* 2013(9).
28. 31. Ng SS, Lak DC, Lee SC, et al. Concurrent validation of a neurocognitive assessment protocol for clients with mental illness in job matching as shop sales in supported employment. *East Asian Arch Psychiatry.* 2015;25:21–28.
29. Cancro R. The introduction of neuroleptics: A psychiatric revolution. *Psychiatric Services.* 2000 Mar;51(3):333–335.
30. Liberman RP, Hilty DM, Drake RE, Tsang HW. Requirements for multidisciplinary teamwork in psychiatric rehabilitation. *Psychiatric Services.* 2001 Oct;52(10):1331–1342.
31. Dencker SJ, Liberman RP. From compliance to collaboration in the treatment of schizophrenia. *International Clinical Psychopharmacology.* 1995 Jan.

32. Eckman TA, Liberman RP, Phipps CC, et al. Teaching medication management skills to schizophrenic patients. *J Clin Psychopharmacol.* 1990;10:33–38.
33. Liberman RP, Glick ID. Rehab rounds: Drug and psychosocial curricula for psychiatry residents for treatment of schizophrenia: Part I. Psychiatric services. 2004 Nov;55(11):1217–1219.
34. Nordt C, Rössler W, Lauber C. Attitudes of mental health professionals toward people with schizophrenia and major depression. *Schizophrenia Bulletin.* 2006 Oct 1;32(4):709–714.

51
Optimising Patient Care in Psychiatry – Impact of the COVID-19 Pandemic

Karishma Rupani, Sushma Sonavane, Avinash De Sousa

Introduction	557
Looking at the Current State of Affairs in the Pandemic	*557*
Why Discuss Mental Health During the COVID-19 Pandemic?	*558*
Continuing Mental Health Care in COVID 19	559
What Are the Ways of Providing and Optimising Care?	*559*

INTRODUCTION

Looking at the Current State of Affairs in the Pandemic

COVID containment strategies, we all know, were implemented in the form of physical distancing, including total lockdowns. This made it difficult for people to adapt to the 'new normal'. Treatment or prevention of other diseases as morbid as COVID-19 (including mental health disorders) has taken a back seat when compared with treatment of SARS COV-2. This happened even though these other non-COVID illnesses continue to cause high rates of morbidity and mortality in the population. COVID has had unprecedented repercussions on the mental health of the population at large. A study in China found that in the first 2 months of 2020, patients with COVID-19 suffered from anxiety, depression and other stress-related symptoms (1).

The fear of contracting COVID whilst visiting the doctors for non-COVID ailments took precedence, and patients were therefore reluctant to visit their physicians, resulting in worsening of their pre-existing disorders (including mental health disorders). The irony is that the incidence of psychiatric disorders has increased during this pandemic; however, help seeking for the same is at an all-time low. The other options we could see available were providing consultation on the phone. Other resources such as social media platforms were an option; however, middle-income countries were caught unaware because our pre-existing online telemedicine services were in their infancy, at least as far as psychiatry was concerned, thereby compounding the deleterious effects of the pandemic on mental health. Included in this challenge was dealing with patients with existing psychiatric illnesses who tested positive for SARS COV-2, needing medical and psychiatric intervention at the same time and vice versa (2).

Why Discuss Mental Health During the COVID-19 Pandemic?

Lockdowns have led to loss of livelihood for many, especially daily wage workers. Afflicted with multiple waves, it was seen that the longer the lockdown, the greater the financial strain, leading to depression, anxiety and uncertainty about the future, which culminated in panic and anxiety disorders. Persons with financial liabilities succumbed more during the lockdown period, and this led to an increase in the severity of depressive symptoms and an increased frequency of panic attacks (3).

Thus, we know now how public health emergencies affect the safety and well-being of people at large by causing insecurity, confusion, emotional isolation, stigma, economic loss and inadequate resources for medical response. These translate into a range of emotional reactions (such as distress or psychiatric conditions) and unhealthy behaviours (such as excessive substance use, increased screen time).

Research from countries afflicted by COVID-19 early on indicated that 8.4% of the general population reported severe to extremely severe anxiety, while 4.3% reported severe to extremely severe depression. Reactions due to catastrophic events have adverse effects on physical recovery as well. (4)

On the other hand, those who already had a psychiatric disorder prior to the pandemic had to face yet another challenge in getting their routine appointments and medications during the lockdown (5).

Hurdles Along the Way While Treating Psychiatric Disorders During the Pandemic

Those suffering from non-communicable diseases (especially psychiatric disorders) were afraid of visiting and seeking help from health professionals, lest they get infected with SARS COV-2. Psychiatric services have traditionally been delivered in person, so before the COVID-19 pandemic, there were not many advances in alternative modalities of providing care and treatment in psychiatry (6).

Thus it became difficult to provide mental healthcare in the way we were traditionally accustomed to. In countries which had been impacted early on in the pandemic, psychiatric care had to be scaled back and was decreased in order to free up resources for COVID-19 patients (7). A higher risk of morbidity and mortality due to COVID-19 was seen amongst patients with co-morbid psychiatric disorders due to several contributory factors, including a high rate of smoking, lung disease, cardiovascular disease and obesity. Thus, many of our patients who do contract COVID-19 are at a higher risk of a grave prognosis.

Treatment of those with comorbid psychiatric disorders and COVID-19 presents yet another challenge because, per a study done by Zhu et al. (8), the wards in psychiatric hospitals are not designed to match the standards of isolation wards designed for infectious respiratory diseases with high contagion like COVID-19, and psychiatric medical staff have little experience of dealing with infectious diseases. On the other hand, activities to 'stabilise' psychiatric patients in medical wards may not be compatible with the standard protocols for preventing diseases such as COVID-19. Nosocomial spread in outpatient psychiatric clinics is another challenge we face in everyday practice.

Difficulties in Using Psychopharmacological and Other Treatments

One of the major challenges in this pandemic has been the availability of psychiatric medications. Procuring medications has been difficult in the lockdown due to short supply. This has resulted in relapses of psychiatric illnesses and de-stabilising patients well maintained on treatment (9).

Mental Health of Frontline Healthcare Personnel

The healthcare personnel working in hospitals and isolation wards are not an exception to the deleterious effect the pandemic has had on their mental health and also deserve optimum mental health services. The stress of the work they do takes a toll on their mental health, and it will be difficult for them to bear the brunt of the rising number of cases (10).

Another hurdle is the gap between rural and urban mental health services in low- and middle-income countries, which prevails because of poor knowledge and stigmatising beliefs among the general population (11).

To conclude, we foresee an increasing mismatch between existing psychiatric care and the overall impact of COVID-19 on mental health. In spite of the high prevalence of mental health disorders, if the necessary contingency strategies are unplanned for and not in place, traditional support systems will fall short.

Thus, the challenge is now to be able to provide optimal psychiatric services whilst preventing the spread of infection. Let us look at the various options that can be utilised for optimising psychiatric services as a means of not only treating but also preventing psychiatric disorders.

CONTINUING MENTAL HEALTH CARE IN COVID 19

What Are the Ways of Providing and Optimising Care?

Adapting Existing Treatment Models to the 'New Norm'

While, due to the lack of better options for providing mental health services in the lockdown, telephonic services, which were earlier used mainly for emergency services, are now being made use of even for routine care, and although considering our profession wherein nothing matches 'in person' assessment for building a rapport and for various therapies, lockdowns have forced us to adapt existing communication services, and we have had to shift our focus onto telemedicine.

What Is Telemedicine?

Telemedicine encompasses the 'use of information and communications technology to provide health care services to individuals who are some distance from the health care provider' (6).

Under the umbrella of telemedicine comes telepsychiatry, which is a method where online psychiatric consultations, e-prescriptions and therapies can be practised. Thus, telemedicine is now helping us to adapt to the 'new norm'.

What Do We Mean by Technology-Based Interventions?

A SUBSET OF TELEMEDICINE

Safire et al. (12) did a scoping review of telemedicine interventions to optimise mental health outcomes to find that three technology-based interventions could be explored for providing mental health prevention, promotion, assessment and treatment on a large scale whilst following the rules of social distancing. These were:

- Smartphone-based applications
- TV-based platforms
- Video call interventions

SMARTPHONE-BASED INTERVENTIONS

A study of smart phone-based applications has found that they facilitated telemedicine and prescription management. Amongst the apps are health and fitness apps prepared by health experts that provide strategies to prevent mental disorders by providing a plethora of customised apps depending on the specific needs of individuals. Apps to support visually and hearing impaired individuals (13) have been introduced to increase inclusivity.

On the other hand, internet-based integrated interventions designed for COVID-19 patients with technical know-how, focusing on relaxation, self-care and developing a sense of security, have been developed. These adapted interventions were found to be significantly associated with decreased levels of anxiety and depressive symptoms (13). Another review studied smartphone applications to connect individuals with mental healthcare service providers (14). Some of the applications provided adaptations to existing service provision (such as telemedicine) and also provided new, innovative ways of connecting older adults with service providers 24/7 through different platforms.

Another intervention is using television platforms, which can be designed and used to assist older adults to obtain authentic information related to COVID-19 to explain and demonstrate COVID-appropriate behaviours in simple terms and visuals. These can also be used for performing memory exercises specific to the elderly. (15). One of the ways that clinicians may be able to cater to patients' mental health during this pandemic is by providing health education and supporting health literacy. This can be done by providing accurate and relevant information to patients as well as directing them to reliable sources to remain updated on news relating to COVID-19. Research shows that information overload contributes to the worsening of mental health (16, 17), and therefore these measures would go a long way in preventing new onset of psychiatric disorders.

Video calls providing home support during COVID-19 for community-dwelling, older adults with mild cognitive impairment or mild dementia have been implemented at various levels. A study done during earlier pandemics showed that video calls for older adults in nursing homes were helpful in preventing loneliness and depression and improved overall quality of life (18).

Applications of Technology-Based Interventions

USING TECHNOLOGY-BASED INTERVENTIONS TO TRAIN HEALTH PERSONNEL

A review of expert opinions suggested that new interventions could be considered for training community health personnel so that they could be deployed to provide basic mental healthcare to the masses (19). One of the ways that clinicians may be able to cater to patients' mental health during this pandemic is by providing health education and supporting health literacy. This can be done by providing accurate and relevant information to patients as well as directing them to reliable sources for consultation and thus helping them to remain updated with news related to COVID-19, as research shows that information overload contributes to the worsening of mental health (16).

Studies done also suggest that physical activity may be positively associated with improved mental health. Clinicians may consider encouraging patients to engage in daily physical activities (20).

The lack of use of digital means in the elderly may affect their access to mental healthcare and young adults shall have to take the lead and help them (Yang et al., 2020; Johnson et al., 2015). A study found that respondents reported that spending time with family and talking with friends or partners online were the best ways to cope with COVID-19-related anxiety (21).

UTILISING CAREGIVERS AS HELPING HANDS

During the COVID-19 pandemic lockdown, emotion-focused coping seemed to increase anxiety and depressive symptoms, probably due to the uncontrollable nature of the stressful event and the high emotional response. Family support, which reduces the sense of loneliness, has a major role in mitigating depressive symptoms. These results highlight the importance of promoting psychological strategies to improve emotional regulation skills by reducing isolation from family.

While past research has indicated that telemedicine is not necessarily as effective in each field, it has demonstrated effectiveness in psychiatry (6). Technology can be utilised not only as a means of treatment and providing care but also as a means preventing mental health issues (13).

CREATING TOOLS TO SUSTAIN TECHNOLOGY-BASED INTERVENTIONS

By training community health personnel in basic aspects of mental healthcare, technology-based interventions (TBI) could be used assess the scope of mental health problems, and accordingly, online materials for mental health education (22) can be tailored. Considering a high mortality rate, the provision of online counselling, with a special reference to grief counselling, should be provided (22). Thus, TBI can be explored by community health workers, general practitioners and psychiatrists to gather and increase manpower to reach the masses and help set straight the mismatch between the demand and supply in mental healthcare. Beyond the regular provision of care delivered through technological platforms, physicians may incorporate additional treatment methods, including mind-body modalities (i.e., mindfulness meditation) and psychological first aid (23).

TACKLING PROBLEMS WITH LIMITED RESOURCES

The availability of psychiatrists in many rural areas is also a challenge, and there is a need to train local doctors there to rise to the occasion (24).

Mental healthcare can be optimised by the involvement of village elders, panchayat heads, district health officers and traditional healthcare providers along with religious heads in rural areas in training and implementation of basic health services. The availability of psychiatrists in many rural areas is also a challenge, and there is a need to train local doctors there to match the deficit (25).

WORLD HEALTH ORGANIZATION GUIDELINES

To prevent or mitigate the risk of negative psychological outcomes caused by COVID-19, the World Health Organization (WHO) Department of Mental Health and Substance Use published a document, "Mental Health and Psychosocial Consideration During COVID-19 Outbreak." It is a way of supporting mental health and psychosocial well-being of different population groups during this pandemic by providing information on strengthening preparedness and response plans with regard to mental health and the psychosocial consequences of the COVID-19 outbreak, wherein particular mention of psychological first aid (PFA) is made (26).

WHAT IS PSYCHOLOGICAL FIRST AID?

PFA involves humane, supportive and practical assistance for people who are distressed in ways that respect their dignity, culture and abilities.

PFA is an initial disaster response intervention with the goal to promote safety, stabilise survivors of disasters and connect individuals to help and resources. PFA is delivered to affected individuals by mental health professionals and other first responders. The purpose of PFA is to assess the immediate concerns and needs of an individual in the aftermath of a disaster and not to provide on-site therapy. PFA is important, first-line psychosocial support for people affected by crisis events (27) (WHO publication www.who.int/mental_heal th/emergencies/en/).

Let Us Look at Some of the Systems in Place

Let us have a look at contingency measures taken until now. China, being one of the first-hit countries, started taking steps to ameliorate the mental health toll that COVID-19 took on its citizens. Some of these are, for example, a mental health surveillance system (MHSS), which enabled systematic data collection, analysis, interpretation and timely dissemination of the data to those responsible for prevention and control of the epidemic; thereafter, they conducted training of volunteers and healthcare workers in psychological first aid skills and designated special clinics for mental health (also a shift to telepsychiatry).

The role of PFA in the COVID-19 outbreak is crucial and significant in managing the intensifying mental stress originating from enormous impacts promoted by the infection in various facets of socioeconomic activities (28). The growing mortality and morbidity across many populations may instil fear, helplessness and horror in both infected and uninfected populations.

BENEFITS OF PFA

In the past, international organisations like the World Health Organization have shown benefits by implementing PFA to reduce panic and anxiety in pandemic-stricken locations, such as during the Ebola pandemic in Liberia and Sierra Leone. Local and international organisations should play an imperative role in increasing government efforts to safeguard the health of people (29).

Training of additional staff in hospitals and trauma centres to deal with the panic induced by the pandemic is among the first steps in realising the benefits of PFA. One of the current gaps challenging the effectiveness of PFA is the scarcity of skilled personnel with PFA skills to facilitate psychological intervention (30–36).

Given the rising infection rates and statistics concerning COVID-19, many people will need psychological intervention to help conform and cope in the new environment.

Health workers at the forefront in fighting the infection will also receive family support using PFA measures, without the risk of infecting their loved ones, thus reducing their stress while enhancing positive coping mechanisms. Forming support groups through digital chatrooms and social media will enhance recovery and coping by keeping the population connected and socially active despite isolation measures like quarantine. PFA administered through technology will enhance people's coping during the COVID-19 crisis and resiliency during and after the resolution of the pandemic.

Lessons From Previous Pandemics

PFA's application was effective during past outbreaks such as severe acute respiratory syndrome (SARS), where the population was fearful and anxious about the severe infection. According to Gillespie (1963), PFA is a crucial psychological intervention tool for mitigating the adverse impacts of traumatic events of persons witnessing or surviving humanitarian disasters (37). Severe acute respiratory syndrome outbreaks in the past caused significant distress for healthcare workers and the general population for similar reasons as now (38).

CONTINGENCY MEASURES PUT IN PLACE IN THE PAST AND THEIR EFFICACY

Results from the past implementation of PFA during past epidemics provided significant benefits in aiding people with emotional distress. The extensive measures imposed at the time to curb the spread of the infection in the population caused mental stress across the community. PFA helped in coping with stressors by enabling people to solve problems and take control of the situation.

The PFA training program ensured the responders' availability to provide timely counselling and physiological intervention to both medical personnel and the community (36).

It helped in coping with stressors by providing coping strategies. The emotional support provided to health workers was vital in reducing stress and alleviating anxiety stemming from interpersonal separation induced by the pandemic (37).

COPING SKILLS

The training program on modifiable coping strategies ensured timely counselling and psychological intervention to both medical personnel and the community. Two cross-sectional studies analysed modifiable coping mechanisms for decreasing anxiety and stress during COVID-19 and found promising results (38).

Another study of individuals with self-reported disabilities or chronic conditions found that modifiable coping strategies accounted for 54% of variance in well-being (Umucu and Lee 2020). Active coping, use of emotional support, humour and religion were associated with higher well-being scores (39).

USE OF TBI FOR PREVENTIVE MEASURES

Mariani studied the relationship among coping styles, perceived social support and depressive/anxious symptoms. A correlational analysis showed that depressive symptoms positively correlated with emotional coping style, avoidant coping style and low social support, specifically related to family support (40).

COVID-19 and Psychopharmacology: Critical Issues to Be Kept in Mind for Providing Optimum Care

It is plain to see that in reducing the burden of psychiatric disorders in this pandemic, while PFA acts as a stopgap, very often therapy, including pharmacotherapy, is required. However, this comes with a risk of drug-drug interactions that can jeopardise the overall mental and physical health of the people. Additionally, neuropsychiatric manifestations of COVID-19 can complicate the picture. We know that antipsychotics affecting the immune system would increase the risk of infection. Similarly, antidepressants such as fluoxetine and fluvoxamine can decrease metabolism of other medications, increasing their levels dangerously. Also benzodiazepines can cause respiratory depression in already compromised lung function secondary to COVID-19 infection.

If there is moderate to severe renal impairment, it is better to avoid psychotropics highly dependent on renal excretion like lithium, gabapentin and topiramate.

COVID-19 can produce myocarditis and arrhythmias, so it would be better to avoid psychotropics with a propensity to the prolong QT interval (42). One must also be vigilant about psychiatric side effects that may come up with corticosteroid use in COVID patients. These include depression, mania, agitation, mood lability, anxiety, insomnia, catatonia and psychosis. The majority of these side effects occur early in treatment within days and are usually seen at high doses (prednisolone equivalents of >40 mg/day) (43).

Clozapine needs monitoring along with absolute neutrophil count (ANC) monitoring, which may be difficult due to the movement restrictions and lockdown caused by the pandemic (44).

Hydroxychloroquine is recommended by some researchers as treatment in COVID-19. Chloroquine and hydroxychloroquine can rarely produce behavioural side effects, lightheadedness, sleep disturbances, irritability, confusional states and psychosis (45). Ritonavir was found to be a potent inhibitor of CYP3A-mediated biotransformation. Ritonavir is also an inducer of CYP1A4, glucuronosyl transferase (GT) and possibly CYP2C9 and CYP2C19. Agents that increase CYP3A activity, such as carbamazepine, phenobarbital and phenytoin, increase ritonavir clearance, resulting in decreased ritonavir plasma levels. Alprazolam, diazepam, estazolam, flurazepam, midazolam, triazolam and zolpidem may cause extreme sedation and respiratory depression when used together. Bupropion and clozapine, when used together with ritonavir, may increase plasma levels of these drugs, thus increasing the patient's risk of arrhythmias, hematologic abnormalities, seizures or other potentially serious adverse effects. Ritonavir formulations contain alcohol that can produce disulfiram-like reactions when used with metronidazole or disulfiram. Ritonvir may increase statin levels in patients as well (46, 47). A patient who tests positive for COVID-19 and has an acute psychiatric illness or is suffering from acute substance withdrawal is a unique challenge in all settings. It may be a difficult task, especially in low-resource countries, to manage such patients in a medical intensive care unit. The staff are ill equipped to handle psychiatric emergencies, and there may be a risk of violence on the part of the patient. Team management by a combination of both medical and psychiatric units is required in such cases. The patient would need admission in a restrictive environment such as an in-patient psychiatric unit and at the same time would need intensive care backup if available (48). COVID-19-positive psychiatric patients would ideally need input from psychiatrists and internal medicine experts working in the same unit. At any point in time, either the psychiatric disorder or the medical disorder could take priority, and there may be instances where both conditions should be treated simultaneously. Some patients need isolation and primary medical treatment, whereas others need medical monitoring while the primary management is delivered by psychiatrists. Many patients will need individual psychotherapy, occupational therapy and help from a psychiatric social worker, so all these professions should ideally contribute to the staffing of such units (49).

Many stable ambulatory patients with schizophrenia may be prescribed long-acting injectable antipsychotics to maintain antipsychotic levels and reduce withdrawal psychosis, as may be seen with abrupt stoppage of antipsychotic drugs.

Management of Critical Cases

We know that even during the pandemic, cases of patients with suicidal ideation, suicide attempts and catatonia to continue to seek treatment. In spite of being in the midst of a pandemic, it is imperative for us to provide evidence-based treatment, that is, electro-convulsive therapy, which in these cases would be life saving.

However, how does one manage a hospital procedure requiring anaesthesia and generating aerosols without causing nosocomial infections, and cross-contamination (50)? An article by Yeole et al. describes how a team of psychiatrists, anaesthetists and paramedical staff worked together to deliver nine to ten ECTs per day in the midst of a pandemic, providing an optimum level and standard of care (51).

Many countries have reached a consensus on the significance of psychological assistance during disasters, including pandemics. This assistance should be flexible according to the accessibility of medical resources. The outbreak of the COVID-19 pandemic is a gap between the resources available related to psychological services and the need. Along with offline services, online assistance can be used for efficient psychological interventions for promoting psychological first aid, coping skills, rehabilitation and preventive measures. Non-psychiatric medics such as paramedics can be trained in delivering psychological assistance and serve the masses. Use of e-prescriptions can help patients with their medications and improve compliance. It is critical to keep drug-drug interactions in mind whilst prescribing medications, and finally, it is equally important to take care of the psychological health of our brethren at work.

References

1. Ryder AL, Azcarate PM, Cohen BE. Ptsd and physical health. *Curr Psychiatry Rep*. 2018;20:116.
2. Duan L, Zhu G. Psychological interventions for people affected by the COVID-19 epidemic. *Lancet Psychiatry*. 2020;7(4):300–302.
3. Sood S. Psychological effects of the Coronavirus disease-2019 pandemic. *Res Hum Med Educ*. 2020;7:23–26.
4. Rajkumar RP. COVID-19 and mental health: A review of the existing literature. *Asian Journal of Psychiatry*. 2020;52:102066. doi: 10.1016/j.ajp.2020.102066
5. Avinash De Sousa, Sai Krishna. Psychosocial impact of the lockdown and COVID-19 Avinash De Sousa1*, Sai Krishna P2. *Telangana Journal of Psychiatry*. 2020 Jan–Jun;6(1):4–6.
6. Roine R, Ohinmaa A, Hailey D. Assessing telemedicine: A systematic review of the literature. *Cmaj*. 2001;165(6):765–771.
7. Arango C. Lessons learned from the coronavirus health crisis in Madrid, Spain: How COVID-19 has changed our lives in the last two weeks. *Biol Psychiat*. 2020. [Epub ahead of print] https://doi.org/10.1016/j.biopsych.2020.04.003
8. Zhu Y, Chen L, Ji H, Xi M, Fang Y, Li Y. The risk and prevention of novel coronavirus pneumonia infections among inpatients in psychiatric hospitals. *Neurosci Bulletin*. 2020;36(3):299–302.
10. Adams JG, Walls RM. Supporting the health care workforce during the COVID-19 global epidemic. *JAMA*. 2020;323(15):1439–1440.
11. De Sousa, ME, Javed A. A critical issues in treating COVID-19-positive psychiatric patients in low- and middle-income countries. *Bjpsych International*. 2020 Jul 20 at 13:35:34.
12. Safieh et al. Interventions to optimise mental health outcomes during the COVID-19 pandemic: A scoping review. *International Journal of Mental Health and Addiction*. https://doi.org/10.1007/s11469-021-00558-3
13. Banskota S, Healy M, Goldberg EM. 15 smartphone apps for older adults to use while in isolation during the COVID-19 pandemic. *The Western Journal of Emergency Medicine*. 2020;21(3):514–525. https://doi.org/10.5811/westjem.2020.4.47372.
14. Goodman-Casanova JM, Dura-Perez E, Guzman-Parra J, Cuesta-Vargas A, Mayoral-Cleries F. Telehealth home support during COVID-19 confinement for community-dwelling older adults with mild cognitive impairment or mild dementia: Survey study. *Journal of Medical Internet Research*. 2020;22(5):e19434.
15. Wei N, Huang BC, Lu SJ, Hu JB, Zhou XY, Hu CC, et al. Efficacy of internet-based integrated intervention on depression and anxiety symptoms in patients with COVID-19. *Journal of Zhejiang University SCIENCE B*. 2020;21(5):400–404.
16. Ahmad AR, Murad HR. The impact of social media on panic during the covid-19 pandemic in Iraqi Kurdistan: Online questionnaire study. *Journal of Medical Internet Research*. 2020;22(5):e19556. https://doi.org/10.2196/19556.
17. Olagoke AA, Olagoke OO, Hughes AM. Exposure to coronavirus news on mainstream media: The role of risk perceptions and depression. *British Journal of Health Psychology*. 2020;10:865–874. https://doi.org/10.1111/bjhp.12427.
18. Noone C, McSharry J, Smalle M, Burns A, Dwan K, Devane D, Morrissey EC. Video calls for reducing social isolation and loneliness in older people: A rapid review. *The Cochrane Database of Systematic Reviews*. 2020;5(5):CD013632. https://doi.org/10.1002/14651858.CD013632.
19. Rajkumar RP. COVID-19 and mental health: A review of the existing literature. *Asian Journal of Psychiatry*. 2020;52:102066. https://doi.org/10.1016/j.ajp.2020.102066.
20. Goethals L, Barth N, Guyot J, Hupin D, Celarier T, Bongue B. Impact of home quarantine on physical activity among older adults living at home during the COVID-19 pandemic: Qualitative interview study. *JMIR Aging*. 2020;3(1):e19007.

21. Talidong KJB, Toquero CMD. Philippine teachers' practices to deal with anxiety amid covid-19. *Journal of Loss and Trauma.* 2020;25:573–579. https://doi.org/10.1080/15325024.2020.1759225.
22. Liu X, Luo WT, Li Y, Li CN, Hong ZS, Chen HL, Xiao F, Xia JY. Psychological status and behavior changes of the public during the COVID-19 epidemic in China. *Infectious Diseases of Poverty.* 2020d;9(1):58.
23. Cheng W, Zhang F, Hua Y, Yang Z, Liu J. Development of a psychological first-aid model in inpatients with COVID-19 in Wuhan, China. *General Psychiatry.* 2020;33(3):e100292.
24. Hoeft TJ, Fortney JC, Patel V, Unützer J. Task-sharing approaches to improve mental health care in rural and other low-resource settings: A systematic review. *J. Rural Health.* 2018;34(1):48–62.
25. Maulik PK, Devarapalli S, Kallakuri S, Tewari A, Chilappagari S, Koschorke M, Thornicroft G. Evaluation of an anti-stigma campaign related to common mental disorders in rural India: A mixed methods approach. *Psychol. Med.* 2017;47(3):565–575.
26. World Health Organization. Mental health and psychosocial considerations during COVID-19 outbreak. World Health Organization. (2020). Available online at: www.who.int/docs/default-source/coronaviruse/mental-health-considerations.pdf.
27. WHO publication. www.who.int/mental_health/emergencies/en/.
28. Shah K, Kamrai D, Mekala H, Mann B, Desai K, Patel RS. Focus on mental health during the coronavirus (COVID-19) pandemic: Applying learnings from the past outbreaks. *Cureus.* 2020;12:e7405. doi: 10.7759/cureus.7405.
29. Gispen F, Wu AW. Psychological first aid: CPR for mental health crises in healthcare. *J PatientSaf Risk Manag.* 2018;23:51–53. doi: 10.1177/2516043518762826.
30. Ruzek JI, Brymer MJ, Jacobs AK, Layne CM, Vernberg EM, Watson PJ. Psychological first aid. *JMent Health Couns.* 2007;29:17–49. doi: 10.17744/mehc.29.1.5racqxjueafabgwp.
31. Everly GS Jr, Barnett DJ, Sperry NL, Links JM. The use of psychological first aid (PFA) training among nurses to enhance population resiliency. *Int J Emerg Ment Health.* 2010;12:21–31.
32. Psychological first aid for schools: Field operations guide. (2017). Accessed: May 15, 2020. www.nctsn.org/resources/psychological-first-aid-schools-pfa-s-field-operations-guide.
33. Taylor M, Wells G, Howell G, Raphael B. The role of social media as psychological first aid as a support to community resilience building: A Facebook study from 'cyclone Yasi update'. *Austr J Emergency Manag.* 2012;27:20–26.
34. Jacobs GA, Gray BL, Erickson SE, Gonzalez ED, Quevillon RP. Disaster mental health and community-based psychological first aid: Concepts and education/training. *J Clin Psychol.* 2016;72:1307–1317. doi: 10.1002/jclp.22316.
35. Horn R, O'May F, Esliker R, Gwaikolo W, Woensdregt L, Ruttenberg L, Ager A. The myth of the 1-day training: The effectiveness of psychosocial support capacity-building during the ebola outbreak in West Africa. *Global Mental Health.* 2019;6:e5. doi: 10.1017/gmh.2019.2.
36. McCabe OL, Everly GS Jr, Brown LM, Wendelboe AM, Abd Hamid NH, Tallchief VL, Links JM. Psychological first aid: A consensus-derived, empirically supported, competency-based training model. *Am J Public Health.* 2014;104:621–628. doi: 10.2105/AJPH.2013.301219.
37. Gillespie DK. Psychological first aid. *J Sch Health.* 1963;33:391–395. doi: 10.1111/j.1746-1561.1963.tb00427.x. 37 Matsuishi K, Kawazoe A, Imai H, Ito A, Mouri K, Kitamura N, Miyake K, Mino K, Isobe M, Takamiya S, Hitokoto H, Mita T. Psychological impact of the pandemic (H1N1) 2009 on general hospital workers in Kobe. *Psychiatry Clin Neurosci.* 2012 Jun;66(4):353–360. doi: 10.1111/j.1440-1819.2012.02336.x. PMID: 22624741.
38. Maunder RG, Leszcz M, Savage D, et al. Applying the lessons of SARS to pandemic influenza. *Can J Public Health.* 2008;99:486–488. doi: 10.1007/BF03403782.
39. Umucu E, Lee B. Examining the impact of COVID-19 on stress and coping strategies in individuals with disabilities and chronic conditions. *Rehabil Psychol.* 2020 Aug;65(3):193–198. doi: 10.1037/rep0000328. Epub 2020 May 14. PMID: 32406739.
40. Mariani R, Renzi A, Di Trani M, Trabucchi G, Danskin K, Tambelli R. The impact of coping strategies and perceived family support on depressive and anxious symptomatology during the coronavirus pandemic (COVID-19) lockdown. *Front. Psychiatry.* 2020;11:587724. doi: 10.3389/fpsyt.2020.587724.
41. World Health Organization. Mental health and psychosocial considerations during COVID-19 outbreak. World Health Organization. (2020). Available online at: www.who.int/docs/default-source/coronaviruse/mental-health considerations.pdf.
42. Bessière F, Roccia H, Delinière A, et al. Assessment of QT intervals in a case series of patients with coronavirus disease 2019 (COVID-19) infection treated with hydroxychloroquine alone or in combination with azithromycin in an intensive care unit. *JAMA Cardiol.* 2020;5(9):1067–1069. doi: 10.1001/jamacardio.2020.1787.

43. Dubovsky AN, Arvikar S, Stern TA, Axelrod L. The neuropsychiatric complications of glucocorticoid use: Steroid psychosis revisited. *Psychosomatics*. 2012;53(2):103–115.
44. Vermeulen JM, van Rooijen G, van de Kerkhof MP, Sutterland AL, Correll CU, de Haan L. Clozapine and long-term mortality risk in patients with schizophrenia: A systematic review and meta-analysis of studies lasting 1.1–12.5 years. *Schizophr Bull*. 2019;45(2):315–329.
45. Vermeulen JM, van Rooijen G, van de Kerkhof MP, Sutterland AL, Correll CU, de Haan L. Clozapine and long-term mortality risk in patients with schizophrenia: A systematic review and meta-analysis of studies lasting 1.1–12.5 years. *Schizophr Bull*. 2019;45(2):315–329.
46. Wang Y, Zhang D, Du G, Du R, Zhao J, Jin Y, Fu S, Gao L, Cheng Z, Lu Q, Hu Y. Remdesivir in adults with severe COVID-19: A randomised, double-blind, placebo-controlled, multicentre trial. *Lancet*. 2020;Apr 29. (Epub ahead of print).
47. Stebbing J, Phelan A, Griffin I, Tucker C, Oechsle O, Smith D, et al. COVID-19: Combining antiviral and anti-inflammatory treatments. *Lancet Infect Dis*. 2020;20(4):400–402.
48. Fagiolini A, Cuomo A, Frank E. COVID-19 diary from a psychiatry department in Italy. *J Clin Psychiatry*. 2020; 81:20com13357.
49. Bojdani E, Rajagopalan A, Chen A, Gearin P, Olcott W, Shankar V, et al. COVID-19 pandemic: Impact on psychiatric care in the United States, a review. *Psychiatr Res*. 2020;289:113069.
50. Bernardo M, González-Pinto A, Urretavizcaya M, eds. Consenso Español Sobre La Terapia Electroconvulsiva. Madrid: Sociedad. Española de Psiquiatría Biológica; 2018. Available at: www.sepsiq.org/file/Enlaces/SEPB%20-%20Consenso%20Espa%C3%B1ol%20sobre%20la%20Terapia%.
51. Yeole S, et al. Electroconvulsive therapy administered during the COVID-19 pandemic. *The Journal of ECT*. 2021; 37(1):e2–e3. doi: 10.1097/YCT.0000000000000734.

Index

Note: Page numbers in *italics* indicate figures and those in **bold** indicate tables.

AAN (American Academy of Neurology) 234
abnormal anxiety 259
Abnormal Involuntary Movement Scale 209
abnormal swallowing syndrome, sleep-related 283
Academy of Consultation Liaison Psychiatry 334
acamprosate (calcium homotaurinate) 157–158
acetaldehyde dehydrogenase (ALDH) inhibitors 293; *see also* disulfiram
acrophobia 261, 270
ACT (Assertive Community Treatment) 211, 430, 549, 553
actuarial methods of risk assessment 93–94
adaptive functioning, in QoL 19
ADHD *see* attention-deficit/hyperactivity disorder (ADHD)
ADR *see* adverse drug reaction (ADR)
advance directives (ADs) 113
adverse drug reaction (ADR): in COVID-19 563–564; CPZ-induced EPS and 530, 532–533; with disulfiram 295–296; scales for, in geriatric psychiatry 209
Affymetrix Gene Chip System 3000 Dx 526
Africa: Africa Mental Health Foundation (AMFH) in Kenya 462; AMFH in Kenya 462; children whose mothers had postnatal depression in 86; Friendship Bench in Zimbabwe 462; group IPT for depression in 387
Africa Mental Health Foundation (AMFH) 462
African-American patients, buprenorphine and 157
aggression: causes of 349–350; in dementia 240; in mood disorders 350; in neurotic disorders 350; overview of 349; in personality disorders 350; in psychotic disorders 350; in substance abuse 350
agitation: causes of 344–345; C-L psychiatry and 334; in dementia 240; in mood disorders 345; in neurotic disorders 345; overview of 344; in personality disorders 345; in psychotic disorders 345; in substance abuse 344
agoraphobia 262–264: biopsychosocial management of 263; CBT for 264; clinical features of 263; comorbidities in 263; course and prognosis in 264; definition of 263–264; diagnostic criteria for 263; differential diagnosis in 263; epidemiology for 263; pharmacotherapy in 264; psychoeducation in 264; virtual therapy in 264
ailurophobia 270
akathesia 352
alcohol dependence: disulfiram therapy in 292–298; pharmacogenetics in 155–156, 157–160, 161
alcoholism, definition of 292
alcohol-related QoL (AL QoL) 25, 28
ALDH (acetaldehyde dehydrogenase) inhibitors 293; *see also* disulfiram
α-adrenergic receptors 528
AL QoL (alcohol-related QoL) 25, 28
Alzheimer's dementia 233, 236–238
American Academy of Neurology (AAN) 234
American Neuropsychiatric Association 334
American Psychiatric Association (APA) 234–235; *see also* DSM-5; DSM IV-TR
American Psychosomatic Society 334
AMFH (Africa Mental Health Foundation) 462
amitriptyline 186
AmpliChip CYP450 526
amygdala: aggression and 349; behavioral addictions and 170; BPD and 217–218; GAD and 268; major depression and 519; panic disorder and 261; PTSD and 520; resilience and 51, 52, 53, 54; schizophrenia and 519; sexual response cycle and 101, 103; specific phobias and 271

anorexia nervosa 183; OCD with 288; pharmacological treatment of 185–186
Anti Cholinergic Cognitive Burden Scale 209
antidepressants 80, 209; *see also* selective serotonin reuptake inhibitors (SSRIs); for alcohol use disorder 156; for anxiety disorders 267; for BDNF 52; for BPD 223–224; contraindicated for COVID-19 563; for eating disorders 186; in gene sight psychotropic algorithm 527; medication counseling and 440; for nicotine dependence 162; for sexual dysfunction 104, 105, 106; for sleep disorders 276, 281, 282, 283; for suicide prevention 46, 324, 325
antipsychotics (AS) 80, 209, 209; for agitation and aggression in PWD 240, 334; akathesia and 352; for Alzheimer's disease 212; AP-induced EPS 528–532; for APS 250, 251, 253; for BPD 223–224; for BPSD in COVID-19 243; for COVID-19 563, 564; CPZ 527–530; decreased bone mineral density and 139; for delirium in PWD 241, 334; in gene sight psychotropic algorithm 527; medication counselling and 440; sexual dysfunction and 102–103, 105, 106
anxiety disorders 258–272; *see also individual anxiety disorders*; abnormal anxiety and 259; agoraphobia 262–264; BPD with 221–222; CBT for 362; cognitive changes in 259; concepts of 259; differentiating 259; disease-specific scales for 24, 25, 27; fear and 259; GAD 267–270; generalized anxiety disorder 267–270; overview of 258; panic disorder 259–262; physiological responses and 259; QoL of patients with 27; sexual response cycle in 105–106; social anxiety disorder 264–267; specific phobias 270–272
APA (American Psychiatric Association) 234–235; *see also* DSM-5; DSM IV-TR; of behavioral addictions 175–176, 177; of suicide 321–322
apnea 278–279
apprehension in GAD 267
APS *see* attenuated psychosis syndrome (APS)
ARFID (avoidant/restrictive food intake disorder) 184–185
Argentina, community psychiatry in 475–479; for addiction treatment 478; for child and adolescent care 478; for elderly patients 479; for family or domestic violence 479; overview of 475–478
arthritis, sleep disorders and 283
AS *see* antipsychotics (AS)
Asha, halfway home 444–445
Asia: disulfiram and Asian flush in 163; ECT in Malaysia 371–375; poor metabolizers in 530; slum dwellers in India from 192; suicide prevention in 46; suicide rates in 318; VAW in 66
Assertive Community Treatment (ACT) 211, 430, 549, 553
assessment and screening: of behavioral addictions 175–176, 177; of social anxiety disorder 266; of suicide 321–322
Assisted Decision-Making (Capacity) Act, Ireland's 37, 114

assisted living facilities (ALFs) 213
asthma, sleep-related 283
attention-deficit/hyperactivity disorder (ADHD): BPD with 222–223; fMRI in 520–521; fNIRS in 543
attenuated psychosis syndrome (APS) 247–255; conclusion and future implications of 254–255; evidence-based interventions in 250–252; historical background and current understanding of 247–248; integrated treatment in 254; management interventions in 249–250; need for optimization of care in 248–249; overview of 247; pharmacological interventions in 250–251; psychosocial interventions in 251–252; recommendations for optimization of treatment in 252–254; risk assessment in 249; treatment in, aims of 249–250
Australia: COPMI in 86; guidelines for diagnosis and management of dementia in 236; mental health of Aboriginal Australianism 381; NTX or OAM in, studies on patients treated with 301, 313; QualityRights Initiative in 115; RF facilities in 443; studies on CPT in 389; three-tiered risk framework in Queensland 95–96
Austria, schizophrenia in 56
autism spectrum disorders 266, 444, 466
automation in bipolar disorder 153
autonomic nervous system in HD, damage to 137–139; cardiovascular system impairments 138–139; gastrointestinal disorders 139; sleep disturbances 138
autonomic overactivity in GAD 267
autonomy and choice; *see also* coercive practices: ADs and 113; in Argentina 475; in CRPD 111; decision-making and 115; as ethical principle in mental healthcare 39, 111; informed consent and 112; involuntary treatment and 116; motivational interviewing and 380; nominated representatives and 114; in psychosocial rehabilitation 545, 547, 553, 554; safety and quality of service delivery and 381; stigma associated with mental illnesses and 43; VAW and 74; women's reproductive and sexual health and 118
avoidant/restrictive food intake disorder (ARFID) 184–185

baclofen 160
BBB (blood brain barrier) 529
BDD *see* body dysmorphic disorder (BDD)
BDNF (brain-derived neurotrophic factor) 52
BED (bing eating disorder) 184
behavioral addictions 169–178; assessment and screening of 175–176, 177; internet addiction 172–175; interventional modalities in 176–178; other 171, *171*; pathological gambling 169, 170–171; psychopharmacological treatments for 176; substance use disorder compared to 169–170
behavioural and psychological symptoms of dementia (BPSD) 239–241; agitation and aggression 240; COVID-19 and 243–244; delirium 241; frailty 240–241; overview of 239

570 • INDEX

benzodiazepines: aggression in abuse of 350; for agitation and aggression in PWD 240; for alcohol dependence 294; for anxiety disorders 262, 264, 267, 268, 272; for BPSD in COVID-19 244; contraindicated in COVID-19 563; for delirium in PWD 241; during ECT 374; excitement and missed use of 347; medication review and 336; psychomotor retardation in abuse of 348; seizures and 439; for sexual dysfunction 104; for sleep disorders 276, 276, 280, 281, 282; for suicide prevention 323, 324
β-adrenergic receptor antagonists 53, 271–272
β-adrenergic receptor blockade 53
bing eating disorder (BED) 184, 186
biological factors that determine resilience 54–55
biopsychosocial management: of agoraphobia 263; of dementia 236, *237*, *238*
bipolar disorder 151–154; automation in 153; BPD with 221, 222; disease-specific scales for 25, 27; fMRI in 519–520; managing, effective methods of 151–152; motivational pharmacotherapy in 152; OCD with 288; overview of 151; patient engagement in therapeutic alliance, effective 153–154; QoL of patients with 26–27; sexual response cycle in 105; telepsychiatry in 153
bizarre behaviour: causes of 345; in mood disorders 346; in neurotic disorders 346; overview of 345; in personality disorders 346; in psychotic disorders 345; in substance abuse 345
blood brain barrier (BBB) 529
blood investigations in geriatric psychiatry 207–208
body dysmorphic disorder (BDD): CBT for 362; eating disorders with 182; OCD and habit disorders with 288; social anxiety disorder with 266
borderline personality disorder (BPD) 216–227; ADHD and 222–223; adolescent treatment in 224; adulthood treatment in 225; bipolar disorder and 222; child and adolescent temperament and personality factors in 218–219; in childhood, factors associated with 219–221; clinical features and comorbidities of 221–222; DBT for 391; epidemiology of 217; overview of 216; pathogenesis of 217–218; trauma history and 222; treatment 223–224; treatment course 224–225; treatment implications 225–227
BPD *see* borderline personality disorder (BPD)
BPSD *see* behavioural and psychological symptoms of dementia (BPSD)
brain-derived neurotrophic factor (BDNF) 52
brain development, child and adolescent psychiatry and 466
brain oximetry in fNIRS 539–541
breathing-related sleep disorders 278–279
bulimia nervosa 184; pharmacological treatment of 186
bulimia nervosa, OCD with 288
buprenorphine, for opioid dependence 157

bupropion 162; adverse drug effects in 564; for behavioral addictions 176; for depressive disorders 27; for nicotine dependence 156, 162; sexual dysfunction and 104

calcium homotaurinate (acamprosate) 157–158
Canada: abstinence-based substance use disorder programs in 427; COVID-19 in 396; guidelines for diagnosis and management of dementia in 235; MHEN intervention in 408–409; NCRMD in 422–423; smartphone technology in 406; telepsychiatry in 396, 398
Canadian Consensus Conference (CCC) 234, 235
capacity: assessments 112; coercive practices and 111–112
carbamazepine 105, 209, 209, 240, 281, 282, 564
cardiovascular symptoms, sleep-related 283
cardiovascular system impairments in HD 138–139
carers and caregivers of patients: with dementia 241, 242, 243, 244; disease-specific scales for 25; of patients with psychiatric disorders 25; in psychopharmacology 437–438; QoL research in 28; support for 241, 242, 243; technology-based interventions to support 561
CARMHA (Centre for Applied Research in Mental Health and Addictions) 462
case management *see* community case managed clients; rehabilitation and recovery
cataplexy 277–278
catatonia: causes of 346; in mood disorders 347; in neurotic disorders 347; overview of 346; in personality disorders 347; in psychotic disorders 347; in substance abuse 346
catechol-O-methyltransferase (COMT) 527
CBGT (cognitive-behavioural group therapy) 365–366
CBT *see* cognitive behavioral therapy (CBT)
CCC (Canadian Consensus Conference) 234, 235
central sleep apnea (CSA) 279
Centre for Applied Research in Mental Health and Addictions (CARMHA) 462
Charles Bonnet syndrome 351
Chetana, day care centre 445, 446, *446*, *449–451*
Cheyne–Stokes breathing 279
child and adolescent psychiatry 465–472; in Argentina 478; barriers in treatment of mental disorders in 467–468; brain development and 466; coercive practices and 119; consequences of mental disorders in 467; mental health issues in children and adolescents 466–467; optimizing treatment and care in 468–472; overview of 465; pandemics and epidemics and 499–500
Child and Adolescent Psychiatry of the World Psychiatric Association (WPA CAP) 468
children of patients with mental illness (COPMI) 84–89; intervention programs for (*see* intervention programs for COPMI); maternal depression and 86; outcomes and their predictors in 86; risks and resilience of 84–85, *86*

CHIME (connectedness, hope and optimism, identity, meaning and purpose and empowerment) framework 382
China: child and adolescent psychiatry in 469; COVID-19 outbreak in 401, 557, 562; sterilisation of individuals with mental illness in 118
chlorpromazine (CPZ) 527–533, *531*, 532–533
chlorpromazine nitric oxide (CPZNO) 528
chlorpromazine sulfoxide (CPZSO) 528
choice *see* autonomy and choice
chronic paroxysmal hemicrania 283
CHRR (Collaborative Healthcare) Platform 409
circadian rhythm sleep disorders 279–280
claustrophobia 261, 270
Clinical Pharmacogenetics Implementation Consortium (CPIC) 534
clozapine 103, 209, 239, 564
C-L psychiatry *see* consultation liaison (C-L) psychiatry
cluster headaches, sleep-related 283
cocaine addiction, pharmacogenetics in management of 162–163
coercive practices, limiting 110–120; ADs and 113; capacity and 111–112; capacity assessments and 112; decision-making and 114–115; general principles of 111–113; for individuals receiving involuntary treatment 115–118; informed consent and 112–113; minors and 119; NRs and 114; for severe illness 113–115; Ulysses clause and 113–114; women's reproductive and sexual health and 118–119
cognitive behavioral therapy (CBT): A-B-C of 358–359; agoraphobia in 264; approach to psychiatric illnesses 361; for APS 251–252; CBGT and 365–366; with children and adolescents 367; in community mental health approach 363–364; core principles of 359, *359*; crisis intervention and 364–365; criticism of 367–368; for eating disorders 187; examples of techniques used in *360*; for GAD 269; NSHW-delivered 458–459; overview of 357–358; for panic disorder 262, 365; plurality and effectiveness of 366; psychiatric disorders and 361–363; for psychoeducation 252, 360–361; REBT and 358; sessions 359–360; for specific phobias 271–272; strategies in 359; third wave of 367
cognitive-behavioural group therapy (CBGT) 365–366
cognitive impairment, sexual response cycle in 106
cognitive processing therapy (CPT) 384, 387–389
cognitive remediation therapy 376–382; *see also* rehabilitation and recovery
cognitive restructuring in insomnia disorder 276
cognitive theories in specific phobias 271
cognitive therapy (CT) 358; *see also* cognitive behavioral therapy (CBT)
cognitive training in NCRP 127–129; cognitive training stimulates 127; sessions 127–129
Collaborative Healthcare (CHRR) Platform 409

community case managed clients 91–98; case management and risks 91–92; duty to disclose and 97; firearms and 96; forensic patients 92–93; implications of better risk management 97–98; management of risks 96–97; newer developments in 96; prevalence of mental illnesses and associated risks 92; risk assessments (*see* risk assessment); risk framework in Queensland, Australia 95–96; risk prediction *vs.* prevention 93; safety culture and, developing 97
community mental healthcare: components of 458; forensic outreach in 429–432; global 457–463; innovations needed in 460–461; interventions in PSR 453; model examples in 462; models of community care in 430; principles and practices in 457; psychopharmacology in 436–441; task sharing in 458–460
community psychiatry 198–201; in Argentina 475–479; challenges faced in, possible solutions for 200–201; Indian scenario for rural psychiatry 199–200; intervention for 88; overview of 198; principles of 198; problem of 199
compulsive sexual behavior/sex addiction 174–175; assessment and screening of 175; criteria for sexual addiction 174; interventional modalities for 178; pharmacotherapy for 176
compulsive shopping and buying 172–173; assessment and screening for 175; interventional modalities for 178; pharmacotherapy for 176; research criteria for 173
computed tomography (CT): in C-L psychiatry 337; in dementia 234, 235; in geriatric psychiatry 208
COMT (catechol-O-methyltransferase) 527
confusion 334
connectedness, hope and optimism, identity, meaning and purpose and empowerment (CHIME) framework 382
consultation liaison (C-L) psychiatry 333–339; benefits of 339; in general hospital 334–333; historical background of 333–334; MSE in 336–337; optimising 335–338; in outpatient setting 339; practice guidelines for 339; problems encountered in 334–335; role of other providers in 338–339; tests ordered in 337–338
continuous measurement (CW) in fNIRS 539–540, *540*
Convention on the Rights of Persons with Disabilities (CRPD): autonomy and patient choice 111, 119; capacity 112; decision-making 114–115; involuntary treatment 39, 111, 115, 116; Mental Healthcare Act (India) 37–40; minors 119; women's reproductive and sexual health 118
conversion disorder 193, 335, 347
COPMI *see* children of patients with mental illness (COPMI)
corticosteroid use in COVID patients 563
corticotropin-releasing hormone (CRH) 51, 52, 261
cortisol: BPD and 217; panic disorder and 261; PTSD and 520; resilience and 51, 55

COVID-19 557–565; *see also* pandemics and epidemics; in Canada 396; in China 401, 557, 562; containment strategies in 557; continuing mental health care in 559–565; critical cases of 564–565; dementia and 243–244; ECT in Malaysia and 374; e-NCRP and, in Moscow 132; fear of contracting 557; frontline healthcare personnel in, mental health of 559; in India 47; mental health during 558–559; psychological first aid in 561–563; psychopharmacology for 558, 563–565; state of affairs in, current 557; suicide and 47; technology-based interventions in 559–563; telemedicine in 559; telepsychiatry in 200, 396, 399, 557, 559; treatment models adapted to the 'new norm' in 559; in United Kingdom 244; in United States 399
CPIC (Clinical Pharmacogenetics Implementation Consortium) 534
CPT (cognitive processing therapy) 384, 387–389
CPZ (chlorpromazine) 527–533, *531*, 532–533
CPZNO (chlorpromazine nitric oxide) 528
CPZSO (chlorpromazine sulfoxide) 528
CRH (corticotropin-releasing hormone) 51, 52, 261
crisis intervention, CBT and 364–365
CRPD *see* Convention on the Rights of Persons with Disabilities (CRPD)
CSA (central sleep apnea) 279
CT *see* computed tomography (CT)
CT (cognitive therapy) 358; *see also* cognitive behavioral therapy (CBT)
CW (continuous measurement) in fNIRS 539–540, *540*
cynophobia 270
CYP (cytochrome 450) 529, 530
CYP1A2 (enzyme 1A2 of cytochrome 450) 527, 529, 530
CYP2B6 (enzyme 2B6 of cytochrome 450) 162, 527
CYP2C9 (enzyme 2C9 of cytochrome 450) 527, 564
CYP2C19 (enzyme 2C19 of cytochrome 450) 160, 526, 527, 564
CYP2D6 (enzyme 2D6 of cytochrome 450) 157, 526, 527, 529–532, 532–533
CYP3A4 (enzyme 3A4 of cytochrome 450) 157, 527
cyproheptadine 186
cytochrome 450 (CYP) 529, 530
cytochrome P450 genes 526–527

DBT (dialectical behavior therapy) 389–391
decision-making, coercive practices and 114–115
dehydroepiandrosterone (DHEA) 51, 55, 105
deletion (Del) 529
deliberate self harm (DSH) 334, 363
delirium: C-L psychiatry and 334; dementia and 241, 242
dementia 233–244; agitation and aggression in 240; Alzheimer's dementia 233, 236–238; biopsychosocial approach to 236, *237*, *238*; BPSD (*see* behavioural and psychological symptoms of dementia (BPSD)); care for, basis of 234; carers and caregiver burden in, support for 241, 242, 243; comorbidities in, management of 240–241; COVID-19 and, impact of 234, 243–244; delirium and 241, 242; frailty in 240–241; frontotemporal dementia 233, 239; guidelines for diagnosis and management of 234, 234–236; Lewy body dementia 233, 238–239; overview of 233; Parkinson's disease dementia 233, 239; pharmacological management of 236–239; social support and carer stress and, impact of 244; vascular dementia 233, 238
Dementia Mood Assessment Scale 210
Denmark, disulfiram introduced in 293
DEOR model of sexual response cycle 101
deoxyribonucleic acid (DNA) 52, 525, 527
depressive disorders: BPD with 221–222; C-L psychiatry and 334; disease-specific scales for 24, 27; fMRI in 519; fNIRS in 543; group IPT for 387; in homeless 193; MDD 222, 225, 437, 543; OCD with 288; QoL of patients with 27; REBT for 392; scales for, in geriatric psychiatry 209; sexual functioning and 103; sexual response cycle in 103–106
DHEA (dehydroepiandrosterone) 51, 55, 105
Diagnostic and Statistical Manual of Mental Disorders *see* DSM-5; DSM IV-TR
dialectical behavior therapy (DBT) 389–391
differential awareness of psychiatric presentations 341–353; aggression 349–350; agitation 344–345; bizarre behaviour 345–346; catatonia 346–347; excitement 347–348; hallucinations 350–351; psychomotor retardation 348–349; self-neglect 343–344; suicide, attempted 351–352; unexplained somatic symptoms 352–353
disease-specific scales for bipolar disorder 25, 27
disorder-specific scales in measurement of QoL 22, 24–25
distal-level intervention 70–73; global and interventional level of 70; service enhancement in 71–73, *72*–*73*; social transformation in 71; structural interventions in 71
disulfiram: for alcohol dependence 156, 157, 292–298; for cocaine addiction 162–163; consent for 297; drug interactions with 294–295; history of 293; mode of action and 293–294; overview of 292–293; psychoeducation and 297–298; side effects and precautions in 295–296; usage of, in special groups 296–297; use of 295
DNA (deoxyribonucleic acid) 52, 525, 527
dopaminergic receptor D2 (DRD2) 158, 159, 162, 527, 529, 530
dopaminergic receptor D3 (DRD3) 529, 530
dopaminergic system 51
DPWG (Dutch Pharmacogenetics Working Group) 534
DRD2 (dopaminergic receptor D2) 158, 159, 162, 527, 529, 530
DRD3 (dopaminergic receptor D3) 529, 530

drug-induced movement disorders 209
DSH (deliberate self harm) 334, 363
DSM-5: agoraphobia in 263; alcohol use disorder in 292; anxiety disorders in 266; APS in 247; BPD in 221, 224; categorical diagnosis in 471; cluster B personality disorders and 425; compulsive buying in 171; compulsive sexual behavior/sex addiction in 174; on differential diagnosis 343; eating disorders in 181, 183; gambling disorder in 169; impulse control disorders in 169; OCD in 287, 288; paraphilias defined and described in 428, 428; sleep disorders in 275, 283
DSM IV-TR 169
Dutch Pharmacogenetics Working Group (DPWG) 534
dysphoria 163, 169, 239

eating disorders 180–187; anorexia nervosa 183; avoidant/restrictive food intake disorder 184–185; bing eating disorder 184; bulimia nervosa 184; causes of 181–182; CBT for 362; child maltreatment and 182; classification and types of 183–185; complications of 182–183; developmental influences and 181; environmental influences and 182; epidemiology of 181; genetics and 181; night eating syndrome 185; non-pharmacological treatment of 186–187; other psychiatric illnesses and 182; overview of 180–181; parental influence and 182; peer and internet pressure and 182; pharmacological treatment of 185–186; pica 185; purging disorder 185; sleep-related 281; social isolation and 182
ECT *see* electro-convulsive therapy (ECT)
educational strategies: addressing the "how" 4–5; design process, summary of 10; example from practice (*see* practice, example from); learning objectives 5; models of learning 6–10, 11; pedagogical strategies 5–6; transfer of learning into practice 10; what healthcare professionals need to know 4
EEG *see* electroencephalogram (EEG)
EFT (emotional freedom technique) 290
Ekbom syndrome (restless legs syndrome) 282
elderly patients, psychiatric care in *see* geriatric psychiatry
elderly patients in pandemics and epidemics 499
electro-convulsive therapy (ECT): in geriatric psychiatry 206; in India 38; in Ireland 26; in Malaysia 371–375
electroencephalogram (EEG): in Malaysia 371; placement of electrodes on scalp 541; in REM/Nonrem sleep 274–275; in seizure 338
electronic neurocognitive rehabilitation program (e-NCRP) 132
emotional dysregulation 74, 169, 217, 221
emotional freedom technique (EFT) 290
emotion regulation, neural circuitry of 54
employment: place and train paradigms in 552–553; train and place approaches in 551–552
e-NCRP (electronic neurocognitive rehabilitation program) 132

endocrine disorders in HD 136–137; hypothalamic dysfunction 136; impaired glucose tolerance 136–137; lesion of the sex glands 137; metabolic disorders, weight loss and 137
England: involuntary care in 36; Mental Health Act 34
environmental factors that determine resilience 55
environment domain of QoL 20
enzyme 1A2 of cytochrome 450 (CYP1A2) 527, 529, 530
enzyme 2B6 of cytochrome 450 (CYP2B6) 162, 527
enzyme 2C9 of cytochrome 450 (CYP2C9) 527, 564
enzyme 2C19 of cytochrome 450 (CYP2C19) 160, 526, 527, 564
enzyme 2D6 of cytochrome 450 (CYP2D6) 157, 526, 527, 529–532, 532–533
enzyme 3A4 of cytochrome 450 (CYP3A4) 157, 527
epidemics *see* pandemics and epidemics
epigenetic mechanisms of resilience 52
epilepsy, progressive myoclonus type 2A (EPM2A) 529, 530
epileptic seizures, sleep-related 283
EPM2A (epilepsy, progressive myoclonus type 2A) 529, 530
EPS (extrapyramidal syndrome) 528–532; AP-induced 531–532, 532–533
EQ-5D (EuroQoL five-dimension) 24, 28
ERP-based psychotherapy 287
escitalopram 27, 104, 176, 262, 267
ethanol consumption/abuse *see* alcohol dependence
Europe: APS in 253; internet addiction in 177–178; risperidone for use in treatment of BPSD in 240; schizophrenia in, resilience and 56; suicide prevention in 46; work cooperatives in 552
European Association for Psychosomatic Medicine 334
European Psychiatric Association 253
European Union (EU), CPZ discontinued in 528
EuroQoL five-dimension (EQ-5D) 24, 28
excitement: causes of 347–348; in mood disorders 348; in neurotic disorders 348; overview of 347; in personality disorders 348; in psychotic disorders 347; in substance abuse 347
excoriation disorder 288
exhibitionistic disorder 428
exposure and response prevention (ERP)-based psychotherapy 287
extensive metabolizer (EM) 529, 530, 532
extrapyramidal syndrome (EPS) 528–532; AP-induced 531–532, 532–533
eye movements and disturbances in HD 141–142

FACT (forensic assertive community treatment) 430
factitious disorder 335, 343
family or domestic violence, psychiatric care in 479
family therapy: for APS 252; for eating disorders 187
farmer suicides and their survivors 198–201; *see also* community psychiatry

574 • INDEX

FDA (Food and Drug Administration) 293, 302, 526
FD (frequency domain) in fNIRS 540, *540*
fear: in anxiety disorders 259; neural circuitry of 53; in specific phobias 270
fetishistic disorder 428
Finland, assistance and open dialogue in 115
firearms, violence risk assessment and 96
5HT2C (5-hydroxytryptamine 2C receptor) 527
5-hydroxytryptamine 2C receptor (5HT2C) 527
fixations in HD 141
fMRI *see* functional MRI (fMRI)
fNIRS *see* functional near-infrared spectroscopy (fNIRS)
Food and Drug Administration (FDA) 293, 302, 526
forensic assertive community treatment (FACT) 430
forensic patients 92–93
forensic psychiatry 421–432; actuarial *vs.* structured professional judgment instruments 423–425; compulsory nature of forensic mental healthcare and 431; forensic outreach in community 429–432; forensic outreach service delivery and 430–431; forensic system and 422–423; insanity defense and 422; models of community care in 430; overview of 421–423; personality disorder and psychopathy and 425; risk for violence, assessing 422–425; sexual behaviour problems and 427–429, 428; substance use disorders and 425–427; transition in forensic mental healthcare and 431–432; unstructured *vs.* structured risk assessment 423
forensic risk assessment *see* community case managed clients
frailty in dementia 240–241
France, sexual dysfunction and, cross-sectional study on 104
frequency domain (FD) in fNIRS 540, *540*
Friendship Bench 462
frontotemporal dementia 233, 239
frotteuristic disorder 428
functional MRI (fMRI) 515–522; in ADHD 520–521; advantages/disadvantages of 518; basics of 515–516; in bipolar disorder 519–520; cerebral blood flow in 517; future clinical applications of 521–522; guidelines for patient training 516; guidelines for scanning 516–517; in major depression 519; in OCD 520; overview of 515; PET 518–521; post-processing guidelines in 517–518; in PTSD 520; resting state in 517; in schizophrenia 519; studies in psychiatric diseases 517; in substance abuse 521; task-based scans in 517
functional near-infrared spectroscopy (fNIRS) 538–543; applications of 542–543; components of 539; continuous measurement in 539–540, *540*; frequency domain in 540, *540*; future directions in 543–544; MRI for validation study with 541; NIRS instrumentation and brain oximetry in 539–541; optode placement in 541; other neuroimaging modalities compared to 541–542, *542*; overview of 538; principles of 538–539; studies of 543; time-domain in 540, *540*

GABA *see* gamma-aminobutyric acid (GABA)
GABA B-receptor (GABBR1) 160
gabapentin 156, 563
GABBR1 (GABA B-receptor) 160
GAD *see* generalized anxiety disorder (GAD)
Gambler's fallacy 170–171
gambling disorder 170–171; fallacies observed in gamblers 170–171; formal diagnosis in ICD 11 171; overview of 170
gamma-aminobutyric acid (GABA): alcohol dependence and 157–158, 159, 160; GAD and 268; HD and 135; resilience and 51; sleep disorders and 274, 276
gastroesophageal reflux, sleep-related 283
gastrointestinal disorders in HD 139
Gatekeeper model 211
GDS (Geriatric Depression Scale) 210, 409
gene cept assay 527
generalized anxiety disorder (GAD) 267–270; CBT for 269; clinical features of 267; comorbidities in 268; definition of 267; early experiences and 269; epidemiology of 268; genetic factors in 269; in homeless 193; neurological basis of 268; OCD with 288; personality and 268; prognosis in 269; psychoanalytic theory in 269; stressful events and 269; treatment in 269
generic scales in measurement of quality of life (QoL) 22, 23–24
gene sight psychotropic algorithm 527
genetic engineering in chemical addiction treatment 156, 163–164
genetic factors: in eating disorders 181; in GAD 269; in social anxiety disorder 264; in specific phobias 271
genetic methods to personalise pharmacotherapy 156–163; for alcohol dependence 157–160, 161; for cocaine addiction 162–163; for nicotine dependence 162; for opioid dependence 156–157
Geriatric Depression Scale (GDS) 210, 409
geriatric psychiatry 204–214; blood investigations in 207–208; diagnostic possibilities coexisting with psychiatric disorders in 207; history taking in 205–207; HOPES model in 211; IMPACT model in 210; integrated and multi-disciplinary approaches in 213–214; models for older nursing home residents 212–214; PATCH program in 211; patient interview in 204–205; PEARLS in 210; physical examination in 207; PRISM-E study model in 210–211; psychosocial rehabilitation in 548; psychotropic drug monitoring in 209, 209; scales for use in 209–210; WRAP program in 211–212
Geriatric Resources for Assessment and Care of Elders (GRACE) model 214
Germany, internet addiction in 178
Ghana's Mental Health Act 35
global mental health approaches 457–463
GQOL (Geriatric Quality of Life) 210

GRACE (Geriatric Resources for Assessment and Care of Elders) model 214
green skilling activity 445, *447*, 447–448, 449
group IPT 386–387
group psychotherapy in NCRP 129–130

habit disorders 286–290; *see also* obsessive-compulsive disorder (OCD)
habit reversal therapy (HRT) 289
hair-pulling disorder (trichotillomania) 288
hallucinations: causes of 350–351; hypnagogic and hypnopompic 278; in mood disorders 351; in neurotic disorders 351; overview of 350; in personality disorders 351; in psychotic disorders 351; sleep-related 281; in substance abuse 350–351
HD *see* Huntington's disease (HD)
healthcare workers in pandemics and epidemics 498–499
health promotion and disease prevention in mental health 44–45
health-related QoL (HRQoL) 20; *see also* quality of life (QoL)
Helping Older People Experience Success (HOPES) model 211
hemolysis, sleep-related 283
hippocampus: behavioral addictions and 170; BPD and 217–218; GAD and 268; HD and 136; panic disorder and 261; PTSD and 519; resilience and 51, 52, 53, 54; schizophrenia and 519
history taking in geriatric psychiatry 205–207; medical complaints 205–206; past psychiatric history 206; personality assessment 206; presenting complaints 205; social history 206; substance use history 206–207
hoarding disorder 288
homeless mentally ill patients in India 191–196; administration and policy factors in 193; challenges in 194–195; context of 192; delivery of service factors in 193–194; factors contributing to 193–194; future directions for optimizing care for 196; illness factors in 194; overview of 191–192; policies and programmes in 195–196; prevalence of 192–193; rehabilitation services in 195; societal factors in 194
HOPES (Helping Older People Experience Success) model 211
hormones in sexual response cycle 101
House Tree Person (HTP) Test 481–494, *484*, *485*, *486*, *487–488*, *489*, *490–491*, *492–493*
HPA (hypothalamus-pituitary-adrenal) axis 51, 136, 217, 265
HRQoL (health-related QoL) 20; *see also* quality of life (QoL)
HRT (habit reversal therapy) 289
HTP (House Tree Person) Test 481–494, *484*, *485*, *486*, *487–488*, *489*, *490–491*, *492–493*

Huntington's disease (HD) 134–143; autonomic nervous system in, damage to (*see* autonomic nervous system in HD, damage to); endocrine disorders in 136–137; haematological disorders in 140; huntingtin and 135; ophthalmic manifestations of (*see* ophthalmic manifestations of HD); overview of 135; skeletal muscle atrophy in 140–141; skeletal system in, damage to 139–140
hydrophobia 270
hydroxychloroquine 564
hypersomnia 277, 283
hypersomnolence disorders 277
hyperventilation in GAD 267
hypnagogic and hypnopompic hallucinations 278
hypothalamic dysfunction 136
hypothalamic dysfunction in HD 136
hypothalamus: BPD and 218; HD and 136, 138; resilience and 51, 52; sexual response cycle and 101, 103; sleep disorders and 274
hypothalamus-pituitary-adrenal (HPA) axis 51, 136, 217, 265

IACAPAP (International Association for Child and Adolescent Psychiatry and Allied Professions) 468
ICD-10 275
ICD-11: alcohol use disorder in 292; anxiety disorders in 266; categorical diagnosis in 471; compulsive sexual behavior/sex addiction in 174, 175; disorders due to addictive behaviors in 172; gambling disorder in 171
ID (intellectual disability) 26
idiopathic CSA 279
idiopathic hypersomnia 277
IDUQoL (Injection Drug User QoL Scale) 25, 28
IGD *see* internet gaming disorder (IGD)
IMPACT (Improving Mood-Promoting Access to Collaborative Treatment) 210
impaired glucose tolerance in HD 136–137
Improving Mood-Promoting Access to Collaborative Treatment (IMPACT) 210
impulse-control disorders 171, *171*, 288
India; *see also* Richmond Fellowship Society (RFS), Bangalore: ADs in 113; community psychiatry in 198–201; COVID-19–related suicide cases in 47; disulfiram for alcohol dependence in 295, 297; farmer suicides in 198–201; group IPT for depression in 387; health budget allocated to mental health in 199, 470; health promotion and disease prevention in mental health in 44; homelessness in 192–196; HTP Test in 481–494, *484*, *485*, *486*, *487–488*, *489*, *490–491*, *492–493*; human resources in, shortage of 38; innovations in community mental health in 461; MCHA in 37–39, 114, 117–118, 195–196; mental health legislation in 37–39; Mental Health Review Boards in 37; NIMHANS in 472; optimising mental health care in 196; place and

train paradigms in 552–553; policies and programmes for mental health care in 195–196; rehabilitation services in 195; rural psychiatry in 199–200; school counselors in 418, 419; sexually active older adults in 106; Special Marriage Act in 118; stigma surrounding mental illnesses in 43; train and place approaches in 551; treatment gap for mental health care in 436–437; urban population of, mental health services and 79; work cooperatives in 552–553

informed consent, coercive practices and 112–113
Injection Drug User QoL Scale (IDUQoL) 25, 28
inpatient programs for eating disorders 187
insanity defense 422
insertion (Ins) 529
insomnia disorder 275–276; cognitive restructuring in 276; definition of 275; history and physical examination in 275–276; pharmacological treatment in 276; sleep hygiene measures (non-pharmacological) in 276
Inspector of Mental Health Services, Ireland's 36
instructivism 6, 11
integrated treatment in APS 254
intellectual disability (ID) 26
intermediate metabolizer (IM) 529, 531, 532
International Association for Child and Adolescent Psychiatry and Allied Professions (IACAPAP) 468
International Classification of Diseases *see* ICD-10; ICD-11
International College of Psychosomatic Medicine 334
International Organization for Consultation-Liaison Psychiatry 334
internet addiction 172–175; adverse effects of 172; assessment and screening 175–176; compulsive sexual behavior/sex addiction 174, 174–175, 176; compulsive shopping and buying 172–173, 173, 175; internet gaming disorder 172, 175; interventional modalities for 177; in South Korea 177–178
internet gaming disorder (IGD) 172; assessment and screening of 175; pharmacotherapy for 176
interpersonal psychotherapy (IPT) 384, 385–386; for depression 387; group 386–387; NSHW-delivered 459; for OCD 289; overview of 385–386; phases of treatment in 385–386; principles of 386; strategies for key problems and 386
intervention programs for COPMI 86–88; combined and integrated intervention program 88; intervention for community 88; interventions for children 87–88; interventions for professionals 88; for parents with mental illness 87; summary of domains and types of 89
involuntary treatment: case for 115–116; limiting coercion for individuals receiving 116–118
IPT *see* interpersonal psychotherapy (IPT)
IPT-GU (Group IPT in Uganda) 387
IPT Model of Depression 386

Ireland: Assisted Decision-Making (Capacity) Act 37, 114; Inspector of Mental Health Services 36; mental capacity legislation in 114; Mental Health Act 35, 36; mental health legislation in 35–37
Israel: child and adolescent psychiatry in 469; Ultra-Rapid Opiate Detoxification (UROD) in 312
Italy: internet addiction in 172; sexually active older adults in, cognitive functioning and 106; work cooperatives in 552

jactatio capitis nocturna (sleep rhythmic movement disorder) 282
Japan: fasting camps in 177–178; fNIRS approved in 543; resilience among patients of schizophrenia in 56
Japanese Health Ministry 543
job clubs 552
job coach 552
job maintenance 552
job training 551
Jyothi, long stay home 445

Kleine–Levin syndrome 277
kleptomania 169, 170
KLH (Kuala Lumpur Hospital) 372–373
Korsakoff syndrome 293
Kuala Lumpur Hospital (KLH) 372–373

Lancashire Quality of Life Profile (LQoLP) 24, 26, 28
Lawson Health Research Institute (LHRI) 408
learning: models of 6–10, 11; objectives 11; transfer of, into practice 10
leg cramps, sleep-related 282
Lehman Quality of Life Interview and Quality of Life Scale 26
lesion of the cortical part of the visual pathway in HD 142
lesion of the sex glands in HD 137
level of independence domain of QoL 19
Lewy body dementia 233, 238–239
LHRI (Lawson Health Research Institute) 408
life satisfaction, in QoL 19
Life Satisfaction Index 27
lithium: for bipolar disorder 105; contraindicated for COVID-19 563; drug-monitoring parameters when prescribing psychotropics in the elderly 209; during ECT 374; for hypersomnia 277; for pathological gambling 176; for suicide prevention in BPD 223
LQoLP (Lancashire Quality of Life Profile) 24, 26, 28

magnetic resonance imaging (MRI): in C-L psychiatry 337; in dementia 234, 235; functional (*see* functional MRI (fMRI)); in geriatric psychiatry 208; mobile scanners in telepsychiatry 401; in schizophrenia 443; for validation study in fNIRS 541
major depressive disorder (MDD) 222, 225, 437, 543

INDEX • 577

Malaysia, ECT in 371–375; CIVID-19 and 374; future directions of 374–375; laws governing mental healthcare in 371; Nationwide ECT Survey 2020 and 373–374; neuropsychiatry in KLH 372–373
malingering 335, 343, 353, 436
massively multiplayer online role-playing game (MMORPG) 172
MCI *see* mild cognitive impairment (MCI)
McNaughton Rules 422
MDD (major depressive disorder) 222, 225, 437, 543
MDS (Minimum Data Set) 213
measurement of quality of life (QoL) 20–22; commonly used instruments to assess QoL 23–25; evaluation in patients with psychiatric disorders, role of 21–22; generic scales *vs.* disorder-specific scales 22; impact of time on QoL assessment 22; subjective *vs.* objective assessment of QoL 21
mechanical ventilation 279
medical gymnastics in NCRP 130–131
medical management in NCRP 131
Medical Outcomes Study Short Form – 36 items (SF-36) 23, 26, 27, 28
medication; *see also* pharmacological interventions: administration of, in Ireland 36; CTOs and 117; errors 438; medication optimization approach for bipolar mood disorder 152; in NCRP 131; neuroleptic 56; open dialogue to reduce use of 115; prescribed by PCPs 80; for psychoactive drug dependence (*see* pharmacogenetics in management of addictions); in research on QoL 22, 26; for sexual dysfunction 102–103; for sexual functioning in cognitive impairment 106; for treating psychiatric consequences of VAW 74
medication compliance: C-L psychiatry and 335; mobile apps and 45; social worker's role in 438–439; suicide and 46, 47
melanocortin 4 receptor (MC4R) 527
memory clinics in Moscow *see* neurocognitive rehabilitation program (NCRP) in Moscow
menstrual-related hypersomnia 277
mental health access to the unreached *see* mobile mental health
Mental Health Act (England and Wales) 34
Mental Health Act (Ireland) 35–37
Mental Healthcare Act (MCHA) in India 37–39, 114, 117–118, 195–196
Mental Health Commission 36
Mental Health Engagement Network (MHEN) 408–409
mental health first aid 45–46
mental health Gap Action Programme (mhGAP) 468
mental health legislation: history of 33–34; in India 37–39; in Ireland 35–37; need for 34; overview 33–35
Mental Health Review Boards 37
mental retardation in homeless 193

mental status examination (MSE) in C-L psychiatry 336–337
metabolic disorders in HD, weight loss and 137
methadone 157
methylphenidate 176, 277, 521
mHealth (mobile health) 45; *see also* mobile mental health
MHEN (Mental Health Engagement Network) 408–409
mhGAP (mental health Gap Action Programme) 468
Middle East, suicide prevention in 46
mild cognitive impairment (MCI) 125–126; *see also* neurocognitive rehabilitation program (NCRP) in Moscow; cognitive psychodrama for 130; memory clinics in Moscow for 125–126
Mini-Mental State Examination (MMSE) 409
Minimum Data Set (MDS) 213
minors *see* child and adolescent psychiatry
mirror neuron system 54
MMORPG (massively multiplayer online role-playing game) 172
MMSE (Mini-Mental State Examination) 409
mobile health (mHealth) 45; *see also* mobile mental health
mobile mental health 45, 79–81; awareness regarding mental health problems and 81; mobile phones in 80–81; policies, plans and laws in 80; primary healthcare in 79–80; in urban population of India 79
mobile phones: role of, in mobile mental health 80–81; smartphone technology and 405–411
models of learning: instructivism 6; situated learning 7–8; social cognitivism 6–7; social constructivism 8; summary of 11
molecular genetics of resilience 52–53
Monte Carlo fallacy 170–171
mood disorders; *see also* anxiety disorders; bipolar disorder: aggression in 350; agitation in 345; bizarre behaviour in 346; BPD with 221; catatonia in 347; CBT for 362; cognitive reappraisal and 54; excitement in 348; hallucinations in 351; psychomotor retardation in 349; self-neglect in 344; suicide in, attempted 352; unexplained somatic symptoms in 353
motivational interviewing for eating disorders 187
motivational pharmacotherapy in bipolar disorder 152
movement disorders: akathesia 352; drug-induced 209; hypothalamic dysfunction and 136; sleep-related 282–283
MRI *see* magnetic resonance imaging (MRI)
MSE (mental status examination) in C-L psychiatry 336–337
muscle tension in GAD 267
mysophobia 270

N-acetyl cysteine 176
N-acetyl homotaurine 157–158
nail-biting (onychophagia) 288, 289
nalmefene 158–159

578 • INDEX

naltrexone (NTX): for alcohol dependence 155–156, 158, 161; for behavioral addictions 176; blockade 308–310; case history 310; challenges 309; future developments 313–314; initiating treatment 311–313; for opiate overdose prevention 310; for opioid use disorders 156, 300–314; overview of 300–303; problems of 308; psychological, pharmacological and educational components of 303–308; sexual function and 310–311

narcolepsy 277–278; cataplexy and 277–278; characteristics of 277; etiology of 278; hypnagogic and hypnopompic hallucinations and 278; sleep-onset REM latency and 278; sleep paralysis and 278; tests in 278; treatment in 278

National Institute for Health and Care Excellence (NICE) 234, 235–236, 237, 238

National Institute of Drug Addiction of the United States (NIDA) 164

National Institute of Mental Health and Neurosciences, Bengaluru (NIMHANS) 193, 443, 448, 472

Nationwide ECT Survey 2020 373–374

NCRMD (not criminally responsible on account of mental disorder) 422

NCRP in Moscow *see* neurocognitive rehabilitation program (NCRP) in Moscow

near misses 171

nefazodone 104

neural circuitry of resilience 53–54; additional relevant neural circuits 54; neural circuitry of emotion regulation 54; neural circuitry of fear 53; neural circuitry of reward 53–54

neural mechanisms in specific phobias 271

neurobiology of sexual response cycle 101

neurochemicals in social anxiety disorder 265

neurocognitive rehabilitation program (NCRP) in Moscow 124–132; characteristics of 126–127; cognitive training in 127–129; COVID-19 and 132; daily schedule in *126*; effectiveness of 131; e-NCRP 132; group psychotherapy in 129–130; medical gymnastics in 130–131; medical management in 131; memory clinics and 125–126

neurodevelopmental disorder, BPD with 221

neuroimaging *see individual techniques*

neurons: alcohol dependence and 157, 159; in developing brain 466; dopaminergic 53–54; GAD and 268; glutamatergic 159; HD and 135, 136, 138; noradrenergic 157, 268; orexinergic 136; resilience and 51, 53–54; sleep disorders and 274

neuropeptide Y (NPY) 52

neuropsychiatric symptoms in dementia 234

neuropsychiatry in KLH 372–373

neurotic disorders: aggression in 350; agitation in 345; bizarre behaviour in 346; catatonia in 347; excitement in 348; hallucinations in 351; psychomotor retardation in 349; self-neglect in 344; suicide in, attempted 352; unexplained somatic symptoms in 353

neuroticism 268

neurotransmitters in sexual response cycle 101

New Zealand's Mental Health (Compulsory Assessment and Treatment) Act 34

NGOs (nongovernmental organisations) 73, 92, 95–96, 115, 196, 200–201, 376, 378–379, 443–446, 469, 470

NICE (National Institute for Health and Care Excellence) 234, 235–236, 237, 238

nicotine dependence 156, 162

nicotine replacement therapy 162

NIDA (National Institute of Drug Addiction of the United States) 164

night eating disorder 185; pharmacological treatment of 186

nightmare disorder 281

NIMHANS (National Institute of Mental Health and Neurosciences, Bengaluru) 193, 443, 448, 472

nocturnal myoclonus 282

nominated representatives (NRs) 114

nongovernmental organisations (NGOs) 73, 92, 95–96, 115, 196, 200–201, 376, 378–379, 443–446, 469, 470

non-paraphilic hypersexuality 169

non-rapid eye movement (NREM) sleep 274–275, 280

non-suicidal self injury 221, 322, 363, 364

noradrenergic system 51

not criminally responsible on account of mental disorder (NCRMD) 422–423

NPY (neuropeptide Y) 52

NREM (non-rapid eye movement) sleep 274–275, 280

NRs (nominated representatives) 114

NTX *see* naltrexone (NTX)

nurses in psychopharmacology 439–440

Nursing Home Reform Act (1987) 213

nursing home residents, models for older 212–214

nutritional rehabilitation for eating disorders 187

objective assessment of QoL 21

obsessive-compulsive disorder (OCD) 286–290; aversion stimulus for 289–290; CBT for 288–289; components of psychiatric management in 287–288; diagnostic criteria for 288; EFT for 290; ERP-based psychotherapy for 287; fMRI in 520; fNIRS in 543; HRT for 289; IPT for 289; nail cosmetics for 289; NICE Guidelines for interventions in 286; OCRDs and 288; overview of 286; self-help techniques for 290; SSRIs in 288; stimulus control for 289

obsessive compulsive related disorders (OCRDs) 288; *see also* obsessive-compulsive disorder (OCD)

obstructive sleep apnea (OSA) 279

OCD *see* obsessive-compulsive disorder (OCD)

oculomotor disorders in HD 141, 141–142

ondansetron 160, 161

online gaming 169, 170
onychophagia (nail-biting) 288, 289
OOD (opiate overdose deaths) 310
ophthalmic manifestations of HD 141–142; eye movements and disturbances in 141–142; lesion of the cortical part of the visual pathway 142; oculomotor disorders 141; retinal changes 142; visual function 141; visual hallucinations 142
opiate overdose deaths (OOD) 310
opioid dependence 156–157
opioid receptor agonists 157
opioid receptor antagonists 156, 158
oppositional defiant disorder (ODD) 470
optokinetic reflex in HD 142
organic causes: of aggression 349; of agitation 344; of bizarre behaviour 345; of catatonia 346; of excitement 347; of hallucinations 350; of psychomotor retardation 348; of self-neglect 343; of suicide, attempted 351; of unexplained somatic symptoms 352
OSA (obstructive sleep apnea) 279
overall QoL and general health beliefs domain of QoL 20
oxytocin in promoting social attachment 54

paedophilic disorder 428
PAIS (Psychosocial Adjustment to Illness Scale, interview version), and Self-Report Version (PAIS-SR) 23
pandemics and epidemics 47, 495–508; see also COVID-19; accommodation needs in 505; addiction in 500; characteristics of outbreaks of 496; children and adolescents in 499–500; community needs and 501; cultural status in 505–506; elderly in 499; formats of interventions and plans in 506; future challenges in 507–508; healthcare workers in 498–499; intervention in 503–507; leaders in 502; mental health during in aftermath of outbreaks 496–498; mental health during outbreaks 496–501; overview of 495; planning in 501–502; prediction of high-risk patients in future 507; preexisting psychiatric disorders and 500–501, 506–507; prevention of 501–502; research on 502; risk factors and vulnerable populations in 498–501; schools and, intervention in 505; social support and safety in 507; special populations in 500; stigma and, education to erase 504; survivors of 498; telepsychiatry in 507–508; training and education in 503–504; vaccination hesitancy in 506
panic disorder 260–262; agoraphobia with 263; CBT for 262, 365; characteristics of 260; clinical features of 261; comorbidities in 262; course and prognosis in 262; definition of 260; diagnostic criteria for 260; differential diagnosis in 261–262; in disaster survivors 497; DSM 5 criteria for 260; epidemiology of 260; excitement with 348; fNIRS in 543; generalized anxiety disorder with 267, 268; genetic factors in 261; in homeless 193; neuroanatomical changes in 261; neurochemistry in 261; OCD with 288; panic attacks in 260; panicogens in 261; pharmacotherapy for 262; psychoeducation for 262; psychotherapy for 262; psychosocial factors in 261; QoL of patients with 27; social anxiety disorder with 266; suicide and, attempted 352; treatment for 262
paraphilic disorders 175, 422, 428, 428
parasomnias 280–282; drug or substance use-related 281–282; medical-related 281–282; nightmare disorder 281; NREM sleep arousal disorders 280; recurrent isolated sleep paralysis 281; REM sleep behavior disorder 281; sleep enuresis 281; sleep-related eating disorder 281; sleep-related hallucinations 281
parents with mental illness, interventions for 87
Parkinson's disease dementia 233, 239
partial opioid receptor agonist-antagonists 157
PASRR (Preadmission Screening and Resident Review Program) 213
PATCH (Psycho-Geriatric Assessment and Treatment in City Housing) 211
pathological gambling (PG) 169, 170–171; assessment and screening of 175, 177; disulfiram for 295; Gambler's fallacy or Monte Carlo fallacy in 170–171; interventional modalities for 176–177, 178; pharmacotherapy for 176
patient engagement in bipolar disorder 153–154
patient interview in geriatric psychiatry 204–205
patient-reported outcome measures (PROs) 20
PCR (polymerase chain reaction) 526
PEARLS (Program to Encourage Active and Rewarding Lives for Seniors) 210
pedagogical strategies 5–6, 11–14
periodic leg movement disorder 282
personal factors that determine resilience 54, 55
personality disorders: aggression in 350; agitation in 345; bizarre behaviour in 346; BPD with 221; catatonia in 347; CBT for 363; excitement in 348; forensic psychiatry in 425; hallucinations in 351; psychomotor retardation in 349; self-neglect in 344; sexual response cycle in 105–106; suicide in, attempted 352; unexplained somatic symptoms in 353
Personal Recovery Framework 379
person with dementia (PWD) 26
Peru's Mental Health Law 29889 35
PET see positron emission tomography (PET)
PFA see psychological first aid (PFA)
PFI (preventive family intervention) 88
PG see pathological gambling (PG)
PGx (pharmacogenetic testing) 525–527, 531–532
pharmacists in psychopharmacology 440–441
pharmacogenetics in management of addictions 155–164, 161; for alcohol dependence 155–156, 157–160, 161; for cocaine addiction 162–163; genetic engineering in chemical addiction treatment 156, 163–164; genetic

methods for personalisation of 156–163; hereditary factors influencing response to 156; for nicotine dependence 156, 162–163; for opioid dependence 156–157

pharmacogenetic testing (PGx) 525–527, 531–532

pharmacological interventions; *see also* medication: for agoraphobia 264; for anxiety disorders 267; for APS 250–251; for behavioral addiction 176; for bipolar disorder 152; for dementia 236–239; genetic methods to personalise 156–163; for insomnia disorder 276; for panic disorder 262; in social anxiety disorder 267

physical domain of QoL 19

physical examination: in C-L psychiatry 336–337; in geriatric psychiatry 207

pica 185

place and train paradigms 552–553; job clubs in 552; job coach in 552; work cooperatives in 552–553

PM (poor metabolizer) 529, 530, 531, 532

polymerase chain reaction (PCR) 526

poor metabolizer (PM) 529, 530, 531, 532

positron emission tomography (PET) 518–521; in ADHD 520–521; in bipolar disorder 519–520; in major depression 519; in OCD 520; overview of 518; in PTSD 520; in schizophrenia 519; in substance abuse 521

post-traumatic stress disorder (PTSD): aggression with 350; agoraphobia with 263; BPD with 218, 222; CBT for 364; CPT for 387, 389; in disaster survivors 497, 498, 502; fMRI in 515, 520; in homeless 193; panic attacks with 262; PET in 518; resilience and 53, 55; suicide with, attempted 352; trauma history and 222; VAW and 74; in victims of sexual assault 389

practice, example from 11–15; context 11; learning objectives 11; overall aim of the teaching session 11; pedagogical strategies and teaching methods 11–14; simulation format 14–15

Preadmission Screening and Resident Review Program (PASRR) 213

pregabalin 159–160

prepared learning in specific phobias 271

PREVENT (Providing Resources Early to Vulnerable Elders Needing Treatment) 212

preventive family intervention (PFI) 88

PRISM-E study model 210–211

professional judgment instruments, actuarial *vs.* structured 423–425

professionals, interventions for 88

Program to Encourage Active and Rewarding Lives for Seniors (PEARLS) 210

PROs (patient-reported outcome measures) 20

Providing Resources Early to Vulnerable Elders Needing Treatment (PREVENT) 212

proximal-level intervention 73–74; for children and family 73; for perpetrators 74

psychiatric disorders, QoL research in caregivers of patients with 28

psychoanalytic theory: for GAD 269; in specific phobias 271

psychobiology of resilience 51–52; BDNF and 52; HPA axis and 51; noradrenergic system and 51; NPY and 52; serotonergic and dopaminergic systems and 51

psychoeducation: for agoraphobia 264; for BPD 223; in CBT 360–361; for disulfiram 297–298; family therapy and 553; for panic disorder 262; in telepsychiatry and self-help 400–401

Psycho-Geriatric Assessment and Treatment in City Housing (PATCH) 211

psychological arousal in GAD 267

psychological domain of QoL 19

psychological first aid (PFA) 561–563; benefits of 562; in COVID-19 562; description of 561–562; in previous pandemics 562–563

psychomotor retardation: causes of 348–349; in mood disorders 349; in neurotic disorders 349; overview of 348; in personality disorders 349; in psychotic disorders 349; in substance abuse 348

psychoneurological diseases 524–534; biomedical products for 525; chlorpromazine for 527–533, *531*, 532–533; new approaches to treatment of 526; personalized medicine in 525; pharmacogenetic testing for 526–527; pharmacogenomics in 525

psychopharmacology 436–441; caregivers in 437–438; for COVID-19 558, 563–565; nurses in 439–440; overview of 436–437; pharmacists in 440–441; social health care workers in 438–439

psychosis; *see also* attenuated psychosis syndrome (APS); schizophrenia: CBT for 363; in children and adolescents 467; in COPMI 86; disulfiram-induced 293, 296; in geriatric patient 207; involuntary treatment and 116; neuroimaging for 337–338; psychoeducation and family therapy for 553; psychopharmacology in COVID-19 and 563–564; resilience and 56; telepsychiatry and 400

Psychosocial Adjustment to Illness Scale, interview version (PAIS), and Self-Report Version (PAIS-SR) 23

psychosocial interventions in APS 251–252

psychosocial rehabilitation 545–554; case management in 549; characteristics of 546; cognitive remediation in 550–551; components of 548–553; objectives of 545–546; overview of 545; populations benefiting from 547–548; psychiatrists role in 554; psychoeducation and family therapy in 553; psychotherapeutic interventions in 549–553; self-efficacy and management of illness in 549; skill training and rehabilitation in 549; social skills training in 549–550; strategies of 548; supported employment in 553; symptomatic remission in 548–549; vocational rehabilitation in 551–553 psychotherapy 384–393; CBT 384, 385; CPT 384, 387–389; DBT 384, 389–391; for eating disorders 187; forensic psychiatry and 425; future directions of 392–393; group, in NCRP 129–130; group IPT 386–387; IPT 384, 385–386; for optimizing patient care 384–393; RCTs in 384; REBT 384, 391–392; for social anxiety disorder 266–267; for suicide 327–330; telepsychiatry in 400

psychotic disorders: aggression in 350; agitation in 345; bizarre behaviour in 345; catatonia in 347; disease-specific scales for 24, 26; excitement in 347; hallucinations in 351; psychomotor retardation in 349; QoL of patients with 26–27; self-neglect in 344; suicide in, attempted 352; unexplained somatic symptoms in 352

psychotropic drug monitoring in geriatric psychiatry 209

PTSD *see* post-traumatic stress disorder (PTSD)

public health-mental health integration 45–47; mental health first aid in 45–46; substance abuse education programming in 46–47; suicide prevention programs in 46; Wellness Recovery Action Plan (WRAP) in 46

purging disorder 185

PWD (person with dementia) 26

pyrophobia 270

QLDS (Quality of Life in Depression Scale) 24, 27

Q-LES-Q (Quality of Life Enjoyment & Satisfaction Questionnaire) 23, 27

QLI (Quality of Life Index) 23

QLS (Quality of Life Scale) 24

QoL *see* quality of life (QoL)

QoL-AD-SR (Quality of Life in Alzheimer's Disease Self-Rating scale) 25, 26

QoL-BD (Quality of life in Bipolar Disorder) 25

QOLI (Quality of Life Inventory) 23, 27

QoL Scale for Drug Addicts 28

QUALID (Quality of Life in Late Stage Dementia) 210

quality of life (QoL): concept of 18; defining 19–20; dimensions of 19; measurement of 20–22; research on, in major psychiatric disorders 22–28, 23–25; strategies to improve 28; WHO domains 19, 19–20

Quality of Life Enjoyment & Satisfaction Questionnaire (Q-LES-Q) 23, 27

Quality of Life in Alzheimer's Disease Self-Rating scale (QoL-AD-SR) 25, 26

Quality of life in Bipolar Disorder (QoL-BD) 25

Quality of Life in Depression Scale (QLDS) 24, 27

Quality of Life Index (QLI) 23

Quality of Life Index for Mental Health 26

Quality of Life Inventory (QOLI) 23, 27

Quality of Life Scale (QLS) 24

QualityRights initiative (WHO): ADs 113; autonomy and patient choice 111, 119; capacity 112; decision-making 115; involuntary treatment 39, 116

Queensland University of Technology (QUT) 234, 236

QUT (Queensland University of Technology) 234, 236

rapid eye movement (REM) 274–275; parasomnias associated with 281; sleep behavior disorder 281; sleep-onset REM latency 278

rapid opiate detoxification (ROD) 312

rational emotive behaviour therapy (REBT) 358, 391–392

REBT (rational emotive behaviour therapy) 358, 391–392

recurrent isolated sleep paralysis 281

rehabilitation and recovery 376–382; *see also* psychosocial rehabilitation; alliance between 377; assessment in 379; challenges in 382; CHIME framework for measuring personal recovery in 382; defined 377; for homeless mentally ill patients in India 195; motivational interviewing in 380; needs met in 381; overview of 376–377; partnership in 379–380; personal experience of recovery and 378; Personal Recovery Framework analysis in 379; principles of recovery-oriented practice and 378; recovery-oriented rehabilitation workforce in 378–379; rehabilitation setup in 379–381; safety and quality of service delivery in 381; self-management skills 380; strength-based interventions in 380; supervision and reflective practice in 381; therapeutic relationship in 379; therapeutic use of environment in 380; types of rehabilitation in 378; workforce and professional development in 380–381

REM *see* rapid eye movement (REM)

research on QoL in major psychiatric disorders 22–28, 23–25; anxiety disorders 27; bipolar disorder 27; caregivers of patients with psychiatric disorders 28; depressive disorders 27; intellectual disability 26; patients with dementia 26; schizophrenia/psychotic disorders 26–27; substance abuse disorders 27–28

resilience 50–58; concept of 50–51; epigenetic mechanisms of 52; factors determining 54–55; indicators of 55–56; interventions based on 57; molecular genetics of 52–53; neural circuitry of (*see* neural circuitry of resilience); psychobiology of (*see* psychobiology of resilience); rehospitalization and 56–57; schizophrenia and 56; transcriptional mechanisms of 52–53

Resource Book on Mental Health, Human Rights and Legislation (WHO) 36, 38, 116

restless legs syndrome (Ekbom syndrome) 282

retinal changes in HD 142

reward, neural circuitry of 53–54

RF ASPAC (Richmond Fellowship Asia Pacific Forum) 371–372, 443

RF PG College (Richmond Fellowship Post Graduate College for psychosocial rehabilitation) 448

RFS, Bangalore *see* Richmond Fellowship Society (RFS), Bangalore

Richmond Fellowship Asia Pacific Forum (RF ASPAC) 371–372, 443
Richmond Fellowship Post Graduate College for psychosocial rehabilitation (RF PG College) 448
Richmond Fellowship Society (RFS), Bangalore 442–456; Asha, halfway home and 444–445; branches of 444; challenges of, future 454; community-centred interventions and 453; dignity and, restoring 453–454; family-centred interventions and 452–453; green skilling activity in 445, *447*, 447–448, 449; individual-centred interventions and 452; Jyothi, long stay home and 445; psychological interventions and 451–452; psychosocial rehabilitation and 448–449; registration and other legal formalities and 454–455; rehabilitation components of 452–453; vocational rehabilitation and 449
risk assessment: actuarial methods of 93–94; in APS 249; forensic (*see* community case managed clients); in schizophrenia 249; in suicide *vs.* suicide prediction 318–319; tools 93–95; unstructured *vs.* structured 423; violence and firearms 96
ROD (rapid opiate detoxification) 312
Russia: child and adolescent psychiatry in 469; cognitive function and well-being of patients in 125, 132; CPZ to treat patients with schizophrenia in 528; drug dependence treatments in 155–156, 163, 301–302; memory clinics in (*see* neurocognitive rehabilitation program (NCRP) in Moscow); NTX and opiate overdose protection in 310; NTX injections and, RCTs of 301–302; PGx in, software for decoding 527; "quack" methods of treating alcoholism in 163; resilience-based interventions in 57
Russian Foundation of Basic Research 124, 131, 132, 155

saccades in HD 141
SAMHSA (United States Substance Abuse and Mental Health Services Administration) 46
SARS (severe acute respiratory syndrome) 495, 497, 557, 558, 562–563
Satisfaction with Life Scale 27
scales: in geriatric psychiatry 209–210; in measurement of QoL 22, 23–25
SCARF (Schizophrenia Research Foundation) 201
Scarf Telepsychiatry (STEP) 201
Schalok and Keith's QoL questionnaire 26
schizophrenia: CBT for 362; CPZ for 527–533, *531*, 532–533; disease-specific scales for 24, 26; ECT for 374; fMRI in 519; fNIRS in 543; PET in 519; phobic symptoms with 271; QoL of patients with 26–27; resilience and 56; risk assessment in 249; sexual dysfunction with 102–103; sleep difficulties with 284; social anxiety disorder with 266; suicide and 321
Schizophrenia Research Foundation (SCARF) 201
school mental health services 415–419; age-appropriate interventions in 417; building partnerships with teachers 416–417; future strategies in 418–419; incorporating school counseling in teacher and psychologist training and education 418; maintaining commitment despite poor gains 418; making your presence felt 416; moving away from just the special children 416; overview of 415; in pandemics and epidemics 505; reaching out to all age groups 417–418; school counselor's role in 415–416
SCQoL (Smoking Cessation QoL) Questionnaire 25, 28
screening *see* assessment and screening
seclusion and restraint: in involuntary treatment 117; in Ireland 36
seizures, sleep-related epileptic 283
selective mutism 266
selective serotonin reuptake inhibitors (SSRIs): for alcohol dependence 156, 160; for behavioral addictions 176; for eating disorders 186; for frontotemporal dementia 239; for OCD 288; for problematic sexual behaviours 429; for sleep disorders 278; for suicide prevention 324
self-agency 68, 69, 329
self-help groups for eating disorders 187
self-neglect 343–344
serotonergic system 51
7-HOCPZ (7-hydroxy chlorpromazine) 528
7-hydroxy chlorpromazine (7-HOCPZ) 528
severe acute respiratory syndrome (SARS) 495, 497, 557, 558, 562–563
severe illness, limiting coercion for individuals with 113–115
sex glands in HD, lesion of 137
sexological assessment 428–429
sexual assault, CPT for victims of 389
sexual dysfunction 100–106; CBT for 363; depression and 103; forensic psychiatry and 427–429; mental illness and 102–103; NTX and 310–311; overview of 102; paraphilic disorders described in DSM-5 428; schizophrenia and 102–103; sexological assessment and 428–429; sexual problem *vs.* 101; treatment of problematic sexual behaviours 429
sexuality: multidimensional concept of 100–101; normal or healthy, definition of 101; sexual problem *vs.* sexual dysfunction and 101; WHO definition of 100
sexual masochism disorder 428
sexual response cycle: anxiety disorders and 105–106; bipolar disorders and 105; cognitive impairment and 106; DEOR model of 101; depression and 103–106; neurobiology of 101; personality disorders and 105–106
sexual sadism disorder 428
sheltered employment 552
Short Form Health Survey 27
Simpson-Angus Scale 209
simulation format 14–15
single nucleotide variant (SNV) 526, 529, 530, 533, 534

situated learning 7–8, 11
skeletal muscle atrophy in HD 140–141
skeletal system in HD, damage to 139–140
skin picking 171, 288
SLC6A4 (solute carrier family 6 member 4) 161, 527
sleep: functions of 273–275; NREM sleep and 274; REM sleep and 274–275; requirements for 274; sleep-wake cycles and 274
sleep bruxism (tooth grinding) 282
sleep disorders 273–284; breathing-related 278–279; circadian rhythm 279–280; in clinical practice, significance of 283; in GAD 267; in HD 138; hypersomnolence disorders 277; insomnia disorder 275–276; medical disorders associated with 283; narcolepsy 277–278; overview of 273; parasomnias 280–282; sleep-related movement disorders 282–283
sleep enuresis 281
sleep-onset REM latency 278
sleep paralysis 278; recurrent isolated 281
sleep-related leg cramps 282
sleep-related movement disorders 282–283; due to drug or substance use 282; due to medical condition 282; leg cramps 282; periodic leg movement disorder 282; restless legs syndrome (Ekbom syndrome) 282; sleep bruxism (tooth grinding) 282; sleep rhythmic movement disorder (jactatio capitis nocturna) 282
sleep rhythmic movement disorder (jactatio capitis nocturna) 282
sleep terror disorder 280
sleep-wake cycles 274
sleep-wake disorders 334
sleepwalking disorder (somnambulism) 280
smartphone technology 405–411; CHR app in 409, *410*, 411; in COVID-19 560; enhanced access to psychiatric care and 406; implementation of smartphone-based psychiatric care interventions, examples of 408–411; improvements in clients' engagement and satisfaction with treatment 406–407; optimized community psychiatric care outcomes and 407–408; overview of 405–406
Smoking Cessation QoL (SCQoL) Questionnaire 25, 28
SNV (single nucleotide variant) 526, 529, 530, 533, 534
social anxiety disorder 264–267; assessment instruments in 266; clinical features of 265; comorbidities in 266; course and prognosis in 265–266; definition of 264; diagnostic criteria for 266; differential diagnosis in 266; epidemiology of 264; genetic factors in 264; management of 266; neurochemicals in 265; neuroimaging in 265; pharmacotherapy for 267; psychosocial factors in 265; psychotherapy for 266–267; treatment in 266–267
social attachment, oxytocin in promoting 54
social cognitivism 6–7, 11
social constructivism 8, 11
social health care workers in psychopharmacology 438–439
social phobia, OCD with 288
social relationships domain of QoL 20
social skills training in APS 251–252
social support in QoL 19
sodium valproate 209
solute carrier family 6 member 4 (SLC6A4) 161, 527
somatic symptoms, unexplained: causes of 352–353; in mood disorders 353; in neurotic disorders 353; overview of 351; in personality disorders 353; in psychotic disorders 352; in substance abuse 352
somatoform disorders 283, 362
somnambulism (sleepwalking disorder) 280
South Korea, internet gaming addiction in 177
Spain, ROD in 312
specific phobias 270–272; *see also* agoraphobia; childhood fears and, persistence of 270; clinical features of 270; cognitive theories in 271; differential diagnosis in 271; epidemiology of 270; genetic factors in 271; neural mechanisms in 271; prepared learning in 271; prognosis in 271; psychoanalytical theories in 271; treatment in 271–272
spirituality/religion/personal beliefs domain of QoL 20
Spitzer Quality of Life Index (Spitzer QL-Index) 24
SSRIs *see* selective serotonin reuptake inhibitors (SSRIs)
STEP (Scarf Telepsychiatry) 201
stigma surrounding mental illnesses 43–44
stimulus control 289
structured professional judgement 94–95
subjective assessment of QoL 21
subjective feeling of wellbeing in QoL 19
substance use disorders: abstinence-based programs in 427; addiction in pandemics and epidemics 500; aggression in 350; agitation in 344; behavioral addictions compared to 169–170; bizarre behaviour in 345; BPD with 221; catatonia in 346; disease-specific scales for 28; education programming 46–47; excitement in 347; fMRI in 521; in forensic context 425–427; hallucinations in 350–351; monitoring substance use in 426–427; parasomnias due to 281–282; psychiatric care in 478; psychomotor retardation in 348; QoL of subjects with 27–28; sleep-related movement disorders due to 282; suicide in, attempted 351; unexplained somatic symptoms in 352
suicide 317–330; active therapeutic stance for prevention 327–328; assessment and screening of 321–322; attempted 351–352; CBT for intervention in 363; co-operative patients and 325; *de facto* decriminalization of, in India 37; factors that increase risk of 320–321; farmer suicides and their survivors, in India 198–201 (*see also* community psychiatry); intent to act, assessing 320; lethal and non-lethal suicide intention, differentiation between 330;

managing patients at risk for 322–326; patient's ability to connect actions and feelings and 329–330; patients with a chronic risk for 325–326; patient with a suicide plan and high intent 323; patient with low intent but with serious risk factors 323; patient with suicidal thoughts but no plan 324; prevention 46, 317–330; psychotherapy for 327–330; rates 317–318; risk and protective factors in assessment 318–321; risk assessment *vs.* suicide prediction 318–319; self-agency and 329; self-harm *vs.* suicidality 320; severity of the suicidal intent and, investigating 319–320; specific strategies for prevention of 326; therapist access to supervision and 330; transferring high-risk patient for emergency psychiatric consultation 324–325; treatment model for suicidal patients 327; uncooperative patients and 325; validation and 328–329; Zero Suicide and 318, 327

Sweden: disulfiram introduced in 293; personal ombudsperson in 115

tapping method 290
TBI *see* technology-based interventions (TBI)
TD (time-domain) in fNIRS 540, *540*
technology-based interventions (TBI) 559–563; for caregiver support 561; coping skills and 563; for preventative measures 563; for psychological first aid 561–563; smartphone-based applications 560; to tackle problems with limited resources 561; tools to sustain 561; to train health personnel 560; TV-based platforms 560; video call interventions 560; WHO guidelines for 561
telemedicine; *see also* telepsychiatry: effectiveness of 561; interventions 559–560; licenses 401; overview of 559; smartphone technology in 405–411
Telemedicine and Patient-Reported Outcome Measurement (TELEPROM-Y) 409, 411
Telemedicine and Patient-Reported Outcome Measurement for Geriatric population (TELEPROM-G) 409, 410, 411
TELEPROM-G (Telemedicine and Patient-Reported Outcome Measurement for Geriatric population) 409, 410, 411
TELEPROM-Y (Telemedicine and Patient-Reported Outcome Measurement) 409, 411
telepsychiatry 395–401; in bipolar disorder 153; for bipolar mood disorder 153; challenges of, future 507–508; for clinical assessment 399; costs of 398; COVID-19 and 200, 399, 557, 559; difficulties in 397–398; legal issues and 401; mHealth in 45, 81; mobile applications for 201; mobile phones in 81; outcomes 398; overview of 395–396; in pandemics and epidemics 507–508; psychiatric care optimized by 395–401; for psychiatric epidemiology 399; for psychoeducation and self-help 400–401; psychotherapy in 400; in research 401; smartphone technology in 405–411; for training and supervision of trainees 400; uses of 399–401; video therapy in 396–397
television platforms in COVID-19 560
time-domain (TD) in fNIRS 540, *540*
tooth grinding (sleep bruxism) 282
topiramate 159, 161; for alcohol dependence 156, 159, 161, 295; for behavioral addictions 176; for BPD 223; contraindicated for COVID-19 563; for eating disorders 186
tracking movements in HD 141
train and place approaches 551–552; job maintenance in 552; sheltered employment in 552; training for specific jobs in 551; transitional employment in 552; work adjustment in 551; work skills assessment in 551
transcriptional mechanisms of resilience 52–53
transitional employment 552
transvestic disorder 428
trichotillomania (hair-pulling disorder) 288

Uganda: child and adolescent psychiatry in 469; group IPT for depression in 387
ultra-rapid metabolizer (UM) 529, 530
Ultra-Rapid Opiate Detoxification (UROD) 312
Ulysses clause 113–114
UM (ultra-rapid metabolizer) 529, 530
United Kingdom: AChEIs in management of Alzheimer's disease in 237, 238; antipsychotic prescribing for PWD in 243; Carer's Assessment in 242; COPMI in 86; COVID-19 in, PWD and carers and 244; decision-making in 115; frontotemporal dementia in, pharmacological therapies approved for 239; guidelines for diagnosis and management of dementia in 235–236; internet addiction in 178; pregnancy and legal protections for women in 118; QualityRights Initiative in 115; RFS started in 443; risperidone for use in treatment of BPSD in 240; sexual dysfunction and, cross-sectional study on 104; social cognitivist learning in 7; support for carers in 242, *243*; teaching methodologies in 6; vascular dementia in, licenced treatments for 238
United States: ALF in 213; BPD originated in 216; C-L psychiatry in 333–334; COPMI in 86, 88; CPT in 389; disulfiram approved by FDA in 293; frontotemporal dementia in, pharmacological therapies approved for 239; gene cept assay developed in 527; gene sight psychotropic algorithm in 527; guidelines for diagnosis and management of dementia in 234–235; IMPACT in 210; internet addiction in 172, 178; job clubs in 552; naltrexone for opioid use disorders in 302; Nursing Home Reform Act in 213; OOD in 310; PMs in 530; risperidone for use in treatment of BPSD in 240; simultaneous detoxification and NTX induction in, opposition to 312; stigma surrounding

mental illnesses in 43; suicidal ideation in, screening for 322; teletherapy in, COVID-19 and 399; VAW in 67; Vocational Rehabilitation Act in 545
United States Substance Abuse and Mental Health Services Administration (SAMHSA) 46
unstructured clinical judgement 93
UROD (Ultra-Rapid Opiate Detoxification) 312

vaccination hesitancy in pandemics and epidemics 506
vareniclin 162
vascular dementia 233, 238
VAW *see* violence against women (VAW)
venlafaxine 27, 104, 105, 262, 267
vergences in HD 141
vestibulo-ocular in HD 142
video calls in COVID-19 560
Vietnam: promoting mental health among adults and children in 462; US soldiers addicted to opium and heroin who fought in 302
violence, assessing risk for 422–425
violence against women (VAW) 65–75; consequences of 70; distal factors in 67–68; individual factors in 68, 69; individual-level intervention in 74; multidisciplinary approaches to prevent 72–73; overview of 65–66; proximal factors in 68; strategies and interventions in 70–74 (*see also* distal-level intervention; proximal-level intervention); type of violence in 66–67; wheel of power and control in 68, 69
virtual therapy for agoraphobia 264
visual function in HD 141
visual hallucinations in HD 142
visual pathway, lesion of the cortical part of, in HD 142
vocational rehabilitation: 551-553; place and train paradigms in 552–553; train and place approaches in 551–552

voluntary patients 36–37, 117–118
voyeuristic disorder 428

Wales, Mental Health Act in 34
Wellness Recovery Action Plan (WRAP) 46, 211–212
Wernicke's disorder 293
WHO *see* World Health Organization (WHO)
WHOQOL 24, 26
WHOQOL-BREF 26, 27
WHOQOL-OLD 210
Wisconsin Quality of Life Index (W-QLI) 23
women's reproductive and sexual health, coercive practices and 118–119
work adjustment 551
work cooperatives 552–553
work skills assessment 551
World Association for Infant Mental Health (WAIMH) 468
World Health Organization (WHO) 33, 42, 66, 111, 292, 475, 547, 561; *see also* QualityRights initiative (WHO); QoL defined by 19; QoL domains 19–20; *Resource Book on Mental Health, Human Rights and Legislation* 36, 38, 116; WHOQOL 24, 26; WHOQOL-BREF 26, 27; WHOQOL-OLD 210
World Psychiatric Association-Section of General Hospital Psychiatry 334
worry in GAD 267
WRAP (Wellness Recovery Action Plan) 46, 211–212

xenophobia 270, 504

Yale Geriatric Care Program 214

Zero Suicide 318, 327
zoophobia 270

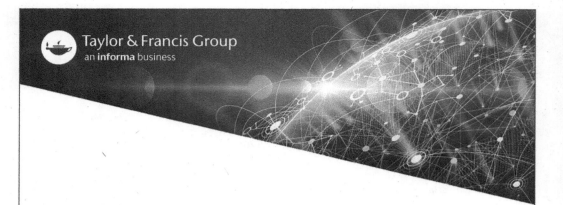